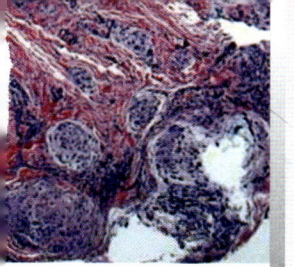

Dermatopathology

with a Clinical Base

Text and Atlas

Contributory authors

Dr Jushya Bhatia, MD (Dermatology), Resident
Dr Ankur Sarin, MD (Dermatology), Resident
Dr Sompal Singh, MD (Pathology), Senior Specialist, Hindu Rao Hospital, New Delhi

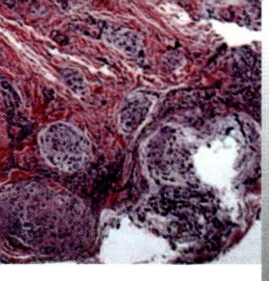

Dermatopathology
with a Clinical Base

Text and Atlas

Priyanka Anand

MBBS, MD (Pathology)

Ex-Senior Resident, Department of Pathology

Hindu Rao Hospital, New Delhi

Sonam Kumar Pruthi

MBBS, MD (Pathology)

Specialist, Department of Pathology

Hindu Rao Hospital, New Delhi

Namrata Sarin

MBBS, MD (Pathology)

Head, Department of Pathology

Hindu Rao Hospital, New Delhi

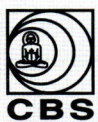

CBS

CBS Publishers & Distributors Pvt Ltd

New Delhi • Bengaluru • Chennai • Kochi • Kolkata • Mumbai

Bhopal • Bhubaneswar • Hyderabad • Jharkhand • Nagpur • Patna • Pune • Uttarakhand • Dhaka (Bangladesh)

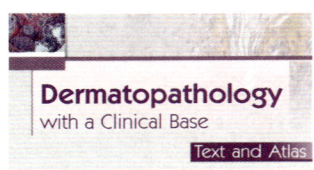

ISBN: 978-93-88902-86-1

First Edition: 2019

Published by Satish Kumar Jain and produced by Varun Jain for
CBS Publishers & Distributors Pvt Ltd
4819/XI Prahlad Street, 24 Ansari Road, Daryaganj, New Delhi 110 002, India
Ph: 23289259, 23266861, 23266867 Website: www.cbspd.com
Fax: 011-23243014   e-mail: delhi@cbspd.com; cbspubs@airtelmail.in

Corporate Office: 204 FIE, Industrial Area, Patparganj, Delhi 110 092
Ph: 4934 4934   Fax: 4934 4935   e-mail: publishing@cbspd.com; publicity@cbspd.com

Branches

- **Bengaluru:** Seema House 2975, 17th Cross, K.R. Road, Banasankari 2nd Stage, Bengaluru 560 070, Karnataka
  Ph: +91-80-26771678/79   Fax: +91-80-26771680   e-mail: bangalore@cbspd.com
- **Chennai:** 7, Subbaraya Street, Shenoy Nagar, Chennai 600 030, Tamil Nadu
  Ph: +91-44-26680620/26681266   Fax: +91-44-42032115   e-mail: chennai@cbspd.com
- **Kochi:** 42/1325, 1326, Power House Road, Opp KSEB Power House, Ernakulam 682 018, Kochi, Kerala
  Ph: +91-484-4059061-65   Fax: +91-484-4059065   e-mail: kochi@cbspd.com
- **Kolkata:** 6/B, Ground Floor, Rameswar Shaw Road, Kolkata 700 014, West Bengal
  Ph: +91-33-22891126, 22891127, 22891128   e-mail: kolkata@cbspd.com
- **Mumbai:** 83-C, Dr E Moses Road, Worli, Mumbai 400018, Maharashtra
  Ph: +91-22-24902340/41   Fax: +91-22-24902342   e-mail: mumbai@cbspd.com

Representatives

• **Bhopal**	0-8319310552	• **Bhubaneswar**	0-9911037372	• **Hyderabad**	0-9885175004	• **Jharkhand**	0-9811541605
• **Nagpur**	0-9421945513	• **Patna**	0-9334159340	• **Pune**	0-9623451994	• **Uttarakhand**	0-9716462459
• **Dhaka (Bangladesh)**	01912-003485				

Printed at: HT Media Ltd., Greater Noida, UP, India

———————●———————

to

my late father **Mr Vinay Kumar**, who always believed in my ability;
that I will be successful in academics. Even though he is not with us anymore,
his belief in me has made this journey possible. His personality not only inspired me,
but also many others. "Great souls leave earth, but their inspirations are immortal."

— Dr Priyanka Anand

my loved ones

— Dr Sonam Kumar Pruthi

my family and friends

— Dr Namrata Sarin

———————●———————

Foreword

My happiness knows no bounds as I write the Foreword for Dr Sonam's fifth book *Dermatopathology with a Clinical Base: Text and Atlas*. Dr Sonam Pruthi is currently working as Specialist Pathologist at Hindu Rao Hospital and NDMC Medical College, New Delhi. He did his MD (Pathology) training at Kasturba Medical College, Mangalore, Manipal Academy of Higher Education. I am proud to be his teacher and a dear friend.

This book is one of its kind written by Indian authors on skin pathology keeping in mind the Indian medical curriculum and disease prevalence. This is a well-planned and executed team project. The other text and reference books by respected and revered foreign authors are either voluminous, costly or unavailable to most of us. This book is simplistic and the content has been laid out in 18 parts with total 116 chapters dedicated to common non-neoplastic and neoplastic skin disorders. The textual matter has been presented under clear headings, sub-headings and bullets. The pointwise description is in a lucid language which makes it easy to read and retain. The histological description in the text has been supplemented with photomicrographs and the features have been uniquely highlighted with arrows for ease of identifying and understanding. The clinical photographs complement the macroscopic description. This book is going to be very useful for students of MD, Pathology, Dermatology and Venereology, as well as a ready reckoner or handbook for practising pathologists and dermatologists.

Sonam is an avid reader, honest researcher and dedicated to his profession of teaching and diagnostics. His unfathomable passion for writing and love for pathology is evident from his more than applaudable feat of publishing five books within six years of completing postgraduate training. His other four books are: *Comprehensive Review of Pathology, Preparatory Manual of Pathology for Undergraduate Students, My Pathology Notes for FMGE and Preparatory Manual of Pathology for Medical Laboratory Technology Students,* have all been good sellers and well-appreciated by the medical student fraternity throughout India and outside India too.

My heartfelt best wishes to Dr Pruthi in this venture and God bless him with continuing success.

Shrijeet Chakraborti
MD, DNB, PDF-Neuropath, DipRCPath, PGDEA, MNAMS
Specialty Doctor, Histopathology, Leighton Hospital, Crewe
Mid Cheshire Hospitals NHS Foundation Trust, Cheshire, United Kingdom
Ex-Associate Professor and in-charge Blood Bank
Department of Pathology, Kasturba Medical College, Mangalore
Manipal University, India

Foreword

Dermatopathology can be a daunting subject for both pathologists and dermatologists. The sheer number of conditions that present with a cutaneous abnormality, the considerable overlap in the findings in a variety of diseases, the thick jungle of terminology and the lack of sufficient attention to this subject in most dermatology and pathology training programmes—all contribute to this situation. There is a need for teaching material that makes the subject accessible to those wanting to learn it because skin biopsy continues to be the most·important diagnostic test in dermatology.

The authors of this book have put together a well-illustrated text supplemented with brief, focused accounts of a variety of common and some rare conditions that are likely to be seen in a dermatopathology practice. The large numbers of images help to visualize the findings and this is supplemented by point-wise text that provides essential information about the condition in a user-friendly format.

I am certain the book will be useful, both to trainees and practitioners of dermatopathology.

M Ramam
President, Dermatopathology Society of India
Professor, Department of Dermatology and Venereology
All India Institute of Medical Sciences
New Delhi

Foreword

Dermatopathology practice requires comprehensive knowledge of each disease entity with respect to its clinical presentation, morphology and differential diagnosis, so that a correct diagnosis can be reached upon.

The subject though challenging, but interesting, requires thorough reading, in conjunction with seeing of the slides. Though a few voluminous reference books are available in dermatopathology, yet good, concise and simplified textbook, is hardly available for reading and reporting purposes.

Dermatopathology with a Clinical Base: Text and Atlas is unique within itself by being concise, well-written, in easy to understand language. This textbook includes high quality, well-explained photomicrographs and clinical images of skin lesions, which will benefit the reader and also will allow an easy grasp of the subject.

My heartfelt best wishes to the authors who have published this textbook that will help pathologists and dermatologists, to learn and practice dermatopathology better.

Kailash Bhatia
Professor and Head, Department of Dermatology
Venereology and Leprosy
Sri Aurobindo Institute of Medical Sciences, Indore
Madhya Pradesh

Foreword

It gives me immense happiness to introduce this dermatopathology textbook, which is first of its own kind, in context to being written by Indian authors. Dermatopathology being a challenging subject to practice, and requires in-depth knowledge of the subject, which has to be gathered by seeing the biopsy slides and also by thorough reading of the text. However, in an ocean of books, there is hardly any book which is written to the point, in simplified language, and also is concise. This textbook provides the reader all these benefits. Apart from the written text, the book includes numerous photomicrographs, which will help the reader to grasp the content easily. Clinical pictures are also diverse and explicit and cover majority of the lesions, which also make this book unique.

I warm-heartedly congratulate the authors for their hard work and also for gifting such an organized textbook of dermatopathology, to the medical fraternity of India and the world.

I am sure that this dermatopathology textbook will be useful not only for pathologists but also for dermatologists globally.

Vinod Kumar Khurana
Head, Department of Dermatology
STI and Leprosy
Hindu Rao Hospital and NDMC Medical College
New Delhi

Preface

Patients, we see daily are the ones, which help us learn the field of medicine, and the books we read, help us to gain more knowledge and experience of that particular disease, we saw in patient and differentiate it with many others, resembling the same.

Dermatopathology, in which 0.5 cm of tissue, teaches us the morphology of disease, which reader will be learning thoroughly in this book.

It requires high skill, lots of patience, experience, knowledge and avid reading to reach to a conclusive diagnosis in dermatopathology.

This book will help the reader to learn about disease entities, which we commonly encounter in department of dermatology.

The role of dermatopathologist is to help the dermatologist, in providing a conclusive diagnosis, so that the best available treatment can be given.

Sometimes, special stains, immunohistochemical markers, immunofluorescence studies and other special tests are required to reach to a conclusive diagnosis. This textbook will make you thorough with all the entities in a different way, due to uniqueness of the text being described, and also the introduction of nearly 500 colored images (including H&E stain, special stains, immunohistochemistry and immunofluorescence) will help the reader, learn the subject, in a much easier way.

The book provides concise and conceptual way to learn and memorize the morphology of common, not so common, difficult and rarely encountered dermatopathology entities.

Long paragraphs, vast description of diseases have been avoided. This has been done purposely, so that when one keeps the slide under microscope, he or she should not be lost in the vast sea of information, while reading.

To learn the differential diagnosis of each entity in dermatopathology is of utmost importance, to reach to a correct diagnosis. Keeping that point in mind, each possible differential of the disease entity has been discussed, concisely.

Photomicrographs of each entity with the best possible morphological description of figures with pointers have been discussed, which will also help the beginner to learn the subject.

Introduction of clinical images of the lesions, with each disease entity, will help dermatologists, to make a strong base in dermatopathology.

We believe and hope that this book of ours will help in transferring our knowledge and love for dermatopathology to the budding and practising pathologists, dermatopathologists, and dermatologists.

Your valuable suggestions, if any, to improve the book are always welcome.

Wishing you all the best for your good future!!

Priyanka Anand
Sonam Kumar Pruthi
Namrata Sarin

Acknowledgements

We would like to thank Dr Jushya Bhatia, MD (Dermatology), Resident and Dr Ankur Sarin, MD (Dermatology), Resident, for providing us the clinical and immunofluorescence photographs.

We would also like to thank our contributory authors, Dr Jushya Bhatia for the chapter "Vesiculobullous disorders" and Dr Ankur Sarin for the chapter "Leprosy".

We also would like to thank Dr Shrijeet Chakraborti, United Kingdom, M Ramam, AIIMS, New Delhi, Dr Kailash Bhatia, Sri Aurobindo Institute of Medical Sciences, Indore and Dr Vinod Kumar Khurana, Hindu Rao Hospital, New Delhi, for taking out their precious time and writing the foreword of our book.

We would also like to express our gratitude towards our teachers, students and colleagues, whose guidance and motivation has helped us to write and finish this book.

We also want to thank our families for their unconditional love and immense support, which cannot be exemplified with words.

We would also like to thank, Mr YN Arjuna, Senior Vice President, Publishing, Editorial and Publicity, CBS Publishers & Distributors, and his team for their constant hard work, which made publication of this book possible.

Priyanka Anand
Sonam Kumar Pruthi
Namrata Sarin

Contents

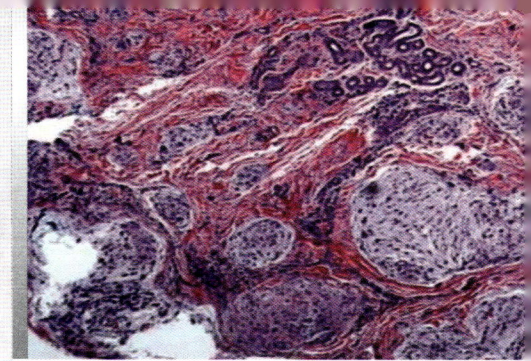

Basics of Dermatopathology

Part 1

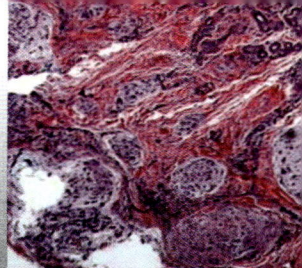

Skin Biopsy

- In dermatopathology, a well-established lesion is preferred for biopsy in order to make a diagnosis
- However, in contrast, biopsy of an early lesion is recommended for vesicobullous disorders, ulcers and pustular lesions
- Clinical details, complete in all respects, in the requisition form, should be provided by dermatologists to the reporting dermatopathologist, along with the biopsy sample

WAYS OF OBTAINING A SKIN BIOPSY

1. *Excision biopsy*
   - For skin tumors, in order to evaluate the margins
   - For inflammatory processes, in order to evaluate the deeper tissue for panniculitis

2. *Punch biopsy*
   - A 4 mm punch biopsy is adequate for histopathological study
   - For diagnosing inflammatory dermatosis

3. *Shave biopsy*
   - Biopsy tissue includes epidermis and papillary dermis
   - Helpful for diagnosis of papillomatous or pedunculated lesions, seborrheic keratosis and verrucous lesions

4. *Deep incisional biopsy*
   - For deep dermal and subcutaneous lesions

5. *Curettage biopsy*
   - Less satisfactory amongst all techniques
   - Superficial and scant tissue is obtained by this technique

Laboratory Methods

Fixation of Skin Biopsy

- For stabilization of proteins and to preserve tissue morphology
- Done in buffered 10% formalin solution for 6–12 hours
- Volume of formalin should be 10–20 times the volume of the specimen

Grossing

- For the specimens, in which margin status is asked, deep and lateral margins, should be painted
- Biopsy of 3 mm or less in size should be processed without bisecting it
- Biopsy of 4 mm and 6 mm should be bisected and fully processed

Processing

- Routine tissue processing steps has to be followed
- After tissue processing, specimens are embedded, with cut-surface facing down
- After the blocks are made, specimens are cut on rotary microtome into 5–7 micrometer thick sections
- Routine sections are stained with hematoxylin and eosin

Histology of Normal Skin

Normal Skin (Fig. 1.1)

- Comprises keratinocytes and dendritic cells
- Keratinocytes are arranged in four layers: Stratum corneum, stratum granulosum, stratum spinosum and stratum basale
- Stratum malpighii—comprises three layers, i.e. stratum spinosum, stratum granulosum and stratum basale

1. *Stratum basalis*
   - Basal cells with basophilic cytoplasm and are columnar with oval to elongated nucleus
   - Most mitotically active cells are present in basalis

2. *Stratum spinosum*
   - Consists of polyhedral cells above the basal cell layer
   - Cells are inter-connected with each other and are tightly clustered

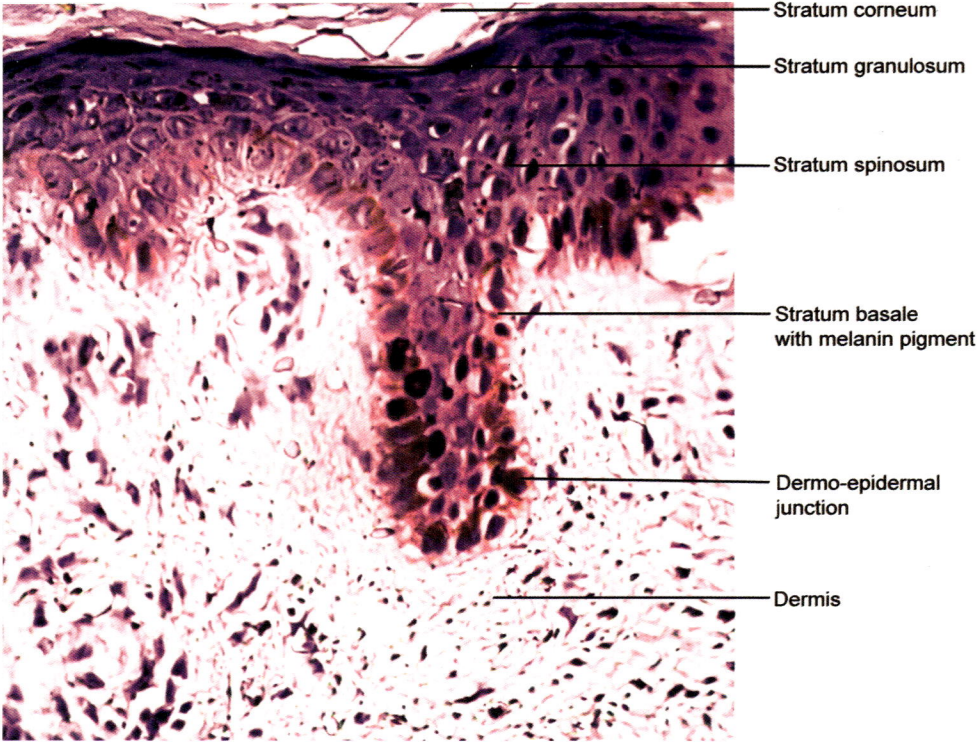

Fig. 1.1: Normal skin

3. *Stratum granulosum*
   - Lined by flattened cells and are filled with kera-tohyaline granules, which are deeply basophilic

4. *Stratum corneum*
   - Anucleate layer
   - Can show basket-weaving
   - Lowest portion of stratum corneum is called stratum lucidum

Melanocytes (Fig. 1.2)

- Comprise melanin and are present in the basal cell layer of the epidermis
- Can be demonstrated with special stains like Masson-Fontana
- Melanin can be removed from the tissue by melanin bleach, which can be done by using strong oxidizing agents such as hydrogen peroxide or potassium permanganate
- Immunohistochemical stain for their identification is S-100

Merkel Cells

- Present within the basal cell layer of the epidermis
- Cannot be demonstrated by hematoxylin and eosin stain
- Immunohistochemical stain for their identification is cytokeratin-20 (CK-20)

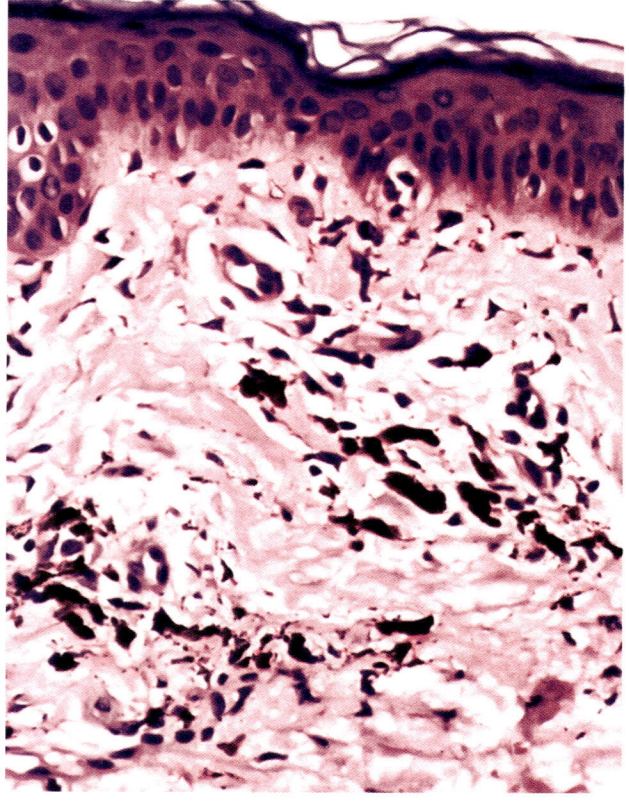

Fig. 1.2: Melanophages in upper dermis

- On electron microscopy—Merkel cells contain neurosecretory granules

Langerhans Cells

- Found in supra-basal epidermis and have antigen presenting capacity
- Nuclear characteristics—nucleus appears kidney shaped and is cleaved with dendritic architecture
- Monoclonal antibody to demonstrate is CD1a
- Electron microscopy—demonstrates characteristic cytoplasmic granules (Langerhans or Birbeck granules, which have a tennis racket appearance)

Basement Membrane Zone

- Can be demonstrated by PAS stain
- Hemidesmosomes, contain bullous pemphigoid antigen-1 and 2 (BPAG-1, BPAG-2)
- BPAGs are demonstrated by immunofluorescence as a smooth linear band that separates epidermal and dermal layers
- Lamina densa (a component of basement membrane zone) comprises type IV collagen which is anchored to the underlying dermis by anchoring fibrils, composed of type VII collagen

Hair Follicles (Fig. 1.3)

- Comprise three parts—lower portion, isthmus and upper portion (infundibulum)
- Bulb region (knob-like area in the lower pole) gives rise to hair shaft within follicular canal
- Stage of hair growth—anagen hair (stage of active growth) → catagen hair (phase of regression/ involutionary stage) → telogen hair (phase of resting period/end stage)
- Follicular isthmus, catagen hairs and telogen hair show trichilemmal keratinization

Sebaceous Glands (Fig. 1.4)

- Comprise multiple sebaceous lobules with a peripheral layer of cuboidal basophilic cells and central sebaceous cells
- Sebaceous cells contain lipid droplets, which can be demonstrated by lipid stains

Eccrine Glands (Fig. 1.5)

- Composed of three segments—intra-epidermal duct, intradermal duct and secretory portion
- Intra-epidermal eccrine duct, called acrosyringium, comprises a single layer of inner or luminal cells and two or three rows of outer cells
- Intra-dermal eccrine duct is composed of two layers of small, cuboidal and basophilic epithelial cells
- Secretory portion of eccrine gland is made up of a single layer of secretory cells

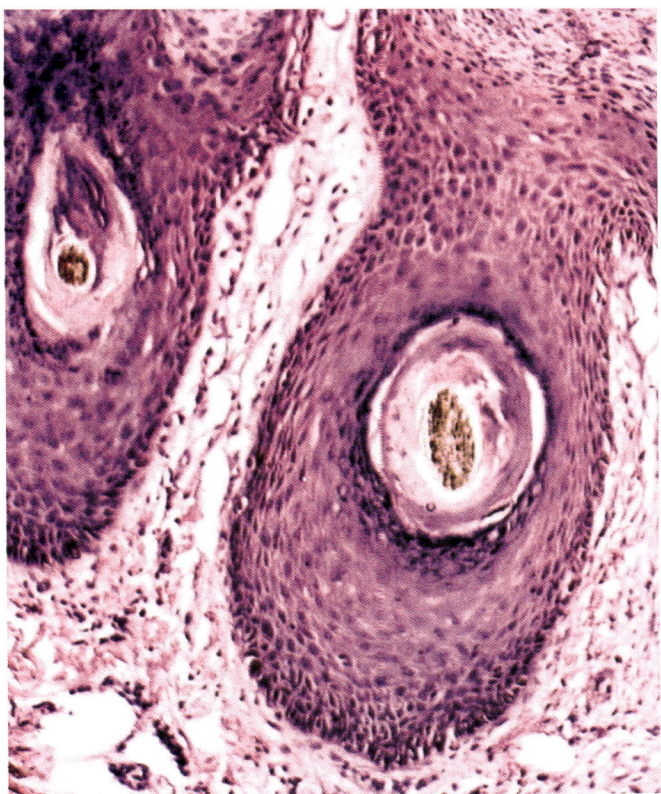

Fig. 1.3: Hair follicle

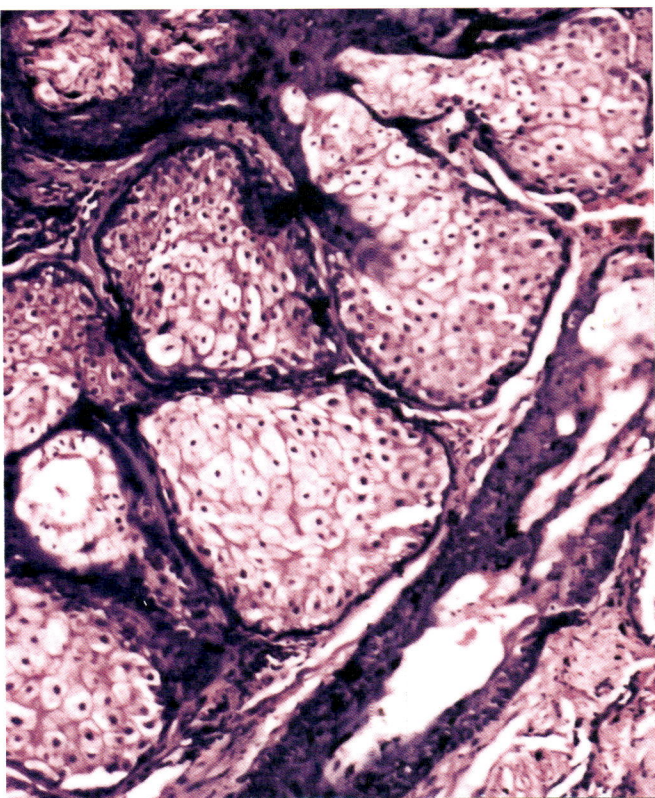

Fig. 1.4: Sebaceous glands

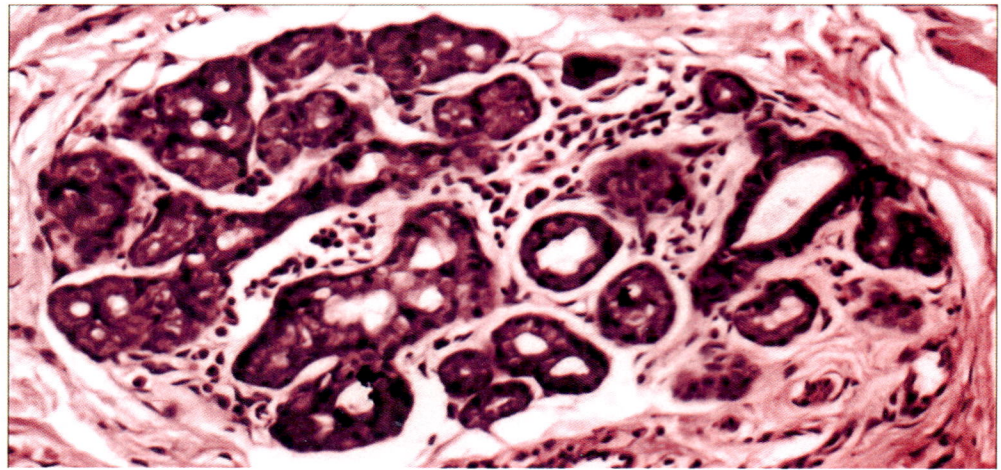

Fig. 1.5: Eccrine glands

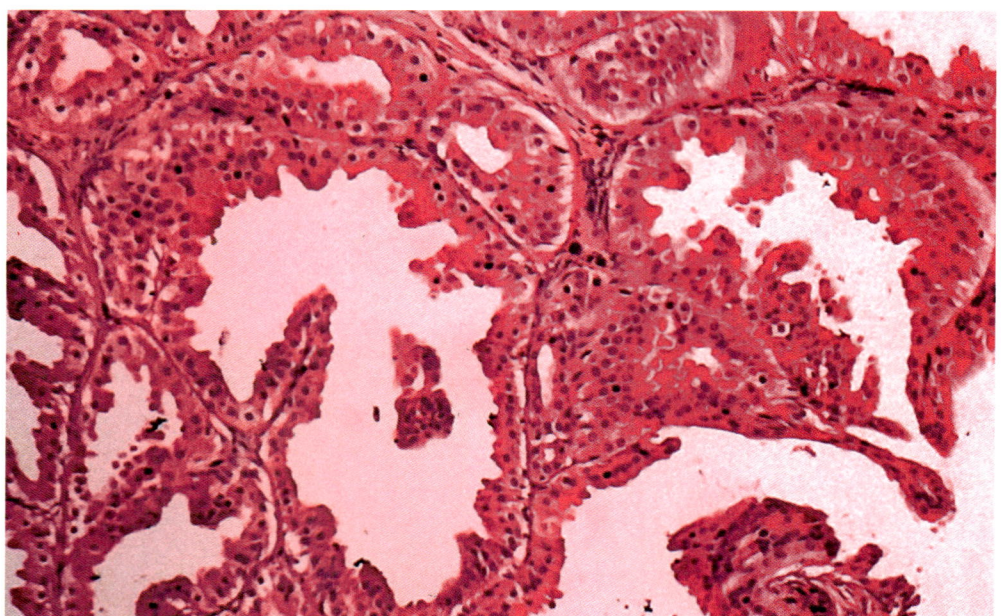

Fig. 1.6: Apocrine glands

- Highlighted by S-100 protein and carcinoembryonic antigen (CEA)
- Function—temperature regulation

Apocrine Glands (Fig. 1.6)

- Are tubular glands with secretory portion of the cell being pinched off during secretion (decapitation secretion), which is PAS positive and contains diastase resistant material (sialomucin)
- Duct of the apocrine glands, opens into the pilosebaceous follicle (in the infundibulum)
- Ductal portion shows double layer of basophilic cells, secretory portion shows a single layer of secretory cells

Dermal Microvascular Unit

- Superficial and deep dermis show numerous small and large vascular channels
- Comprises endothelial cells, basement membrane (highlighted by PAS) and pericytes

Glomus Cells

- Represent arterio-venous shunt and play a role in temperature regulation
- Surround the vessel wall (tunica media) and is arranged in four to six layers
- Each glomus cell is surrounded by a basement membrane

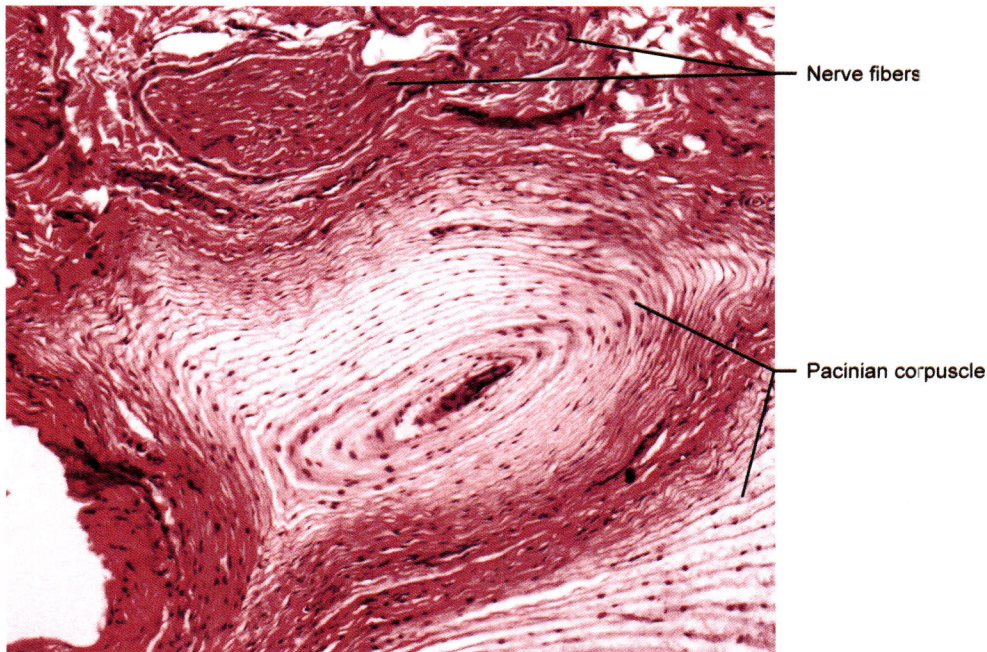

Fig. 1.7: Pacinian corpuscle

Mast Cells

- Can be seen in normal dermis
- Are round to oval cells with centrally located nucleus and granular eosinophilic cytoplasm
- Granules can be highlighted by Giemsa stain, toluidine blue, Alcian blue, methylene blue

Nerve Fibers

- Can be demonstrated by S-100

Nerve End Organs

- Mucocutaneous end organs—seen in hairless skin, at mucocutaneous junction, in the papillary dermis
- Meissner corpuscle—located in dermal papillae, mediates a sense of touch, seen on the ventral aspect of hands and feet
- Pacinian corpuscle—located in subcutis, mediates a sense of pressure, seen on palms and soles (especially at the tips of fingers and toes) (Fig. 1.7)

Dendritic Cells

- Located around the dermal blood vessels
- Express factor XIIIa positivity

Macrophages

- Are transformed monocytes
- Most often seen around the vascular spaces

Inflammatory Cells

- Epidermis and dermis can show inflammatory cells
- Include neutrophils, eosinophils, basophils, lymphocytes and plasma cells

Extracellular Matrix Components

1. *Collagen*
   - Can be thick or thin
   - Type III collagen is predominant in papillary dermis
   - Type I collagen is predominant in reticular dermis

2. *Elastic fibers*
   - Are not demonstrated on hematoxylin and eosin stain
   - Can be demonstrated by elastic tissue stains like orcein

Other Components

- Dermal fibroblasts, dermal smooth muscle and striated muscle cells

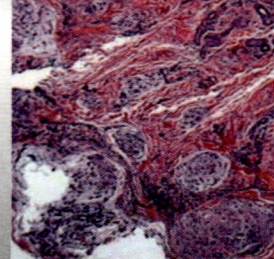

Chapter

Special Stains

2

INTRODUCTION

- Hematoxylin and eosin (H&E) stain is the most common used stain in dermatopathology and it stains nuclei blue and cytoplasm pink
- However, H&E stain cannot highlight all characteristic cellular features
- Thus, histochemical stains are of great value, as these are easily available and less expensive than immunohistochemical stains
- Special stains have rapid turn-around time, are simpler to perform and gives excellent results

HISTOCHEMICAL STAINS

- Utilize chemical reactions to stain and highlight various normal and abnormal components in a tissue biopsy

CARBOHYDRATE STAINS

Periodic Acid–Schiff

Principle

- Periodic acid oxidizes the compounds having free hydroxyl groups
- As a result the -OH bond between the carbon atoms is broken, resulting in production of dialdehyde structure
- This dialdehyde structure reacts strongly with Schiff's reagent to give a magenta colored complex

Result

- A positive stain is perceived as purplish-red or magenta color

Use

- Stains polysaccharides, neutral mucins, basement membrane material and fungus

Periodic Acid–Schiff with Diastase (PAS-D)

- Diastase removes glycogen from the tissue sections and leaves mucopolysaccharides behind
- PAS-D accentuates fungal cell walls

Mucicarmine

- Identifies acid mucopolysaccharides

Results

- Mucin: Deep red (magenta, pink)
- Nuclei: Black
- Other tissue elements: Light yellow

Alcian Blue (pH 2.5)

- Identifies acidic mucins
- Non-sulfated mucins are stained at pH 2.5, e.g. hyaluronic acid (seen normally in papillary dermis and surrounding cutaneous appendage)

Results

- Acidic mucin stains blue with alcian blue

Uses

- Demonstration of acidic mucin in neoplasms and inflammatory conditions
- Demonstration of acidic mucin in dermatoses (e.g. granuloma annulare, lupus erythematosus, scleredema and follicular mucinosis)
- Demonstration of sialomucin in extra-mammary Paget's disease

Alcian Blue (pH 0.5)

- Identifies sulfated mucins like chondroitin sulfate and heparan sulfate
- Produces a bright blue to blue/green color
  Note: Colloidal iron gives equivalent results like Alcian blue

CONNECTIVE TISSUE STAINS

Masson Trichrome

- Differentiates between collagen/connective tissue and soft tissue components
- Collagen and connective tissue stains blue to blue-green
- Muscle stains red and nuclei stains black

Verhoeff-van Gieson

- Demonstrates elastic fibers, which are stained black
- Found in connective tissues, skin, arteries, veins and elastic cartilage
- For example, it can demonstrate thick coarse elastic fibers, parallel to the collagen bundles in Scleroderma

FAT STAINS

Oil Red O and Sudan Black B

- Highlight neutral lipids and stains them red
- Used on frozen section tissues

NERVE STAINS

Silver Nitrate

- Stains nerve fibers and neurofibrils black

Mallory Phosphotungstic Acid-Hematoxylin (PTAH)

- Stains glial fibers—blue
- Stains neurons—salmon-pink
- Stains myelin—blue

STAINS FOR DETECTION OF PIGMENTS, MINERALS AND GRANULES

Prussian Blue

- Highlights ferric iron and stain it deep blue
- Used to distinguish melanin from hemosiderin
- For example, stains hemosiderin in pigmented purpuric dermatosis

Masson-Fontana

- Principle—reduction of silver to form a black precipitate
- Highlights melanin and helps to differentiate melanin from hemosiderin pigment
- Used in evaluation of vitiligo and post-inflammatory hyper-pigmentation

von Kossa

- Used for identification of calcium and calcified structures
- Stains calcium deposits/bone—black
- Useful in confirmation of diagnosis of calcinosis cutis, calciphylaxis, pseudoxanthoma elasticum

Congo Red

- Enhances detection of amyloid in tissue sections
- Stains amyloid brick red on H&E stain, which gives apple-green birefringence under polarized light

Crystal Violet

- Demonstrates amyloid and stains it red-purple color
- Other stains to demonstrate amyloid include Thioflavin-T, Sirius red

STAINS FOR ORGANISM DETECTION

Acid-fast Bacilli

- Ziehl-Neelsen stain is most commonly used in dermatopathology
- Cell wall of acid-fast microorganisms contains mycolic acid, which allows strong binding and retention of carbol-fuchsin dye
- AFB positive organism stains bright red
- Used for confirmation of diagnosis of *Mycobacterium tuberculosis*
- Fite stain is used to identify *Mycobacterium leprosum*
- Auramine-rhodamine stain—modified and most sensitive version of Ziehl-Neelsen stain

Giemsa

- Used to highlight mast cells in conditions like urticaria and urticaria pigmentosum
- Used to demonstrate spirochetes, protozoa and Leishmania
- Positive stain is perceived as bluish-purple color

Warthin-Starry Stain

- Used for identification of spirochetes, e.g. syphilis, Lyme disease, and acrodermatitis chronica atrophicans
- Spirochetes will be stained black

MISCELLANEOUS STAIN

Toluidine Blue

- Highlights mast cells and stains them deep-violet

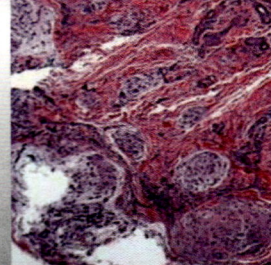

Immunohistochemical Markers

BASIC PRINCIPLES OF IMMUNOHISTOCHEMISTRY (IHC)

- Method of localization of antigen using labeled antibody (visualized by chromogen)
- Performed on formalin fixed paraffin embedded sections
- Formalin fixation can result in masking of antigen sites and thus antigen retrieval is needed
- Antigen retrieval can be done by heating in a microwave oven or by enzyme induced proteolysis
- Chromogen most widely used is Diaminobenzidine (DAB), which imparts a brown color to the reaction site
- IHC has better or equal efficacy than immunofluorescence techniques and has replaced electron microscopy
- For interpretation and correct diagnosis, IHC results should always be correlated with histopathological diagnosis, history and clinical examination

IMPORTANT AND COMMONLY USED IMMUNOHISTOCHEMICAL MARKERS

Cytokeratin/Carcinoembryonic Antigen/Epithelial Membrane Antigen (CEA/EMA)

Positive in

- Normal eccrine and apocrine cells
- Epidermal and appendageal tumors
- Merkel cell carcinoma
- Paget's disease of skin
- Adenocarcinoma
- Squamous cell carcinoma

Neuron Specific Enolase (NSE)

Positive in

- Neuroendocrine cells
- Merkel cell carcinoma

Chromogranin

Positive in

- Neuroendocrine cells
- Merkel cell carcinoma
- Carcinoid tumor

Synaptophysin

Positive in

- Neuroendocrine cells
- Merkel cell carcinoma

S-100

- Used to diagnose and differentiate different melanomas (most sensitive for melanomas)

Positive in

- Melanocytes, Langerhans cell, eccrine and apocrine gland cells, nerves, muscles, Schwann cells, myoepithelial cells, chondrocytes, adipocytes, histiocytes

HMB-45

Positive in

- Melanomas (most specific), melanocytic nevi, spindle cell nevi

Absent in

- Desmoplastic melanomas

Melan-A/MART-1

- Positivity is seen in melanocytes, nevi, Spitz nevi, malignant melanoma

CD-34

Positive in

- Dermatofibrosarcoma protuberans
- Solitary fibrous tumor

- Fibroblastoma
- Neurofibroma
- Spindle cell lipoma
- Hemangioma
- Angiosarcoma
- Kaposi sarcoma

Negative in
- Dermatofibroma

CD-31

Positive in
- Cutaneous angiosarcoma
- Kaposi sarcoma
- Hemangioendothelioma

Factor XIIIa

Positive in
- Dermatofibroma
- Atypical fibroxanthoma
- Juvenile xanthogranuloma
- Epithelioid cell histiocytoma

C-KIT (CD-117)

Positive in
- Mast cells, melanocytes, hematopoietic stem cells, systemic mastocytosis, gastrointestinal stromal tumor

CD-1a

Positive in
- Langerhans cell histiocytosis

CD-45/ Leucocyte common antigen (LCA)

Positive in
- Granulocytes, lymphocytes, monocytes, macrophages, mast cells, Langerhans cell

Vimentin

Positive in
- Non-Hodgkin lymphoma
- Sarcoma
- Melanoma

Desmin

Positive in
- Leiomyoma
- Leiomyosarcoma

Glial–Fibrillary Acid protein (GFAP)

Positive in
- Neurofibroma
- Schwannoma
- Chondroid syringoma

Use of IHC markers to localize primary cancer site (in unknown cutaneous metastasis)

IHC marker	Primary cancer site (in unknown cutaneous metastasis)
Cytokeratin-7	Adenocarcinoma from breast or lung
Cytokeratin-20	Metastatic small cell carcinoma, gastrointestinal carcinoma, mucinous ovarian carcinoma
Epithelial membrane antigen	Carcinoma breast, lungs, stomach, intestine, prostate, kidney, thyroid
Carcinoembryonic antigen	Carcinoma colon, lung, pancreas, breast
Estrogen receptor protein	Metastatic carcinoma breast
Prostate-specific antigen	Metastasis from carcinoma prostate
Thyroglobulin	Metastatic carcinoma thyroid

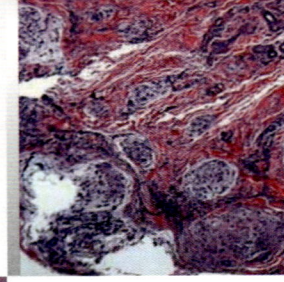

Immunofluorescence in Skin Biopsies

SKIN BIOPSY (STEPS TO BE FOLLOWED BEFORE IMMUNOFLUORESCENCE STAINING)

- 3–4 mm punch biopsy should be taken
- Unfixed tissue is taken for cryostat sections (frozen sections) immediately
- If transportation is required, Michel transport medium at pH 7 is used followed by quick freezing
- Site—peri-lesional skin adjacent to fresh blister in bullous disorders

TWO TYPES OF IMMUNOFLUORESCENCE PATTERNS

Direct Immunofluorescence (DIF)

- To identify immunoglobulin or complement factors on tissue biopsy
- On frozen sections, fluorescence labeled antibodies are applied
- Incubation is done
- On a fluorescent microscope—sites of attachment of IgG, IgM, IgA antibodies on the lesional skin are noted
- Uses—bullous disorders, lupus erythematosus, vasculitis

Indirect Immunofluorescence (IIF)

- Antibodies are detected in patients serum

- Patients serum is applied to the substrate
- Substrate used can be human skin or animal tissue such as esophagus of the monkey
- Antibodies in the serum attach to the tissue antigens on substrate
- Uses—antinuclear antibodies detection (can be detected in serum using Hep-2 as substrate)
- Immuno-mapping/antigen mapping—technique in which patients own skin is used as a substrate

Salt-split skin technique (SSST)

- Skin tissue is incubated in 1 M NaCl solution for 72 hours
- Epidermis is then separated from the dermis with the help of a fine forceps
- Direct and indirect immunofluorescence stains are performed on this tissue

Interpretation of SSST

On indirect immunofluorescence (using the patient's serum)

- Antibodies from bullous pemphigoid patients stain the roof of the blister
- Antibodies from epidermolysis bullosa acquisita patients stain the floor of the blister

Table 4.1: Immunofluorescence interpretation in important skin disorders				
Disease	**Biopsy site**	**DIF**	**IIF**	**SSST**
Lichen planus	Inflamed mucosa/skin	a. Fibrin deposits are present at dermo-epidermal junction b. IgM deposits (granular) and C3 deposits (linear) in basement membrane zone c. IgM positivity of necrotic keratinocytes is seen		
Lichen planopilaris	Inflamed mucosa/skin	a. IgM deposits at infundibulum b. Shaggy fibrin deposits surrounding the affected follicles		

Contd...

Disease	Biopsy site	DIF	IIF	SSST
Lichen planus pemphigoides	Inflamed mucosa/skin	IgG, C3 in linear arrangement along basement membrane zone		
Pemphigus vulgaris	Peri-lesional skin adjacent to the fresh lesion	IgG deposits in squamous intercellular/cell surface areas	Auto-antibodies directed against desmoglein-3	
Pemphigus foliaceus	Same as above	IgG deposits in squamous intercellular space, more pronounced in the upper epidermis	Auto-antibodies directed against desmoglein-1	
Pemphigus vegetans	Same as above	IgG deposits in squamous intercellular space		
Paraneoplastic pemphigus	Same as above	IgG deposits in squamous intercellular space and basement membrane	Auto-antibodies directed against desmoglein-1, 3 and plakins	
IgA pemphigus	Same as above	IgA deposits in squamous intercellular space	Auto-antibodies directed against desmocollin-1, desmoglein-1 and 3	
Bullous pemphigoid	Peri-lesional skin adjacent to the fresh lesion	Linear deposits of IgG and/or C3 at the dermo-epidermal junction (DEJ) or basement membrane zone		IgG antibodies are present on the epidermal roof (blister roof)
Epidermolysis bullosa acquisita	Normal appearing skin of the fresh lesion	Linear IgG deposits at dermo-epidermal junction	Antibodies against type VII collagen in the serum	IgG antibodies bind to the dermal floor
Bullous SLE	Lesional skin and normal skin in sun-exposed area	Linear or granular deposits of IgG and C3 at the dermo-epidermal junction		
Dermatitis herpetiformis		Granular IgA deposits along dermo-epidermal junction and in papillary dermis		
Linear IgA dermatosis		Linear IgA deposits along basement membrane zone		
Erythema multiforme	Normal appearing peri-lesional skin	a. IgM and C3 deposits in the walls of superficial dermal vessels b. Granular deposits of C3, IgM and fibrin along the dermo-epidermal junction		

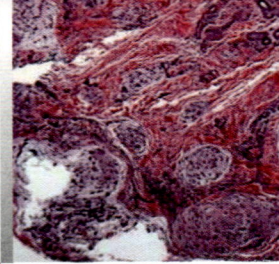

Commonly used Terms in Dermatopathology

Acantholysis
- Loss of adhesion between keratinocytes
- Occurs due to dissolution of intercellular bridges

Acanthosis
- Increase in epidermal thickening (stratum spinosum layer)
- Can be described as regular (rete ridges descend in the papillary dermis at same level) or irregular (rete ridges descend in papillary dermis at different levels)

Apoptosis
- Programmed cell death
- Keratinocyte remnants (i.e. colloid bodies) can be seen in stratum basale and in dermis

Asteroid body
- Stellate shaped intra-cytoplasmic inclusions, present within the giant cells
- Most common associated conditions—Sarcoidosis, Berylliosis, and other granulomatous conditions

Alopecia
- Defined as loss of hair
- Can be of scarring or non-scarring types

Atrophy
- Defined as decrease in epidermal thickening (less than five cell layers thick)

Ballooning degeneration
- Increased intracellular fluid in epidermal keratinocytes with their resultant destruction

Basement membrane
- Defined as a zone on which the epidermis rests and acts as an interface between the epidermis and dermis

Basal cell degeneration
- Appearance of vacuoles in the basal cell layer of epidermis

- Synonyms—vacuolar degeneration or hydropic degeneration or liquefactive degeneration

Cornoid lamella
- Column of parakeratosis, underneath which, there is absence of granular layer

Corps ronds/grains
- Corps ronds—cells with round nucleus and surrounding cytoplasmic halo
- Corps grains—flattened dark blue nucleus with scant cytoplasm

Cowdry-A body
- Also known as the Lipshutz body
- Intra-nuclear eosinophilic inclusions, seen in herpes infection

Cowdry-B body
- Intra-nuclear eosinophilic inclusions, seen in adenovirus and poliovirus infection

Crust
- Stratum corneum showing fluid with inflammatory cells and debris

Donovan body
- Cytoplasm of macrophages, show collections of bacilli
- Seen in granuloma inguinale (donovanosis)

Dutcher body
- Plasma cells with intra-nuclear inclusions of immunoglobulin

Epidermolytic hyperkeratosis
- Irregular hypergranulosis with cell membrane disruption

Epidermotropism
- Lymphocytes are present throughout the dermo-epidermal junction

Exocytosis
- Lymphocytes within the epidermis (migration of lymphocytes from the dermis into the epidermis)

Foam cells
- Lipid laden macrophages

Follicular Mucinosis
- Accumulation of mucin within the hair shaft

Grenz zone
- An area underneath the epidermis, that separates epidermis from the dermis

Guarnieri body
- Eosinophilic cytoplasmic inclusions
- Seen in smallpox

Hyper/hypogranulosis
- Thickened or diminished granular cell layer

Hyper/hypopigmentation
- Increased/decreased melanin pigment

Hyperkeratosis
- Thickening of stratum corneum

Hyper-parakeratosis
- Thickening of stratum corneum with epithelium showing retained nuclei

Ortho-hyperkeratosis
- Thickening of stratum corneum which now resembles a weaved basket

Henderson-Paterson body
- Intra-cytoplasmic eosinophilic inclusions, seen in molluscum contagiosum

Incontinence of pigment
- Deposition of melanin in upper dermis, that occurs following damage to dermo-epidermal junction

Interface dermatitis
- Basal cell layer vacuolization with lymphocytic infiltrate at the dermal-epidermal junction

Koilocyte
- An atypical keratinocyte with hyperchromatic raisin-shaped nuclei and perinuclear halo

Karyorrhexis
- Cellular fragmentation (neutrophilic fragmentation is called leukocytoclasis)

Kamino body
- Eosinophilic globules in epidermis, seen in Spitz nevus

Kogoj pustule
- Collection of neutrophils in stratum spinosum
- Seen in psoriasis

Munro Microabscesses
- Collection of neutrophils in stratum corneum
- Seen in psoriasis

Michaelis-Gutmann body
- Intracellular and extracellular calcified concentric structures within histiocytes
- Seen in malakoplakia

Necrobiosis
- Destruction and necrosis of collagen

Paget cells
- Large cells with abundant clear cytoplasm within the epidermis

Palisading
- Picket-fence like arrangement of cells, at the periphery

Papillomatosis
- Enlargement of the dermal papillae, resulting in exophytic finger-like projections

Pautrier's micro-abscess
- Intra-epidermal collections of atypical lymphocytes
- Seen in mycosis fungoides

Pseudoepitheliomatous hyperplasia
- Hyperplasia of epidermis and adnexal epithelium

Pseudohorn cyst
- Keratotic invaginations within the epidermis

Reticular degeneration
- Epidermal destruction with retained cell membranes in a net-like pattern

Spongiosis
- Intercellular edema of the epidermis

Schaumann body
- Laminated calcified structures, seen in sarcoidosis

Squamatization
- Replacement of cuboidal/columnar epithelial cells with polyhedral squamous cells

Squamous eddies
- Concentric whorled arrangement of squamous cells

Vasculitis
- Damage to the blood vessel wall due to endothelial cell swelling with infiltration by inflammatory cells

Verocay body
- Cellular areas surrounded by nuclear palisades
- Seen in Schwannoma

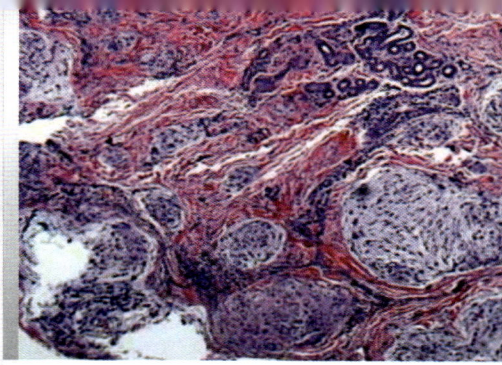

Inflammatory and Infectious Disorders Affecting Epidermis and Dermis

Part 2

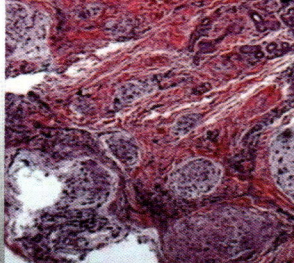

Dermatitis

- It is defined as a dermal reaction, seen in allergies or following a contact with any irritant or toxic substance
- Also called as eczema
- Variants—atopic dermatitis, seborrheic dermatitis, allergic contact dermatitis, stasis dermatitis

ATOPIC DERMATITIS

INTRODUCTION

- Seen in individuals, with a family history of atopy (most commonly allergic rhinitis and asthma)
- Familial predisposition is common
- Age group—affects infants and children and less commonly adults

CLINICAL FEATURES

- Symmetrical, dry, scaly, pruritic patches and plaques
- Most commonly affects extensor surfaces in infants and flexor surface of arms, legs, trunk and face in children
- Chronic lesions show thickening of the skin with abnormal pigmentation
- Remissions and exacerbations are common
- Spontaneous remission can occur in adult life

HISTOPATHOLOGY (Figs 6.1 and 6.2)

Acute variant	Chronic variant
Mild acanthosis	Broad-based acanthosis, hypergranulosis and hyper-parakeratosis with thickened rete ridges
Epidermal spongiosis	Spongiosis is less prominent or absent
Superficial dermis show perivascular lymphohistiocytic infiltrate with or without eosinophils Exocytosis of lymphocytes	Superficial dermis with perivascular lymphocytic infiltrate and occasional eosinophils

DIFFERENTIAL DIAGNOSIS

1. *Contact dermatitis: see below*
2. *Spongiotic drug eruption*
   - Spongiosis
   - Exocytosis of lymphocytes
   - Dyskeratotic cells (cytoid bodies)
   - Perivascular lymphocytic infiltrate in superficial dermis
3. *Dermatophytosis*
   - Neutrophils and fungal elements in the stratum corneum
4. *Pityriasis rosea*
   - Widened dermal papillae
   - Exocytosis of erythrocytes
5. *PLEVA (Pityriasis lichenoides et varioliformis acuta)*
   - Focal basal cell layer vacuolization
   - Apoptotic keratinocytes
   - Wedge-shaped lymphocytic infiltrate in the dermis
   - Extravasation of erythrocytes

SEBORRHEIC DERMATITIS

INTRODUCTION

- Lesions affect sebum rich areas of the body
- Age group—affect individuals around puberty and rarely infants

CLINICAL FEATURES

- Sites—seborrheic areas, i.e. scalp, eyebrows, nose, face, chest wall (around sternum), axillae and groin
- Presents as greasy, scaling erythematous lesions or papules
- Associated with pruritus
- Lesions heal by itself, only to come back again (waxing and waning is common)
- Secondary infection can occur
- Most common cutaneous lesions seen in AIDS patients

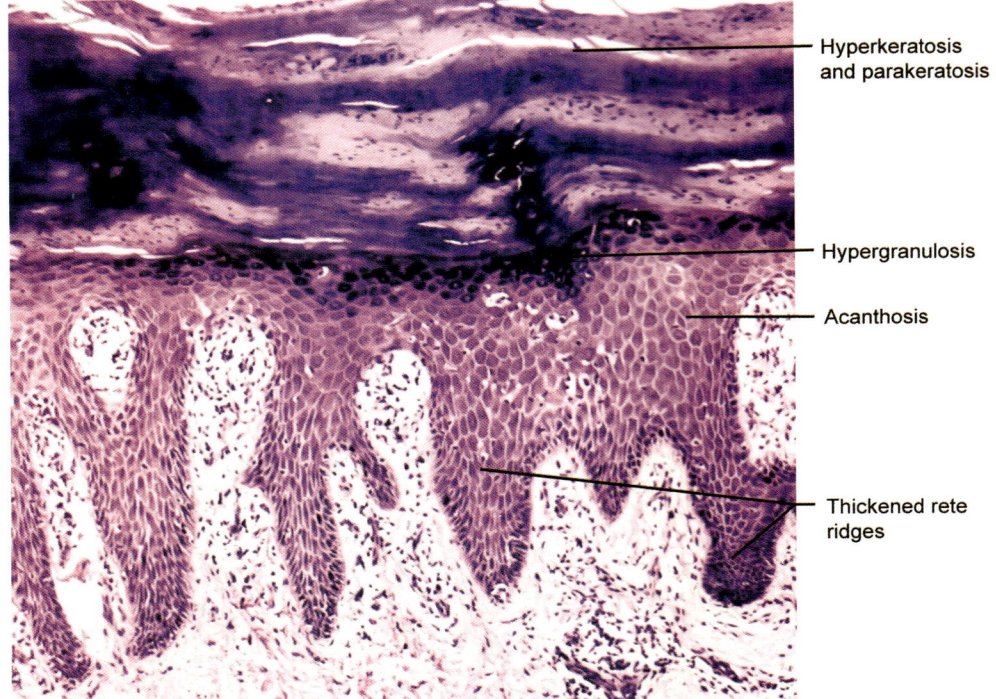

Hyperkeratosis and parakeratosis

Hypergranulosis

Acanthosis

Thickened rete ridges

Fig. 6.1: Dermatitis

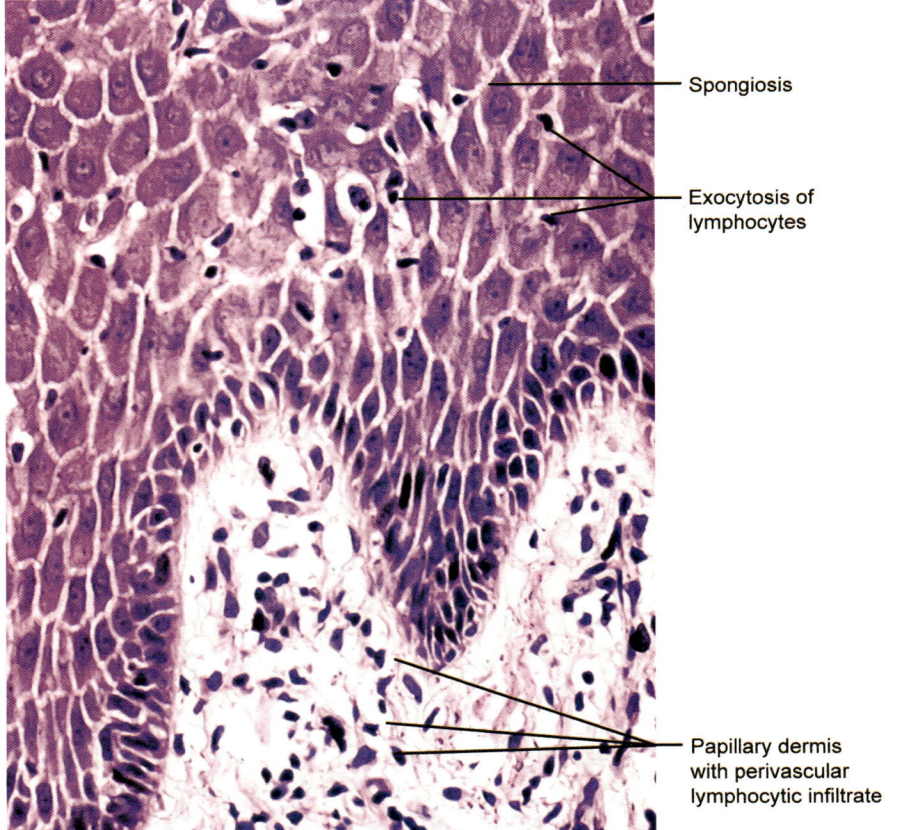

Spongiosis

Exocytosis of lymphocytes

Papillary dermis with perivascular lymphocytic infiltrate

Fig. 6.2: Dermatitis

HISTOPATHOLOGY

- Stratum corneum layer on its top shows a crust containing neutrophilic aggregates (that is often centered on a follicle)
- Mild epidermal spongiosis and irregular acanthosis are seen
- Perifollicular parakeratosis (shoulder parakeratosis)
- Exocytosis of lymphocytes
- Superficial dermis shows perivascular lympho-histiocytic infiltrate

DIFFERENTIAL DIAGNOSIS

Psoriasis

- Neutrophilic aggregates in stratum corneum
- Hyperkeratosis and parakeratosis
- Minimal or no spongiosis

ALLERGIC CONTACT DERMATITIS

INTRODUCTION

- Allergen or irritant mediated delayed hyper-sensitivity reaction
- Common irritants responsible include nickel, uroshiol, perfume, neomycin, formaldehyde

CLINICAL FEATURES (Fig. 6.3)

- Pattern of distribution of the lesion—depends on the area of contact (linear or geometric pattern of eczematous reaction)
- Lesions in initial stage show blisters, erythematous papules and plaques with excoriation

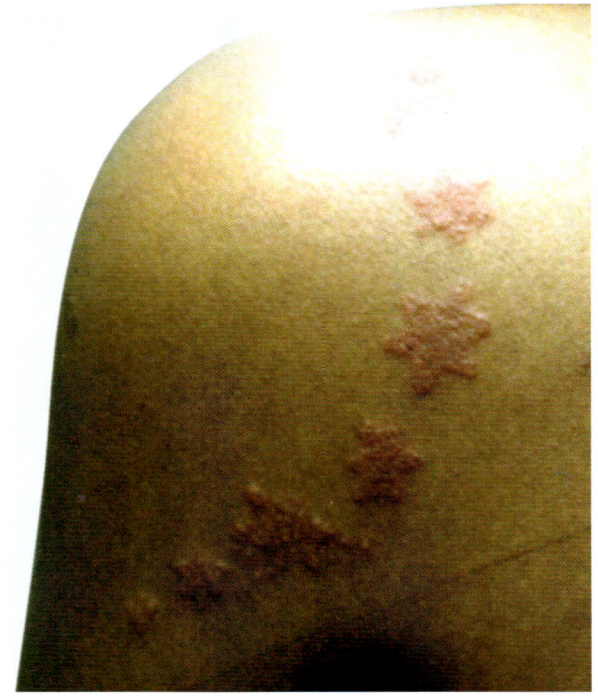

Fig. 6.3: Allergic contact dermatitis to tattoo pigment. Well-demarcated, erythematous, indurated, scaly plaques

- Lesions in later stage shows scaling with post-inflammatory hypo/hyperpigmentation
- Lesions subside within a few days to weeks, after the removal of causative agent.

HISTOPATHOLOGY (Figs 6.4 and 6.5)

Acute Stage

- Epidermal spongiosis
- Exocytosis of lymphocytes

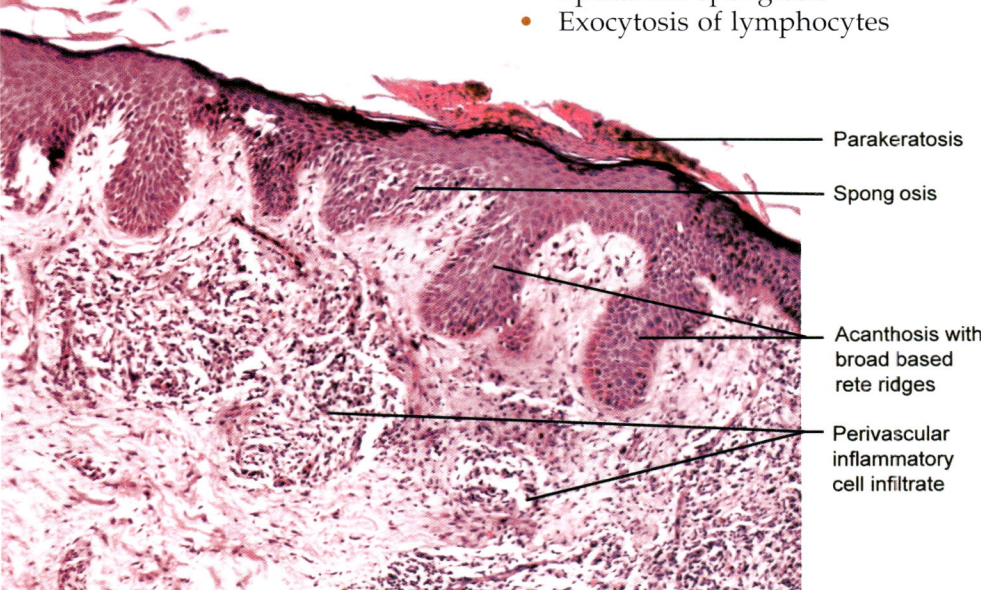

Parakeratosis

Spong osis

Acanthosis with broad based rete ridges

Perivascular inflammatory cell infiltrate

Fig. 6.4: Contact dermatitis

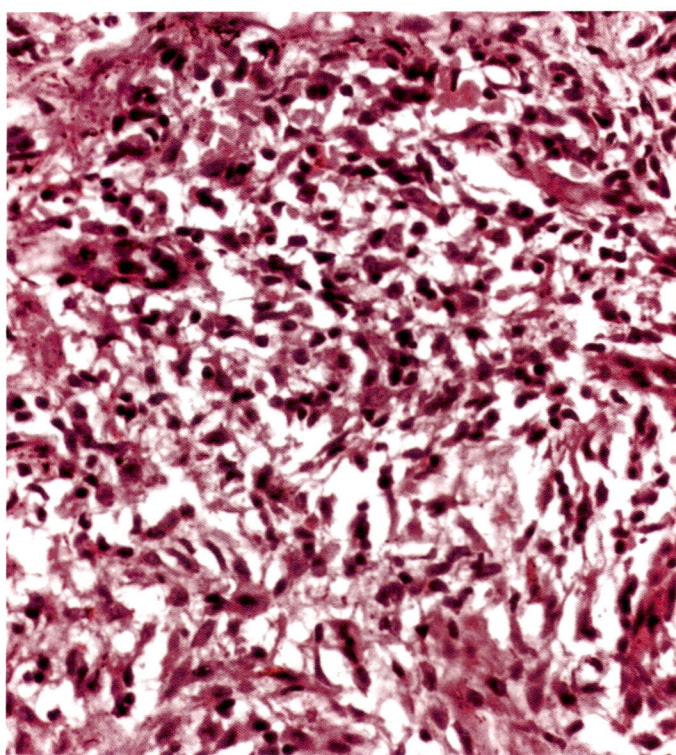

Fig. 6.5: Contact Dermatitis. Perivascular chronic inflammatory cell and histiocytic infiltrate

- Superficial dermal perivascular lymphohistiocytic infiltrate with eosinophils and edema

Chronic Stage
- Little or absent spongiosis
- Focal parakeratosis
- Psoriasiform epidermal hyperplasia
- Fibrosis in the papillary dermis

Differential Diagnosis

1. *Seborrheic dermatitis*
   - Spongiosis and irregular acanthosis
   - Stratum corneum layer with crust on its top containing neutrophils
   - Perifollicular parakeratosis

2. *Insect bite reaction*
   - Epidermal necrosis or ulceration
   - Variable spongiosis
   - Wedge-shaped mixed inflammatory cell infiltrate composed of neutrophils, lymphocytes and eosinophils

3. *Mycosis fungoides*
   - Epidermotropism of atypical lymphocytes

STASIS DERMATITIS

INTRODUCTION
- Eczematous lesions, seen in lower limbs
- Cause—venous stasis, due to varicose veins
- Age group—fifth to sixth decade
- Follows slow progressive course

CLINICAL FEATURES
- Presents as pruritic, painful lesions, localized to lower legs, proximal to the ankles
- Affected lower limb shows edema
- Due to chronic venous stasis, with resultant hemosiderin deposition, skin attains brownish discoloration
- Lichenification and crusting are common
- Secondary infections can occur

HISTOPATHOLOGY
- Variable hyperkeratosis and acanthosis
- Superficial dermis and deep dermis show lobular pattern of new blood vessels
- Surrounding these blood vessels, chronic inflammatory cell infiltrate can be seen
- Dermal fibrosis and hemosiderin deposition can be seen

DIFFERENTIAL DIAGNOSIS

Atopic Dermatitis
- Spongiosis
- Dermis shows perivascular lymphocytes and eosinophils

Table 6.1: Differences between psoriasis, contact dermatitis and seborrheic dermatitis			
Features	Psoriasis	Contact dermatitis	Seborrheic dermatitis
Parakeratosis	Confluent	Focal	Perifollicular
Granular layer	Absent	Present	Present
Spongiosis	Scant	Prominent	Mild
Neutrophils	Present	Absent	Absent
Mitosis	Common	Few	Absent

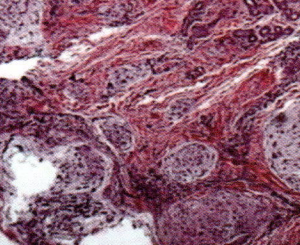

Prurigo

INTRODUCTION

- Reaction pattern, that occurs secondary to chronic exogenous irritation, due to repetitive friction and rubbing
- Age group—fourth to sixth decades
- Females are more commonly affected than males
- Lesions are symmetrical and heal with scarring

CLINICAL FEATURES

Can present as following entities:

1. *Prurigo nodularis* (Fig. 7.1)
   - Thickened erythematous papules or nodules, associated with scarring
   - Single or multiple lesions
   - Most common sites affected—forearms, legs, neck, back

2. *Lichen simplex chronicus*
   - Lesion presents as thickened erythematous plaque
   - End stage lesions of eczema, arthropod bite, folliculitis (similar to prurigo)

3. *Corn/Callus*
   - Occurs in response to friction or pressure
   - Most common site includes palms or soles

4. *Frictional lichenoid dermatitis*
   - Occurs due to repetitive friction
   - Presents as papules or plaques over elbows or knees

5. *Acanthoma fissuratum*
   - Chronic rubbing of spectacles on nose or post-auricular areas

HISTOPATHOLOGY (Figs 7.2 and 7.3)

Prurigo Nodularis

- Hyperkeratosis with acanthosis and hyper-granulosis
- Pseudoepitheliomatous hyperplasia

- Mild spongiosis
- Dermal scarring
- Increased number of dermal blood vessels
- Mixed inflammatory cell infiltrate in the dermis

Lichen Simplex Chronicus

- Hyperkeratosis with hypergranulosis
- Acanthosis with elongation of rete ridges
- Mild spongiosis

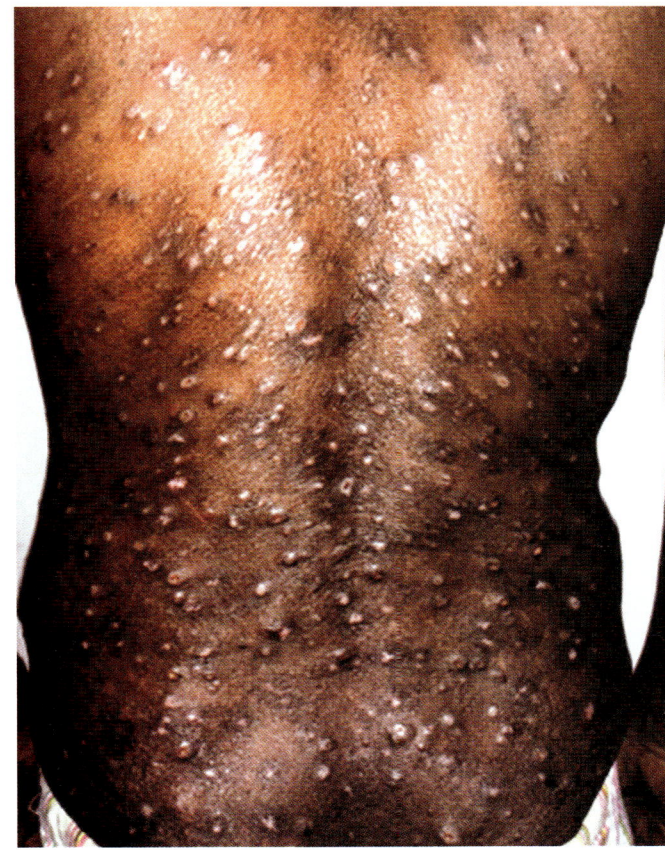

Fig. 7.1: Prurigo nodularis. Firm, dome-shaped, itchy nodules of varying sizes, symmetrically distributed on the trunk

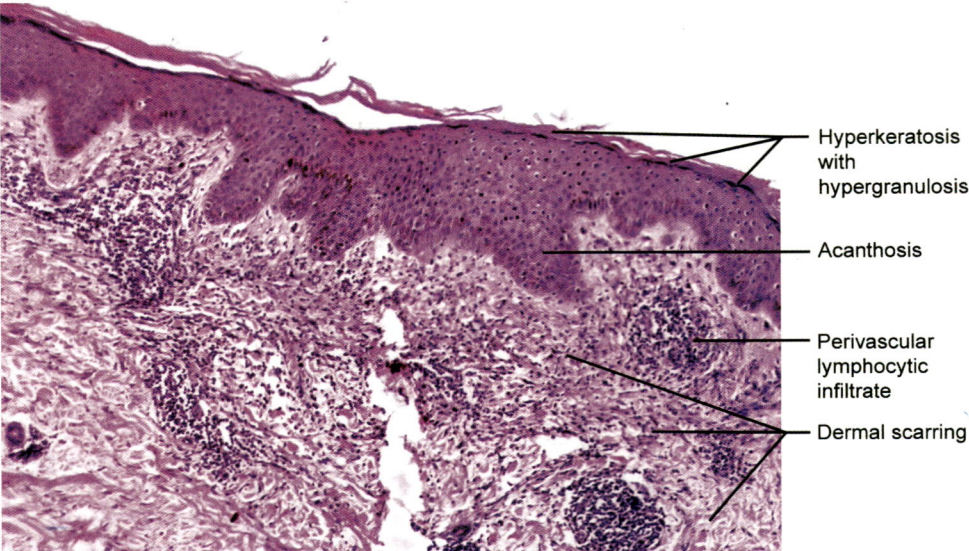

Hyperkeratosis with hypergranulosis

Acanthosis

Perivascular lymphocytic infiltrate

Dermal scarring

Fig. 7.2: Prurigo nodularis

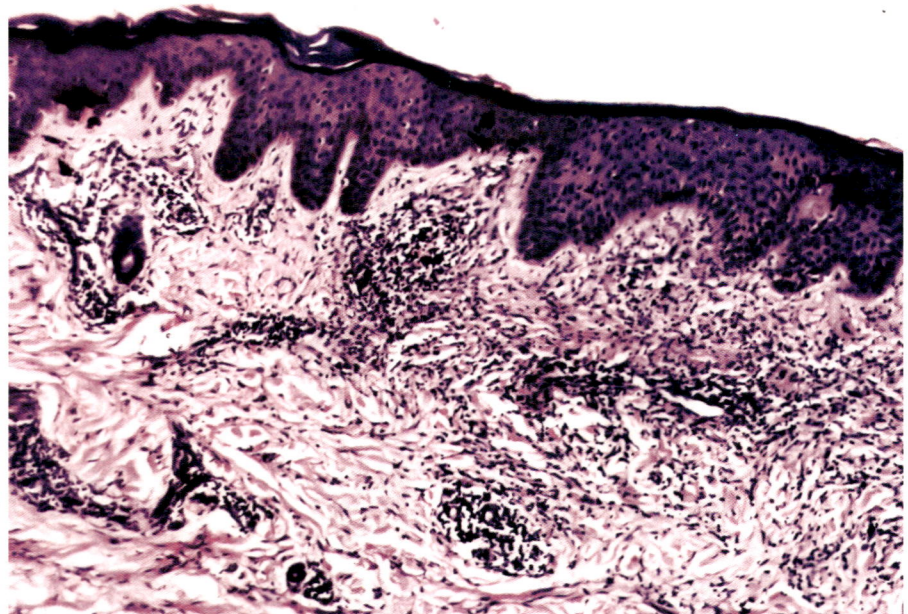

Fig. 7.3: Another case of prurigo nodularis demonstrating hyperkeratosis, acanthosis and dermis showing dense peri-vascular inflammatory cell infiltrate

- Vertical streaks of collagen along the dermal papillae (superficial dermis)
- Perivascular mixed inflammatory cell infiltrate in the superficial dermis

DIFFERENTIAL DIAGNOSIS

Scabies

- Eosinophils form a major part of inflammatory infiltrate
- Diagnosis is made by identification of mite or its eggs

Psoriasis

- Confluent parakeratosis, accumulation of neutrophils in the stratum corneum

Verrucous Lichen Planus

- Interface dermatitis with basal cell vacuolization

Verrucous Carcinoma

- Elongated and broad rete ridges, lined by hyperplastic stratified squamous epithelium showing cytological atypia and pushing or invasive margins

PRURIGO SIMPLEX

- Presents as pruritic papules
- Sites—trunk and extremities

HISTOPATHOLOGY (Figs 7.4 to 7.6)

- Mild acanthosis, spongiosis
- Superficial dermis showing perivascular mixed inflammatory cell infiltrate

DIFFERENTIAL DIAGNOSIS

Dermatitis Herpetiformis

- Neutrophilic microabscesses at the tips of dermal papillae
- Dermis shows mixed inflammatory cell infiltrate

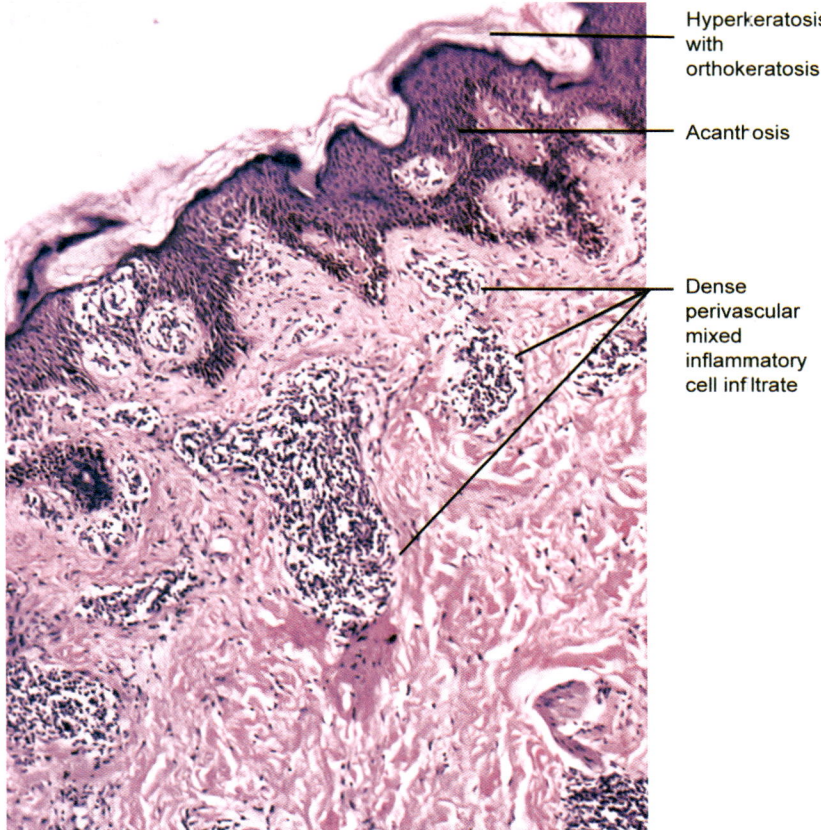

Hyperkeratosis with orthokeratosis

Acanthosis

Dense perivascular mixed inflammatory cell infiltrate

Fig. 7.4: Prurigo simplex

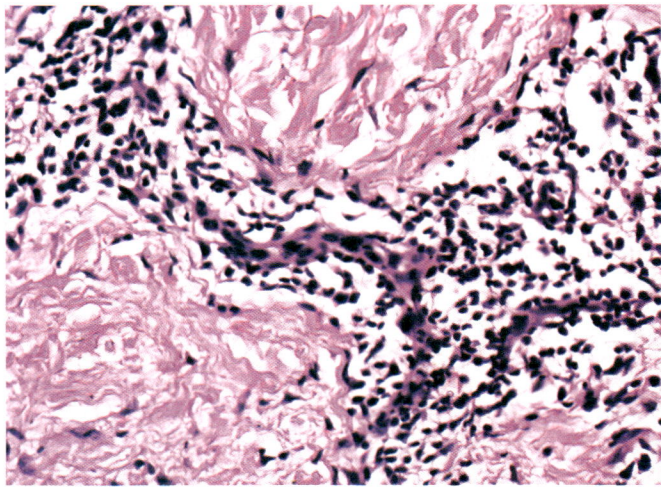

Fig. 7.5: Prurigo simplex. Dense mixed perivascular inflammatory cell infiltrate with plump endothelial cells of the vessel wall

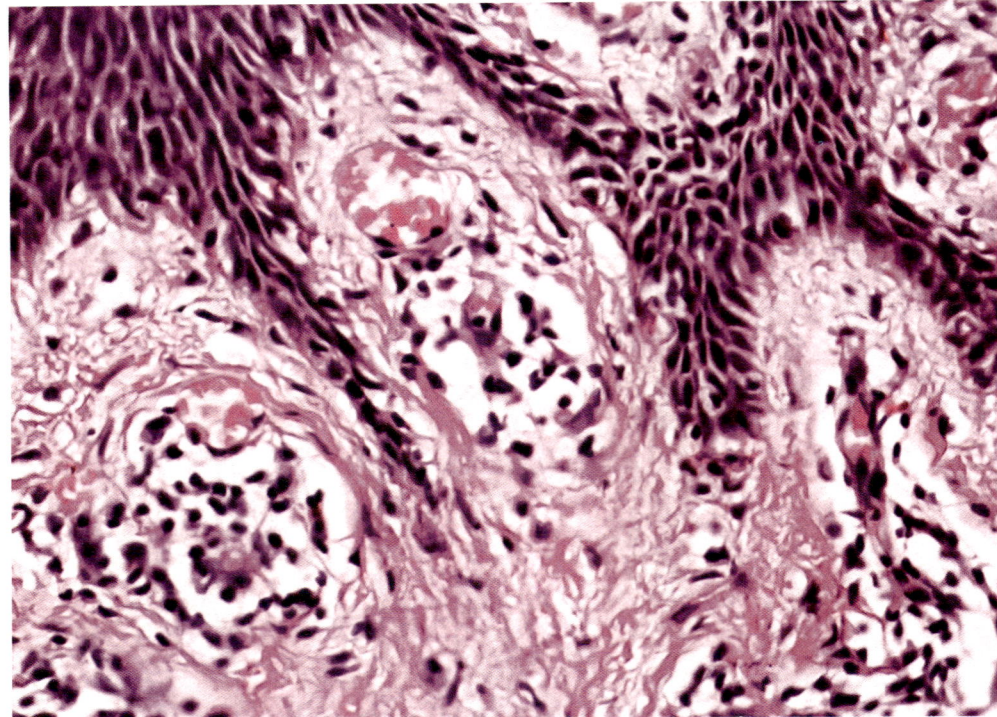

Fig. 7.6: Prurigo simplex. Papillary dermis with mixed perivascular inflammatory cell infiltrate

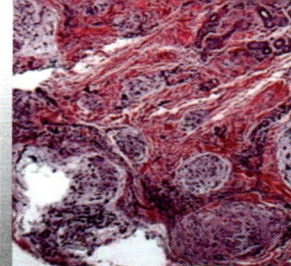

Psoriasis

INTRODUCTION

- It is a chronic inflammatory dermatitis, that has genetic basis
- Age group—most commonly affects children
- Individuals with fair skin are more prone to develop the disease
- Factors exacerbating the disease—beta blockers, lithium, patients suffering from AIDS

CLINICAL FEATURES (Fig. 8.1)

- Lesions are well-circumscribed and symmetrically distributed
- Presents as discrete, erythematous patches or plaques with thick silvery scales

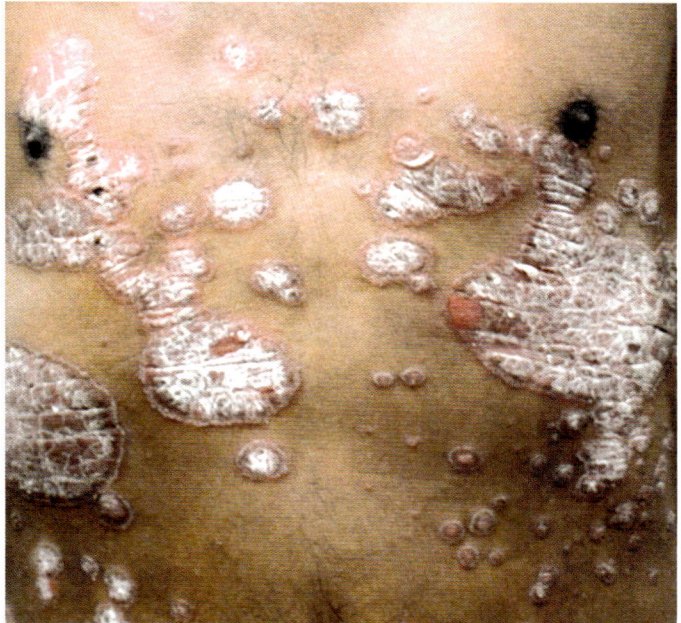

Fig. 8.1: Psoriasis vulgaris. Symmetrically distributed, erythematous papules and plaques with sharp defined edges and silvery white scales

- **Sites affected**—elbows, knees, scalp, umbilicus, buttocks, perianal area
- **Nail changes**—onycholysis, pitting of nails, nail plate thickening
- **Koebner's phenomenon**—development of psoriatic plaques at the site of trauma
- **Auspitz sign**—pinpoint bleeding spots are seen, when the scales are peeled off
- **Tongue**—geographic stomatitis may be seen
- Disease follows a waxing-waning course, with flare ups and remissions
- Patients are at increased risk of developing psoriatic arthritis

VARIANTS

- **Guttate psoriasis**—rapid onset of small papules and plaques, on trunk and extremities, following streptococcal pharyngitis
- **Pustular psoriasis**—generalized small pustules appearing on red and tender skin
- **Inverse psoriasis**—also called flexural psoriasis and involves flexural areas like axilla, perineum and groin
- **Palmoplantar pustulosis**—pustules present on the palms and soles
- **Erythrodermic psoriasis**—generalized erythema with diffuse scaling, administration of steroids can be a precipitating factor
- **Follicular psoriasis**—presents as discrete hyper-keratotic papules, involving thighs

HISTOPATHOLOGY (Figs 8.2 to 8.8)

- **Earliest lesion**—dilatation and congestion of vessels in the papillary dermis with mild perivascular lymphocytic infiltrate
- Confluent parakeratosis, hyper-parakeratosis and hypogranulosis

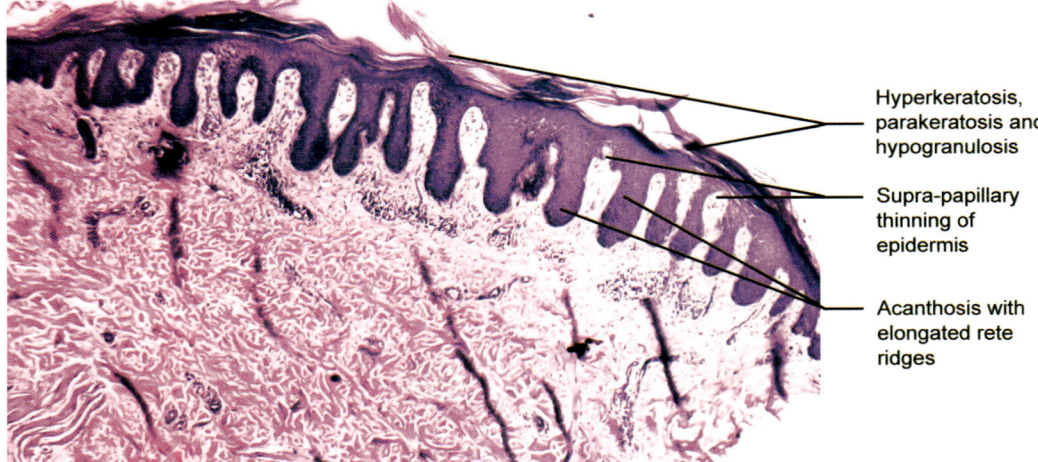

Hyperkeratosis, parakeratosis and hypogranulosis

Supra-papillary thinning of epidermis

Acanthosis with elongated rete ridges

Fig. 8.2: Psoriasis

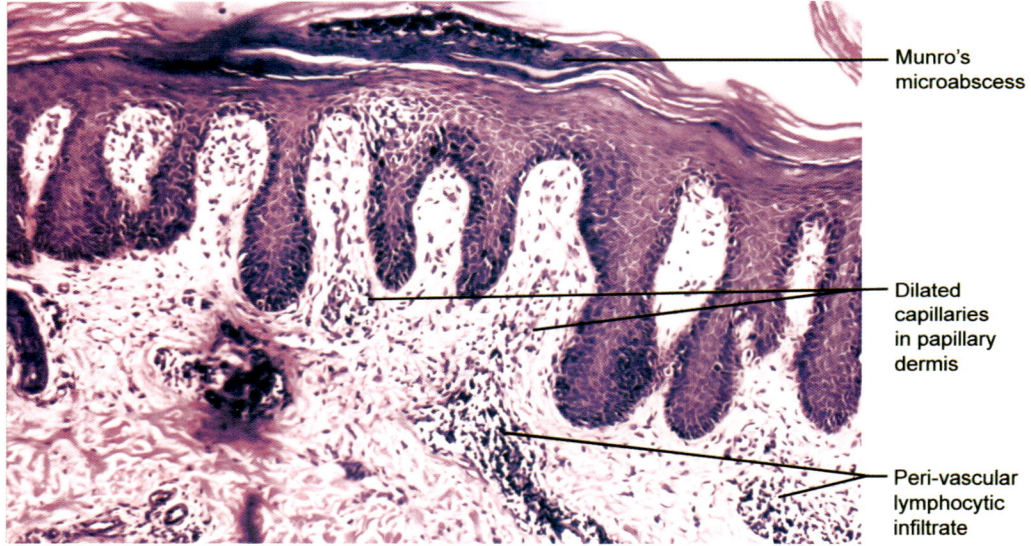

Munro's microabscess

Dilated capillaries in papillary dermis

Peri-vascular lymphocytic infiltrate

Fig. 8.3: Psoriasis

- Epidermal acanthosis, mild spongiosis with elongated rete ridges and suprapapillary thinning of epidermis
- **Munro's microabscesses**—neutrophils in the stratum corneum
- **Spongiform pustules of Kogoj**—neutrophils in stratum spinosum
- **Guttate psoriasis** (Figs 8.5 to 8.8)—absence of epidermal hyperplasia, presence of granular layer, discrete mounds of parakeratosis with collections of neutrophils overlying the epidermis
- **Pustular psoriasis**—less prominent epidermal hyperplasia and prominent neutrophilic abscesses
- **Spongiotic psoriasis**—histopathological features of psoriasis with features of spongiosis in upper dermis

- **Follicular psoriasis** (Figs 8.9 and 8.10)—follicular plugging, parakeratosis, perivascular and peri-follicular inflammatory cell infiltrate

DIFFERENTIAL DIAGNOSIS

Pityriasis Rubra Pilaris (Figs 8.11 and 8.12)

- Presents as follicular papules and peri-follicular erythema which can coalesce to form scaly plaques
- Acanthosis, preserved granular layer, alternating ortho-parakeratosis oriented in both horizontal and vertical directions
- Areas corresponding to follicular papules show dilated infundibulum with orthokeratotic plug

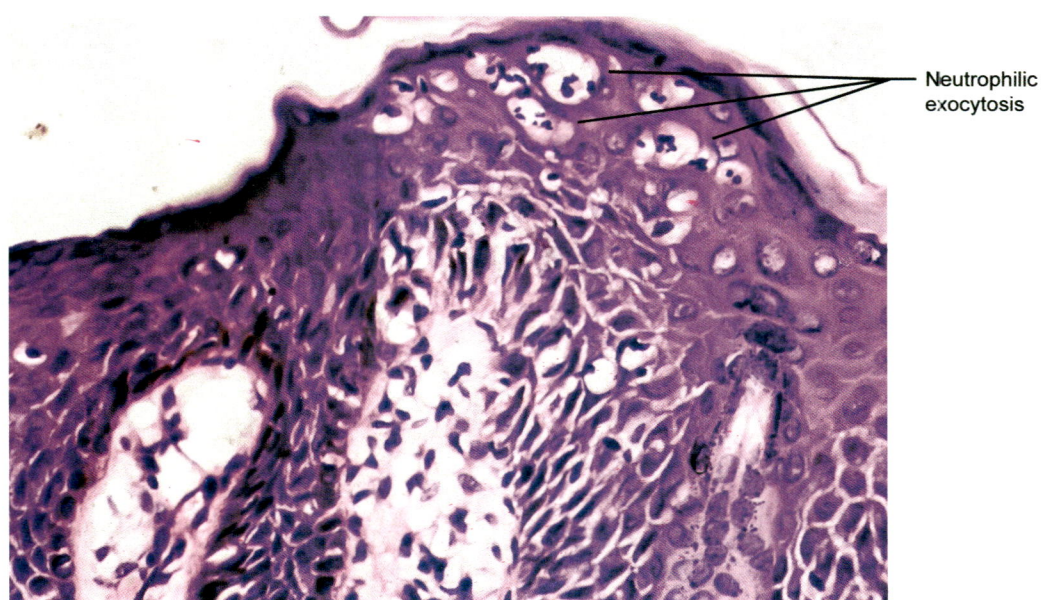

Neutrophilic exocytosis

Fig. 8.4: Psoriasis. A case demonstrating neutrophilic exocytosis in lining epithelium

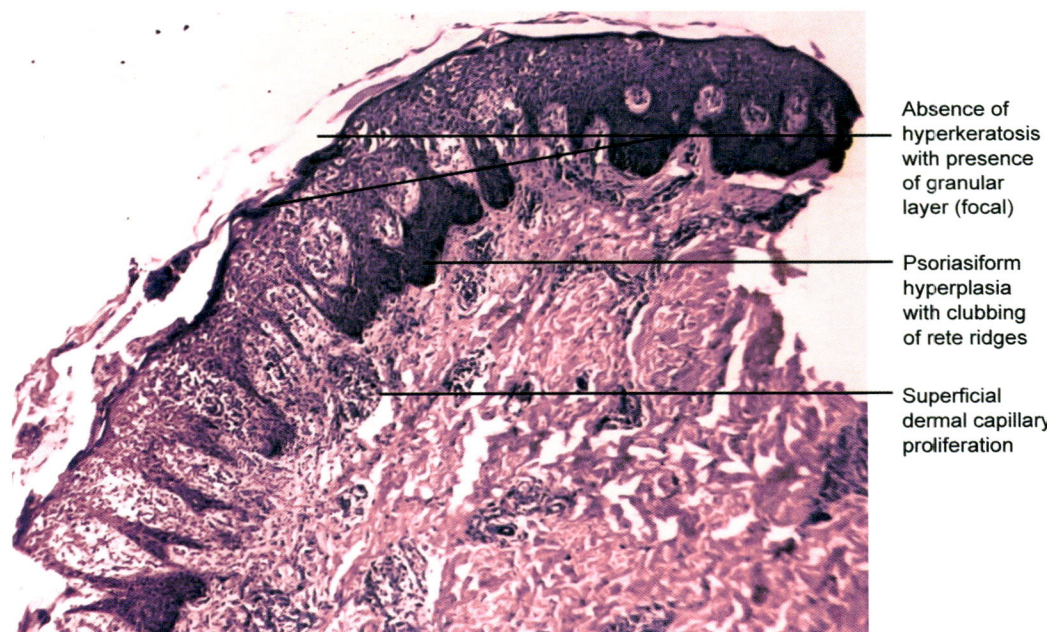

Absence of hyperkeratosis with presence of granular layer (focal)

Psoriasiform hyperplasia with clubbing of rete ridges

Superficial dermal capillary proliferation

Fig. 8.5: Guttate psoriasis

- Superficial perivascular and peri-follicular lymphocytic infiltrate

Dermatophyte Infection
- Parakeratosis, neutrophilic abscesses in stratum corneum, along with eosinophils
- Organism can be demonstrated by periodic acid-Schiff (PAS) or Gomori methenamine silver (GMS) stain

Seborrheic Dermatitis
- Spongiosis, shoulder parakeratosis, irregular acanthosis with preserved granular layer, peri-follicular neutrophilic aggregates

Lichen Simplex Chronicus
- Hyperkeratosis, hypergranulosis
- Vertical streaks of collagen in papillary dermis

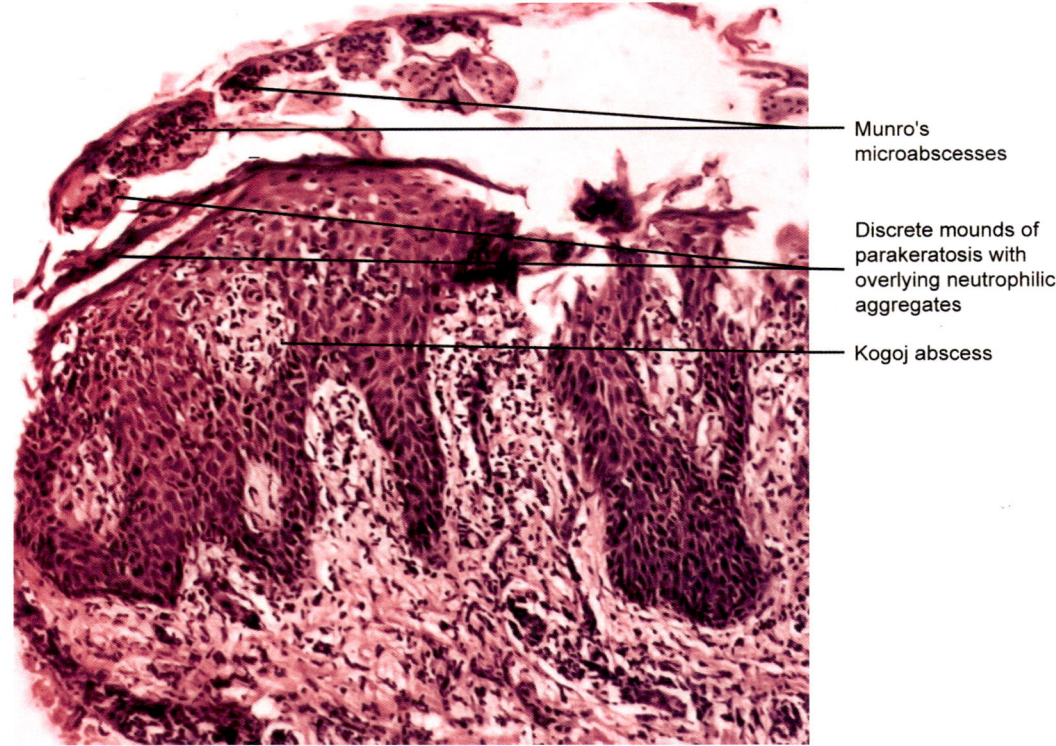

Fig. 8.6: Guttate psoriasis

- Munro's microabscesses
- Discrete mounds of parakeratosis with overlying neutrophilic aggregates
- Kogoj abscess

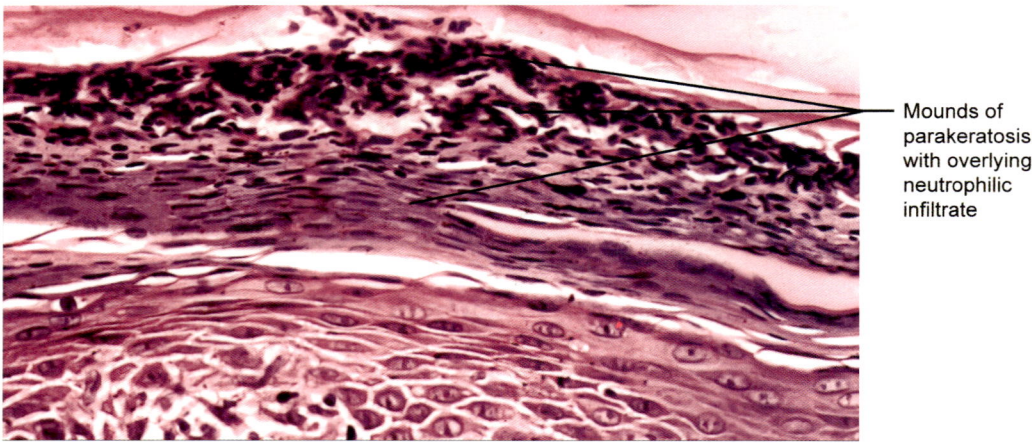

Fig. 8.7: Guttate psoriasis

- Mounds of parakeratosis with overlying neutrophilic infiltrate

IMMUNOPATHOLOGY

- T-cell mediated disorder with CD 8+ T-cells in the epidermis and CD 4+ T-cells in the papillary dermis

PUSTULAR PSORIASIS

INTRODUCTION AND SALIENT FEATURES

- Pustular variant of psoriasis
- Erythematous pustules occurring on palms and soles (Fig. 8.13)

- Can be broadly classified into: **Generalized** and **localized** types

Generalized Pustular Psoriasis

Variants

1. **Acute generalized type of von Zumbusch—** pustular eruptions occur after withdrawal of steroids in patients with pre-existing psoriasis
2. **Impetigo herpetiformis or generalized pustular psoriasis of pregnancy—**pustular eruptions, seen in the last trimester of pregnancy

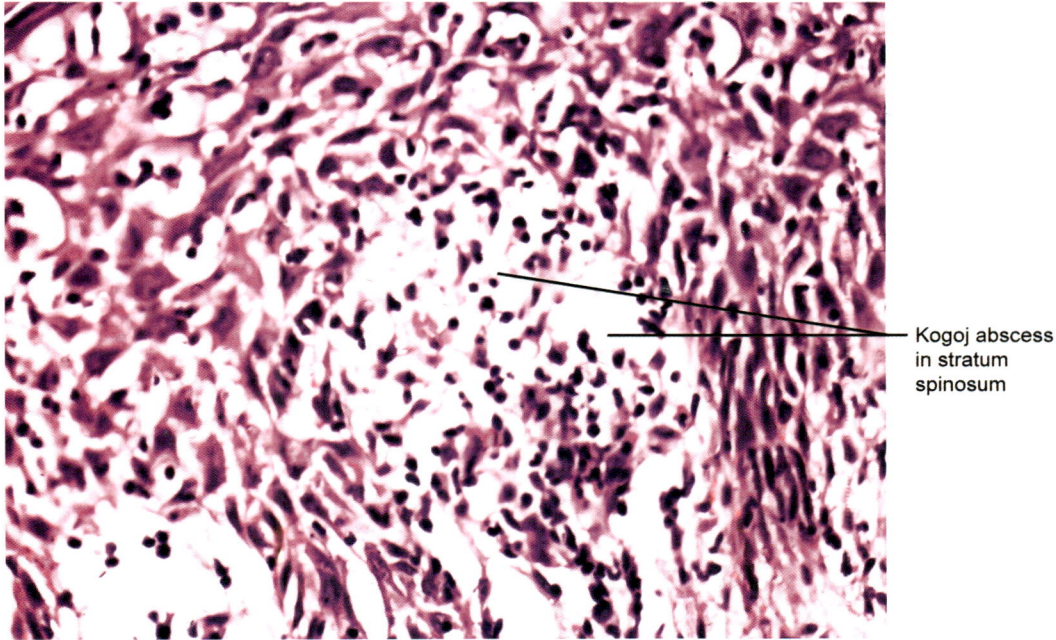

Kogoj abscess
in stratum
spinosum

Fig. 8.8: Guttate psoriasis

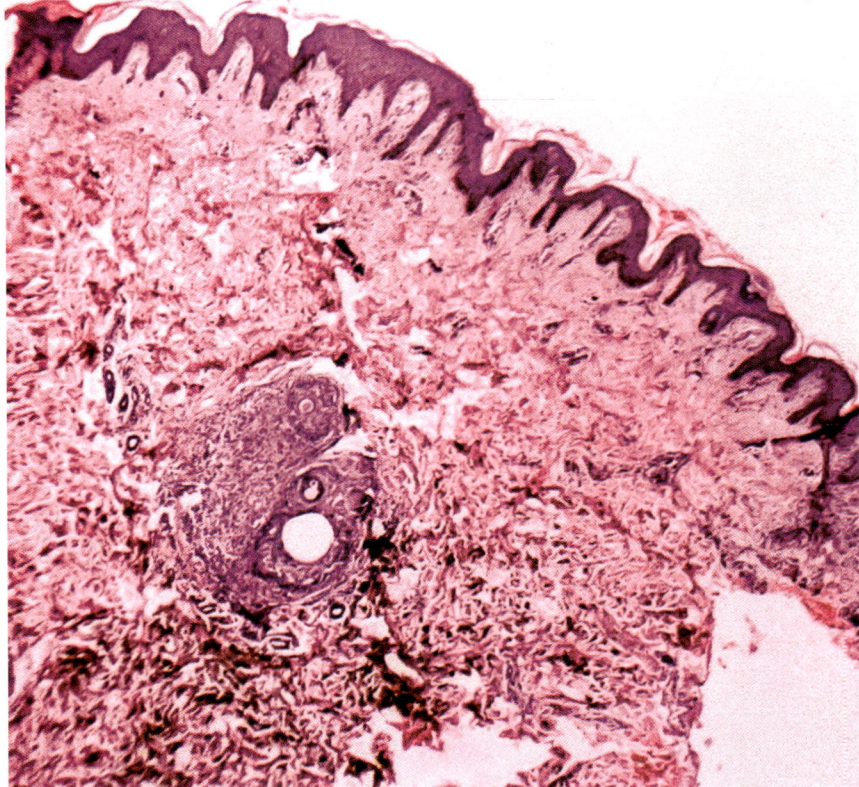

Fig. 8.9: Follicular psoriasis. There is presence of inflammatory cell infiltrate surrounding the follicles

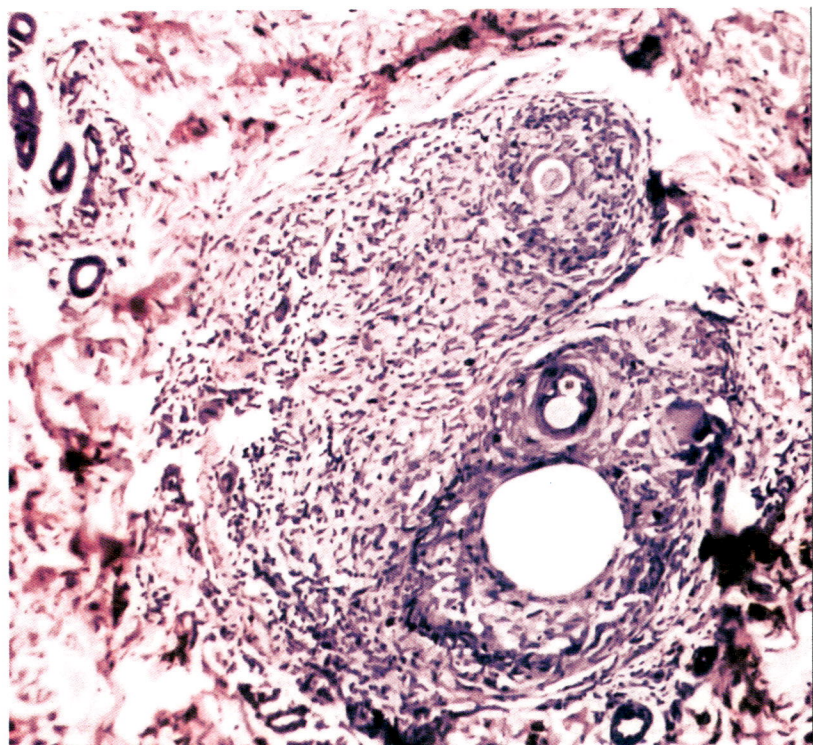

Fig. 8.10: Follicular psoriasis. Inflammatory cell infiltrate surrounding the follicles with presence of giant cells

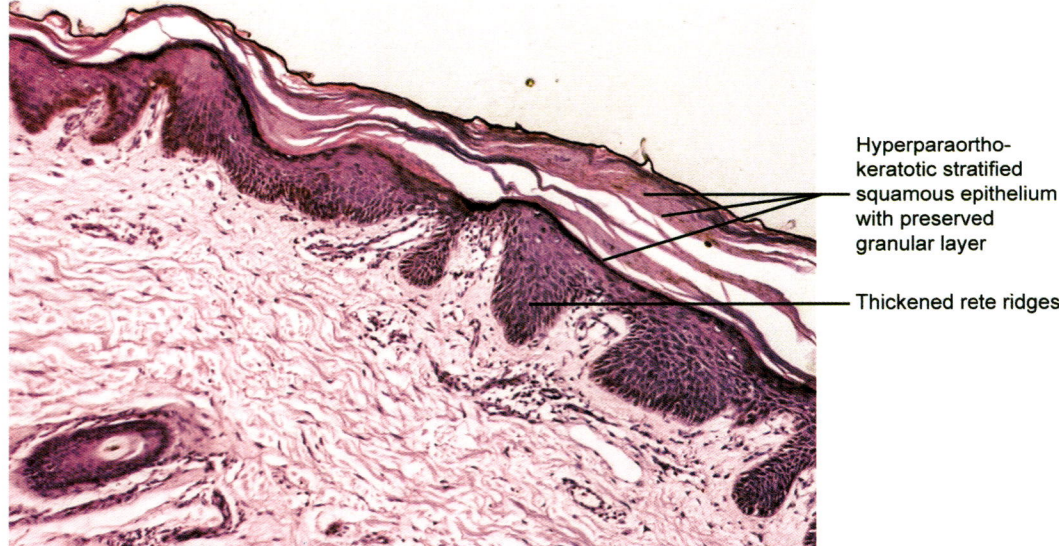

Hyperparaortho-
keratotic stratified
squamous epithelium
with preserved
granular layer

Thickened rete ridges

Fig. 8.11: Pityriasis rubra pilaris

3. **Infantile and juvenile type**—affects children, remissions are commonly seen
4. **Sub-acute annular type**—generalized annular lesions are seen

Histopathology (Figs 8.14 and 8.15)

- Parakeratosis, elongation of rete ridges

- Neutrophilic aggregates forming macroabscesses in the spinosum layer (macropustule of Kogoj) and corneum layer (Munro's abscess)

Localized Pustular Psoriasis

Variants

1. **Psoriasis with pustules**—single or a few affected areas develop pustules

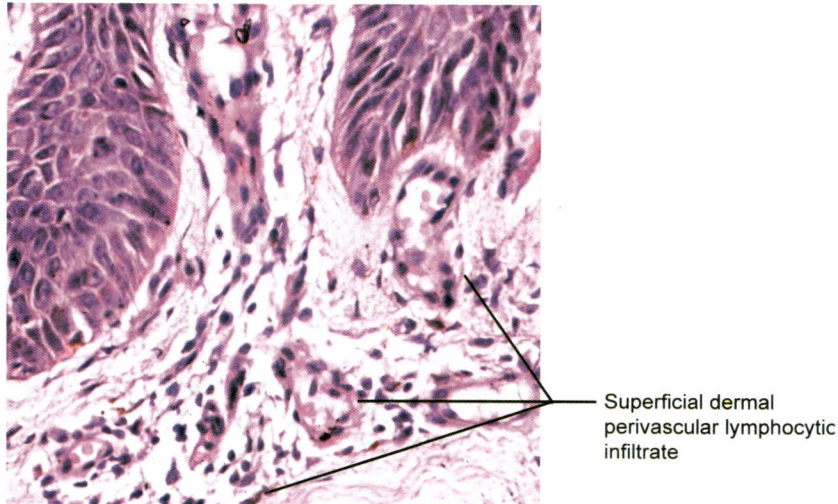

Superficial dermal perivascular lymphocytic infiltrate

Fig. 8.12: Pityriasis rubra pilaris

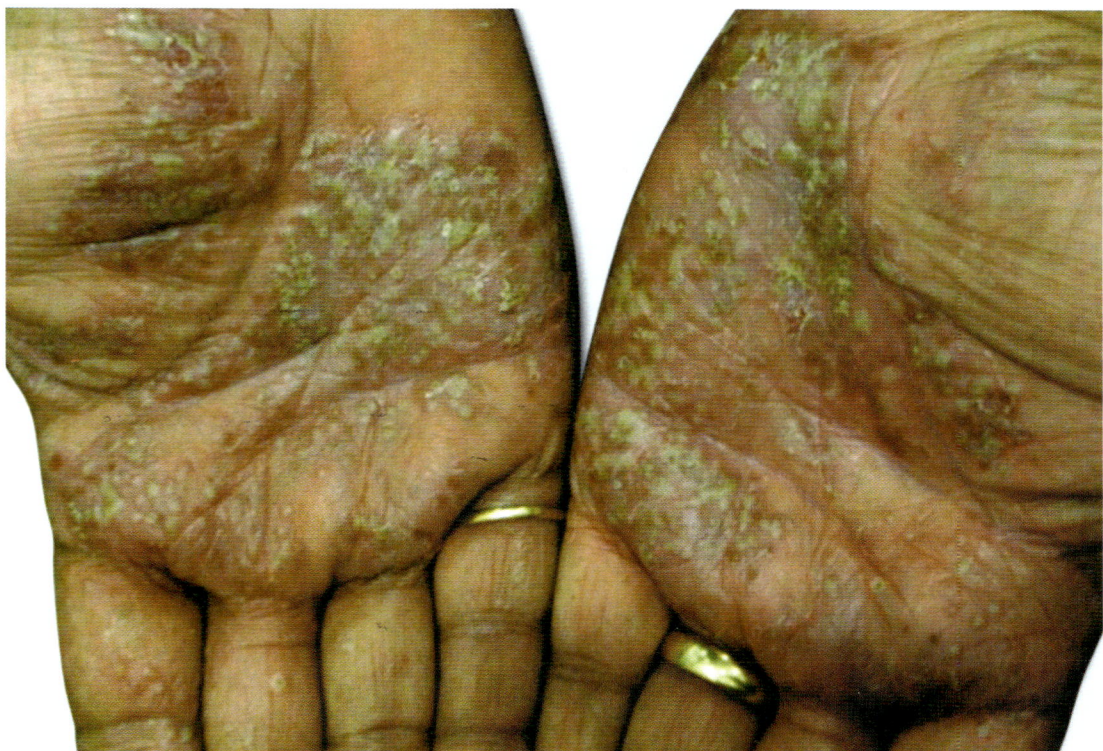

Fig. 8.13: Palmoplantar pustulosis, a type of pustular psoriasis. Clusters of white to yellow-brown sterile pustules with erythema and scaling

2. **Acrodermatitis continua of Hallopeau**—pustules seen on the distal portion of hands and feet
3. **Pustulosis palmaris et plantaris**—lesions involving palms and soles, with acral portions being spared

Histopathology

- Epidermal hyperplasia, orthokeratosis with mounds of parakeratosis and neutrophils
- Pustular cavities containing neutrophils
- Early lesions—spongiosis, exocytosis of lymphocytes in lower epidermis

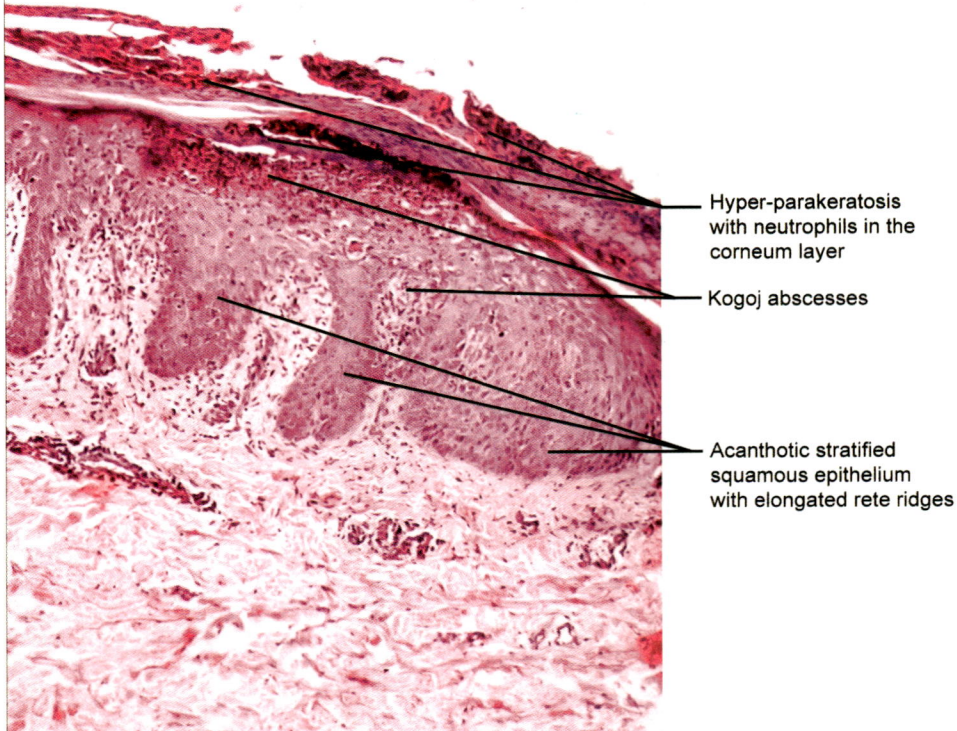

Fig. 8.14: Pustular psoriasis

Hyper-parakeratosis
with neutrophils in the
corneum layer

Kogoj abscesses

Acanthotic stratified
squamous epithelium
with elongated rete ridges

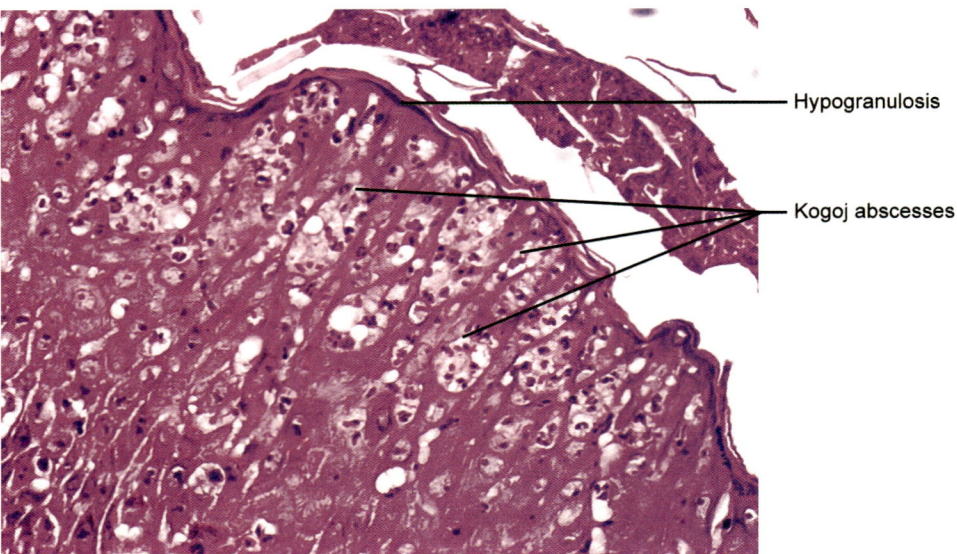

Fig. 8.15: Pustular psoriasis

Hypogranulosis

Kogoj abscesses

DIFFERENTIAL DIAGNOSIS

IgA Pemphigus

- Sub-corneal collection of neutrophils, with acantholysis
- Immunofluorescence demonstrates inter-cellular IgA in upper epidermis

Dermatophyte Infection

- Pustule formation can occur with exocytosis of neutrophils
- PAS stain demonstrates fungal elements in stratum corneum

Impetigo

- Sub-corneal blister with neutrophils as its contents
- Neutrophils can also be seen in stratum corneum
- Gram stain may demonstrate gram-positive cocci in superficial epidermis

Reiter's Syndrome (Figs 8.16 and 8.17)

- Thickened and loosely attached stratum corneum layer
- Large size pustules
- Thicker supra-papillary plate of epidermis

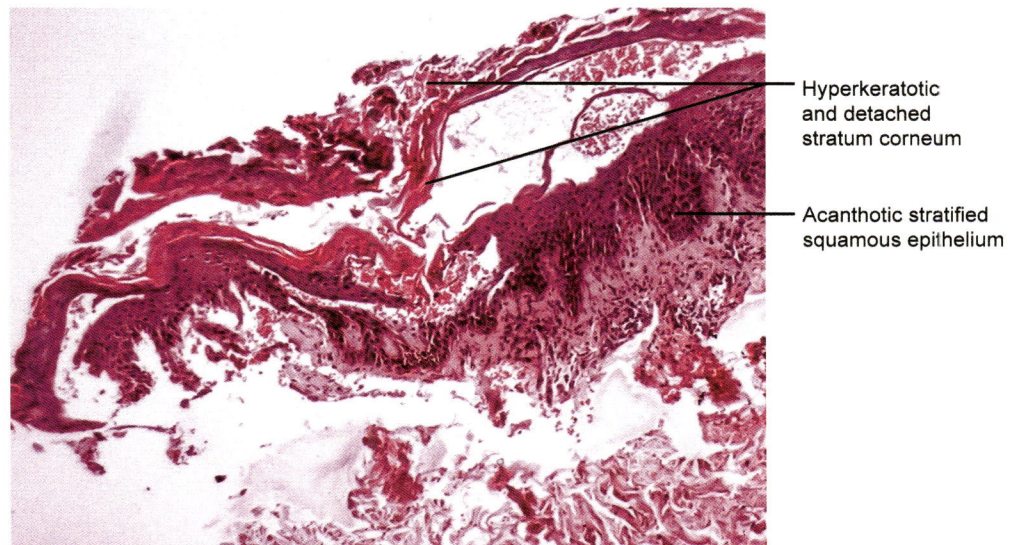

Hyperkeratotic and detached stratum corneum

Acanthotic stratified squamous epithelium

Fig. 8.16: Reiter's syndrome

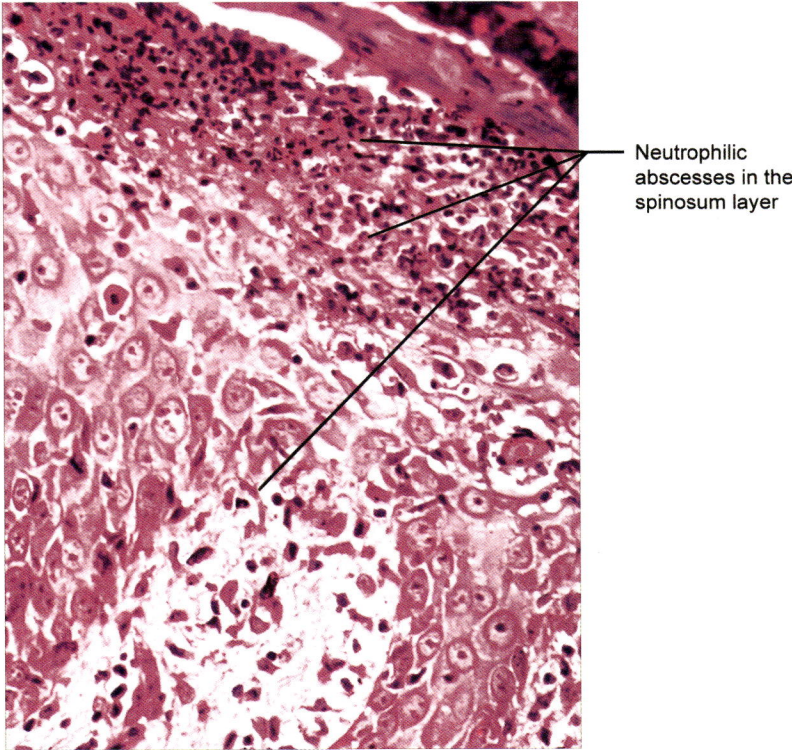

Neutrophilic abscesses in the spinosum layer

Fig. 8.17: Reiter's syndrome

Pityriasis Rosea

INTRODUCTION

- Self-limited disorder
- Clinical presentation—papule or plaque with scaling
- Etiology—human herpes virus (HHV-7) infection, *Chlamydia pneumoniae*, *Mycoplasma pneumoniae*, *Legionella pneumophilia* infections
- Age group—10–35 years, more common in females

CAN PRESENT AS (Fig. 9.1)

Herald Patch

- Single, round to oval, pink to salmon-colored scaly plaque with raised borders

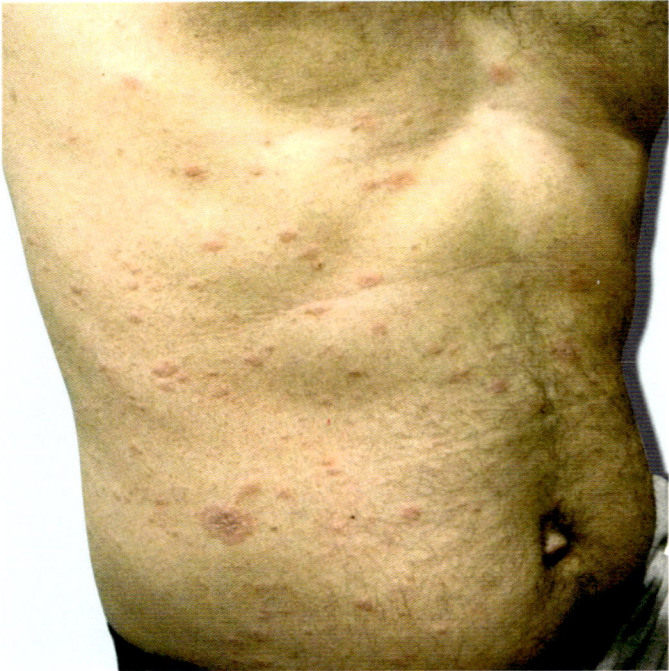

Fig. 9.1: Pityriasis rosea. A single herald patch seen which is round to oval, sharply demarcated, salmon colored lesion along with other smaller lesions with a collarette of scale at the periphery

Generalized Eruption

- Numerous salmon-colored, round to oval papules with a characteristic collarette of scale
- Most commonly affects trunk and proximal extremities
- Face, palms and soles are spared
- Christmas tree pattern—oval papules on the trunk and sacrum, distribution of lesions resemble branches of the tree

HISTOPATHOLOGY (Figs 9.2 and 9.3)

- Mild acanthosis, spongiosis with occasional mounds of parakeratosis
- Hypogranulosis (reduced granular layer)
- Mild perivascular lymphohistiocytic and eosinophilic infiltrate with exocytosis of lymphocytes
- Red blood cell extravasation in papillary dermis and in epidermis
- Late lesions can show psoriasiform pattern with increased eosinophils in the infiltrate

DIFFERENTIAL DIAGNOSIS

Erythema Annulare Centrifugum

- Characterized by ring-shaped lesions, with central clearing
- Spongiosis, parakeratosis, superficial perivascular lymphohistiocytic infiltrate

Pigmented Purpuric Dermatosis

- Discrete purpuric macular lesions, seen in the lower extremities
- Superficial dermis shows perivascular lymphocytic infiltrate
- Variable spongiosis and focal parakeratosis

Guttate Psoriasis

- Presents clinically as multiple discrete drop like papules with a salmon pink hue

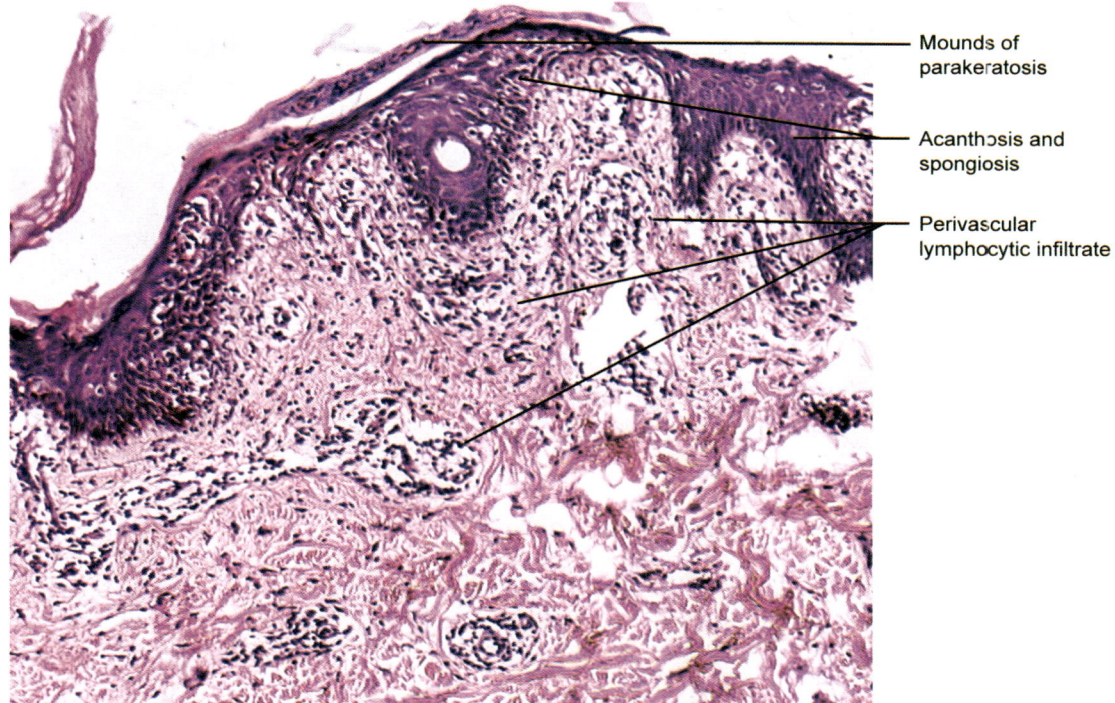

Mounds of parakeratosis

Acanthosis and spongiosis

Perivascular lymphocytic infiltrate

Fig. 9.2: Pityriasis rosea

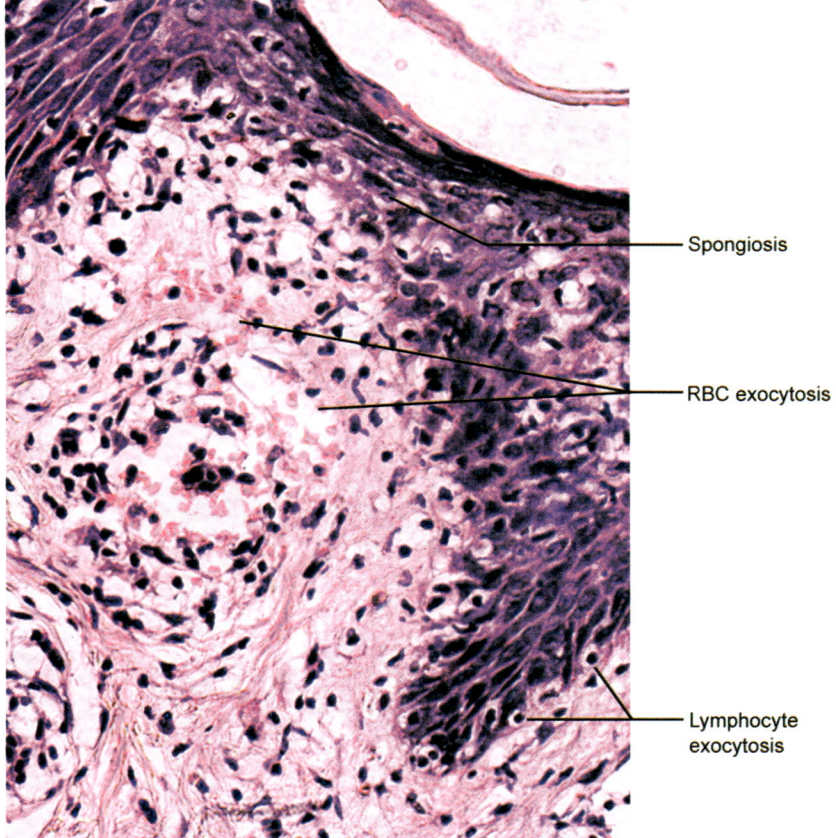

Spongiosis

RBC exocytosis

Lymphocyte exocytosis

Fig. 9.3: Pityriasis rosea

- Foci of neutrophils within or over the mounds of parakeratosis
- Mild spongiosis and perivascular lymphocytic infiltrate

Pityriasis Rosea-like Drug Eruption

- History of drug intake
- Presence of eosinophils in the infiltrate

Dermatophytosis

- Narrow zone of compact orthokeratosis above the granular layer
- Presence of neutrophils in stratum corneum
- PAS stain highlights hyphae in the stratum corneum

Pityriasis Lichenoides Chronica

- Interface dermatitis with vacuolar degeneration of the basal layer
- Red blood cell extravasation

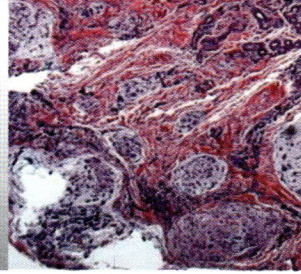

Cutaneous Fungal Infections

DERMATOPHYTOSIS

INTRODUCTION

- **Tinea**—clinical term that describes superficial cutaneous fungal infections (Dermatophytosis)
- Dermatophytes comprises *Trichophyton, Epidermophyton and Microsporum*
- Dermatophytes can infect skin, hair and/or nails
- **Predisposing factors**—immunocompromised conditions, diabetes mellitus, local injury, poor circulation, Cushing syndrome

CAUSAL DERMATOPHYTES ON THE BASIS OF THEIR LOCATION

- **Tinea corporis or Tinea cruris**—erythematous patch with central clearing and scaly border (*Trichophyton rubrum* is the most common causative agent) (Fig. 10.1)
- **Majocchi's granuloma**—presents as nodular plaque like lesions, most commonly affects lower limbs (*Trichophyton rubrum* is most common causative agent), seen in immunocompromised individuals. Nodular granulomatous perifolliculitis (affects calf region)
- **Tinea pedis**—most common dermatophytic infection, presenting as erythematous scaly or vesiculobullous lesions (*Trichophyton rubrum* is most common causative agent), seen in swimmers, runners and malignancies
- **Tinea capitis**—infection of skin and hair of the scalp, can result in patchy alopecia in adults (causative species—*Trichophyton tonsurans, Microsporum canis*)
- **Tinea barbae**—infects hair bearing beard and moustache areas of men
- **Tinea unguium**—dermatophytic infection of the nails
- **Tinea imbricata**—produces concentric erythematous lesions on the trunk (*Trichophyton concentricum* is most common causative agent)

- **Favus**—affects the scalp with formation of yellow-crust like areas (*Trichophyton schoenleinii* is the most common causative agent), associated with disseminated cancer
- **Onychomycosis**—fungal infection of the nail; affects most commonly diabetics; *Trichophyton rubrum* is most common causative agent; can result in thickening, discoloration and splitting of nails

HISTOPATHOLOGY

Tinea Corporis

- Mild acanthosis, compact orthokeratosis, parakeratosis and focal spongiosis

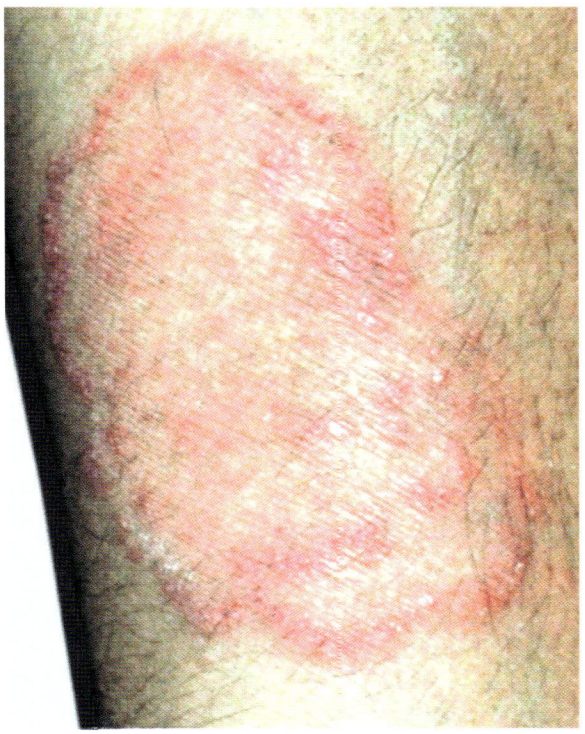

Fig. 10.1: Tinea corporis. Pruritic, round to oval, erythematous, scaly patch that spreads centrifugally

- Neutrophils in stratum corneum
- Sandwich sign —fungal hyphae seen between upper orthokeratotic and underlying parakeratotic stratum corneum layer
- Upper dermis shows perivascular lymphocytic infiltrate with occasional neutrophils or eosinophils

Tinea Capitis (Figs 10.2 and 10.3)

- Hyphae can be seen in the stratum corneum
- Hyphae are commonly found outside the hair follicle but can show invasion inside the follicle

Majocchi's Granuloma

- Perifollicular and dermal granulomas
- Fungal hyphae and spores are found within hairs and hair follicles
- Dermis shows dense mixed infiltrate of lymphocytes, macrophages, epithelioid cells and multinucleate giant cells with central necrosis

Tinea Unguium

- Hyphae seen in the parakeratotic nail plate or in the subungual debris

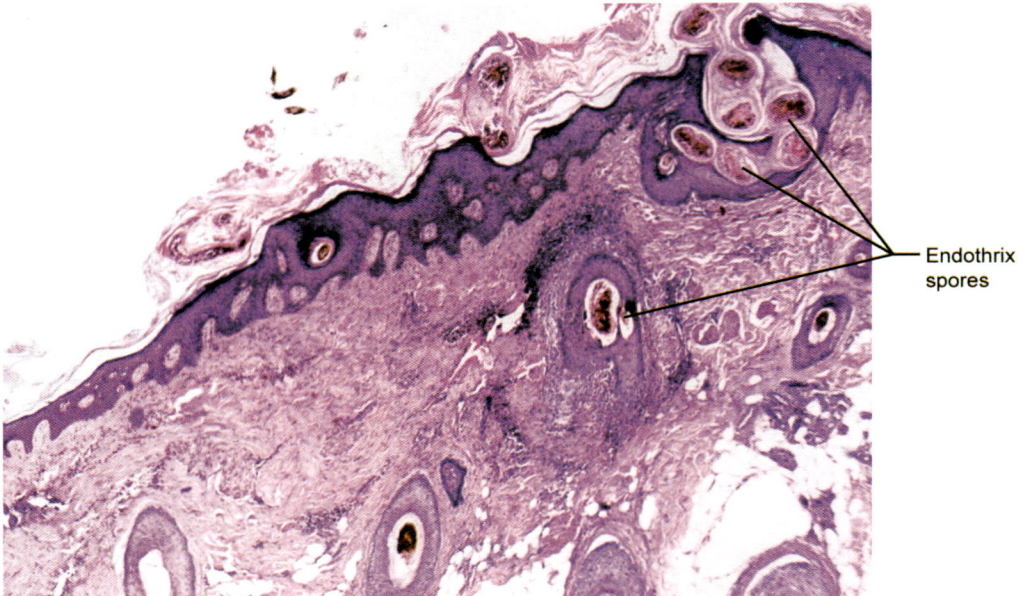

Endothrix spores

Fig. 10.2: Tinea capitis. Endothrix infection

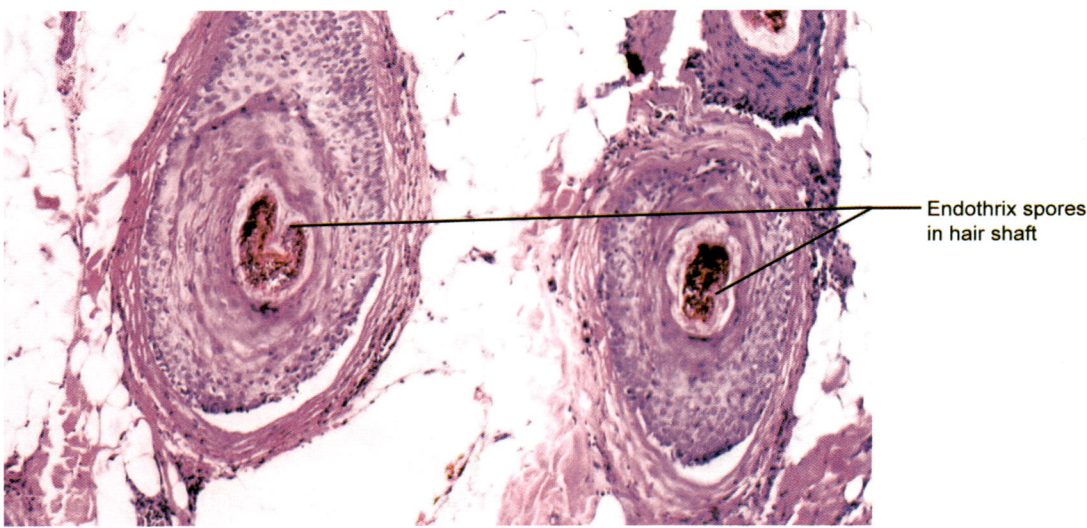

Endothrix spores in hair shaft

Fig. 10.3: Tinea capitis. Endothrix infection

Special Stains

- Periodic acid–Schiff with diastase (PAS-D) and Gomori methenamine silver highlights fungal hyphae and spores

DIFFERENTIAL DIAGNOSIS

1. Acute and sub-acute dermatitis
2. Psoriasis
3. Impetigo
4. Folliculitis

MALASSEZIA FURFUR

- Malassezia are normal commensals of the skin and becomes pathogenic when yeast form transforms into mycelia
- Predisposing factors—heat, sweating, oily skin or immunosuppression
- Includes pityriasis versicolor and *Pityrosporum folliculitis*

1. *Pityriasis Versicolor*
   - Presents as multiple pink to light brown patches with fine white scales
   - Sites—affect trunk and upper extremities (Fig. 10.4)
   - Age group—adolescents and adults
   - **Microscopy**—budding yeasts can be seen in the stratum corneum (Figs 10.5 and 10.6)

2. *Pityrosporum folliculitis*
   - Presents as papules and pustules

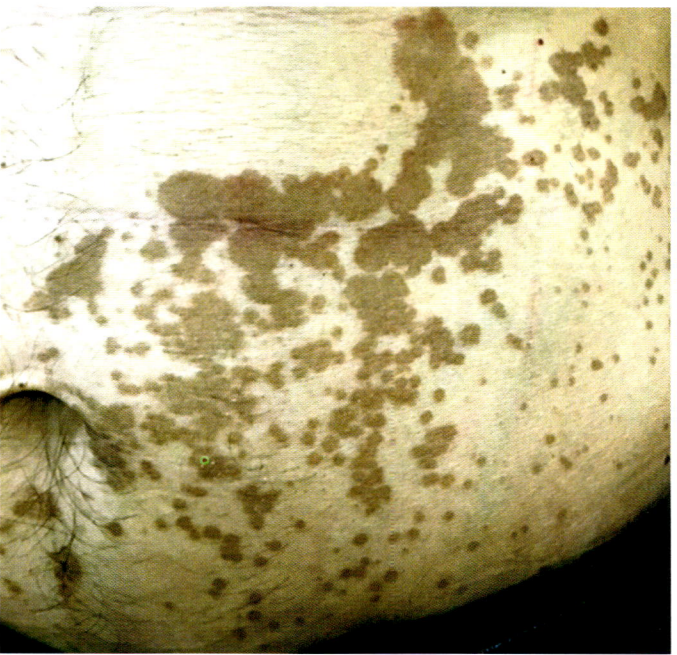

Fig. 10.4: Pityriasis versicolor, caused by *Malassezia furfur.* Hyperpigmented and hypopigmented patches with smaller lesions coalesce to form larger lesion

   - Seen in patients, who are on antibiotics or on corticosteroid treatment
   - Sites—trunk and arms
   - **Microscopy**—follicular dilatation and plugging, fungal hyphae and yeast forms (spores) produces

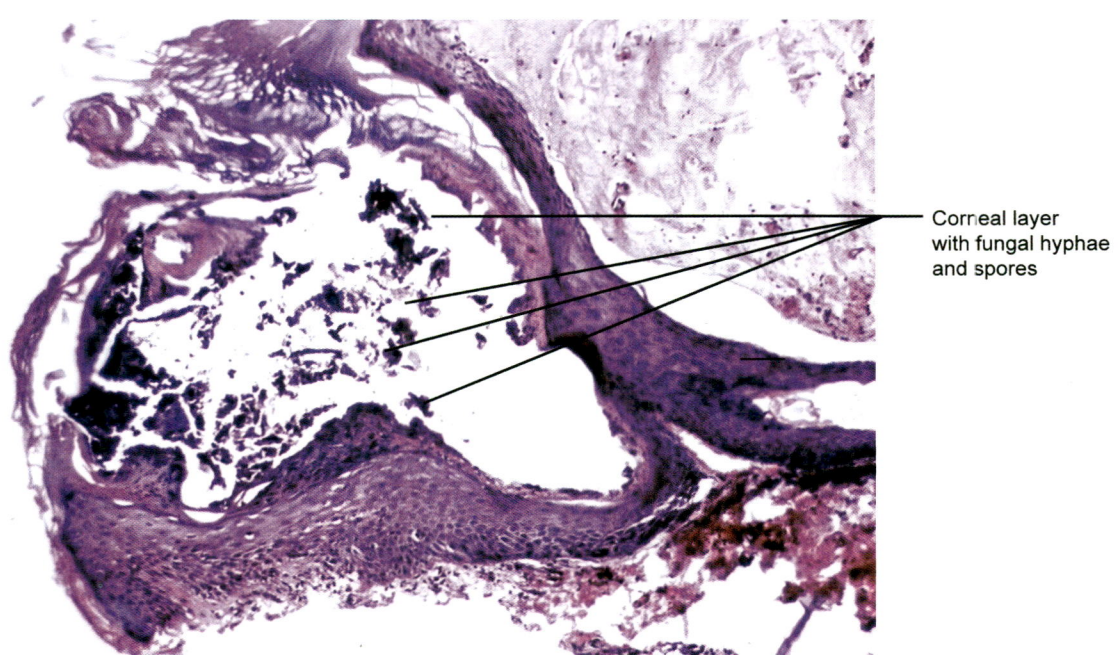

Corneal layer with fungal hyphae and spores

Fig. 10.5: Dermatophyte infection

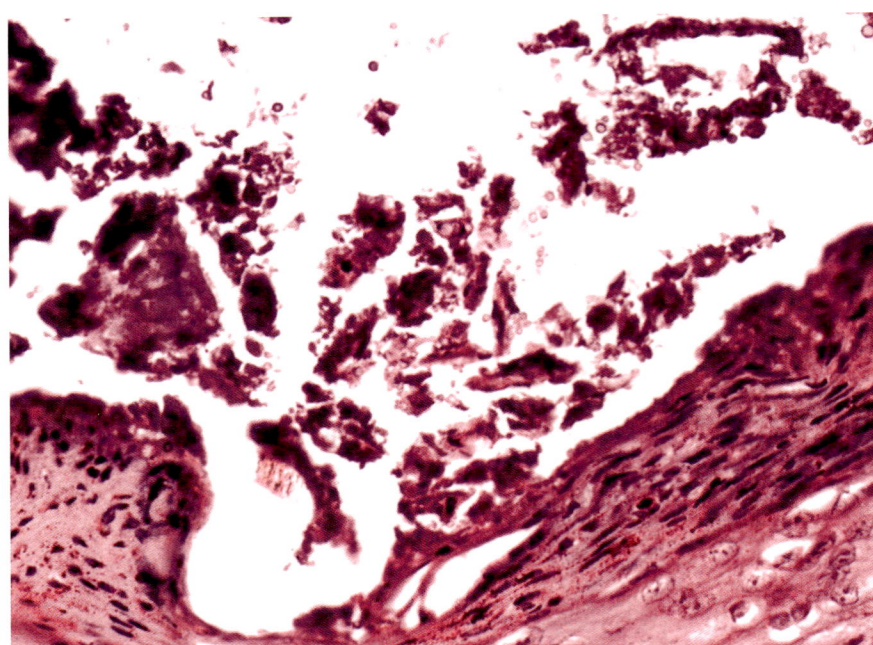

Fig. 10.6: Dermatophyte infection. Fungal spores and hyphae in parakeratotic stratum corneum

'Spaghetti and meatball' appearance in the stratum corneum

Special stains
– PAS with diastase stain demonstrates round to oval budding yeast forms within the infundibulum or in the follicular lumen

DIFFERENTIAL DIAGNOSIS

1. *Dermatophytosis*
   – Neutrophils in stratum corneum
   – Spongiosis
   – Fungal hyphae in stratum corneum without spores
2. *Candidiasis*
   – Psuedohyphae and yeast within the stratum corneum

CANDIDIASIS

INTRODUCTION

- **Causative organism**—*Candida albicans*, a dimorphic fungus with both yeast and filamentous forms
- *Candida albicans* affects superficial skin and mucous membranes
- Most commonly affects immunocompromised patients
- **Predisposing factors**—immunocompromised state, malnutrition, diabetes mellitus, malignancy

CLINICAL MANIFESTATIONS

1. *Acute mucocutaneous candidiasis*—Candida can affect vulvar and vaginal areas (vulvo-vaginal candidiasis), nail folds (candidal paronychia), buccal mucosa, tongue, palate, gingivae (oral thrush)

2. *Chronic mucocutaneous candidiasis* —characterized by chronic superficial candidal infections of skin, nail and oropharynx

3. *Disseminated candidiasis*—affects immuno-compromised patients with trunk and proximal extremities being most common sites

4. *Congenital candidiasis*—occurs due to ascending intrauterine infection from vaginal candidiasis at the time of birth

HISTOPATHOLOGY

Mucocutaneous Candidiasis

- Acanthosis of epidermis
- Stratum corneum showing neutrophilic aggregates with accompanying pseudohyphae and spores
- Dermis shows perivascular and interstitial mixed inflammatory cell infiltrate

Chronic Mucocutaneous Candidiasis

- Epidermal acanthosis
- Compact orthokeratosis
- Stratum corneum shows neutrophils with accompanying hyphae and spores

Disseminated Candidiasis

- Dermis shows microabscesses and mild perivascular mixed inflammatory cell infiltrate
- Leukocytoclastic vasculitis can be seen
- Candidal hyphae and spores, can be seen in vessel walls or within dermal microabscesses

Special Stains (Fig. 10.7)

- PAS (Periodic acid–Schiff) stain and GMS (Gomori methenamine silver) can highlight fungal elements

DIFFERENTIAL DIAGNOSIS

Dermatophytosis

- Septate and branching hyphae in zones of compact orthokeratosis (sandwich sign)

Tinea Versicolor

- Shorter hyphae and round or oval spores ("spaghetti and meatballs") in the stratum corneum

DEEP MYCOSIS

BLASTOMYCOSIS

Introduction

- Causative agent—*Blastomyces dermatitidis*
- Presents as cutaneous disease, or systemic disease with pulmonary involvement
- Cutaneous disease can present as verrucous or ulcerative lesions

Histopathology (Fig. 10.8)

- Pseudoepitheliomatous hyperplasia with intra-epidermal and dermal abscesses
- Abscesses comprise neutrophilic inflammatory cell infiltrate with multinucleated giant cells
- Thick walled spores can be seen either in abscesses or in multinucleated giant cells and require thorough search

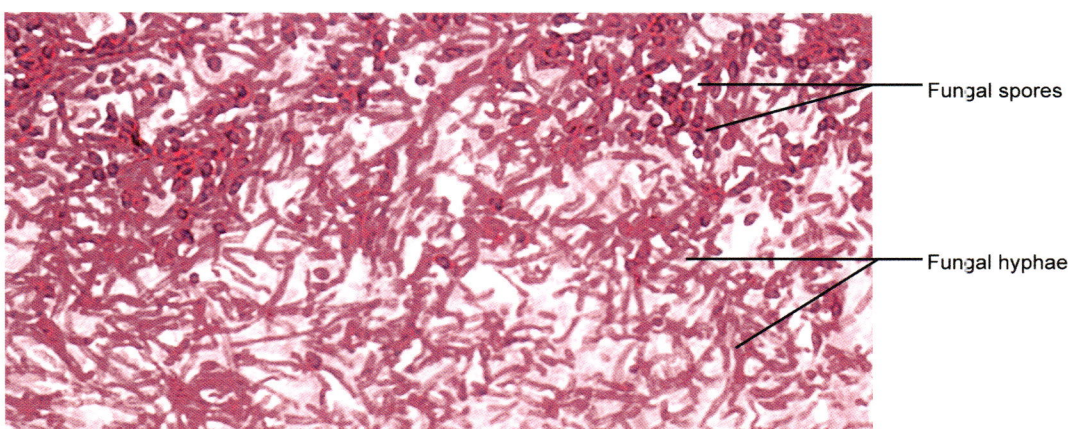

Fungal spores

Fungal hyphae

Fig. 10.7: Fungal hyphae and spores (PAS stain)

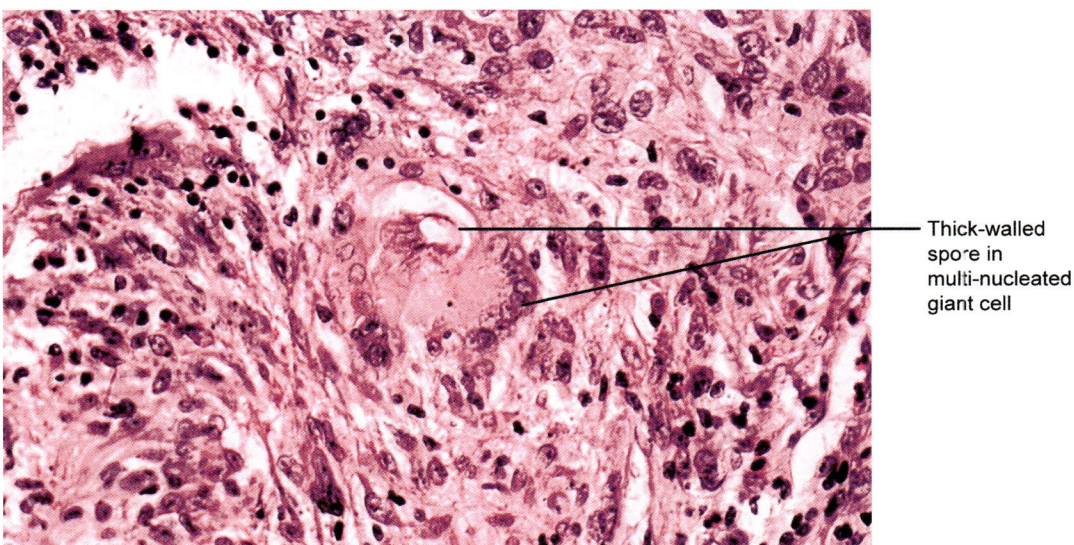

Thick-walled spore in multi-nucleated giant cell

Fig. 10.8: Blastomycosis

- Spores show a characteristic broad-based budding pattern

Special Stain

- Methenamine silver or PAS stain is used to highlight spores

Differential Diagnosis

1. *Deep fungal infections* with Pseudoepitheliomatous hyperplasia—histoplasmosis, coccidioidomycosis, chromomycosis

2. *Tuberculosis verrucosa cutis (TBVC)*
   - Absence of fungal spores
   - Presence of caseation necrosis

3. *Squamous cell carcinoma*
   - Infiltrative and pushing borders
   - Presence of cytological atypia
   - Nuclear pleomorphism

4. *Keratoacanthoma*
   - Keratin filled crater
   - Mature squamous epithelium showing hyperplastic features

PARACOCCIDIOIDOMYCOSIS

Introduction

- Causative agent—*Paracoccidioides brasiliensis*
- Age group—30–60 years
- First clinical manifestation—lesions in the oropharynx and gingivae and can spread to the nasal cavity, nasopharynx, larynx and lungs
- Presents as papules and nodules
- Later stage—progression to granulomatous lesions

Histopathology

- Pseudoepitheliomatous hyperplasia
- Abscesses localized to the dermis and epidermis
- Granulomatous infiltrate with epithelioid cells and giant cells
- Fungal spores can be found in abscess or in giant cells
- Fungal spores show multiple, minute, narrow based budding forms surrounded by large round fungal forms

Differential Diagnosis

1. *Histoplasmosis*
   - Yeasts surrounded by clear space within macrophages
2. *Coccidioidomycosis*
   - Spores are numerous and thick walled
3. *Chromoblastomycosis*
   - Characteristic medlar bodies or copper pennies

4. *North American Blastomycosis*
   - Thick-walled spores with broad-based budding

CHROMOBLASTOMYCOSIS

Introduction

- Fungal implantation on skin occurs at the site of trauma
- Fungi are found in soil or wood

Histopathology

- Hyperkeratosis with pseudo-epitheliomatous hyperplasia
- Dermis shows epithelioid histiocytic granulomas, multinucleated giant cells and abscesses
- Pigmented fungi (medlar bodies or copper pennies) appear as dark brown, thick walled spores, that may be seen singly or in chains

COCCIDIOIDOMYCOSIS

Introduction

- **Causative agent**—*Coccidioides immitis* (dimorphic fungi) is present in soil
- **Pulmonary coccidioidomycosis** – most common form of the infection
- **Cutaneous form**—presents as a nodule (at the site of the inoculation of the fungus), that transforms into an ulcerated plaque
- Disseminated coccidioidomycosis—seen in immune-suppressed patients

Histopathology

- Epidermis—pseudoepitheliomatous hyperplasia
- Dermis—dermal abscess with necrosis and surrounding granulomatous inflammation
- Fungal spores are present within the giant cells or in tissue
- Spores are round and thick-walled with granular cytoplasm

Differential Diagnosis

1. Granulomatous skin diseases
2. Rhinosporidiosis
   - Fungal spherules are larger, with thicker walls

CRYPTOCOCCOSIS

Introduction

- **Causative agent**—*Cryptococcus neoformans* (*C. neoformans*)
- **Predisposing factor**—immunocompromised states of the host
- **Sites**—most commonly affects lungs, central nervous system and rarely cutaneous lesions (consequence of dissemination)

- Cutaneous lesions present as papules, pustules, vesicles, nodules, ulcers, plaques, erythematous swelling and cellulitis

Histopathology

- *C. neoformans* organisms are round, oval with a characteristic peripheral capsular halo

Two histopathological patterns

1. *Gelatinous tissue reaction*
- Aggregates of organisms/spores without inflammatory response
- Fungal organisms are surrounded by broad capsule
- Capsule can be demonstrated by methylene blue (capsule stains purple) or alcian blue (capsule stains blue)

2. *Granulomatous tissue reaction*
- Fungal organisms/spores within histiocytes forming granulomas which also comprise lymphocytes and giant cells
- Fungal organisms are not surrounded by broad capsule

Special stain
- Fungal spores (cell wall) stain with PAS and methenamine silver

Differential Diagnosis

1. *Histoplasmosis*
- Yeasts surrounded by pseudo capsule (clear space) within macrophages

2. *Paracoccidioidomycosis*
- Fungal spores with multiple, minute, narrow based budding forms

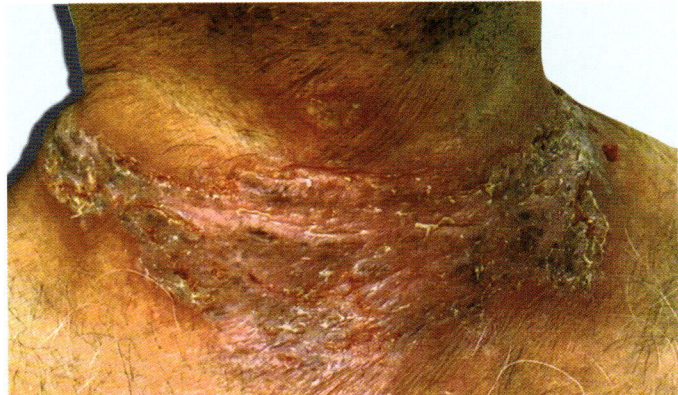

Fig. 10.9: Disseminated histoplasmosis. Plaques, ulcers, vesicles, pustules are seen

3. *Blastomycosis*
- Thick-walled spores with a characteristic broad-based budding

HISTOPLASMOSIS

Introduction

- **Causative agent**—*Histoplasma capsulatum* (dimorphic fungus)
- **Predisposing factor**—immunocompromised state
- **Three forms**—cutaneous, pulmonary and disseminated
- **Cutaneous lesions**—rare and occur secondarily to lung involvement. Present as an ulcer with heaped up borders or as papules, nodules or plaques (Fig. 10.9)

Histopathology (Figs 10.10 and 10.11)

- Show spores of fungi, which appear as round or oval yeast forms, surrounded by clear space (pseudo-capsule) within macrophages
- Spores can be highlighted by Methanamine silver stain (GMS)
- Granulomatous inflammatory response is absent in dermis, but can be seen in lungs

Differential diagnosis

1. *Leishmaniasis*
- Macrophages with round to oval basophilic structures (amastigotes) with bar-shaped paranuclear kinetoplast

2. *Granuloma inguinale*
- Foamy macrophages with intra-cytoplasmic organisms called Donovan bodies, which can be demonstrated by silver stains or giemsa stain

3. *Rhinoscleroma*
- Gram-negative bacilli within large foamy macrophages (Mikulicz cells)

4. *Cryptococcosis*
- Macrophages show fungal organisms with capsule, the latter stains with mucicarmine or Alcian blue

5. *Blastomycosis*
- Pseudoepitheliomatous hyperplasia with broad-based budding yeast forms

SPOROTRICHOSIS

Introduction

- **Causative organism**—*Sporothrix schenckii* (dimorphic fungi)

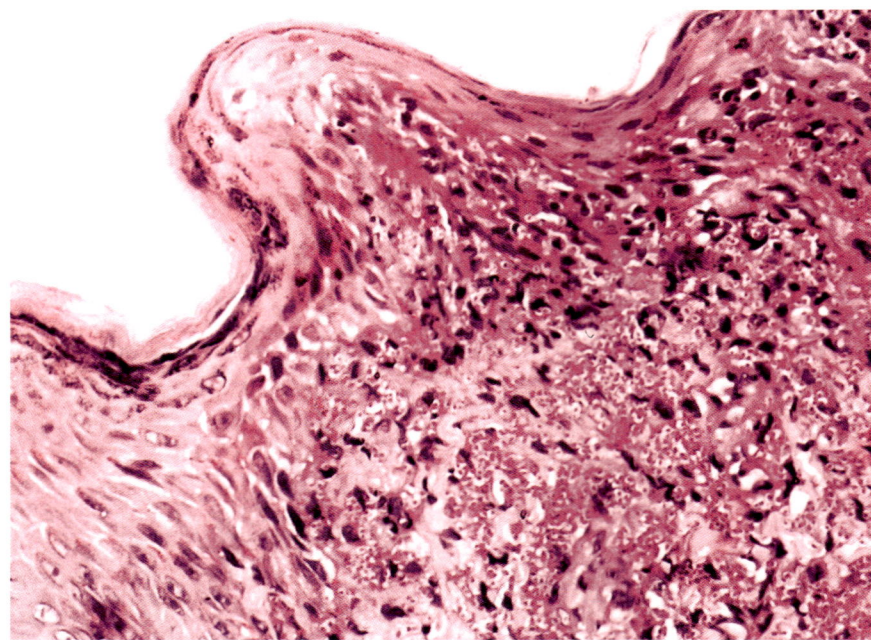

Fig. 10.10: Histoplasmosis. Dermis shows aggregates of macrophages containing histoplasma within its cytoplasm

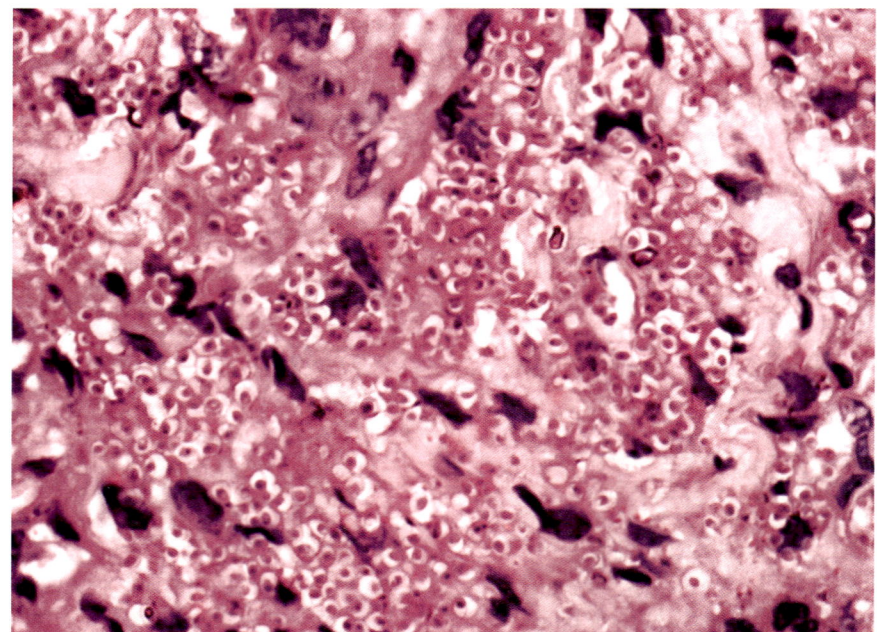

Fig. 10.11: Histoplasmosis. Round to oval yeast forms with a pale halo surrounding them

- Fungus grows as a mycelial form with conidia at the tip, and as yeast form at 37°C
- **Route of transmission**—traumatic inoculation of fungus by thorns, splinters, scratches
- **Types** – cutaneous form, lymphocutaneous form, pulmonary form and systemic form
- Commonly affects upper limbs

Histopathology

- Skin shows hyperplastic epidermis with epidermal and intradermal abscess
- Surrounding these abscesses, epithelioid histiocytes, multinucleated histiocytes, lymphoid cells and plasma cells can be seen
- Fungal spores appear round to oval bodies

- **Sporothrix asteroid body**—15–35 microns in diameter, extracellular structure composed of a central yeast/spore surrounded by radiating eosinophilic spicules
  Culture—gold standard for definitive diagnosis

Differential Diagnosis

1. *Mycobacterium marinum*
   - Positive culture for Sporothrix helps in excluding this atypical mycobacterium

EUMYCETOMA

Introduction

- Includes Actinomycetoma and Eumycetoma
- Actinomycetoma—due to filamentous bacteria from the class Actinobacteria. For example, *Nocardia brasiliensis* and *Actinomadura madurae*
- Eumycetoma—most common causative agent is *Madurella mycetomatis*. The disease starts as subcutaneous nodule on the foot, thus called Madura foot or Maduramycosis (Fig. 10.12)
- Age group—20–40 years
- Clinical presentation—swollen tissues, draining sinuses with sulfur granules or grains, commonly seen in the discharge
- Dark colored (black) grains—characteristic of Eumycetoma
- White/yellow-colored grains (pale grains)—can be seen in both Eumycetoma and Actinomycetoma

Histopathology

- Extensive granulation tissue with granules
- Eumycetoma granules—show 4–5 µm thick, septate, fungal hyphae

- Actinomycetoma granules—show 1 µm thick, fine, branching filaments (Figs 10.13 and 10.14)
- PAS positivity is seen in hyphae and filaments of Eumycetoma and Actinomycetoma species, respectively
- Gram stain helps to differentiate the filaments of Actinomycetoma, which are gram-positive from hyphae of Eumycetoma, which are gram negative
- Splendore-Hoeppli phenomenon—amorphous, eosinophilic, radially arranged material surrounding the mass of hyphae or filamentous bacteria

Special Stain

- PAS and GMS stain
- **Gram stain** – eumycetes granules are gram-negative and Actinomycete granules are gram-positive

Differential Diagnosis

1. *Sporotrichosis*
   - Pseudoepitheliomatous hyperplasia with dermal granulomatous inflammation

2. *Chromoblastomycosis*
   - Pseudoepitheliomatous hyperplasia
   - Granulomatous chronic inflammation
   - Characteristic medlar bodies

ASPERGILLOSIS

Introduction

- **Causative agent**—Aspergillus
- **Predisposing condition**—immunocompromised states
- **Most common species**—*Aspergillus fumigatus, Aspergillus flavus, Aspergillus niger*

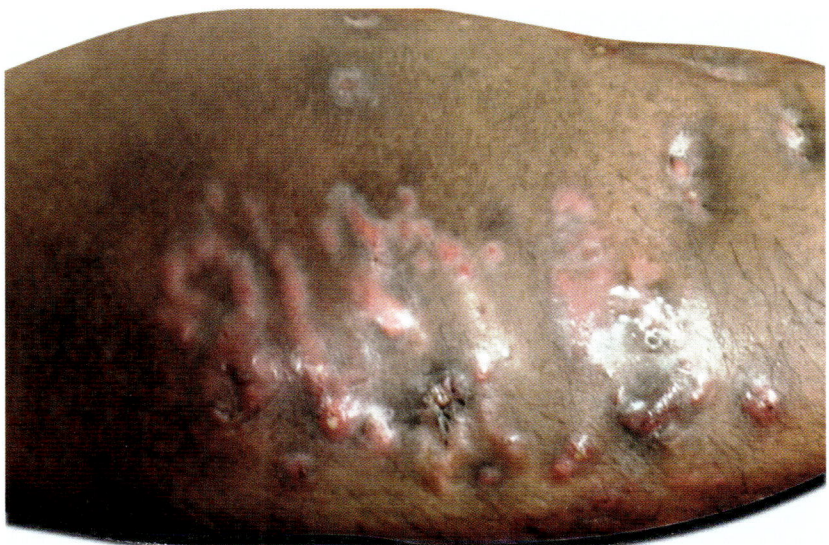

Fig. 10.12: Eumycetoma. Characteristic triad consists of swollen tissue, sinus tracts, and macroscopic grains

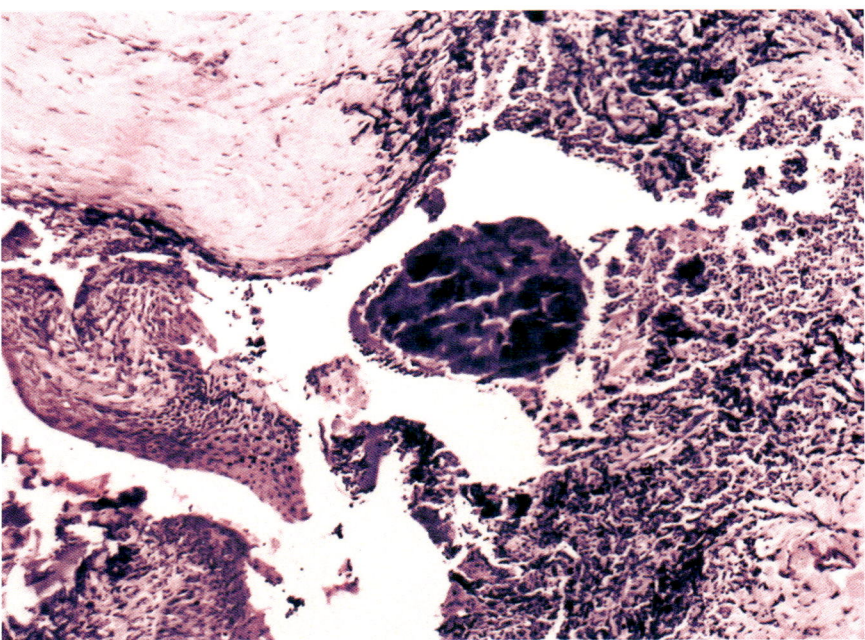

Fig. 10.13: Actinomyces

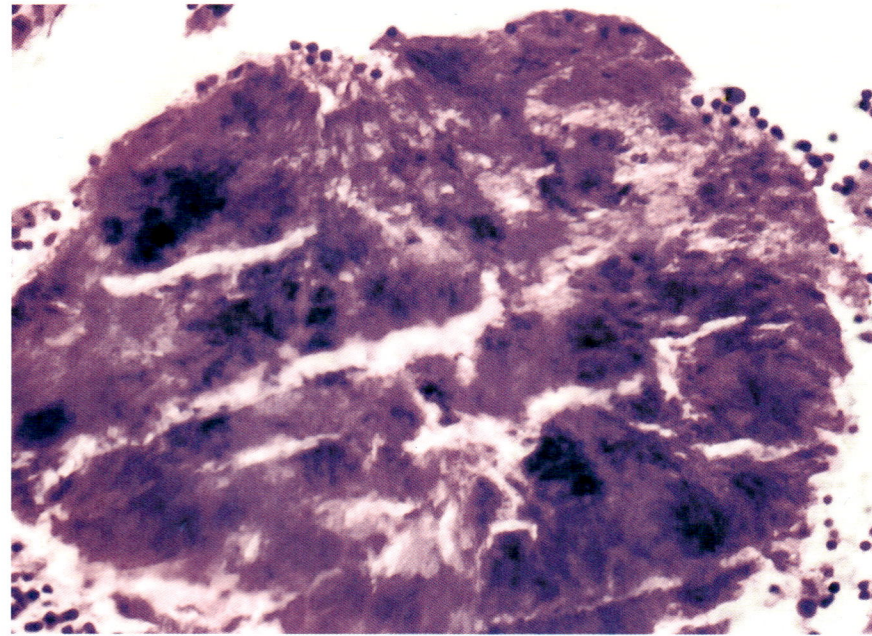

Fig. 10.14: Actinomyces colony with filamentous bacteria arranged in a rosette-shaped pattern with surrounding inflammatory cells

- Can present as primary cutaneous lesion or a complication of disseminated Aspergillosis
- In the primary cutaneous form, patient presents as erythematous papules or plaques

Histopathology (Fig. 10.15)

- Septate hyphae that show branching at 45°
- PAS and silver methenamine stain are used to highlight hyphae
- Spores are characteristically absent

- In disseminated type, hyphae can be seen invading the blood vessels
- Infiltrate of eosinophils, can be seen surrounding fungal hyphae

Differential Diagnosis

1. *Ecthyma gangrenosum*
   - Numerous gram-negative bacilli, surrounding the necrotic vessel wall

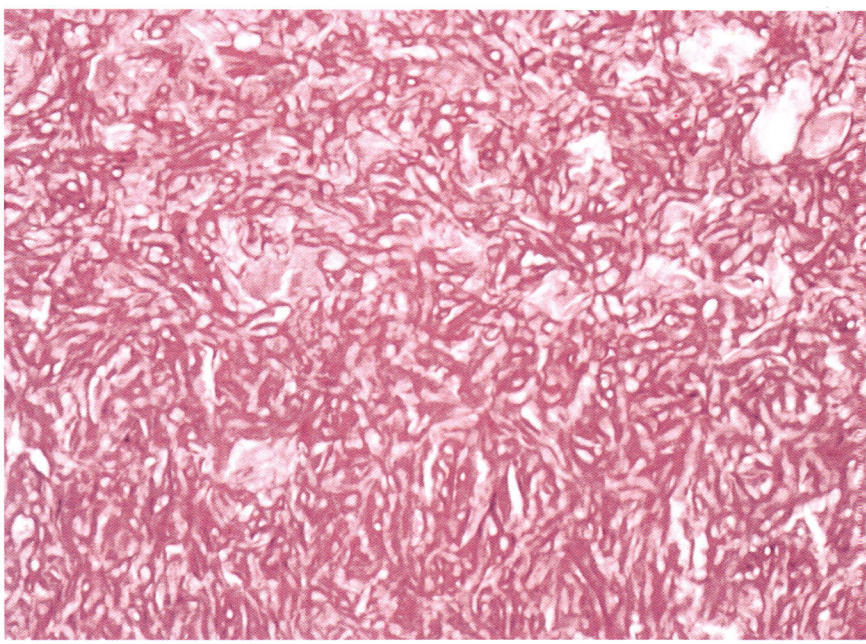

Fig. 10.15: Aspergillosis

2. *Zygomycosis/Mucormycosis*
- Non-septate and broader hyphae with 90° branching

3. Candidiasis
- Psuedohyphae with spores

ZYGOMYCOSIS

Introduction
- Includes Mucormycosis, i.e. Rhizopus and Mucor species
- **Predisposing conditions**—immunocompromised state, transplant patients, leukemia patients, individuals on systemic corticosteroids, HIV patients
- **Rhinocerebral zygomyces**—fulminant infection of the paranasal sinuses, which can spread to brain
- **Cutaneous lesions**—can present as erythematous macules or nodules

Histopathology
- Non-septate, broad hyphae with characteristic right angle branching
- Angioinvasion can be seen
- Spores are rarely seen

Differential Diagnosis

1. *Aspergillosis and Fusarium*
- Septate hyphae with characteristic acute angle branching

RHINOSPORIDIOSIS

Introduction
- **Causative agent**—*Rhinosporidium seeberi*
- Lesions start as papule and transform into a polypoidal mass
- On these polypoidal masses, small cysts develop
- These cysts discharge mucus, pus and organisms, and show tiny white dots on their surface (Strawberry-like lesions)

Histopathology (Figs 10.16 and 10.17)
- Hyperplastic epidermis with papillomatosis
- Spherical sporangium with numerous endospores inside them
- Sporangium have thick, PAS-positive chitinous wall
- Endospores are spherical to oval and measure 6–12 µm
- Surrounding the sporangium, granulomatous inflammation and granulation tissue reaction can be seen

Differential Diagnosis

1. *Coccidioidomycosis*
- Coccidioidal spores are much smaller and endospores are not seen

2. *Myospherulosis*
- Spherules contain altered red blood cells

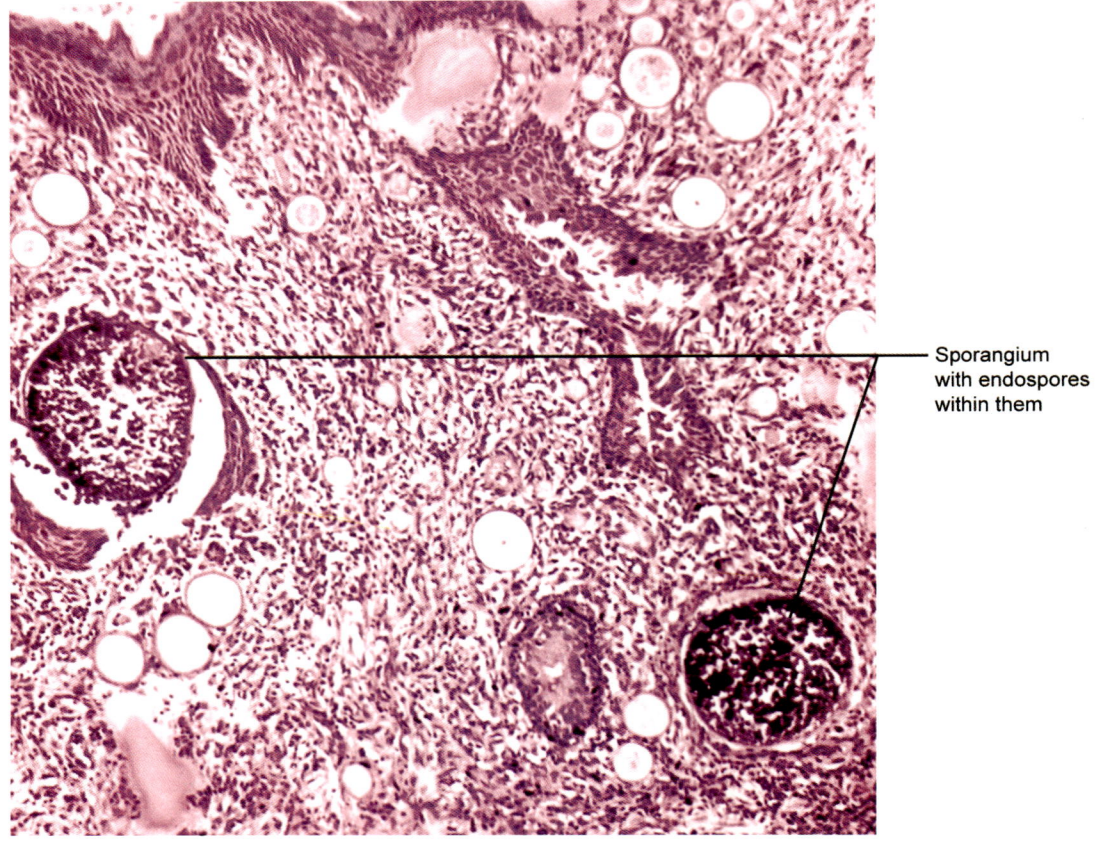

Sporangium with endospores within them

Fig. 10.16: Rhinosporidiosis

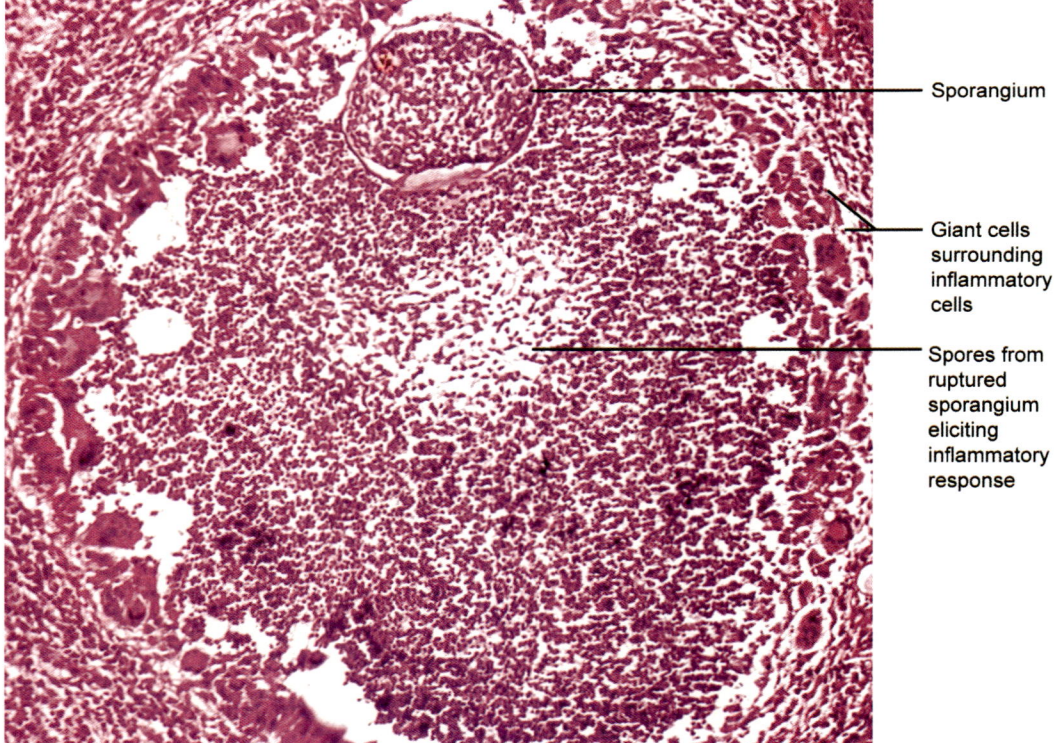

Sporangium

Giant cells surrounding inflammatory cells

Spores from ruptured sporangium eliciting inflammatory response

Fig. 10.17: Rhinosporidiosis

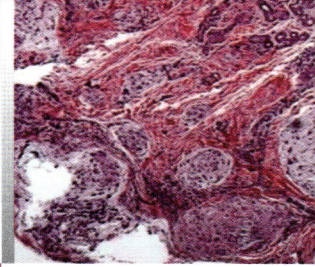

Diseases Caused by Viruses

MOLLUSCUM CONTAGIOSUM

INTRODUCTION

- Causative agent—poxvirus
- Age group—most commonly affects young children
- Clinical presentation—small, waxy, skin colored, dome-shaped papules (Fig. 11.1)
- Sites—face, trunk, extremities of children and anogenital regions in adults

HISTOPATHOLOGY (Figs 11.2 and 11.3)

- Acanthotic epidermis with distinct molluscum bodies
- Epidermal cells contain large eosinophilic to basophilic intra-cytoplasmic inclusions that push aside the nucleus (Henderson-Paterson bodies/ Molluscum bodies)

- Molluscum bodies increase in size as they move towards the surface
- Associated mixed or lymphocytic infiltrate can be seen

HERPES VIRUS

INTRODUCTION

- Causative agents—herpes simplex virus (HSV-1, HSV-2)
- HSV-1 infects oral cavity and face, HSV-2 infects genital areas
- Clinical presentation—clear vesicles with a red base
- Recurrent infection can occur either due to re-infection or re-activation of the virus in the dormant stage, residing in the regional sensory ganglion
- Predisposing factor—immune compromised state

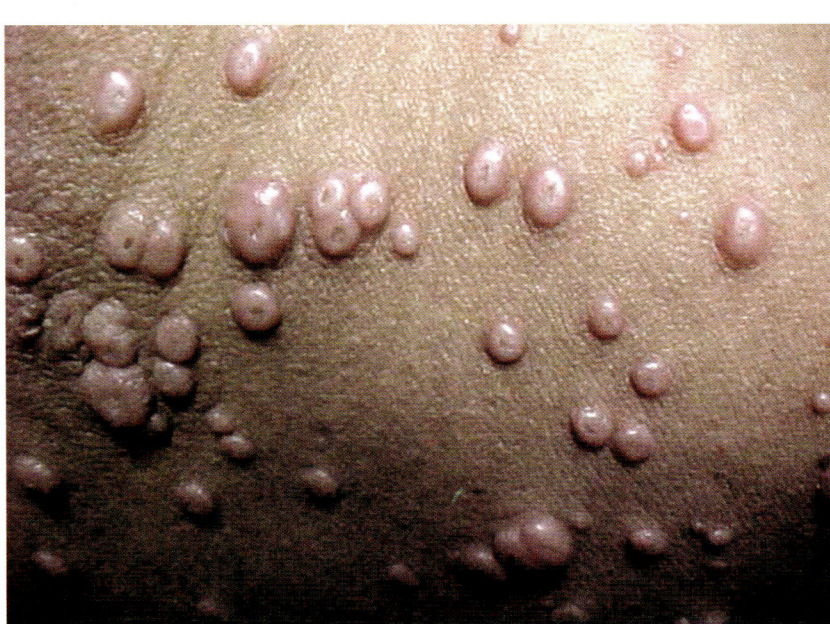

Fig. 11.1: Molluscum contagiosum. Firm, dome-shaped papules with shiny surface and central umbilication

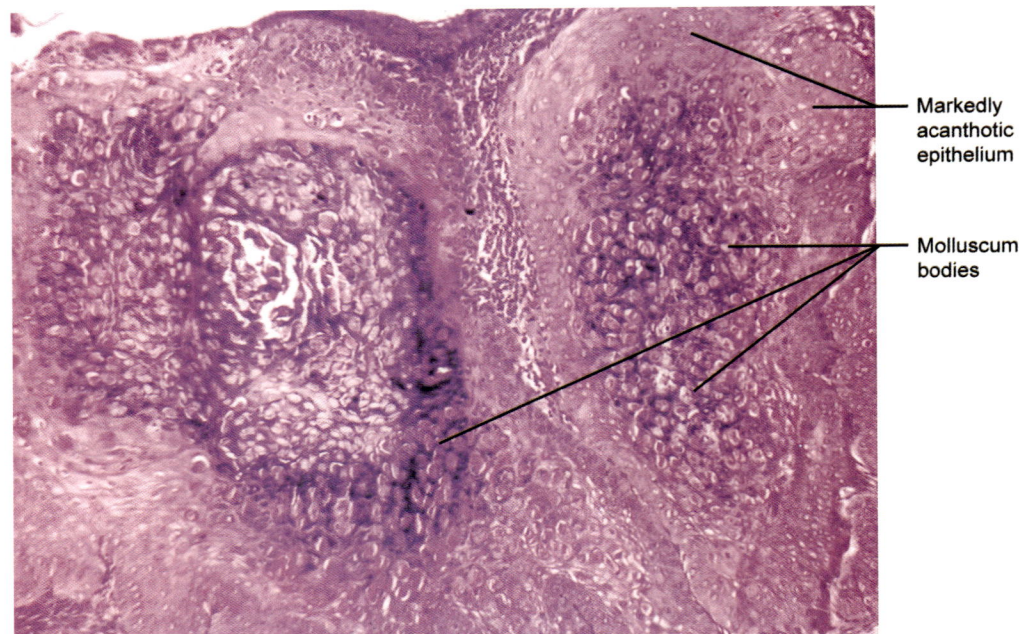

Markedly acanthotic epithelium

Molluscum bodies

Fig. 11.2: Molluscum contagiosum

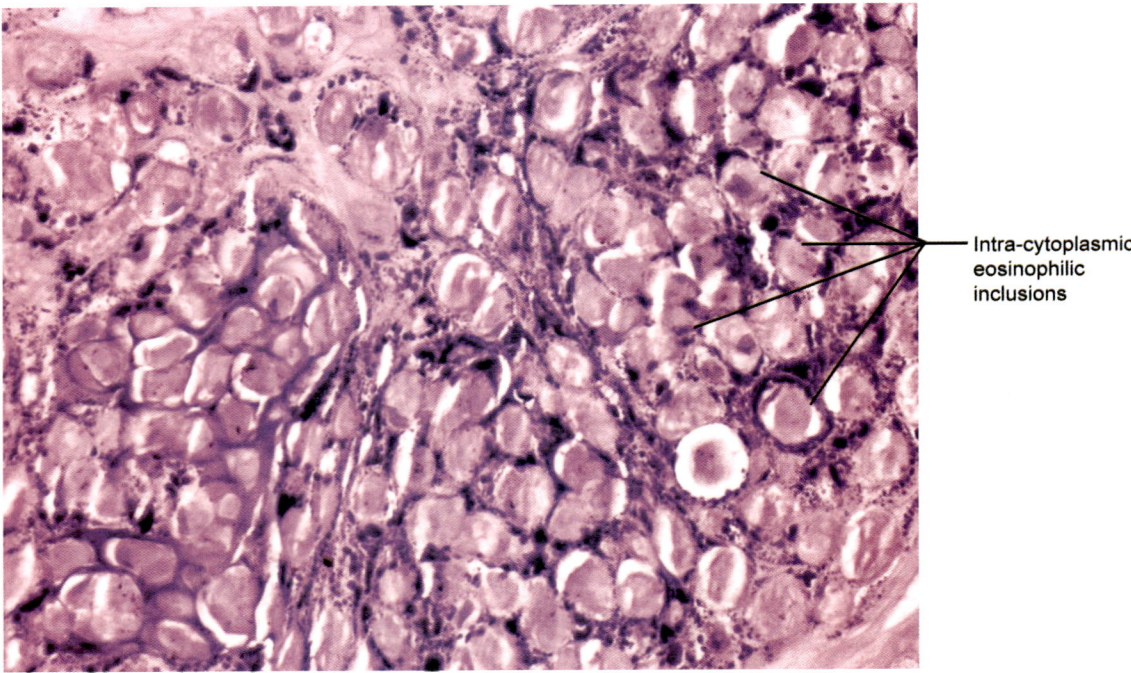

Intra-cytoplasmic eosinophilic inclusions

Fig. 11.3: Molluscum bodies in molluscum contagiosum

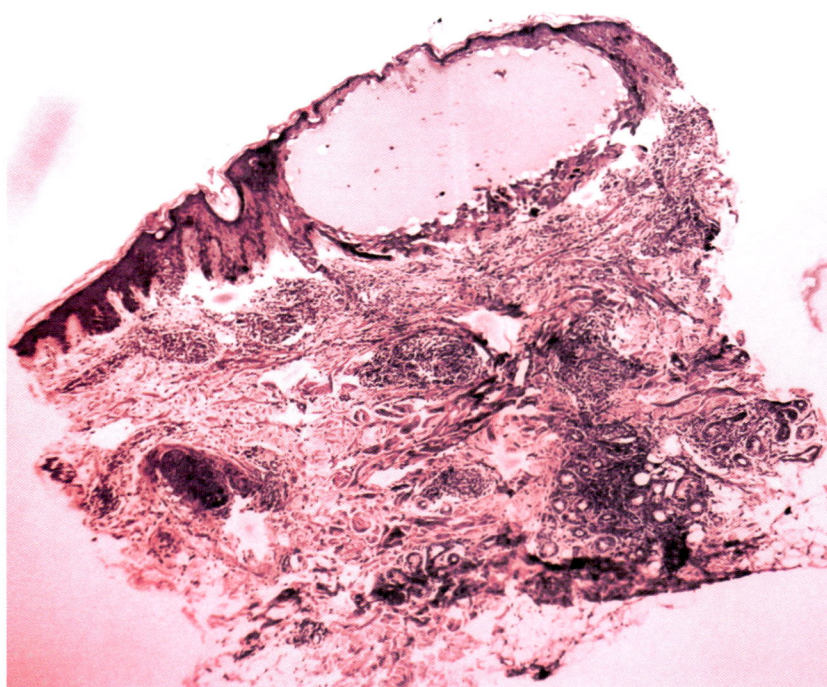

Fig. 11.4: Herpes virus blister

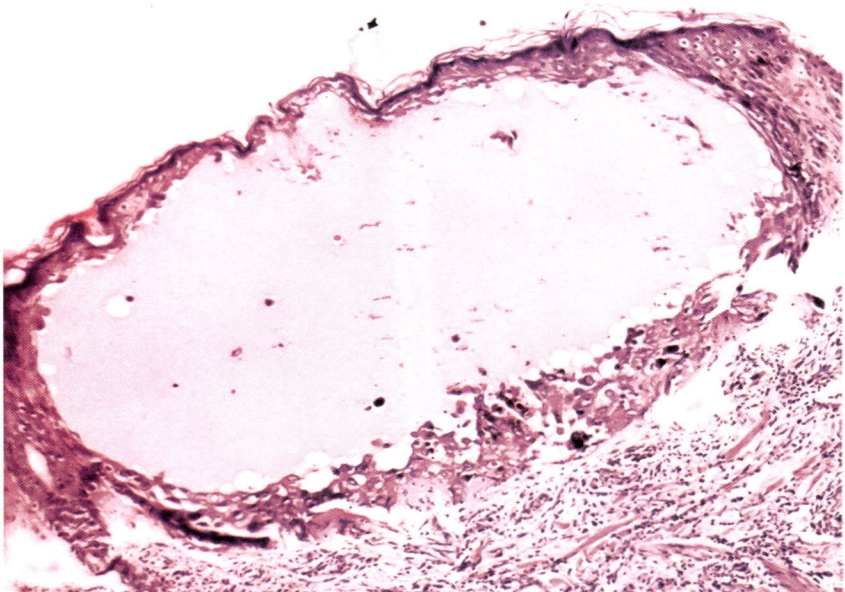

Fig. 11.5: Herpes virus infection of the skin with an intraepidermal blister

HISTOPATHOLOGY (Figs 11.4 to 11.7)

- Intraepidermal blister, keratinocytes showing acantholysis with blister cavity showing solitary keratinocytes
- Keratinocytes infected with the virus show homogenous eosinophilic cytoplasm and can show multi-nucleation
- Intranuclear eosinophilic inclusions (ground glass appearance) surrounded by a halo can be seen
- Dermis shows peri-vascular and peri-adnexal lymphocytic infiltrate

ANCILLARY TESTS

- Immunohistochemistry and *in situ* hybridization studies for identification of the subtype, i.e. HSV-1, HSV-2
- Direct immunofluorescence for viral antigen detection

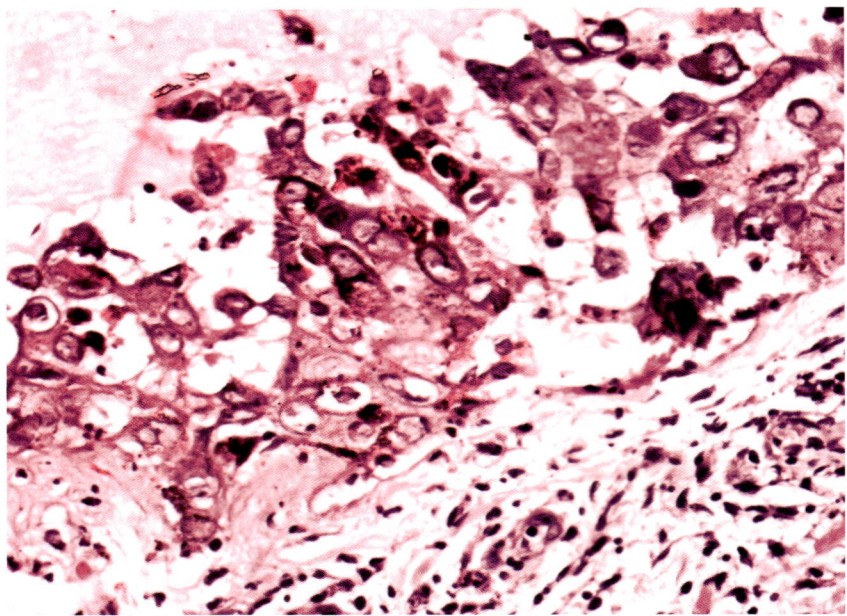

Fig. 11.6: Base of the blister cavity with acantholytic cells showing ballooning degeneration

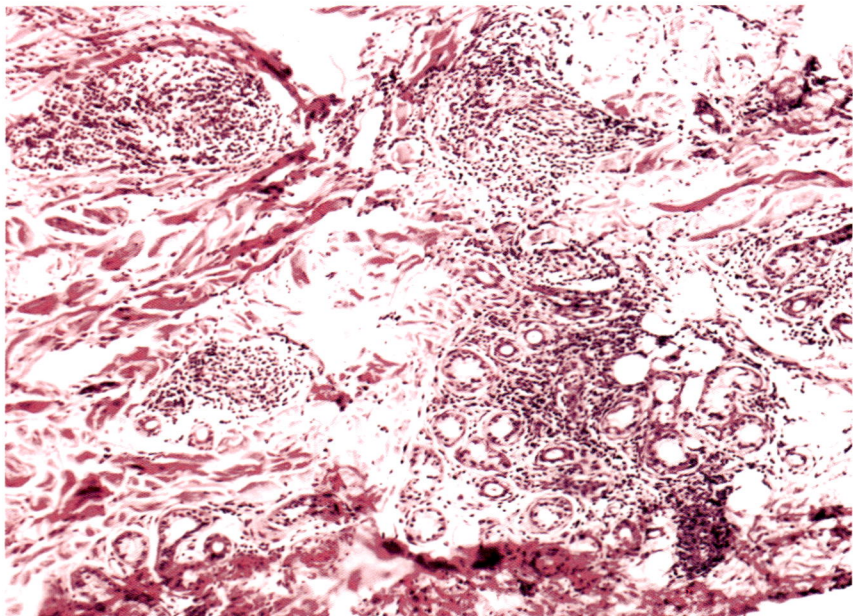

Fig. 11.7: Perivascular and peri-adnexal lymphocytic infiltrate

DIFFERENTIAL DIAGNOSIS

Erythema Multiforme

- Spongiosis, apoptotic keratinocytes, interface epidermal changes
- Absence of multinucleated cells or inclusions
- Dermis shows features of lymphocytic vasculitis

Cytomegalovirus

- Large nuclear inclusions, that can be seen in endothelial cells, fibroblasts, and macrophages
- Cytoplasmic inclusions can also be seen

Varicella/Herpes Zoster

- Lesions present as small vesicles with clear serous fluid surrounded by red halo ("dew drops on rose petal")
- Intraepidermal blister with acantholytic keratinocytes within it
- Ballooning degeneration of keratinocytes with nuclear Cowdry type A inclusions

CYTOMEGALOVIRUS

INTRODUCTION

- Predisposing factor—affects predominantly immunocompromised individuals
- Skin manifestations—can present as maculopapular rash, ulcers, urticaria, blisters
- Blueberry muffin baby—newborn baby with magenta-colored skin lesions, which signifies extramedullary hematopoiesis

HISTOPATHOLOGY

- Dermal vessels appear to be dilated
- Endothelial cells, lining these vessels have large hyperchromatic nucleus, basophilic intra-nuclear and intra-cytoplasmic inclusions (halo may be seen around these inclusions)
- Mixed dermal inflammatory cell infiltrate

EPSTEIN-BARR VIRUS

CAUSATIVE AGENT FOR

1. *Infectious mononucleosis*
   - Triad of fever, pharyngitis, and lymphadenopathy
   - Histopathology: Parakeratosis, spongiosis with sparse, superficial, perivascular lymphocytic infiltrate

2. *Oral hairy leukoplakia*
   - Seen in immunocompromised patients
   - Presents as an adherent, white plaque on the lateral border of tongue
   - Histopathology: Acanthosis with parakeratosis and ballooned koilocyte like cells (pyknotic nuclei with intranuclear inclusions and ground glass appearance of cytoplasm)

3. *Nasopharyngeal carcinoma*
4. *B and T-cell lymphomas*

ANCILLARY TESTS FOR DIAGNOSIS

- Heterophile antibody test (monospot test)
- Serological tests
- Polymerase chain reaction

DIFFERENTIAL DIAGNOSIS

Viral Exanthemas

- Parakeratosis, sparse, superficial, perivascular and interstitial lymphocytic infiltrate
- Can show necrotic keratinocytes, vacuolar interface dermatitis, papillary dermal edema

Drug Eruption

- Parakeratosis, spongiosis and sparse, superficial, perivascular and interstitial infiltrate of lymphocytes and eosinophils
- Can show necrotic keratinocytes and vacuolar interface dermatitis

Cytomegalovirus

- Superficial perivascular infiltrate
- Blood vessel lined endothelial cells show characteristic intra-nuclear and intra-cytoplasmic inclusion body

VIRAL PAPILLOMAS

INTRODUCTION

- Causative agent—human papillomavirus
- Clinical variants—verruca vulgaris, deep palmoplantar warts, verruca plana, condyloma acuminatum
- Single or multiple, circumscribed, firm, elevated papules with verrucous surface (Fig. 11.8)

Condyloma Acuminatum

- In males, penis and anus are most commonly affected
- In females, vulva, vagina, perianal area and cervix are most commonly affected
- Causative agent—human papillomavirus (HPV) 6 and 11
- Presents as verrucous papules, which can coalesce to form cauliflower like masses (Fig. 11.9)

Histopathology (Figs 11.11 and 11.12)

- Acanthosis, papillomatosis and focal parakeratosis
- Koilocytic atypia—stratum spinosum epithelial cells show hyperchromatic raisin like nucleus with perinuclear halo
- However, absence of koilocytes, does not rule out HPV infection

Verruca Vulgaris

- Most commonly affects the dorsal aspect of fingers and hands
- Associated with HPV-2 infection
- Koebner phenomenon—new warts may form at the site of trauma

Histopathology (Figs 11.10 and 11.12)

- Acanthosis, papillomatosis, hyperkeratosis, and parakeratosis
- Elongated rete ridges, which at periphery appears to be turned inwards at the edge of the lesion

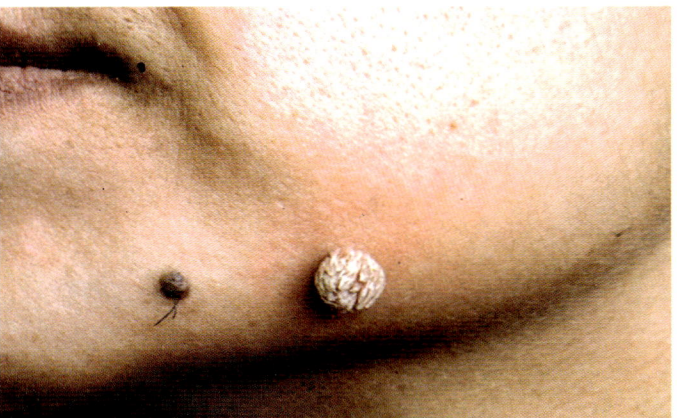

Fig. 11.8: Viral papilloma. A solitary papule with finger-like keratotic projections

- Superficial keratinocytes show koilocytic change and prominent keratohyaline granules

Deep Palmoplantar Wart (Myrmecia)

- Sites—palms, soles, lateral aspect and tips of finger and toes

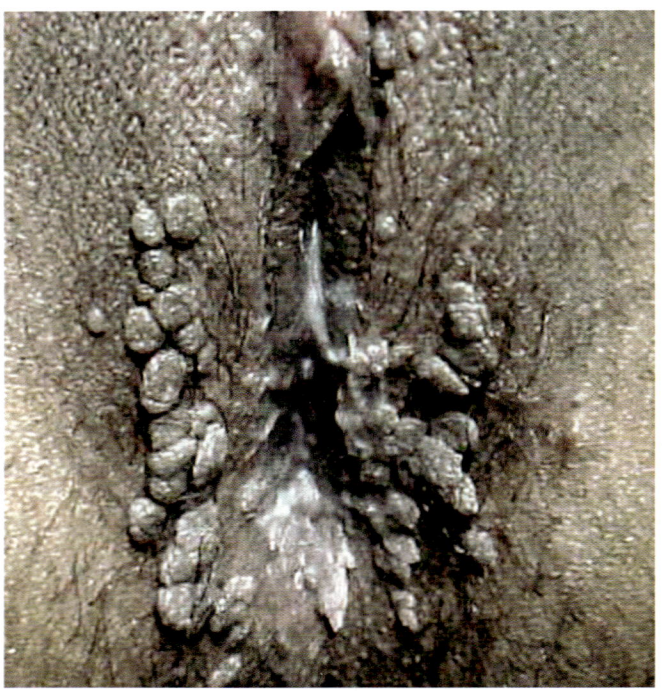

Fig. 11.9: Condyloma acuminata. Multiple, cauliflower-shaped, pedunculated, verrucous papules

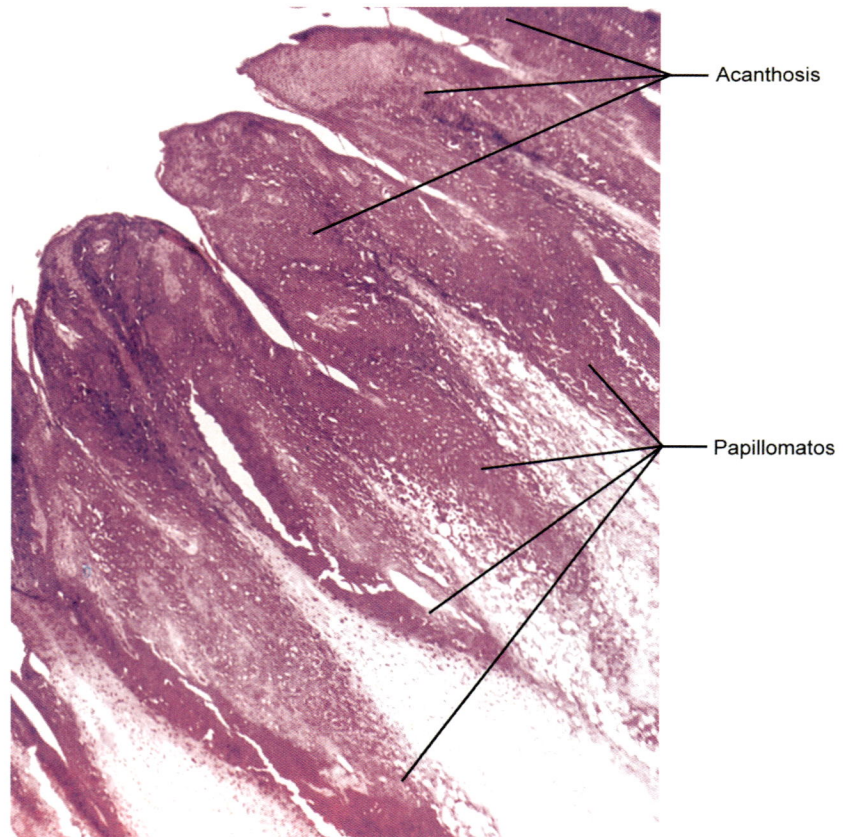

Acanthosis

Papillomatos

Fig. 11.10: Verruca vulgaris

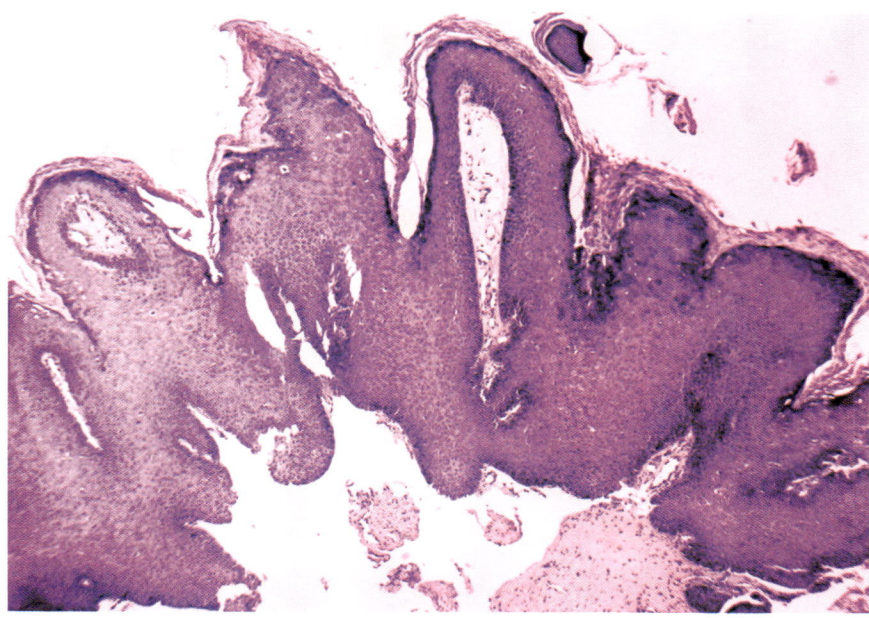

Fig. 11.11: Condyloma accuminata

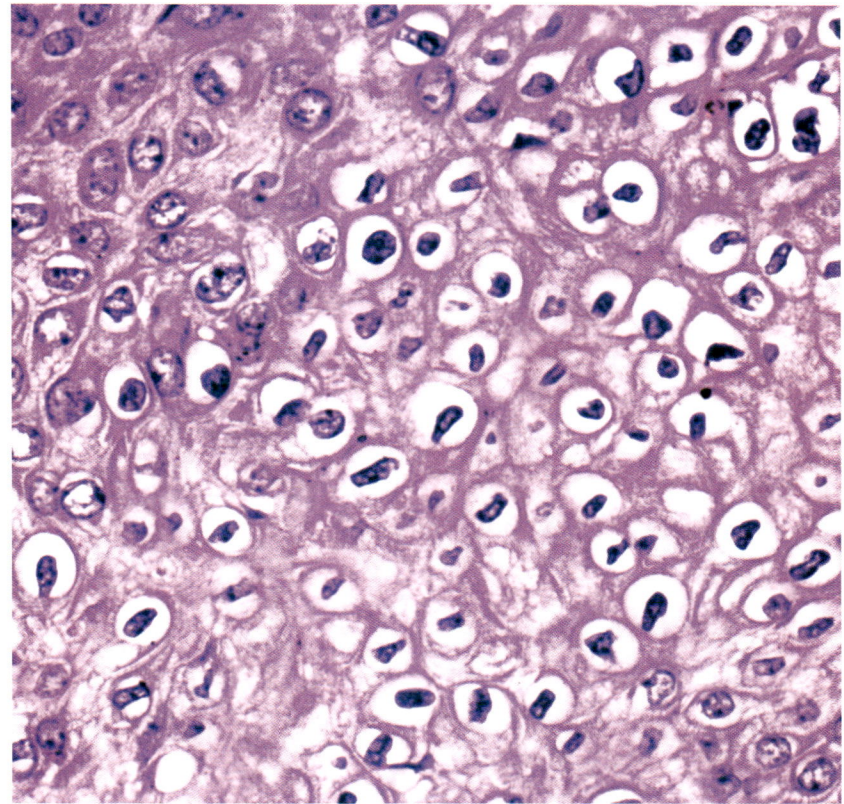

Fig. 11.12: Koilocytic atypia in verruca vulgaris and condyloma accuminata

- Painful lesions
- Associated with HPV-1 infection
- Lesion is covered with thick callus

Histopathology (Figs 11.13 to 11.16)

- Prominent hyperkeratosis
- Keratinocytes and stratum corneum show numerous eosinophilic keratohyaline granules with

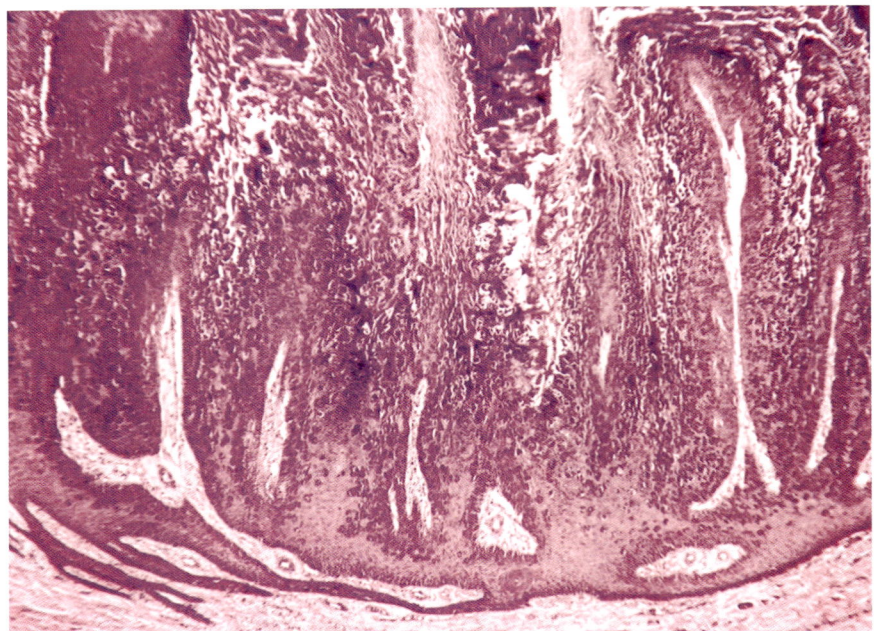

Fig. 11.13: Marked hyperkeratotic and acanthotic epidermis in deep palmoplantar wart

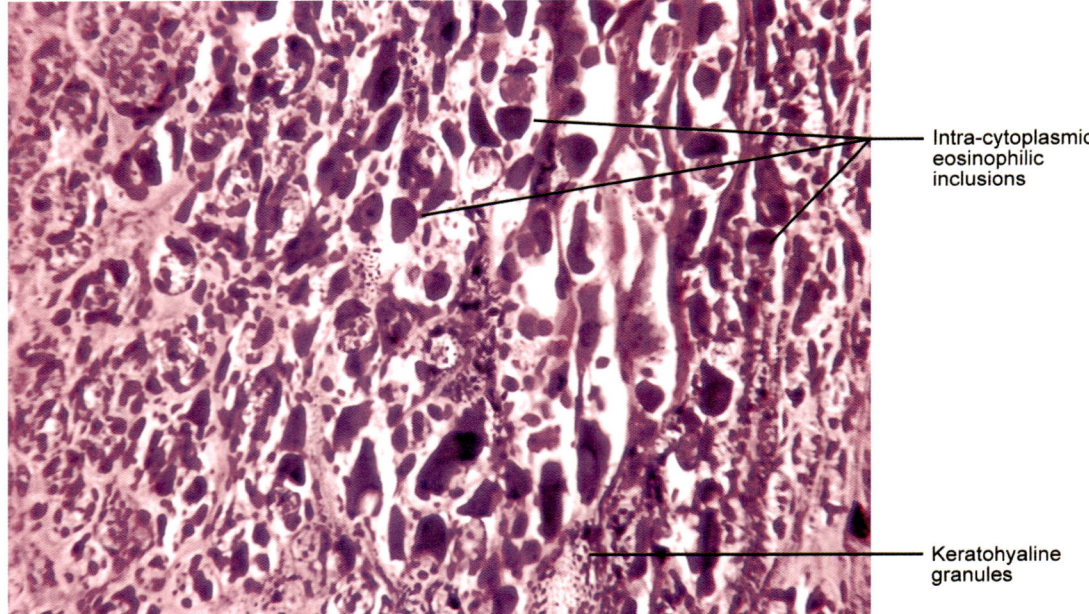

Intra-cytoplasmic eosinophilic inclusions

Keratohyaline granules

Fig. 11.14: Deep palmoplantar wart (high power of Fig. 11.13)

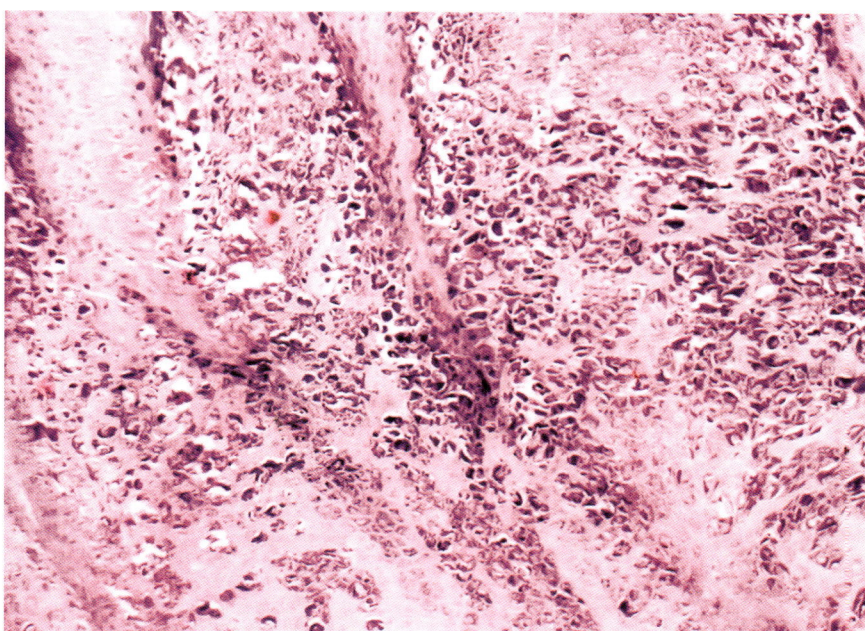

Fig. 11.15: Myrmecia. Numerous intracytoplasmic eosinophilic inclusions (HPV-1 induced)

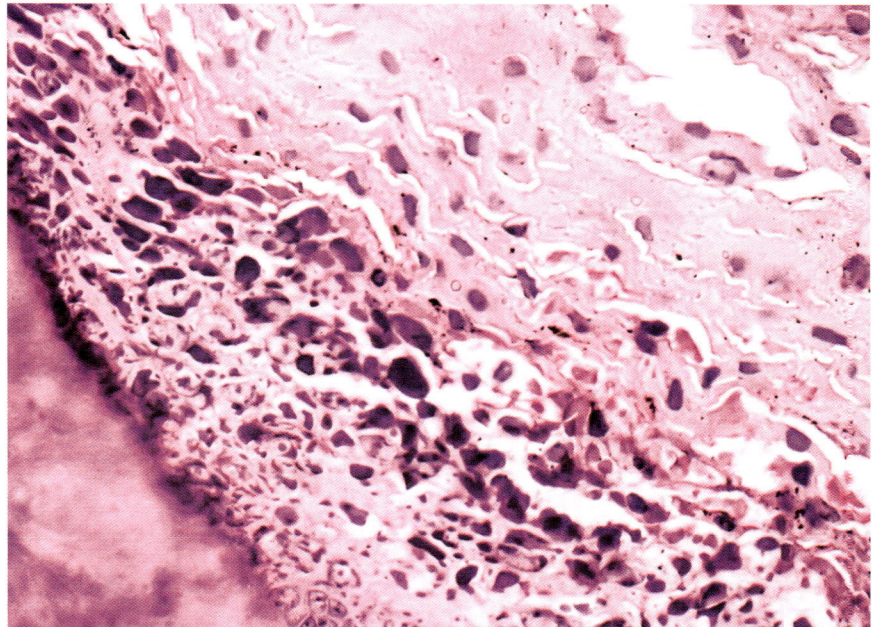

Fig. 11.16: Myrmecia. Numerous intracytoplasmic eosinophilic inclusions (HPV-1 induced)

intracytoplasmic and intranuclear eosinophilic inclusion bodies

Verruca Plana

- Associated with HPV-3 and 10 infection
- Sites—face and dorsum of hands

Histopathology (Figs 11.17 and 11.18)

- Acanthosis, orthokeratosis, hyperkeratosis and lack papillomatosis
- Stratum spinosum, granular layer and corneal layer show vacuolated cells with central basophilic nuclei

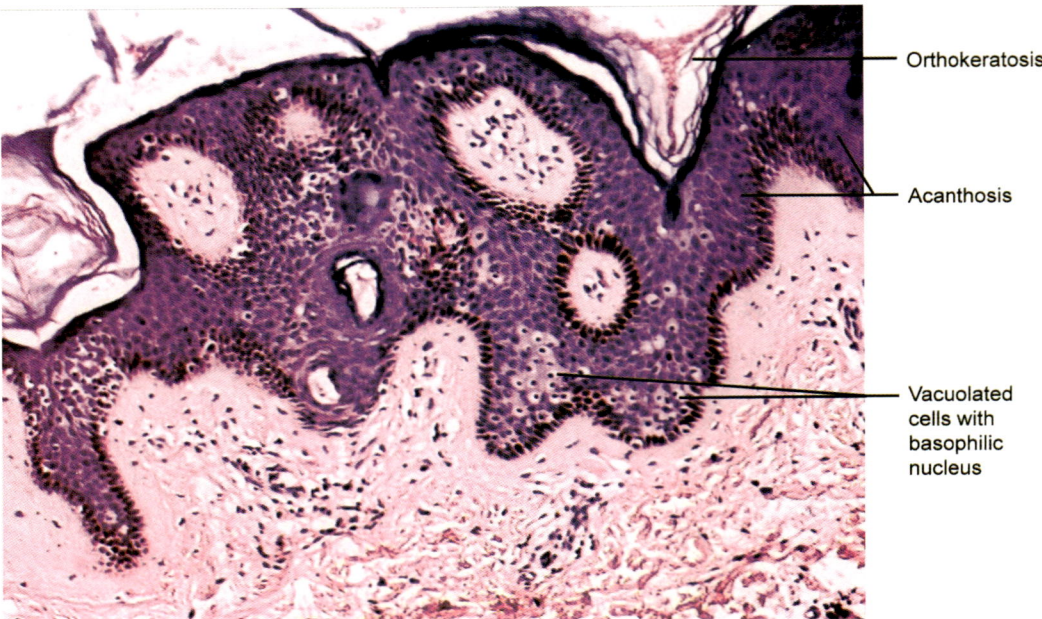

Orthokeratosis

Acanthosis

Vacuolated
cells with
basophilic
nucleus

Fig. 11.17: Verruca plana

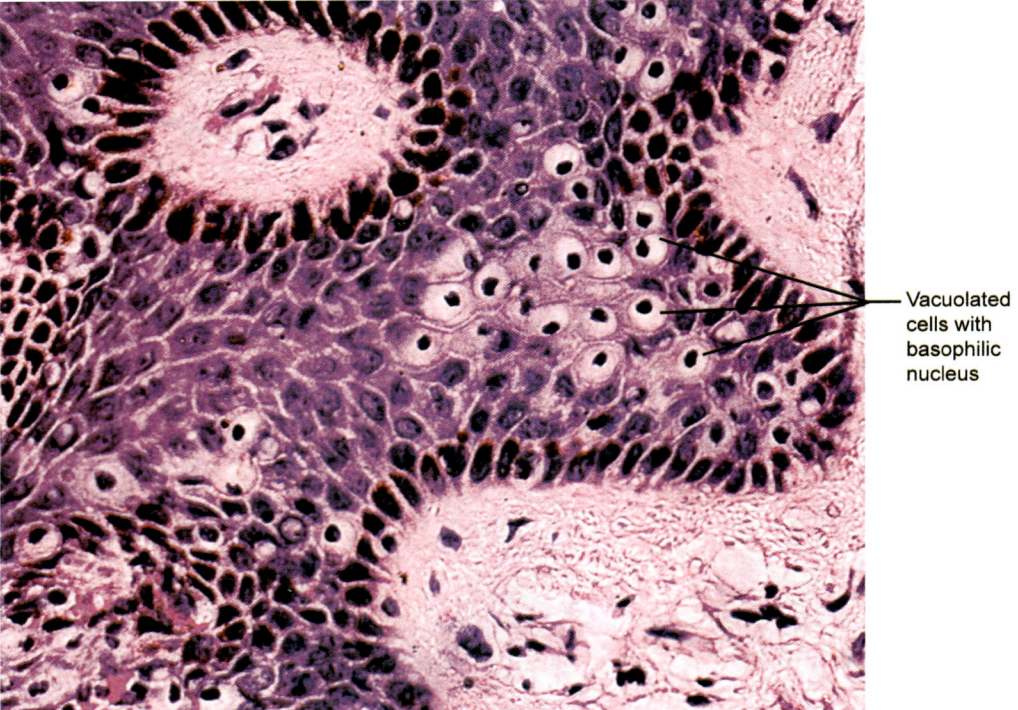

Vacuolated
cells with
basophilic
nucleus

Fig. 11.18: Verruca plana

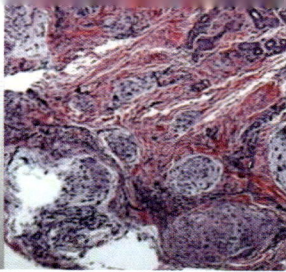

Erythema Multiforme

There are two types of erythema multiforme.

ERYTHEMA MULTIFORME MINOR

Introduction

- Etiology—Herpes simplex virus infection
- Age group—affects young adults
- Sites—most commonly affects extremities
- Presents as red papules (targetoid annular lesions with central epidermal necrosis) (Fig. 12.1)

Histopathology (Figs 12.2 to 12.4)

- Orthokeratotic stratum corneum
- Basal cell layer vacuolization, lymphocytic infiltrate along the dermo-epidermal junction
- Necrotic keratinocytes with eosinophilic cytoplasm and pyknotic nucleus and accompanying lymphocytes

- Superficial dermis show perivascular lymphocytic infiltrate

ERYTHEMA MULTIFORME MAJOR

Introduction

- Includes Stevens Johnson syndrome (SJS) and toxic epidermal necrolysis (TEN)
- Etiology of Stevens-Johnson syndrome—drugs like allopurinol, NSAIDs, sulfonamides, anticonvulsants, penicillin, tetracycline, doxycycline
- Other causes that predispose to erythema multiforme major—herpesvirus infection

Clinical Features

- SJS can present as purpuric macules, which can progress to blister formation and can involve 10% of total body area

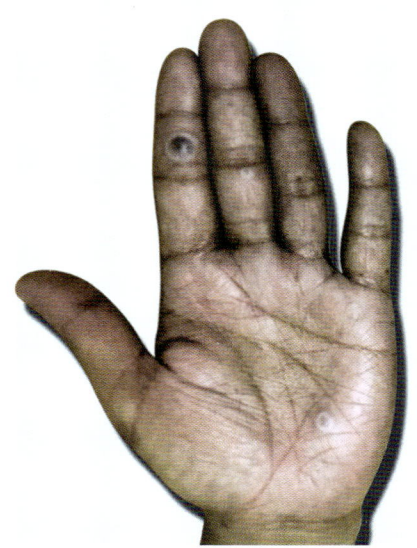
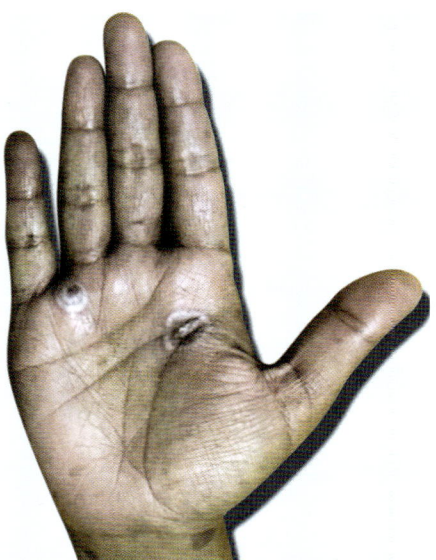

Fig. 12.1: Erythema multiforme. Typical lesion consists of three components—a dusky central area, a dark red inflammatory zone surrounded by a pale ring of edema and an erythematous halo at the periphery

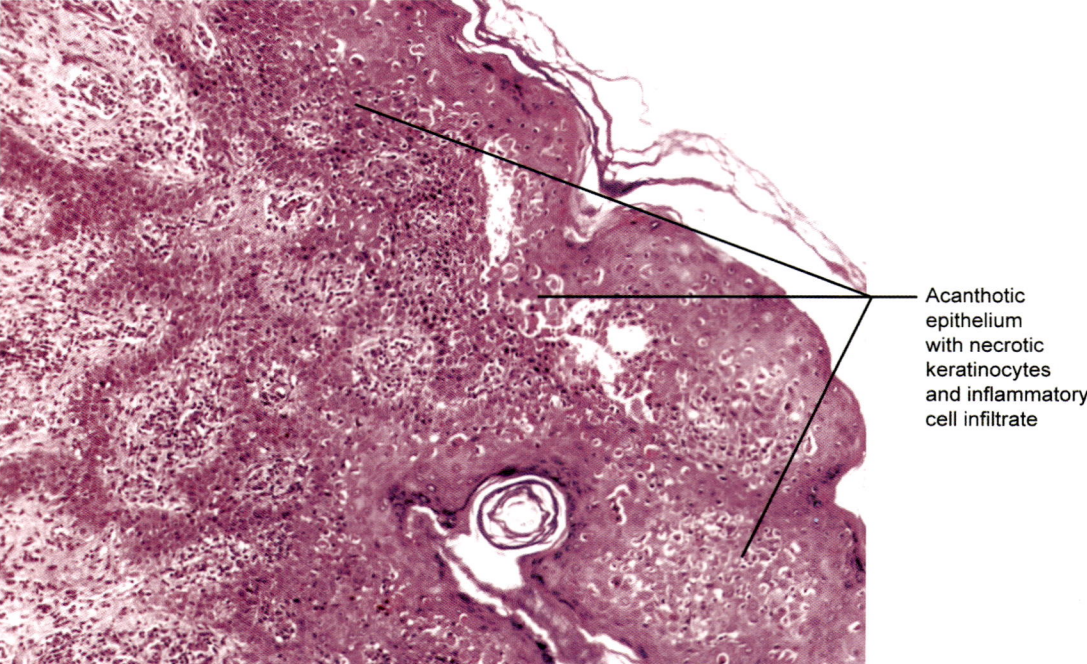

Fig. 12.2: Erythema multiforme

Acanthotic epithelium with necrotic keratinocytes and inflammatory cell infiltrate

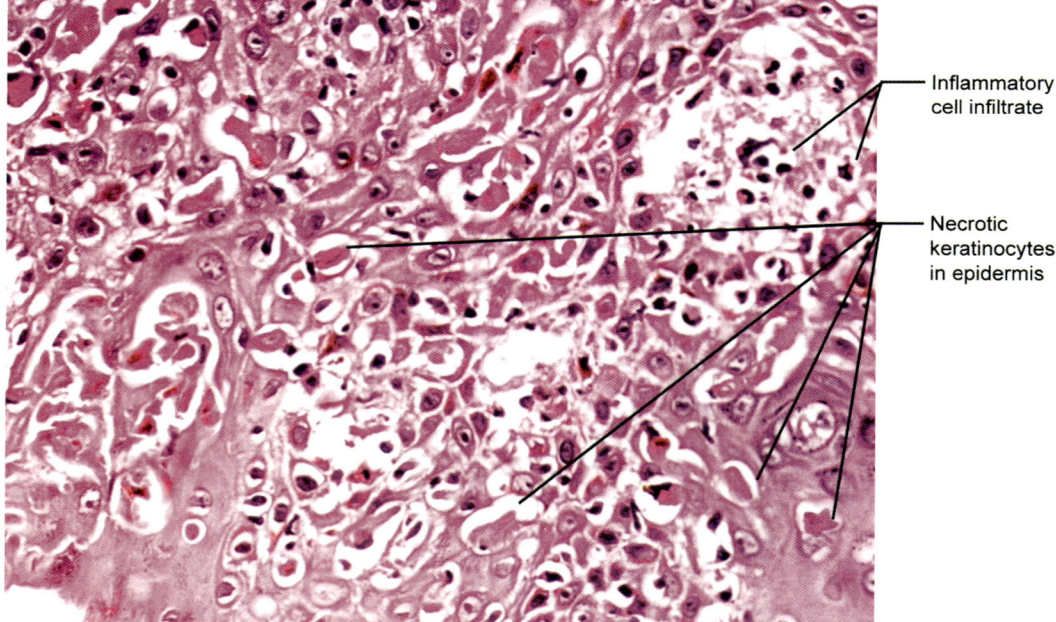

Fig. 12.3: Erythema multiforme

Inflammatory cell infiltrate

Necrotic keratinocytes in epidermis

- Sites of involvement of SJS—most commonly affects trunk, oral involvement can also be seen
- TEN presents as large bullae with epidermal detachment, which is seen more than 30% of total body area

Histopathology

- Sub-epidermal bulla, necrotic keratinocytes which can progress to full thickness epidermal necrosis in TEN
- Extravasated erythrocytes within the blister cavity

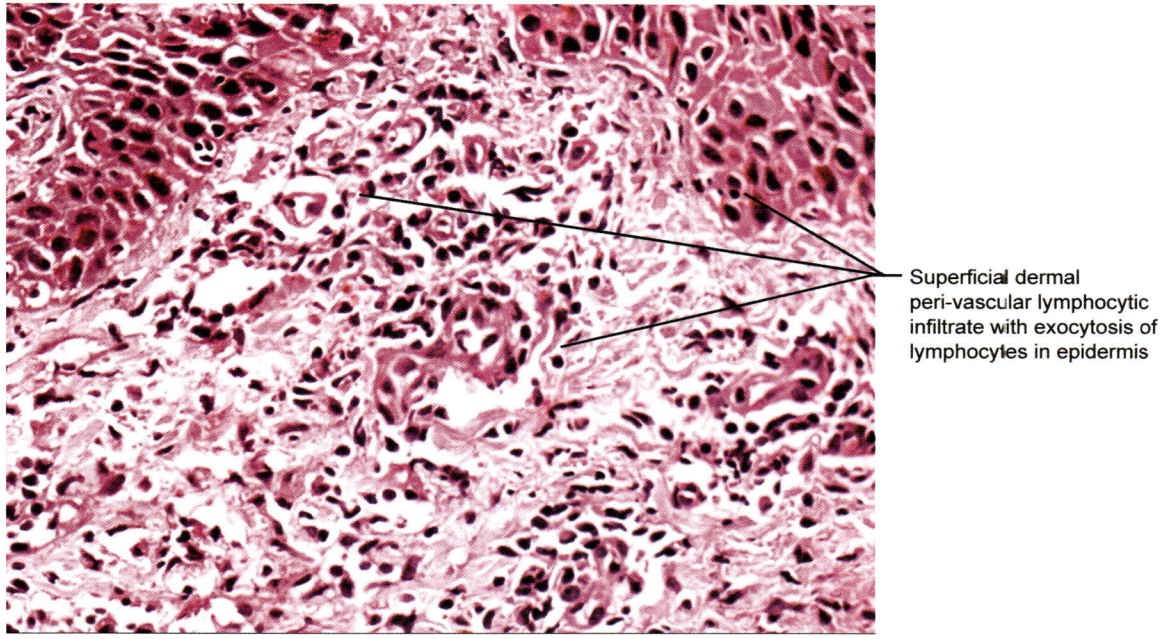

Superficial dermal peri-vascular lymphocytic infiltrate with exocytosis of lymphocytes in epidermis

Fig. 12.4: Erythema multiforme

- Late lesions can show melanophages in papillary dermis

Differential Diagnosis

Fixed Drug Eruption
- Epidermal spongiosis with orthokeratosis
- Interface dermatitis with lymphocytic infiltrate along the dermoepidermal junction
- Basal cell layer vacuolization with keratinocyte necrosis
- Perivascular lymphocytic and eosinophilic infiltrate

Acute Graft Versus Host Disease
- Interface dermatitis and apoptosis of keratinocytes
- Superficial dermal perivascular lymphocytic infiltrate with exocytosis of lymphocytes into the epidermis

- Vacuolar degeneration along the dermal-epidermal junction
- Fibrosis of papillary dermis is seen in chronic cases

Phototoxic Dermatitis
- Spongiosis, necrotic keratinocytes and epidermal necrosis
- Superficial and deep dermal mixed inflammatory cell infiltrate

Porphyria Cutanea Tarda
- Sub-epidermal blister
- Festooning of dermal papillae (preservation of dermal papillae at floor)
- PAS positive diastase-resistant hyaline material deposition in walls of small blood vessels in superficial dermis

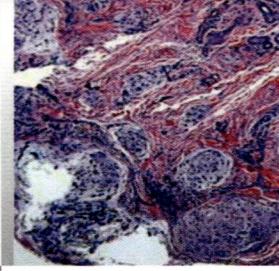

Pityriasis Lichenoides

Pityriasis lichenoides can be presented as follows:

PITYRIASIS LICHENOIDES ET VARIOLIFORMIS ACUTA (PLEVA)

- Acute form
- Sites—trunk and proximal extremities
- Pathogenesis—cytotoxic immune response (CD8+ T-lymphocytes) is responsible for epidermal necrosis

- Presents as erythematous papules, vesicles or nodules, that resolve by itself, within a few weeks or can rarely progress to necrotic ulcers
- Relapse is commonly seen

Histopathology (Fig. 13.1)

- Spongiosis, apoptotic keratinocytes, parakeratosis with neutrophilic abscess
- Basal cell layer vacuolization, exocytosis of lymphocytes and erythrocytes into epidermis

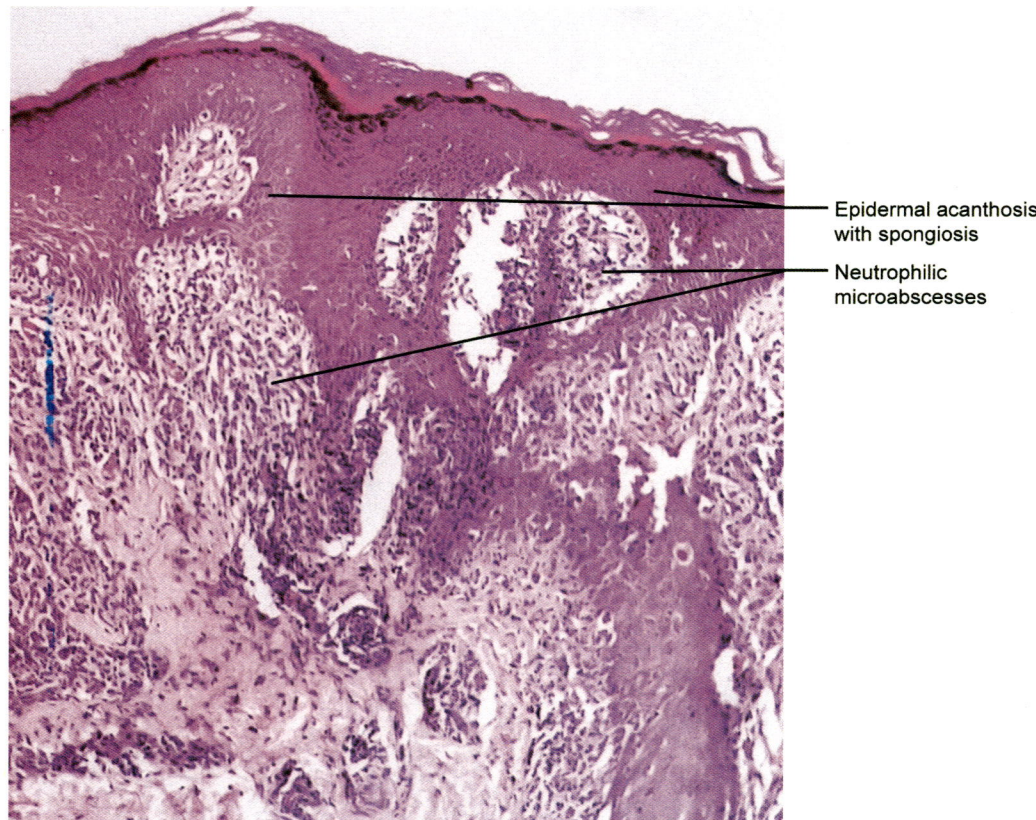

Epidermal acanthosis with spongiosis

Neutrophilic microabscesses

Fig. 13.1: Pityriasis lichenoides

- Band-like infiltrate of lymphocytes along the dermo-epidermal junction
- Lymphocytic infiltrate extends from the papillary dermis into reticular dermis

PITYRIASIS LICHENOIDES CHRONICA (PLC)

- Chronic form
- Etiology—cell-mediated immunity to viral and bacterial infections
- Sites—trunk and extremities
- Presents as red-brown papules and plaques with a characteristic scale (Fig. 13.2)
- Remission followed by relapse is common

Histopathology (Fig. 13.3)

- Epidermis—acanthosis, parakeratosis and spongiosis
- Mild interface change at dermal–epidermal junction
- Superficial dermis shows perivascular lymphocytic infiltrate

Differential Diagnosis

Acute and Sub-acute Dermatitis

- Mild acanthosis, spongiosis
- Exocytosis of lymphocytes
- Superficial dermis shows perivascular lympho-histiocytic and eosinophilic infiltrate

Lymphomatoid Papulosis

- Necrotic keratinocytes
- Atypical lymphoid cells show epidermotropism
- Lymphoid cells can show CD-30 positivity

Fixed Drug Eruption

- Epidermal spongiosis, orthokeratosis, keratinocytic necrosis
- Basal cell layer vacuolization
- Interface dermatitis
- Perivascular lymphocytic and eosinophilic infiltrate

Acute Graft vs Host Disease

- Interface dermatitis and apoptosis of keratinocytes
- Vacuolar degeneration along the dermal–epidermal junction
- Fibrosis of papillary dermis

Guttate Psoriasis

- Mounds of parakeratosis with collections of neutrophils and overlying focal loss of granular layer
- Superficial perivascular lymphohistiocytic infiltrate

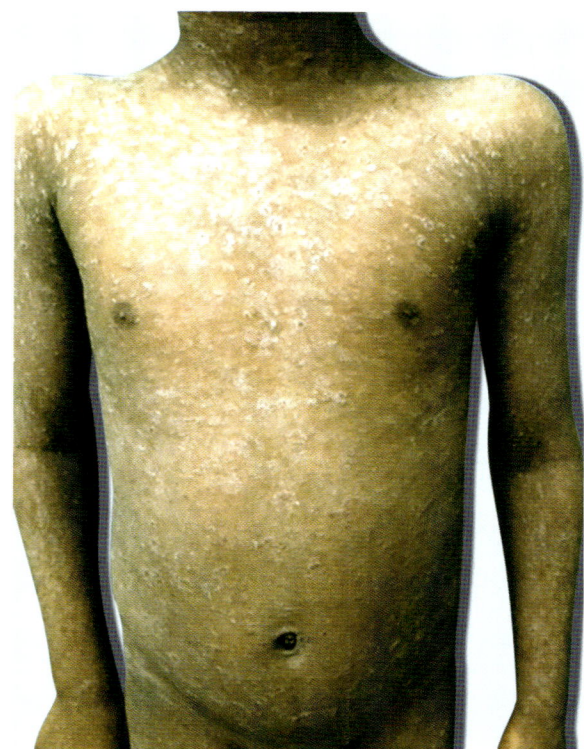

Fig. 13.2: Pityriasis lichenoides chronica. Numerous red brown papules with overlying mica-like scaling

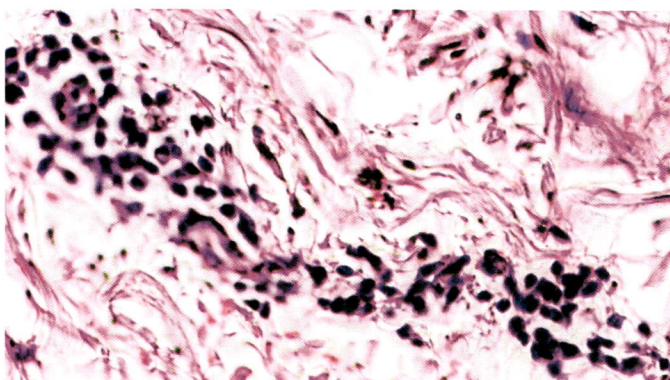

Fig. 13.3: Lymphocytic vasculitis in p tyriasis lichenoides chronica

Pityriasis Rosea

- Focal acanthosis, spongiosis and parakeratosis with hypogranulosis
- Superficial perivascular lymphohistiocytic and eosinophilic infiltrate with exocytosis of lymphocytes
- Red blood cell extravasation in epidermis and papillary dermis

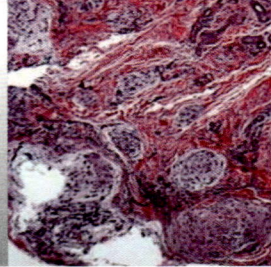

Lichen Planus

INTRODUCTION

- Inflammatory dermatosis, affects more commonly females
- Can affect skin, mucous membranes, hair follicles and nails
- Skin involvement—lesions present as polygonal, violaceous, flat-topped papules that may coalesce into plaques (Fig. 14.1)
- Papules show Wickham's striae (fine white lines)
- Sites—affects wrists, forearm, shin, lumbar region, scalp
- Koebner's phenomenon is commonly seen

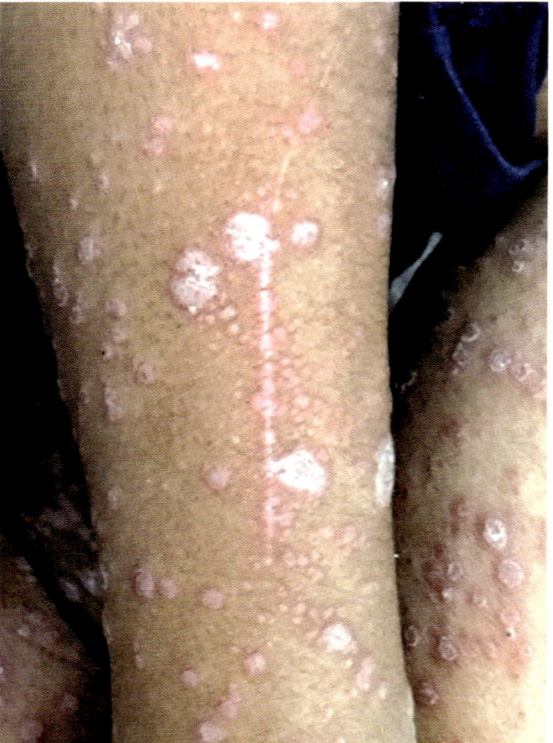

Fig. 14.1: Lichen planus. Flat topped, violaceous papules

- Oral lesions—involve the buccal mucosa, gingivae and tongue
- Nail changes—longitudinal fissures, ridges, destruction and pterygium formation
- Rarely, malignant transformation to squamous cell carcinoma can occur

HISTOPATHOLOGY OF LICHEN PLANUS
(Figs 14.2 and 14.3)

- Compact orthokeratosis, wedge-shaped hyper-granulosis, irregular acanthosis, basal cell layer vacuolization
- Lichenoid interface dermatitis—band-like lympho-cytic infiltrate in the papillary dermis that extends to the epidermis
- Rete ridges appear to be pointed at the lower end, giving it a "saw-toothed" appearance
- Basal cell layer shows vacuolization and necrotic keratinocytes (colloid bodies), which can extend into the dermis
- **Max-Joseph space**—artifactual cleft appears between epidermis and the lichenoid infiltrate, due to damage of basal cell layer due to inflammation
- In hypertrophic variant and in drug-induced lichenoid eruptions, eosinophils may be seen
- **Direct immunofluorescence**—IgM containing colloid bodies in the papillary dermis
- Note: Parakeratosis is not a feature of lichen planus of skin, and it exclude its diagnosis

VARIANTS

Oral Lichen Planus

- Predisposing factor—dental plaques containing mercury

Histopathology (Figs 14.4 and 14.5)

- Shows parakeratosis, less hypergranulosis and band-like infiltrate

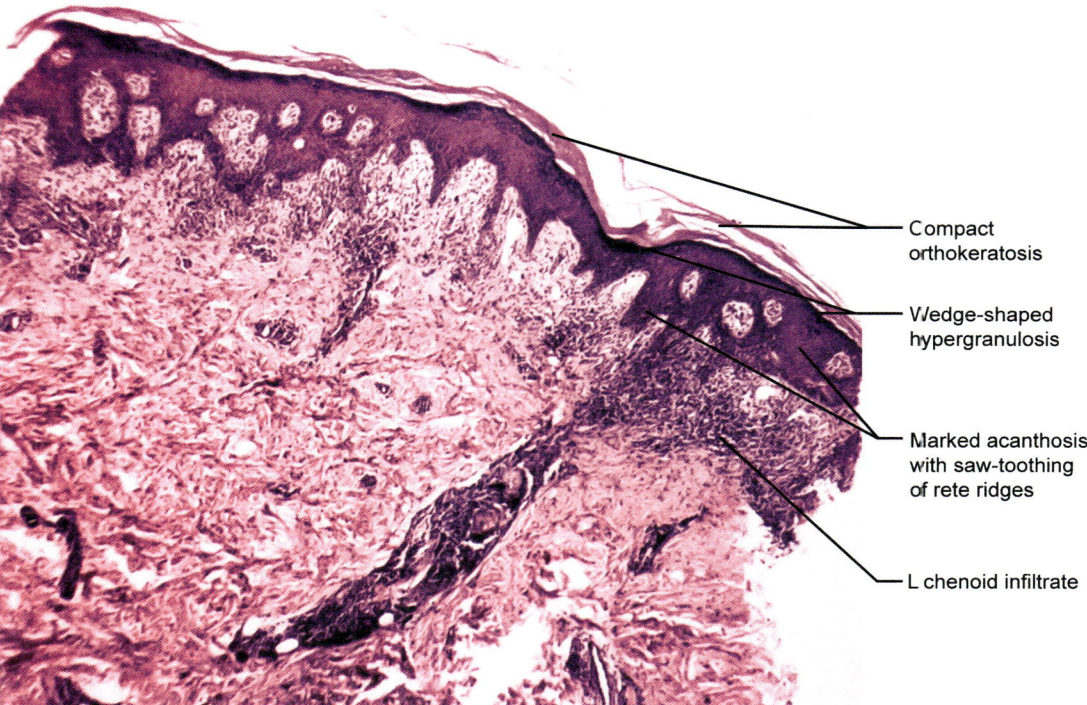

Compact orthokeratosis

Wedge-shaped hypergranulosis

Marked acanthosis with saw-toothing of rete ridges

L chenoid infiltrate

Fig. 14.2: Lichen planus

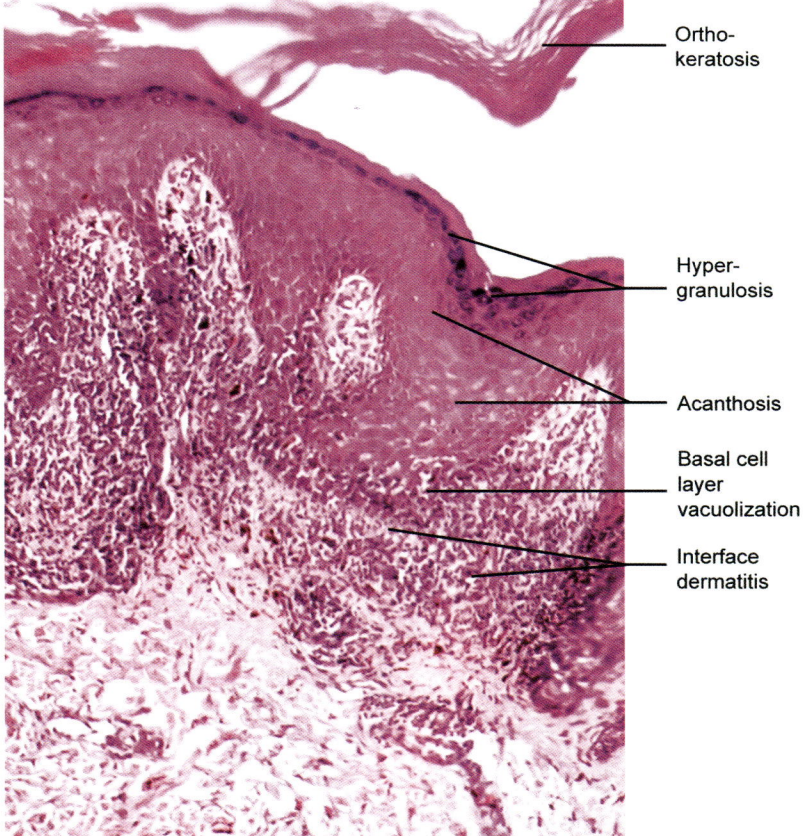

Ortho-keratosis

Hyper-granulosis

Acanthosis

Basal cell layer vacuolization

Interface dermatitis

Fig. 14.3: Lichen planus

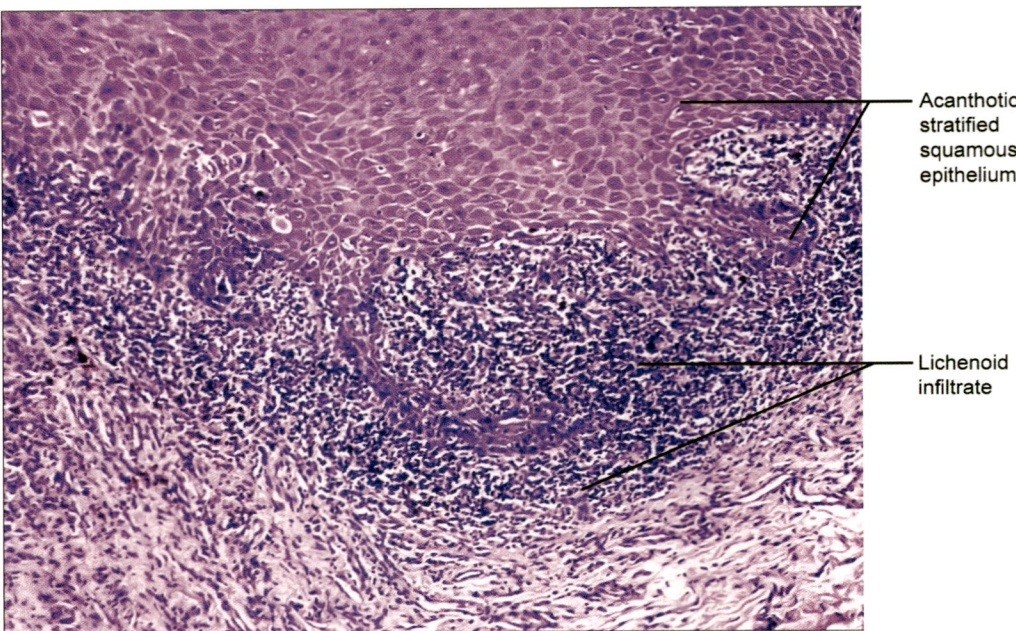

Acanthotic stratified squamous epithelium

Lichenoid infiltrate

Fig. 14.4: Oral lichen planus

Lichen Planopilaris (LPP)
- Affects predominantly females
- Presents as scarring alopecia, follicular keratotic papules and peri-follicular erythema

Histopathology (Figs 14.6 to 14.9)
- Follicular plugging, hypergranulosis, dense peri-follicular band-like lymphocytic infiltrate involving the basal layer of follicular epithelium
- Interfollicular epidermis is not involved
- Hourglass appearance (late stage): Peri-follicular fibrosis, epithelial atrophy around infundibulum with loss of follicles and adnexal structures
- Pseudopelade (of Brocq)—end stage disorder, when all the hair follicles are being destroyed with resultant scarring alopecia
- Direct immunofluorescence shows colloid bodies in the dermis with IgG and IgM antibodies

Actinic Lichen Planus
- Affects sun-exposed areas (face, neck, flexor surfaces of forearms and hands)
- Clinical presentation—lesions appear as red to brown annular plaques or raised areas with surrounding hypo-pigmentation

Annular Lichen Planus
- Annular lesions affecting inter-triginous areas (axilla, groin) and vermilion border of lips

- Size of lesions vary from 0.5 to 2.5 cm in diameter
- Lesions show central clearing

Atrophic Lichen Planus
- Presents as annular violaceous plaques showing central atrophy
- Sites—axilla, glans penis, lower extremities or trunk

Histopathology
- Thinned out epidermis with loss of normal rete ridges
- Less prominent lichenoid infiltrate

Lichen Planus Pemphigoides
- Tense bullae are seen on the extremities
- Resembles bullous pemphigoid

Histopathology
- Sub-epidermal bullae, can show eosinophils as its contents
- Mild perivascular lymphocytic, neutrophilic and eosinophilic infiltrate
- Direct immunofluorescence shows IgG and C3 positivity in the basement membrane zone

Hypertrophic Lichen Planus
- Affects shins and ankles
- Presents as red-brown papules and plaques
- Predisposing factor—persistent scratching

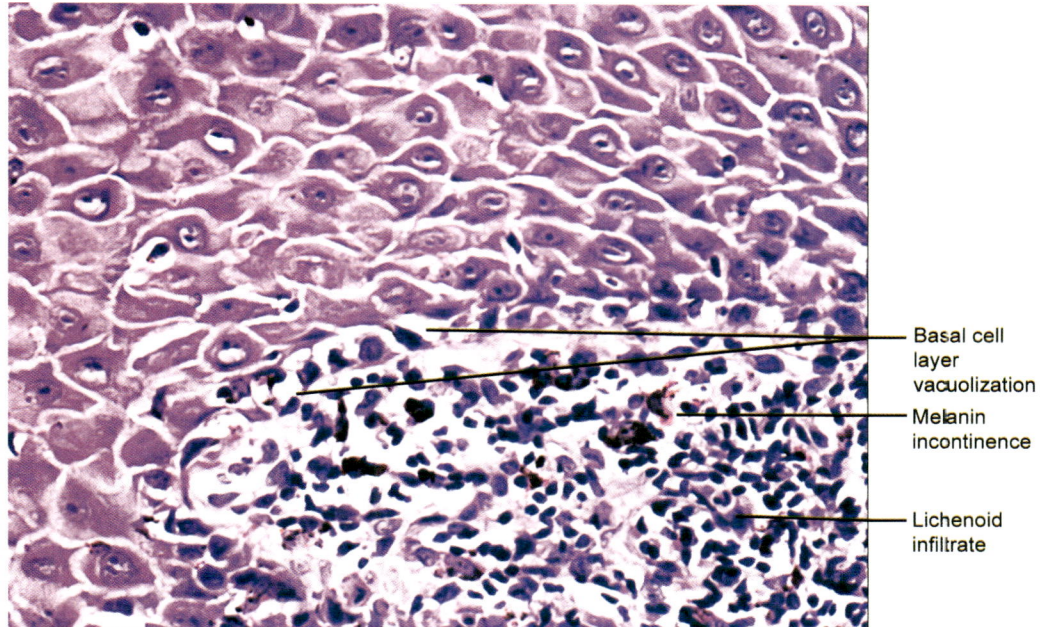

Fig. 14.5: Oral lichen planus

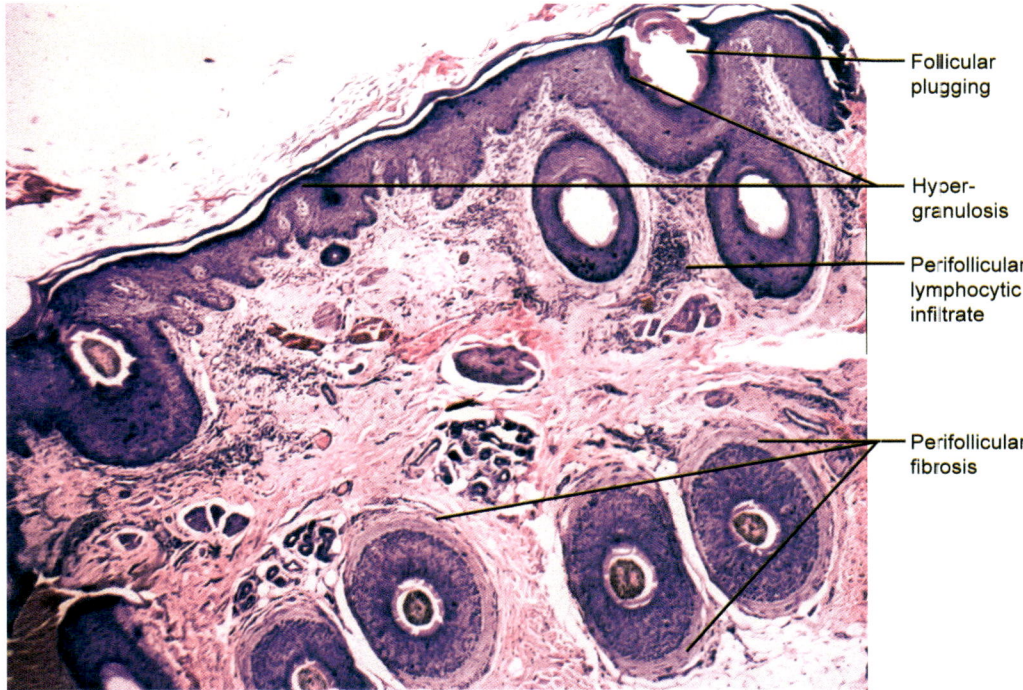

Fig. 14.6: Lichen planopilaris

- Complications—squamous cell carcinoma, verrucous carcinoma, keratoacanthoma

Histopathology (Fig. 14.10)

- Epidermis shows irregular acanthosis, hypergranulosis and compact orthokeratosis
- Basal cell layer shows vacuolization
- Civatte bodies and lymphocytic infiltrate, limited to the tips of rete ridges
- Papillary dermis shows vertically oriented collagen bundles

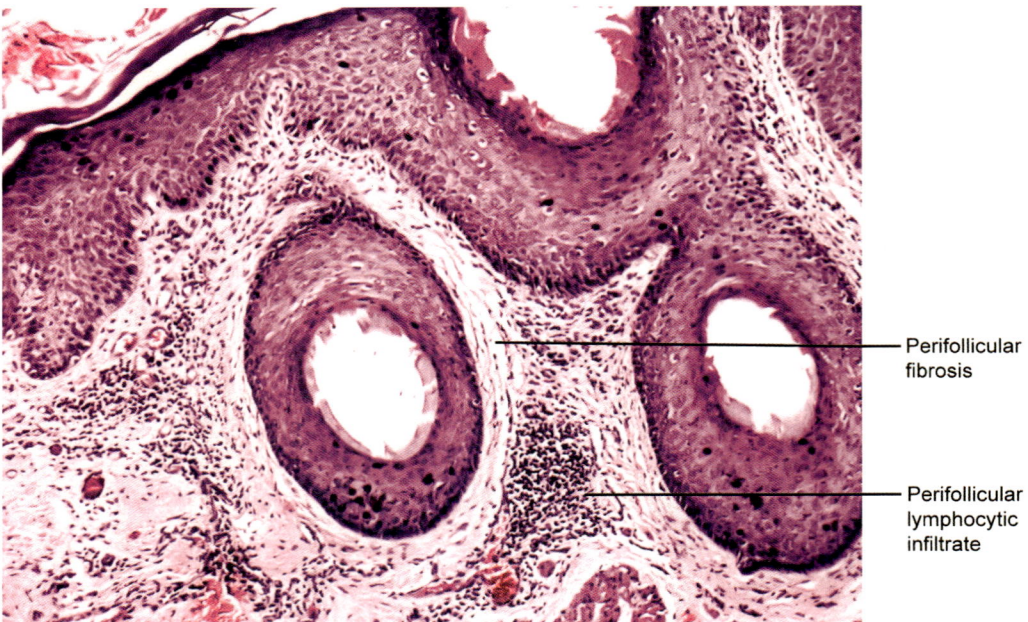

Perifollicular fibrosis

Perifollicular lymphocytic infiltrate

Fig. 14.7: Lichen planopilaris

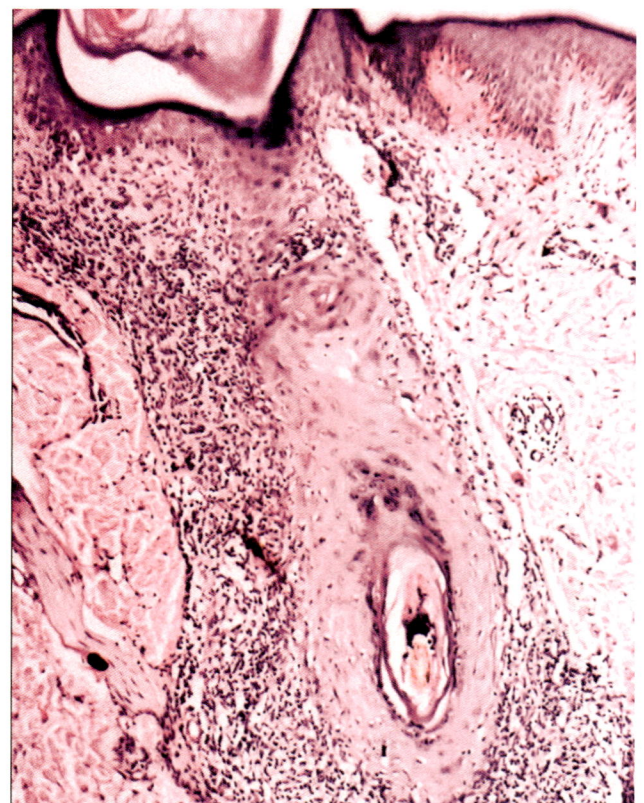

Fig. 14.8: Lichen planopilaris. Perifollicular inflammatory cell infiltrate comprising of lymphocytes

Linear Lichen Planus

- Purple colored papules occurring in a linear or band-like pattern
- Site—lower limbs

Lichen Planus Pigmentosus/Erythema Dyschromicum Perstans/Ashy Dermatosis

- Presents as hyper-pigmented dark brown papules and macules
- Site—sun exposed areas, most commonly affects head and neck
- Erythema dyschromicum perstans—lesions have erythematous borders
- Ashy dermatosis—lesions without erythematous borders

Histopathology (Fig. 14.11)

- Lichenoid infiltrate, basal cell layer vacuolization
- Superficial dermis—melanin incontinence, perivascular lymphocytic infiltrate
- Immunofluorescence—IgM, IgG containing colloid bodies in dermis

Ulcerative Lichen Planus

- Presents as ulcers and erosions
- Sites—palms, soles and mucosal membranes
- Risk factor for development of squamous cell carcinoma

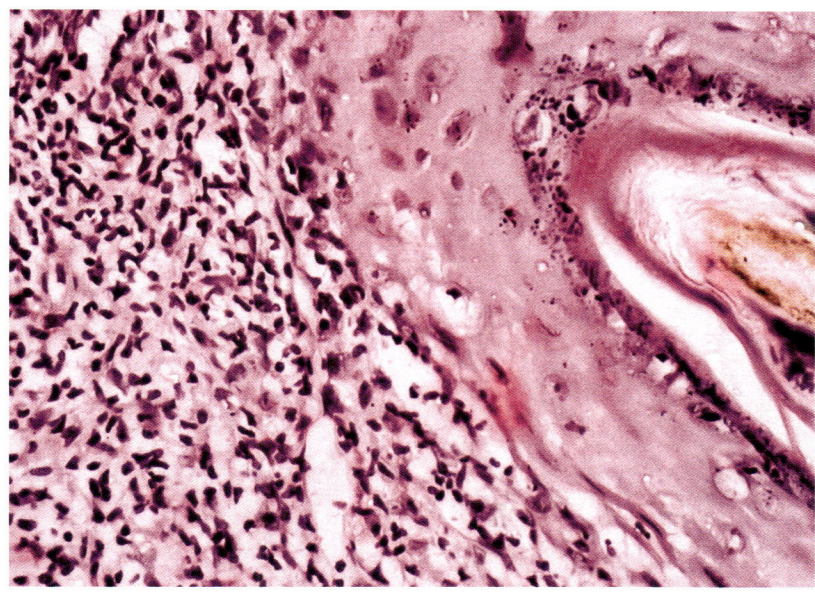

Fig. 14.9: Lichen planopilaris. Peri-follicular mixed inflammatory cell infiltrate

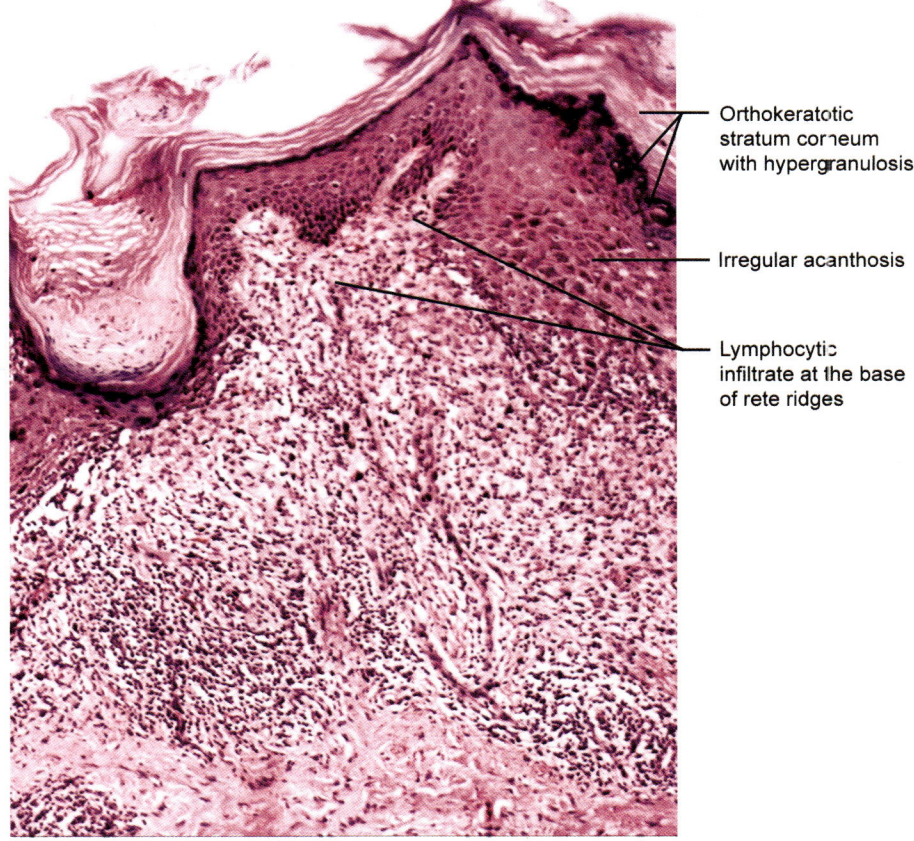

Orthokeratotic stratum corneum with hypergranulosis

Irregular acanthosis

Lymphocytic infiltrate at the base of rete ridges

Fig. 14.10: Hypertrophic lichen planus

DIFFERENTIAL DIAGNOSIS

Lichenoid Drug Eruption

- Focal parakeratosis with absence of granular layer
- Necrotic keratinocytes in the basal and spinosum layers
- Upper epidermis—exocytosis of lymphocytes
- Lichenoid interface dermatitis with eosinophils

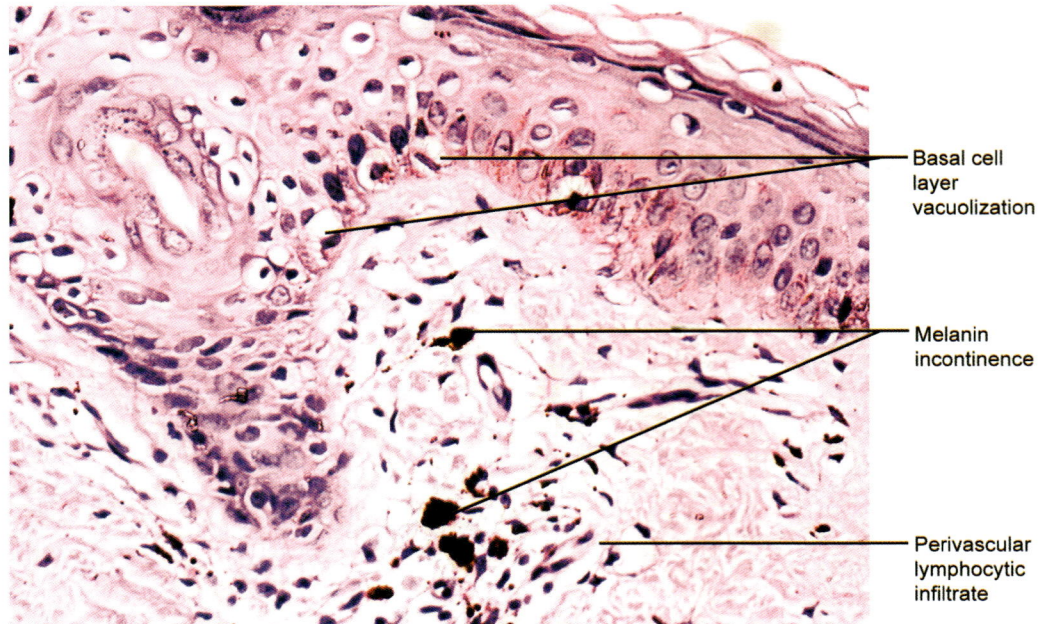

Fig. 14.11: Lichen planus pigmentosus

Chronic Graft-vs-Host Reaction

- Perivascular inflammatory cell infiltrate rather than band-like inflammatory infiltrate
- Langerhans cells are decreased in number
- Note: Langerhans cell number is increased in lichen planus, which shows CD1a and S-100 positivity

Fixed Drug Eruption

- Epidermal spongiosis, orthokeratosis, keratinocytic necrosis
- Basal cell layer vacuolization, pigment incontinence
- Interface dermatitis
- Perivascular lymphocytic and eosinophilic infiltrate

Lichen Sclerosus

- Early stage—lichenoid infiltrate, late stage—epidermal atrophy
- Superficial dermis shows hyalinized collagen with dilated vessels and extravasated erythrocytes

Lichenoid Lupus Erythematosus

- Atrophic epidermis, but can also show acanthosis
- Absence of necrotic keratinocytes in the epidermis
- Lichenoid inflammatory cell infiltrate
- Superficial and deep dermis show perivascular and peri-adnexal lymphocytic infiltrate
- Thickened basement membrane which shows PAS positivity
- Dermis shows mucin deposits

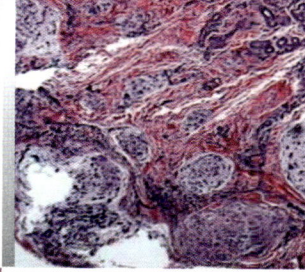

Lichen Nitidus

INTRODUCTION

- Inflammatory dermatosis
- Affects children and young adults
- Site: Flexor aspect of upper extremities, chest, abdomen, or genitals
- Presents as multiple, discrete, flat-topped, flesh-colored papules

HISTOPATHOLOGY (Figs 15.1 and 15.2)

- Sub-epidermal region (dermal papillae) shows mixed inflammatory cell infiltrate comprising of lymphocytes, epithelioid histiocytes, melanophages and occasional giant cells
- Ball in claw appearance (claw clutching a ball)—at each lateral margin of the infiltrate, acanthotic rete ridges, extend downward and seems to clutch the infiltrate (i.e. claw-like epidermal grasp around ball-like inflammatory cell infiltrate)
- Epidermis overlying the inflammatory cell infiltrate is atrophic and shows basal cell hydropic degeneration
- Parakeratotic scale is often present

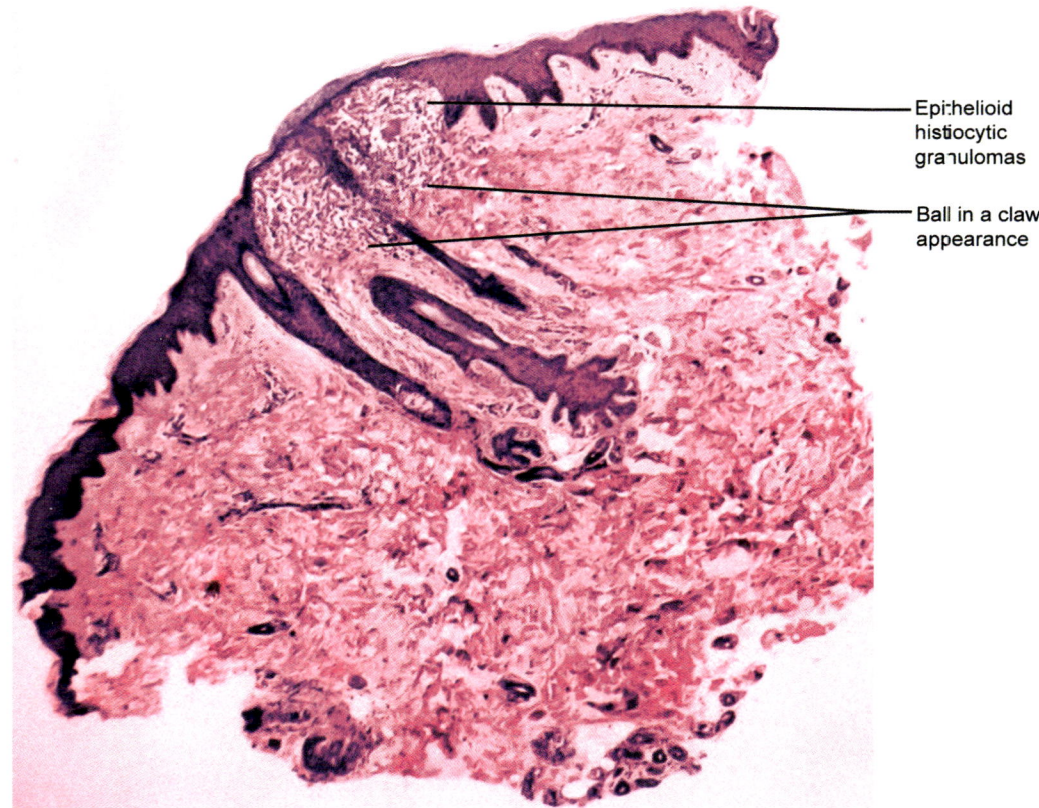

Epithelioid histiocytic granulomas

Ball in a claw appearance

Fig. 15.1: Lichen nitidus

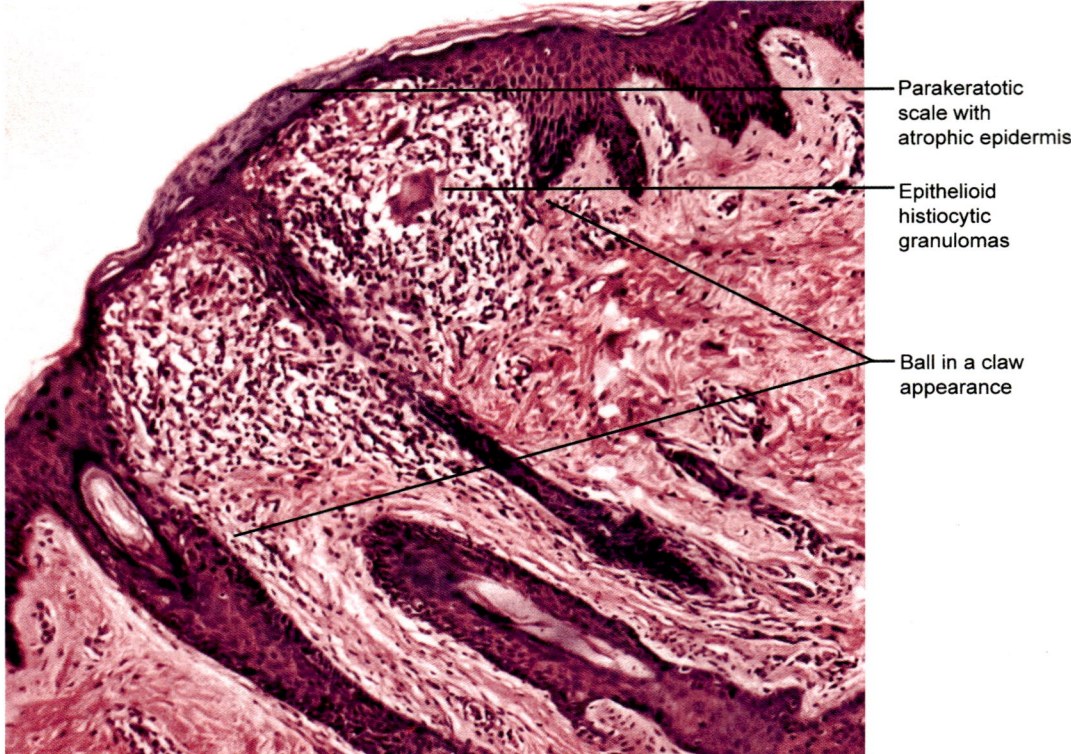

Fig. 15.2: Lichen nitidus

Labels on figure:
- Parakeratotic scale with atrophic epidermis
- Epithelioid histiocytic granulomas
- Ball in a claw appearance

DIFFERENTIAL DIAGNOSIS

Lichen Planus

- Lack parakeratosis
- Shows hypergranulosis and Civatte bodies

- Direct immunofluorescence (DIF) is positive

Lichen Scrofulosorum

- Mild spongiosis
- Exocytosis of neutrophils into the epidermis

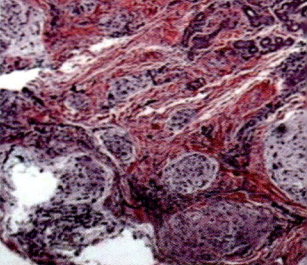

Lichen Striatus

INTRODUCTION

- Present as unilateral erythematous papules
- Papules are arranged in a linear pattern (along the lines of Blaschko)
- Sites—extremities, trunk and neck
- Age group—most commonly affects children
- Spontaneous resolution of the lesions can occur

HISTOPATHOLOGY (Figs16.1 and 16.2)

- Acanthosis, focal parakeratosis, spongiosis, and lymphocytic exocytosis
- Superficial and deep dermis show perivascular, peri-eccrine and peri-follicular inflammatory cell infiltrate comprising of lymphocytes and histiocytes
- Scattered necrotic keratinocytes in the epidermis

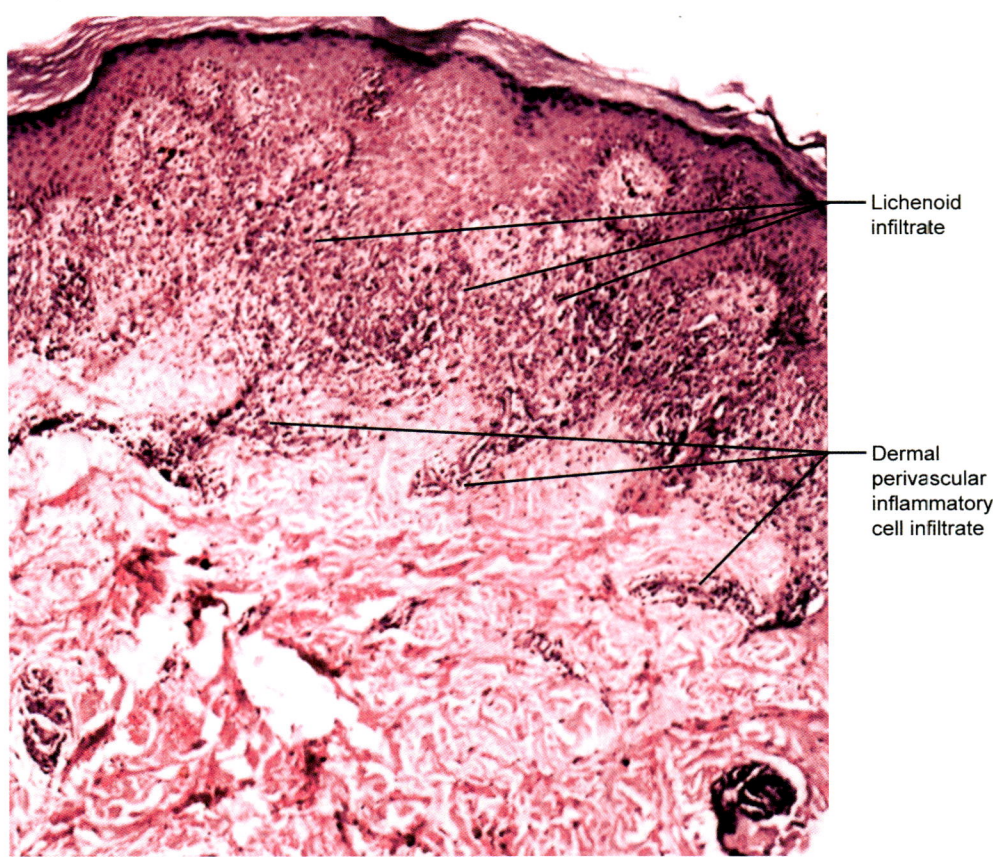

Lichenoid infiltrate

Dermal perivascular inflammatory cell infiltrate

Fig. 16.1: Lichen striatus

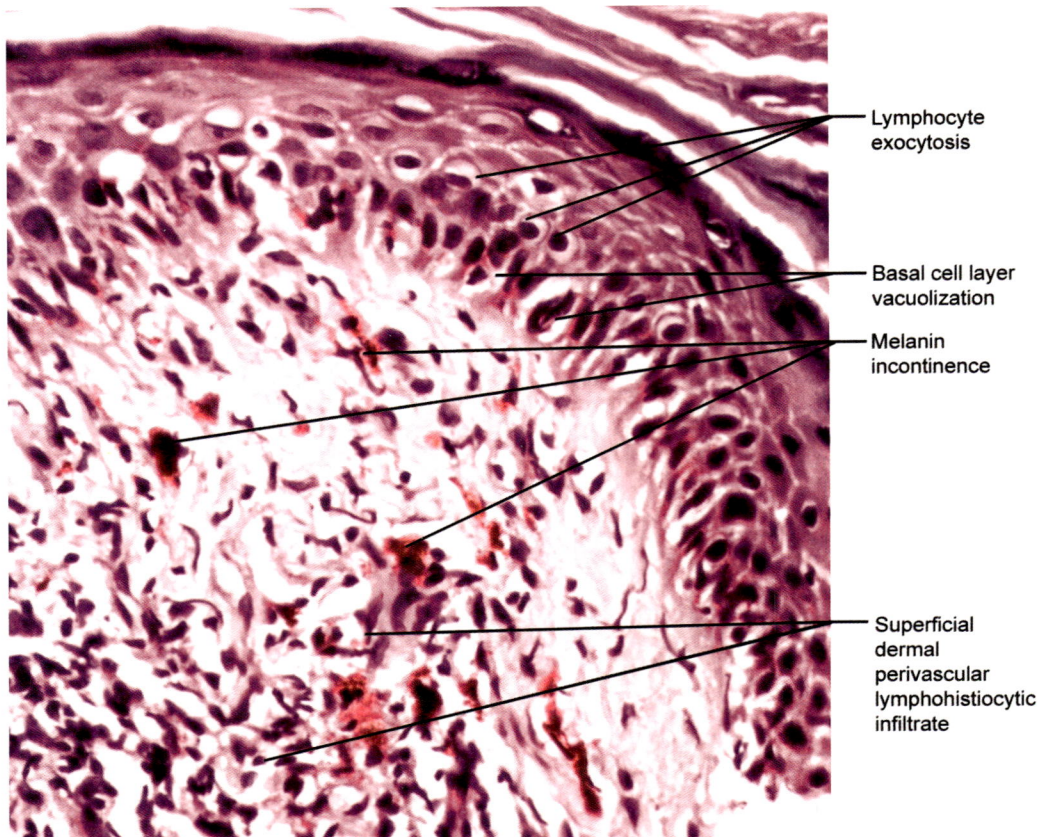

Lymphocyte exocytosis

Basal cell layer vacuolization

Melanin incontinence

Superficial dermal perivascular lymphohistiocytic infiltrate

Fig. 16.2: Lichen striatus

DIFFERENTIAL DIAGNOSIS

Lichen Planus

- Absence of parakeratosis
- Presence of hypergranulosis

Lichen Nitidus

- Papillary dermis shows epithelioid histiocytic granulomas, lymphocytes and giant cells

- Ball in claw appearance of papillary dermis

Graft Versus Host Disease

- Interface dermatitis and apoptosis of keratinocytes
- Vacuolar degeneration along the dermo-epidermal junction
- Superficial dermis—perivascular lymphocytic infiltrate with lymphocytic exocytosis in epidermis
- Chronic—papillary dermal fibrosis

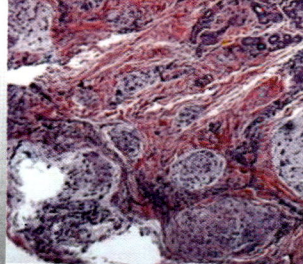

Chapter

17

Lichen Sclerosus

INTRODUCTION

- Includes *lichen sclerosus et atrophicus and balanitis xerotica obliterans*
- Sites—affects ano-genital regions (females and males)
- Presents as white polygonal papules that coalesce into plaques (Fig. 17.1)
- Lesions present with intense pruritis
- *Borrelia burgdorferi* can be demonstrated by silver stain in the lesional skin

- Autoimmune basis—70% of patients may have circulating autoantibodies against extracellular matrix protein 1 (ECM-1)
- Can progress into squamous cell carcinoma

HISTOPATHOLOGY (Figs 17.2 to 17.4)

- Hyper-orthokeratotic atrophic stratified squamous epithelium with pale (white) superficial dermis—giving it a "tri-layered" or "striped appearance"
- Basal cell layer vacuolization can be seen

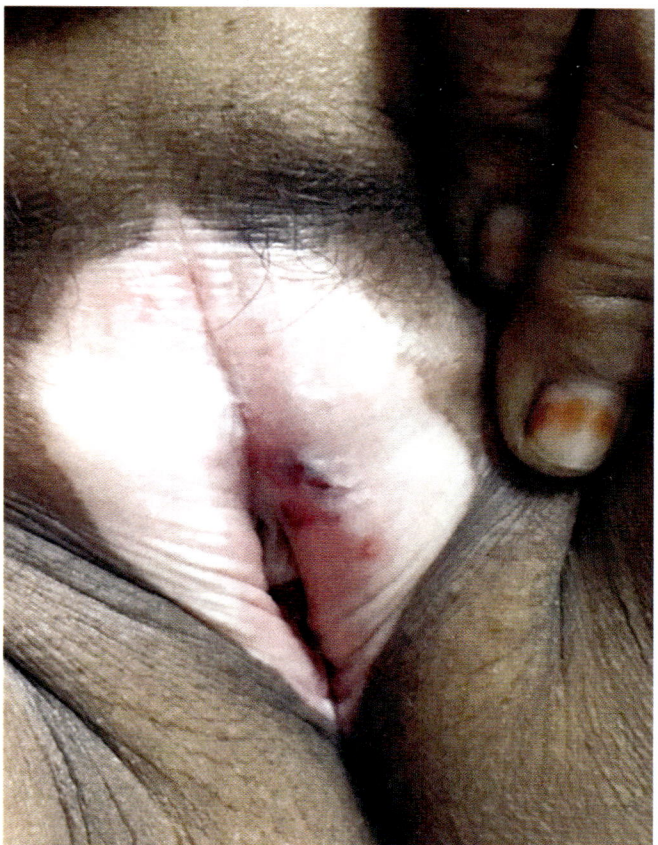

Fig. 17.1: Lichen sclerosus. White atrophic papules that coalesce to form plaques

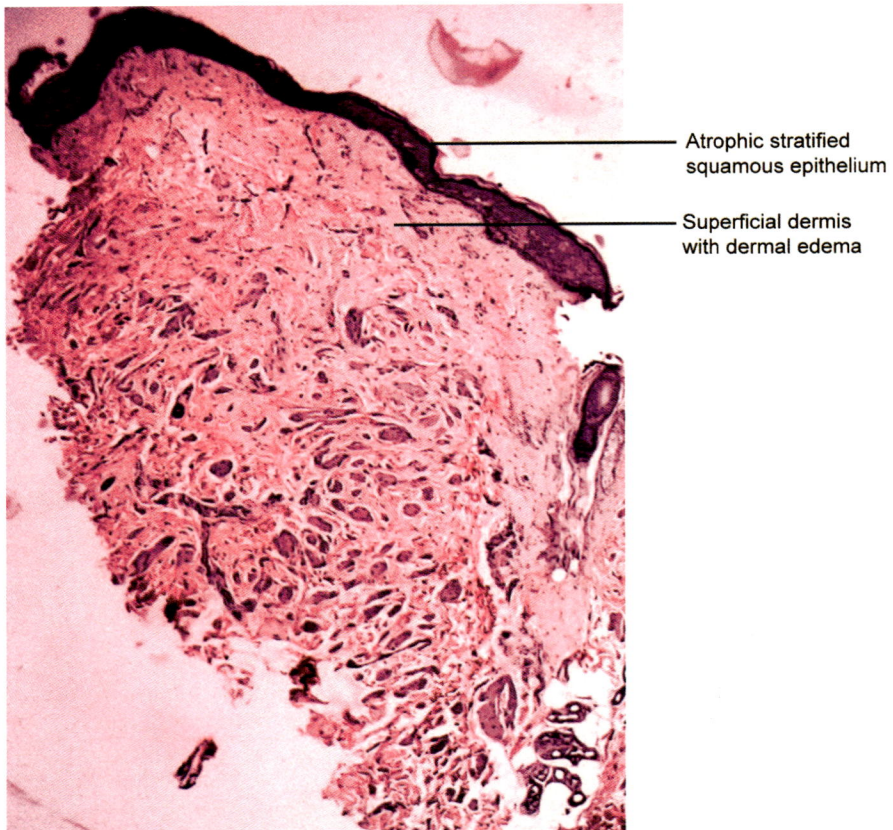

Atrophic stratified squamous epithelium

Superficial dermis with dermal edema

Fig. 17.2: Lichen sclerosus

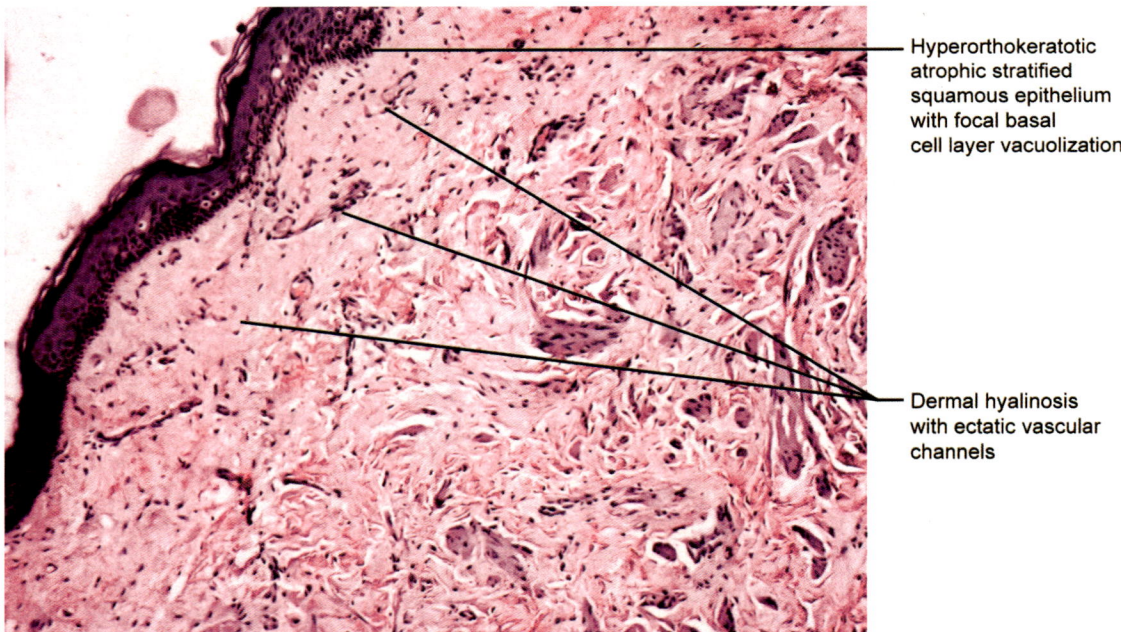

Hyperorthokeratotic atrophic stratified squamous epithelium with focal basal cell layer vacuolization

Dermal hyalinosis with ectatic vascular channels

Fig. 17.3: Lichen sclerosus

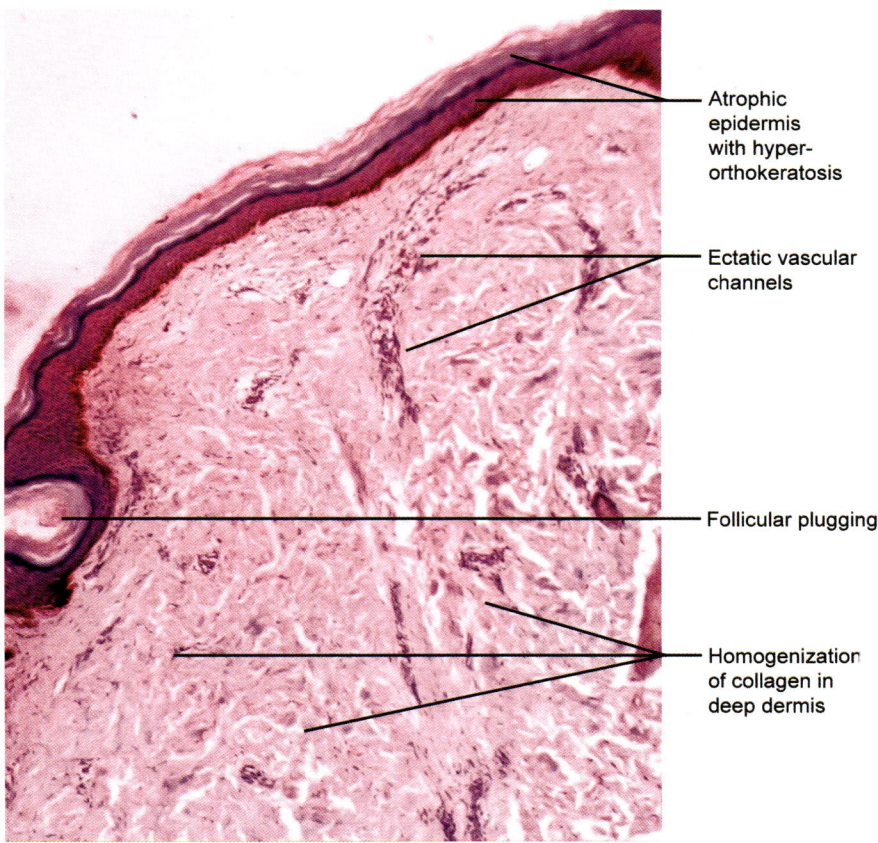

Atrophic epidermis with hyper- orthokeratosis

Ectatic vascular channels

Follicular plugging

Homogenization of collagen in deep dermis

Fig. 17.4: Lichen sclerosus

- Basal cell layer demonstrates epidermotropism of lymphocytes
- Superficial dermis shows edema, deep dermis shows homogenization of collagen
- Early lesions show lymphocytic infiltrate in the superficial dermis and as the lesions age, inflammatory cell infiltrate gets displaced into the deeper dermis

HISTOCHEMISTRY

- Van-Gieson stain shows decreased elastic fibers in the superficial dermis, and an increase in elastic fibers in mid to deep dermis

DIFFERENTIAL DIAGNOSIS

Lichen Planus

- Hyperkeratosis and wedge-shaped hypergranulosis
- Lichenoid infiltrate of lymphocytes
- Presence of Civatte/colloid bodies

Morphea

- Absence of hydropic degeneration of the basal cell layer
- Absence of edema of superficial dermis
- Dermal sclerosis with thickened collagen bundles

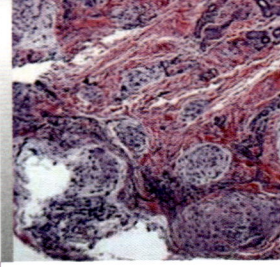

Lupus Erythematosus

- Multisystem autoimmune disorder, which can show involvement of skin
- Affects predominantly young women
- Can be broadly divided into chronic cutaneous, subacute, and systemic lupus erythematosus

CHRONIC CUTANEOUS LUPUS ERYTHEMATOSUS/ DISCOID LUPUS ERYTHEMATOSUS (DLE)

- Well demarcated, erythematous, scaly plaques
- Sites—most commonly affects face (butterfly pattern), scalp, oral cavity, lips

Histopathology (Figs 18.1 to 18.5)

- Hyperkeratotic stratum corneum with follicular plugging
- Atrophic epidermis with loss of rete ridges, hydropic degeneration of the basal layer (most significant finding), colloid bodies (scattered), hydropic change in basal layer of hair follicles
- Thickened basement membrane, which can be highlighted by PAS stain
- Dermis shows perivascular, perifollicular, periadnexal and interstitial dense lymphocytic infiltrate

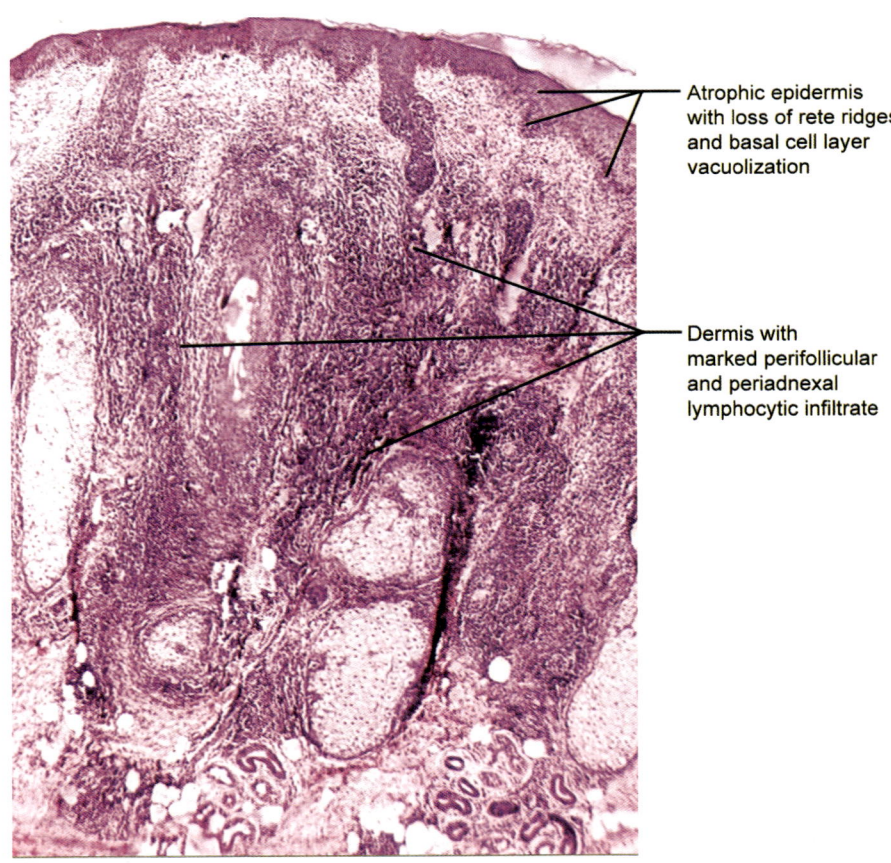

Atrophic epidermis with loss of rete ridges and basal cell layer vacuolization

Dermis with marked perifollicular and periadnexal lymphocytic infiltrate

Fig. 18.1: Discoid lupus erythematosus

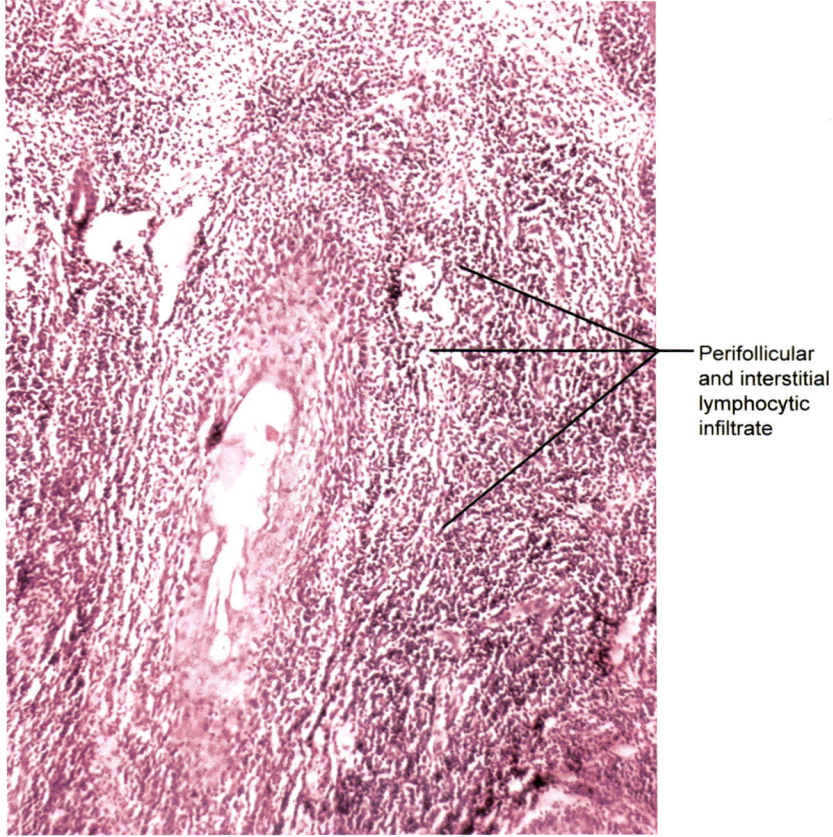

Perifollicular and interstitial lymphocytic infiltrate

Fig. 18.2: Discoid lupus erythematosus

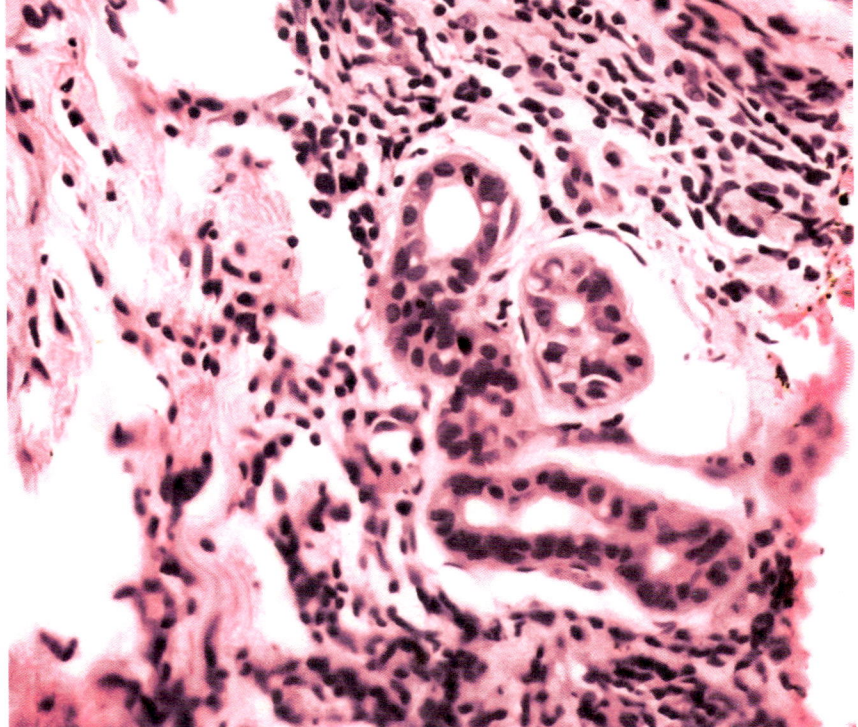

Fig. 18.3: Periadnexal lymphocytic infiltrate in DLE

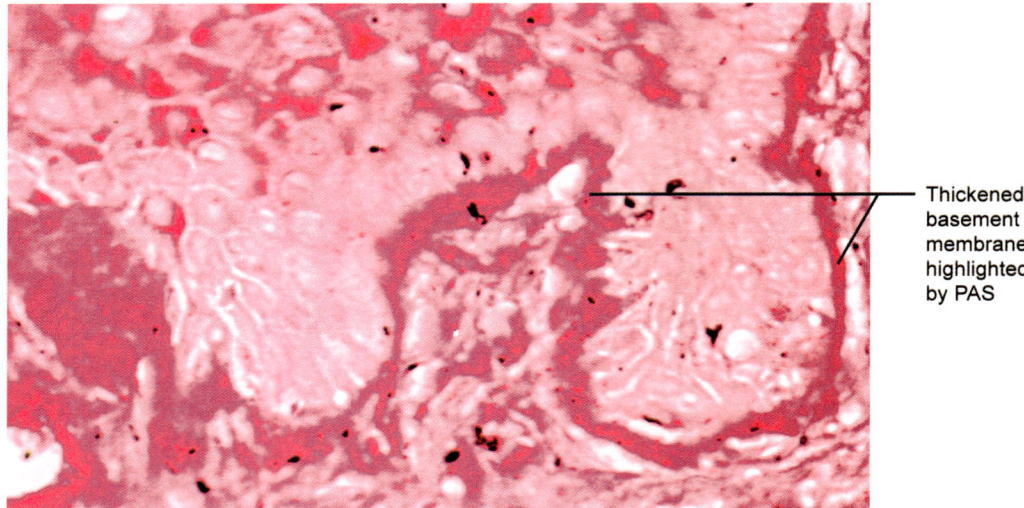

Fig. 18.4: Discoid lupus erythematosus (PAS stain)

Thickened basement membrane highlighted by PAS

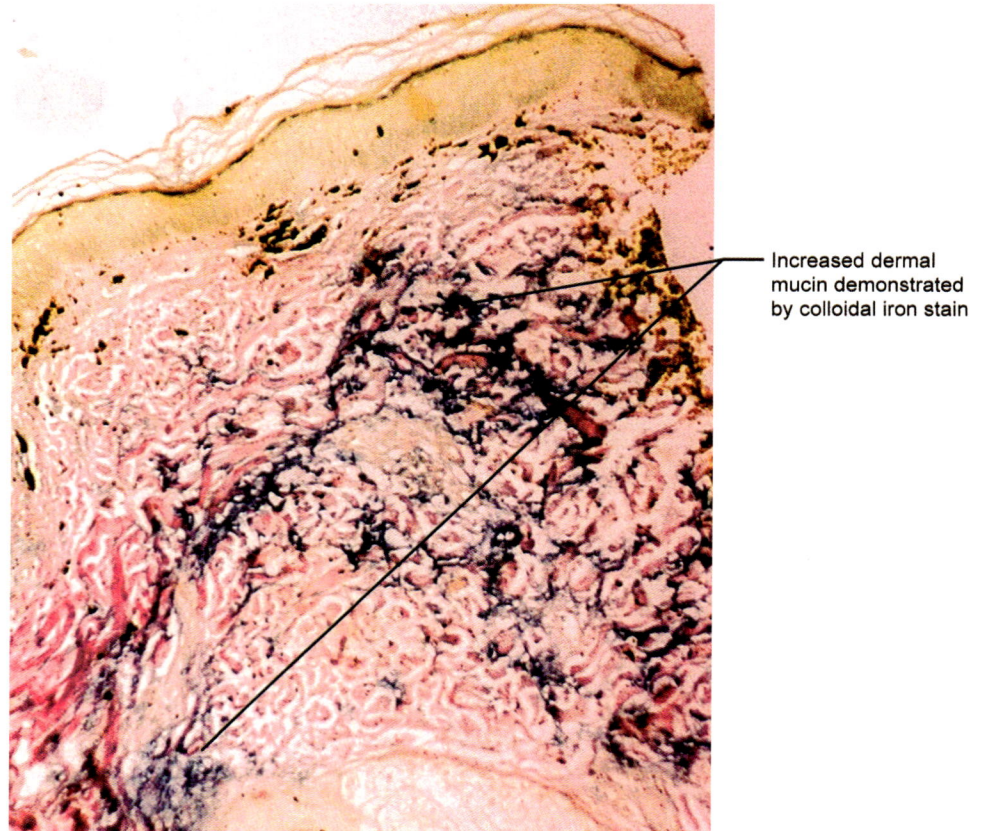

Fig. 18.5: Discoid lupus erythematosus

Increased dermal mucin demonstrated by colloidal iron stain

- Increased dermal mucin between collagen bundles, which can be highlighted by Alcian blue or colloidal iron
- Direct immunofluorescence—linear broad band of C3, IgG or IgM can be seen along the basement membrane zone

Differential Diagnosis

Lichen Planus

- Wedge-shaped hypergranulosis, saw toothed rete ridges, basal cell layer vacuolization
- Dense lichenoid infiltrate obscuring the dermo-epidermal junction

- Numerous civatte bodies in epidermis and/or colloid bodies in superficial dermis
- Absence of periadnexal and deep lymphocytic infiltrate
- Absence of dermal mucin

Lymphocytic Cutis

- Lymphocytic infiltrate forming lymphoid follicles
- Germinal centre formation can be seen
- Lymphocytes does not surround pilo-sebaceous units

Jessner's Lymphocytic Infiltrate of Skin

- Normal epidermis
- Dermis shows perivascular lympho-histiocytic infiltrate, which is also seen surrounding the adnexal structures (focally)
- Interface dermatitis and dermal mucin deposition are not seen

Polymorphous Light Eruption

- Epidermal spongiosis, basal cell layer vacuolization
- Superficial dermal edema
- Superficial perivascular lymphocytic infiltrate
- Lack of dermal mucin

Perniosis or Chilblains

- Acanthosis, hyperkeratosis, epidermal spongiosis
- Marked superficial dermal edema
- Superficial and deep perivascular dense lymphocytic infiltrate
- Fibrinoid change of the vessel wall can be seen

VERRUCOUS/HYPERTROPHIC LUPUS ERYTHEMATOSUS

- Hyperkeratotic scaly plaques (verrucous lesions) with an erythematous base
- Site: Face, arms, dorsum of hands
- Complication—can progress to squamous cell carcinoma

Histopathology

Lichen Planus Type

- Hyperkeratosis, hypergranulosis, acanthosis and papillomatosis
- Lichenoid infiltrate, basement membrane thickening, interstitial mucin deposition
- Perivascular and peri-adnexal lymphocytic infiltrate

Keratoacanthoma Type

- Cup-shaped keratin-filled crater
- Acanthotic epidermis with elongated rete ridges
- Scant mononuclear infiltrate

TUMID LUPUS ERYTHEMATOSUS

- Patient presents as papules, plaques and nodules without erythema or scaling
- Sites—sun-exposed areas, predominantly face and upper body

Histopathology

- Absence of interface dermatitis
- Superficial and deep perivascular and periadnexal lymphocytic infiltrate
- Increased dermal mucin

LUPUS ERYTHEMATOSUS PROFUNDUS OR LUPUS PANNICULITIS

- Presents as multiple, discrete, firm nodules
- Sites—upper extremities and/or upper trunk

Histopathology

- Dermal—sub-cutis interface shows dense lympho-histiocytic infiltrate, which extends deeper into the fat lobules
- Lymphoid follicles with germinal center formation can be seen
- Chronic lesions demonstrate paucity of inflammatory cells with hyalinization of fat lobules
- Stromal mucin can be demonstrated in well-developed lesions

SUB-ACUTE CUTANEOUS LUPUS ERYTHEMATOSUS/ NEONATAL LUPUS ERYTHEMATOSUS

- Presents as symmetrical, erythematous papules or annular lesions
- Sites—upper trunk, face, arms

Histopathology

- Atrophic epidermis
- Vacuolar change of basal cell layer
- Colloid bodies (civatte bodies) in epidermis (most commonly in lower epidermis and papillary dermis)
- Dermis shows edema, increased mucin and focal extravasation of erythrocytes

SYSTEMIC LUPUS ERYTHEMATOSUS (SLE)

Introduction

- 20% of SLE patients present with cutaneous features
- Most common presentation—erythematous malar rash

Histopathology (Figs 18.6 to 18.8)

- Hydropic change of the basal cell layer
- Dermis shows edema, erythrocyte extravasation and fibrinoid deposits

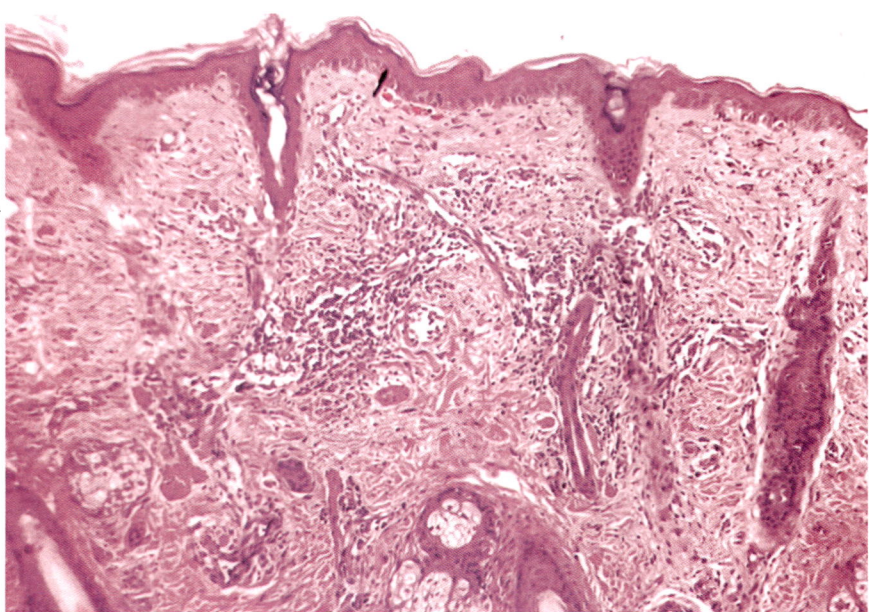

Fig. 18.6: Systemic lupus erythematosus. Dermis shows edema, perivascular lymphocytic infiltrate and fibrinoid material deposits in their vessel walls

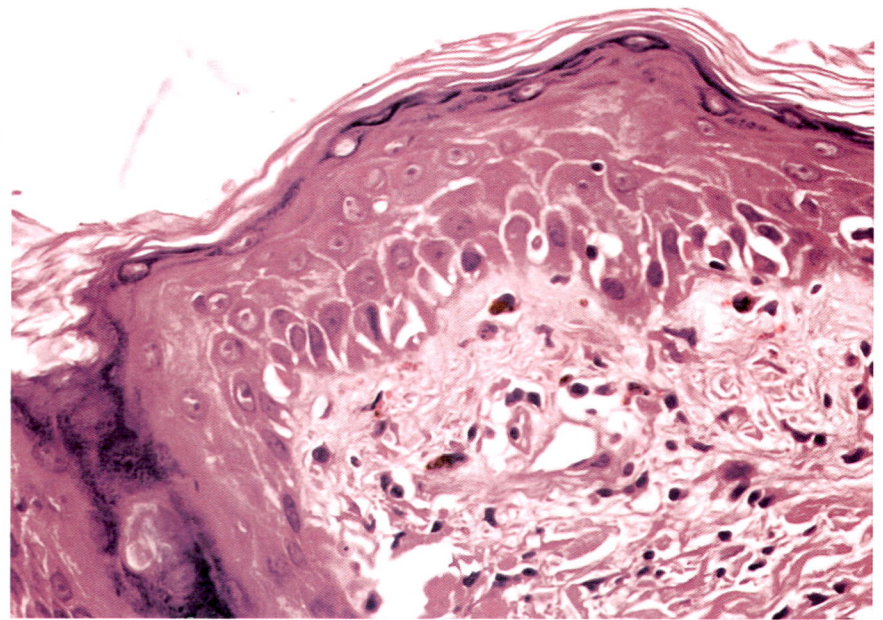

Fig. 18.7: Hydropic change of the basal cell layer in systemic lupus erythematosus

- Fibrinoid deposits are granular, eosinophilic PAS positive deposits, which can be seen within the papillary dermis, basement membrane (can result in thickening of basement membrane zone), collagen bundles, dermal vessel walls

Variant of SLE

Bullous SLE: Can show two patterns

Neutrophilic

- Sub-epidermal blister with neutrophils as its contents, papillary dermal neutrophilic aggregates and edema

Mononuclear

- Sub-epidermal blister with mononuclear cells as its contents

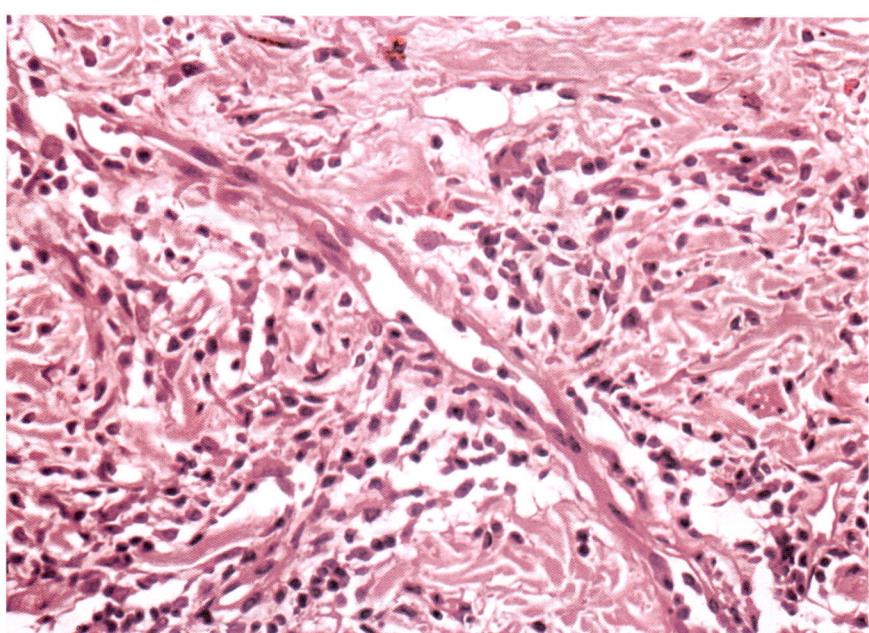

Fig. 18.8: Systemic lupus erythematosus. Perivascular lymphocytic and plasmacytic infiltrate is seen. Vessel wall demonstrates fibrinoid material deposits throughout its circumference

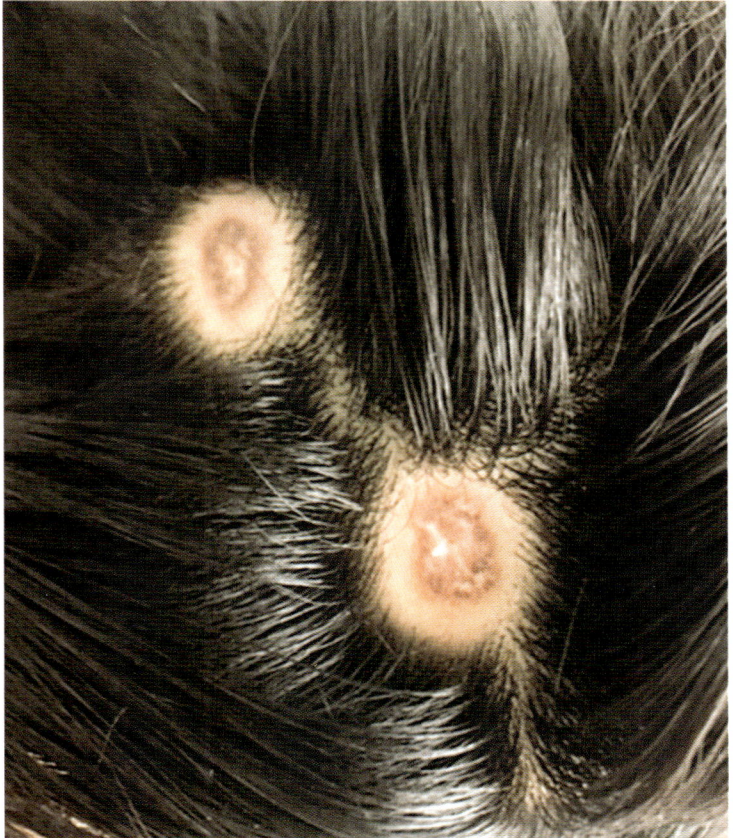

Fig. 18.9: Lupus erythematosus of scalp. Discrete, indurated plaques covered by adherent scale. Healed plaques have central depressed scars with areas of hyperpigmentation

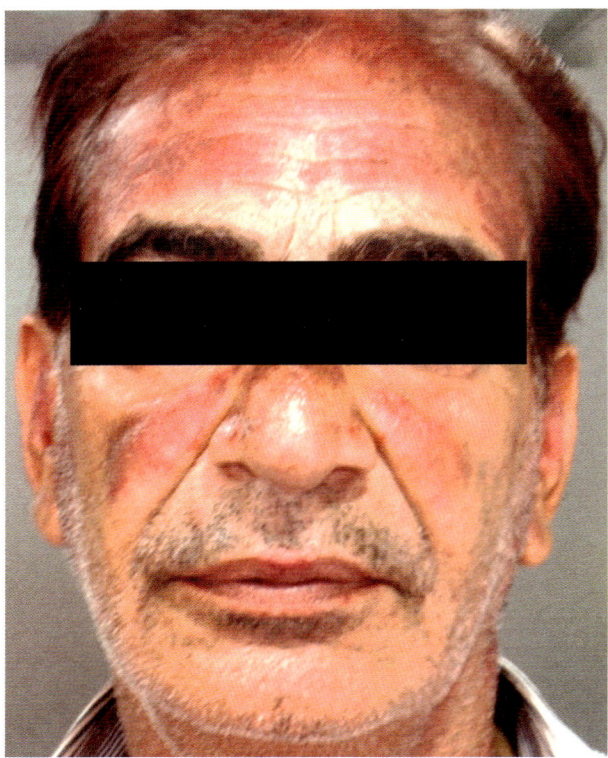

Fig. 18.10: Lupus erythematosus. Erythema in malar distribution with sparing of nasolabial folds

- Perivascular and peri-appendageal lymphocytic infiltrate

CLINICAL ASPECTS OF SLE

For diagnosis of SLE, four of the following eleven criteria should be met (Figs 18.9 and 18.10)

- Malar rash
- Discoid rash
- Photosensitivity
- Oral ulcers
- Nonerosive arthritis
- Pleuritis or pericarditis
- Renal disorder—proteinuria > 0.5 g/day
- Neurological disorder—seizures or psychosis
- Hematologic disorder—hemolytic anemia or leukopenia or lymphocytopenia or thrombocytopenia
- Immunologic disorder—positive anti-dsDNA antibody or anti-Sm antibody or anti-phospholipid antibodies (anti-cardiolipin antibodies)
- Antinuclear antibody (ANA)

Immunofluorescence Studies

- Immunoglobulins and C3 deposits are seen at the dermo-epidermal junction

Lupus Band Test

- Linear homogeneous band of immunoglobulin or complement deposited at the dermo-epidermal junction
- IgM is most commonly deposited (IgG being most specific)

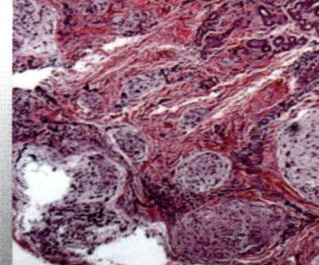

Pigmented Purpuric Dermatoses

INTRODUCTION

- Presents as red brown, pigmented, purpuric lesions
- Age group—third to sixth decade
- More common in males
- Site—bilateral lower extremities
- Associated with hyperlipidemia

VARIANTS

- Schamberg's disease (small, red macules distributed in pre-tibial region)
- Majocchi disease (annular lesions) (Fig. 19.1)
- Gougerot-Blum disease (lichenoid papules, plaques and macules)
- Eczematoid form (papules, scaling and lichenification)
- Granulomatous variant (rare)

HISTOPATHOLOGY (Figs 19.2 and 19.3)

- Epidermis shows variable parakeratosis, slight acanthosis, spongiosis and basal cell layer vacuolization (spongiosis is seen in eczematoid form)
- Perivascular and/or lichenoid lymphocytic infiltrate limited to the dermis (dense band-like infiltrate is seen in Gougerot-Blum disease)
- Extravasated red blood cells and hemosiderin deposits surrounding the capillaries

DIFFERENTIAL DIAGNOSIS

Fixed Drug Reaction

- Epidermal spongiosis with orthokeratosis
- Interface dermatitis with lymphocytic infiltrate along the dermoepidermal junction

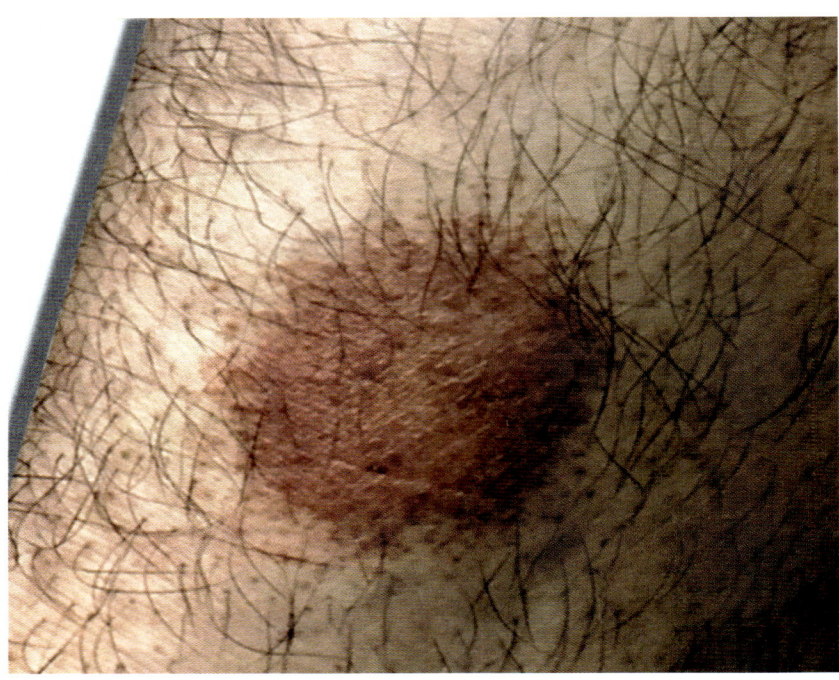

Fig. 19.1: Pigmented purpuric dermatoses (Majocchi's disease/purpura annularis telangiectoides). Nonblanchable, annular, purpuric, telangiectatic patches

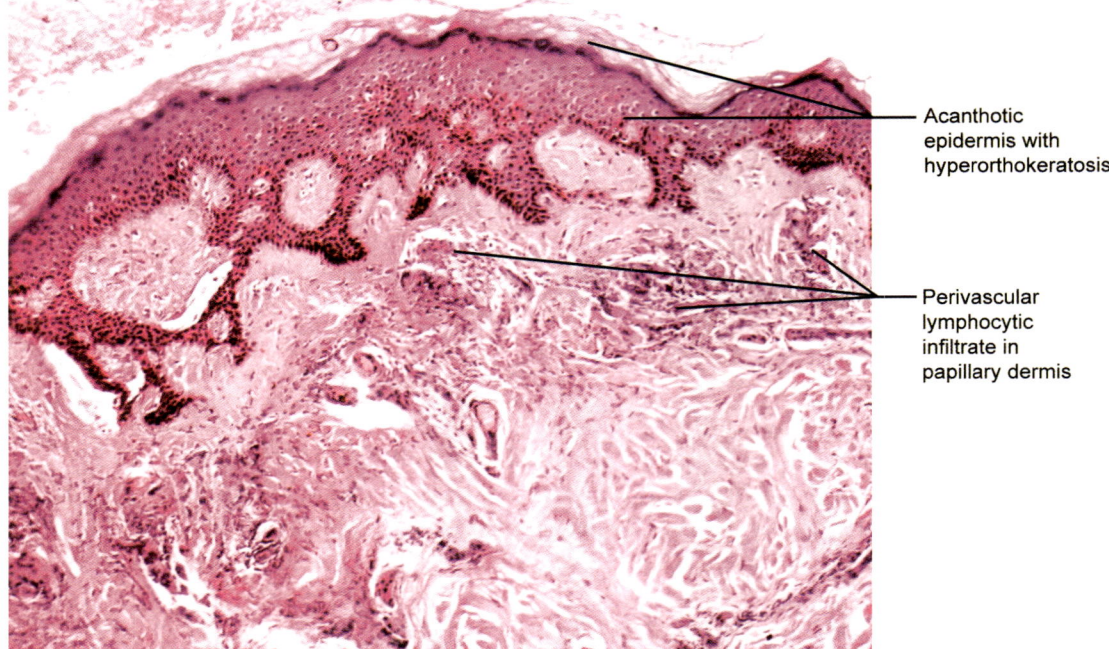

Acanthotic epidermis with hyperorthokeratosis

Perivascular lymphocytic infiltrate in papillary dermis

Fig. 19.2: Pigmented purpuric dermatosis

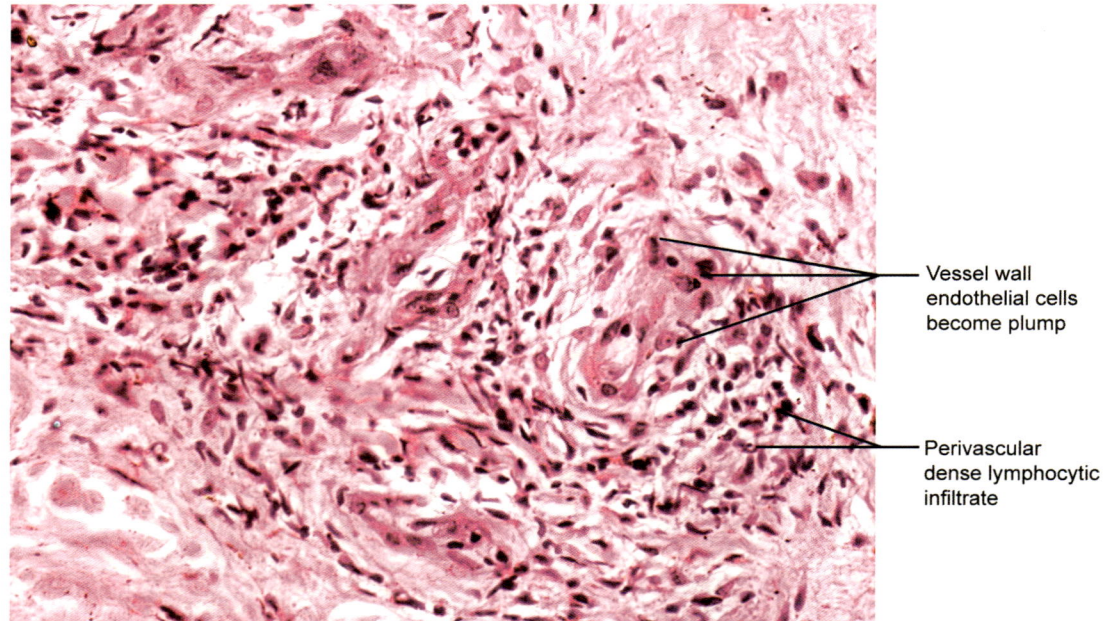

Vessel wall endothelial cells become plump

Perivascular dense lymphocytic infiltrate

Fig. 19.3: Pigmented purpuric dermatosis

- Basal cell layer vacuolization with keratinocyte necrosis
- Perivascular lymphocytic and eosinophilic infiltrate

Acute Graft-vs-Host Reaction
- Interface dermatitis and apoptosis of keratinocytes
- Vacuolar degeneration along the dermal-epidermal junction

- Absence of erythrocyte exocytosis or hemosiderin deposits

Mycosis Fungoides
- Atypical lymphocytes along the dermoepidermal junction (epidermotropism)
- Absence of papillary dermal edema and fibrosis

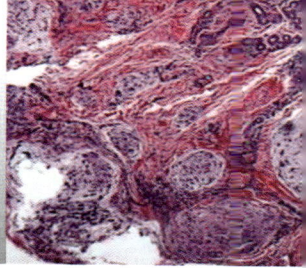

Inflammatory Linear Verrucous Epidermal Nevus (ILVEN)

INTRODUCTION

- Linear, pruritic, erythematous scaly lesion present along the lines of Blaschko
- Site—most commonly affects lower extremities
- Age group—affects infants and children
- Affects females more than males

HISTOPATHOLOGY (Fig. 20.1)

- Acanthosis, hyperkeratosis with alternating orthokeratosis and parakeratosis
- Thickened rete ridges with a psoriasiform appearance

- Absence of granular layer underneath the area of parakeratosis and thickened granular layer underneath the area of orthokeratosis
- Mild spongiosis and lymphocytic exocytosis underneath the area of parakeratosis
- Superficial dermis show mild perivascular lymphocytic infiltrate

DIFFERENTIAL DIAGNOSIS

Lichen Striatus

- Lichenoid infiltrate
- Absence of psoriasiform hyperplasia

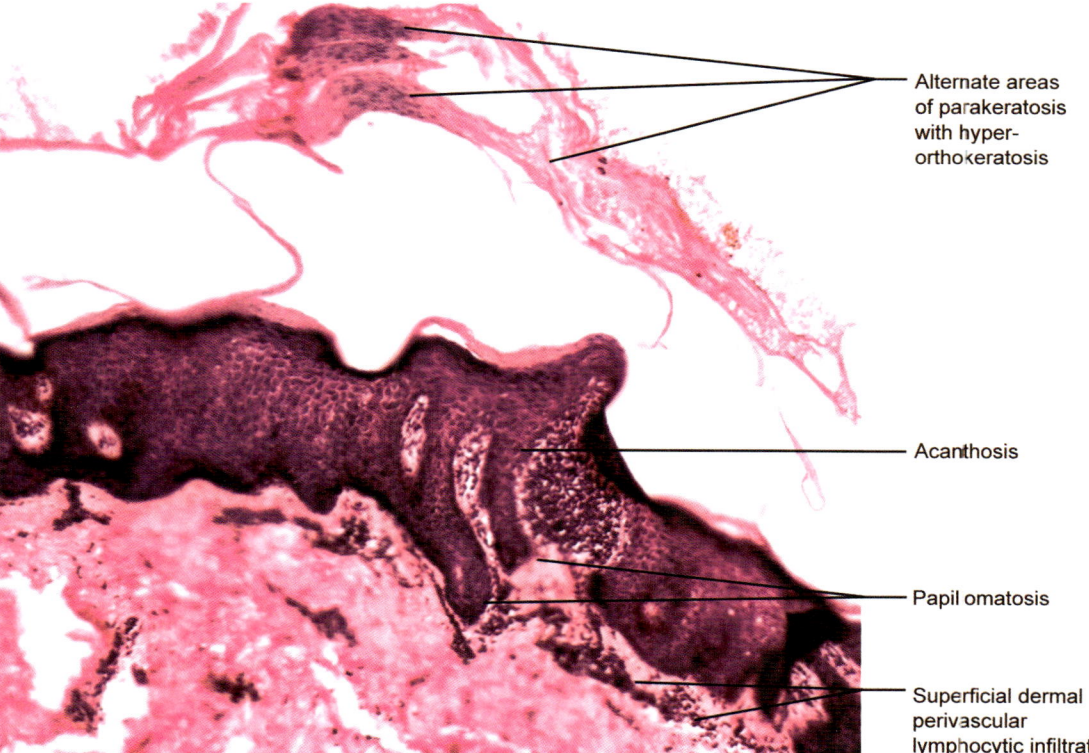

Alternate areas of parakeratosis with hyper-orthokeratosis

Acanthosis

Papillomatosis

Superficial dermal perivascular lymphocytic infiltrate

Fig. 20.1: Inflammatory linear verrucous epidermal nevus

Linear Psoriasis

- Confluent parakeratosis with decreased or absent granular layer
- Psoriasiform hyperplasia with elongation of rete ridges
- Munro's microabscesses
- Involucrin expression is absent in the parakeratotic areas of ILVEN, but is detectable in psoriasis

Epidermal Nevus

- Hyperkeratosis with orthokeratosis
- Elongated rete ridges without psoriasiform hyperplasia
- Absence of alternating parakeratosis and hyper-orthokeratosis

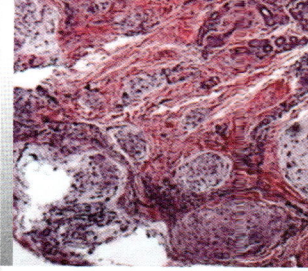

Vesicobullous Disorders

PEMPHIGUS

INTRODUCTION

- Age: Fourth to sixth decade
- Autoimmune disorder, with resultant blisters on skin and mucous membranes
- Etiology—autoantibodies against keratinocyte adhesion antigens result in acantholysis
- **Nikolsky sign:** Slight friction induces new blisters
- **Asboe-Hansen sign:** Gentle pressure can result in lateral extension of intact blister

TYPES OF PEMPHIGUS

Pemphigus Vulgaris

- Most common form of pemphigus
- Autoimmune basis—IgG autoantibodies directed against desmoglein 3 and 1
- Presents with cutaneous and mucosal erosions, can involve oral cavity
- Present as flaccid blisters (Fig. 21.1)
- Associated with other autoimmune disorders like SLE

Histopathology (Figs 21.2 to 21.4)

- Early blister should be sampled
- Eosinophilic spongiosis of the lower epidermis
- Acantholysis (loss of adhesion between keratinocytes) with formation of suprabasal cleft
- Basal keratinocytes remain attached to the basement membrane giving it a "row of tombstone appearance"
- Blister cavity contains acantholytic cells, neutrophils and eosinophils

Direct Immunofluorescence (DIF) (Fig. 21.5)

- Should always be performed on the perilesional skin
- IgG deposits in the intercellular areas of epidermis

Indirect Immunofluorescence

- Detects auto-antibodies against desmoglein-3

Differential Diagnosis

1. ***Hailey-Hailey disease***
   - Site of involvement—neck, axillae, genitals, perianal regions (Figs 21.6 and 21.7)

   Histopathology (Figs 21.8 and 21.9)
   - Suprabasal cleft
   - Full epidermal thickness acantholysis with acantholytic cells retaining some connections giving it an appearance of "dilapidated brick wall"
   - Adnexal structures are not involved
   - Direct immunofluorescence is negative

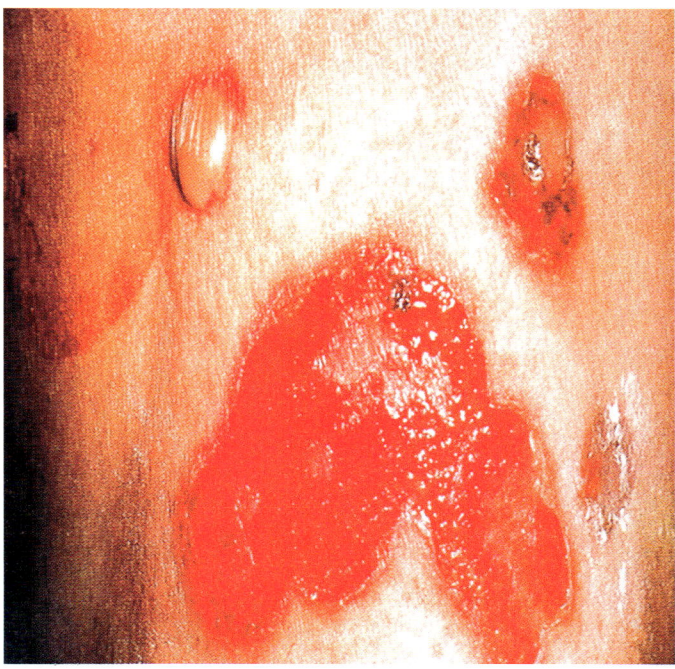

Fig. 21.1: Pemphigus vulgaris. Erosions and bullae over the shin

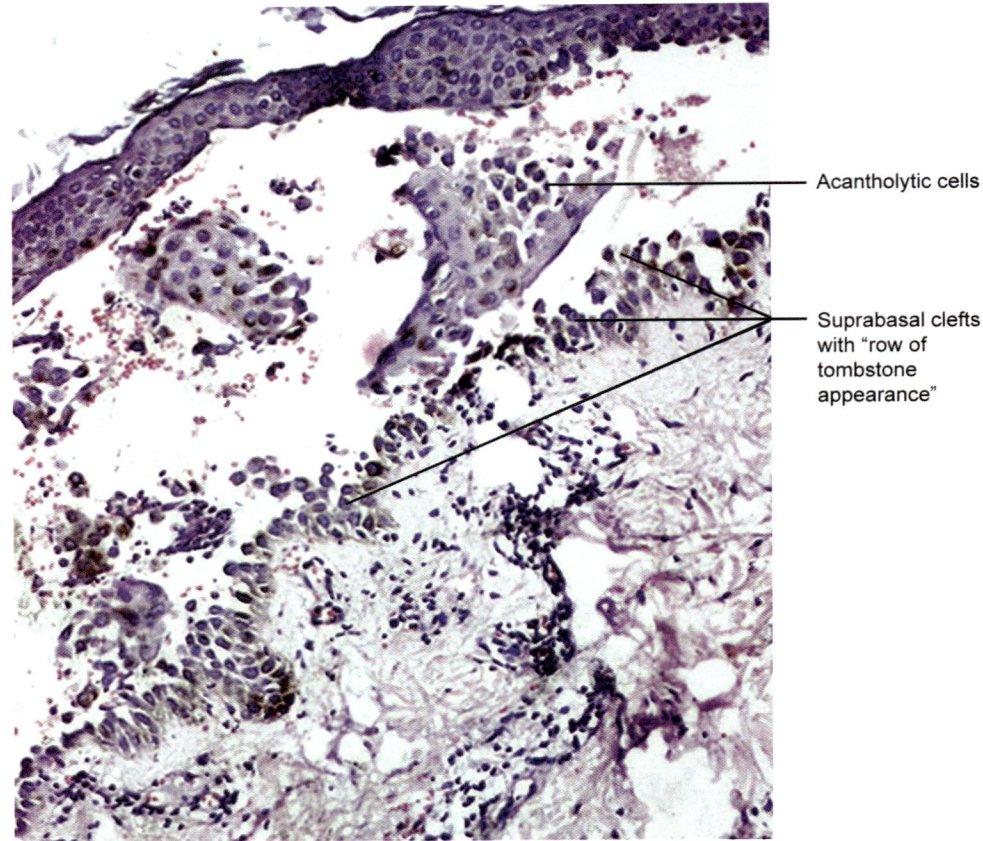

Fig. 21.2: Pemphigus vulgaris

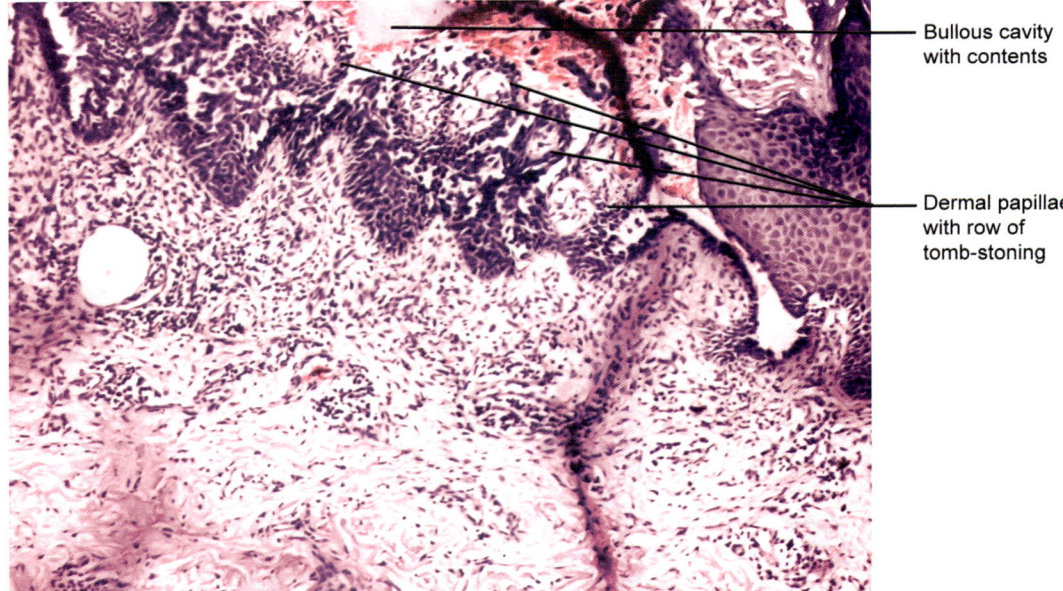

Fig. 21.3: Pemphigus vulgaris

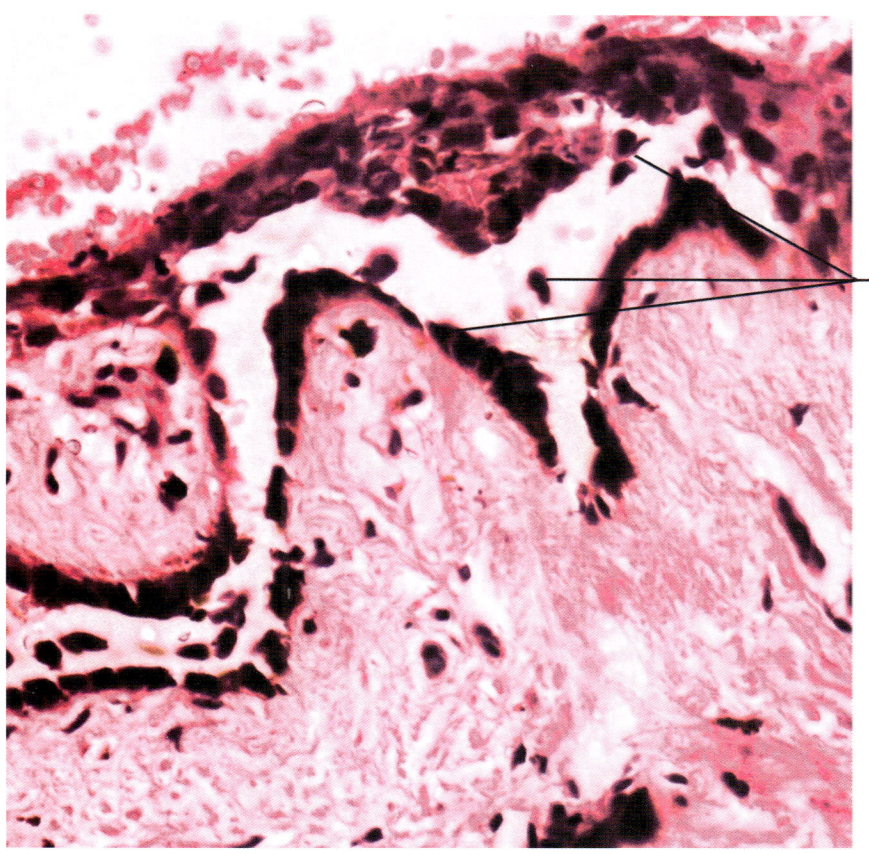

Fig. 21.4: Pemphigus vulgaris

Suprabasal
cleft with
acantholytic cells

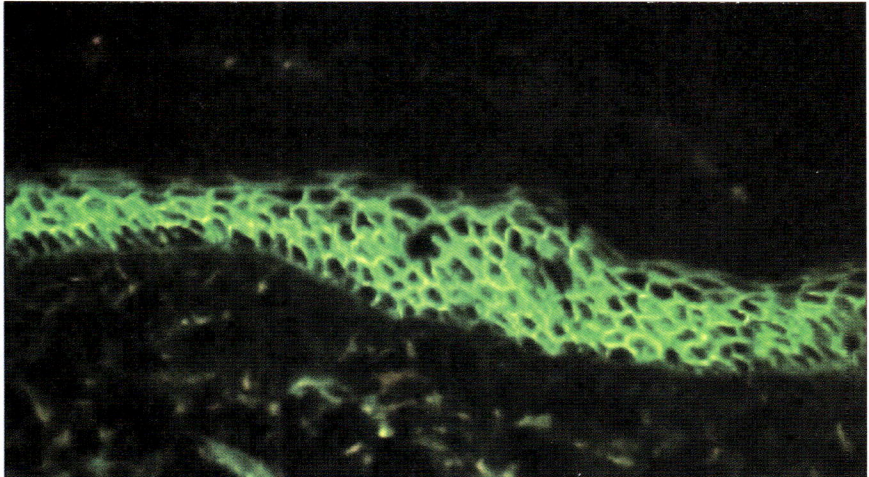

Fig. 21.5: DIF: Intercellular staining/fish net appearance in pemphigus

2. *Darier's disease*
   – Affects seborrheic areas of head, neck and trunk (Fig. 21.10)
   – Lesions appear as greasy, yellow to brown papules

Histopathology (Fig. 21.11)
   – Suprabasal acantholysis with papillary dermis extending into the cleft as villi
   – Dyskeratotic keratinocytes in form of corps ronds (in stratum granulosum and spinosum) and grains of Darier (in horny layers)

3. *Transient acantholytic dermatosis (Grover's disease)*
   – Presents as erythematous papulovesicular lesions
   – Site – trunk

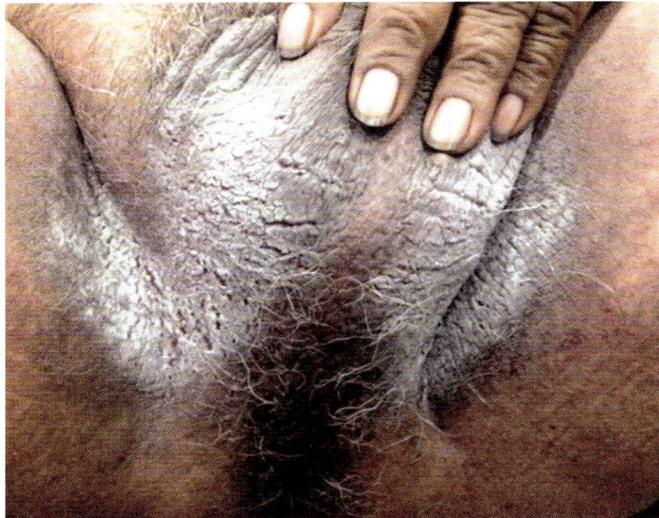

Fig. 21.6: Hailey-Hailey disease. Large, macerated, exudative plaques with crusting

Histopathology
- Suprabasal acantholysis (focal)
- Can present as Darier-like or Hailey-Hailey like or pemphigus vulgaris like pattern

Pemphigus Foliaceus

- Presents as flaccid bullae on an erythematous base
- Most common sites include head, neck and trunk

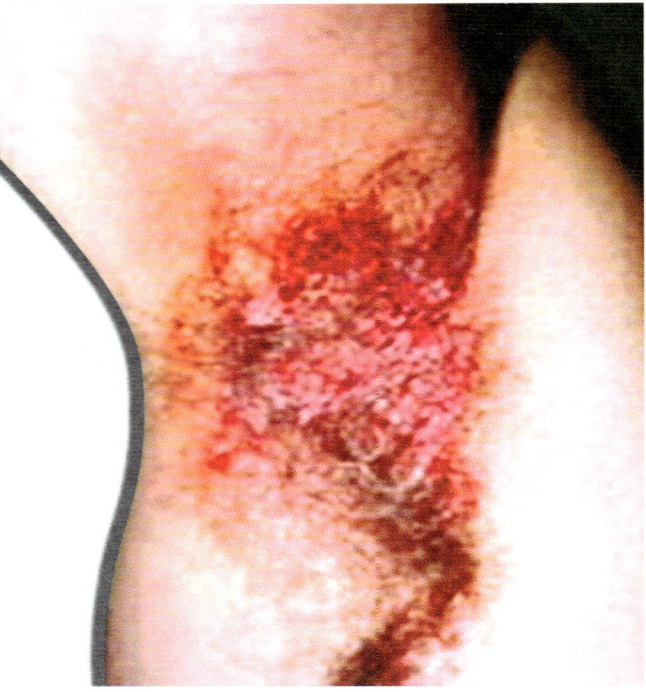

Fig. 21.7: Hailey-Hailey disease. Crusted, eroded plaque in the axilla

- Oral mucosal involvement is not seen
- Autoantibodies directed against desmoglein-1 are seen

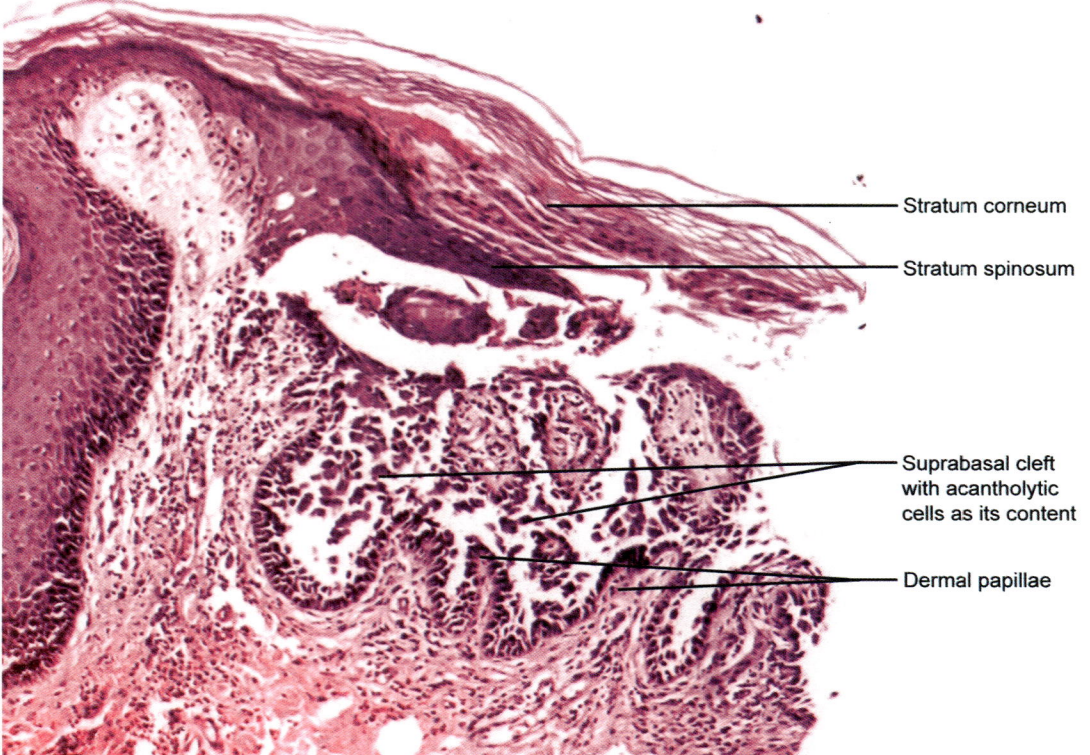

Stratum corneum

Stratum spinosum

Suprabasal cleft with acantholytic cells as its content

Dermal papillae

Fig. 21.8: Hailey-Hailey disease

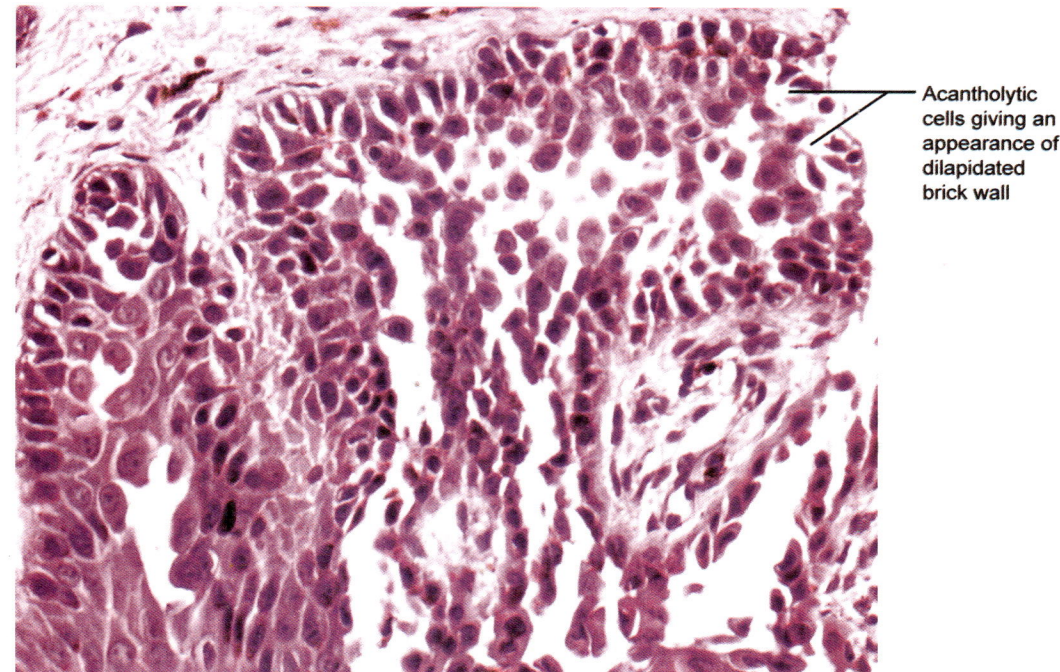

Acantholytic cells giving an appearance of dilapidated brick wall

Fig. 21.9: Hailey-Hailey disease

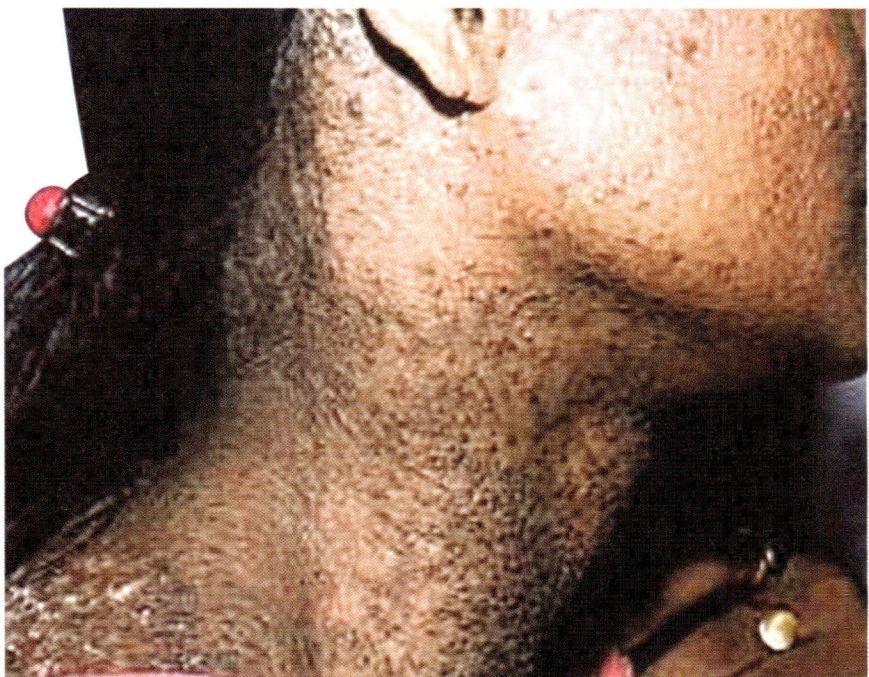

Fig. 21.10: Darier's disease. Dark crusty keratotic papules

- Fogo selvagem—endemic form of pemphigus foliaceus, that affects children and young adults
- Association with other autoimmune disorders and drugs like Penicillamine are seen

Histopathology (Figs 21.12 and 21.13)

- Sub-corneal bullae with separation of stratum corneum and granular layer
- Sub-corneal blister can show acantholytic or dyskeratotic keratinocytes

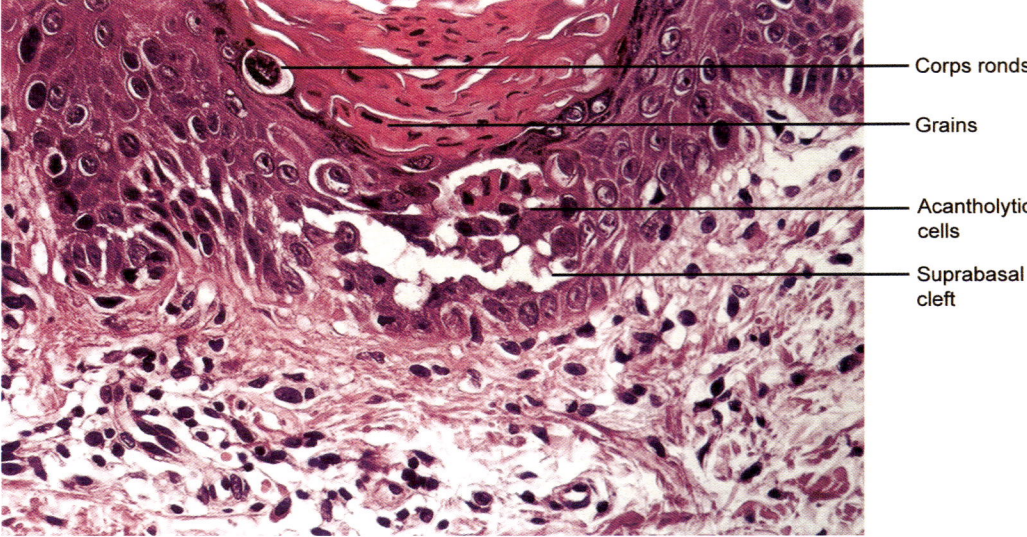

- Corps ronds
- Grains
- Acantholytic cells
- Suprabasal cleft

Fig. 21.11: Darier's disease

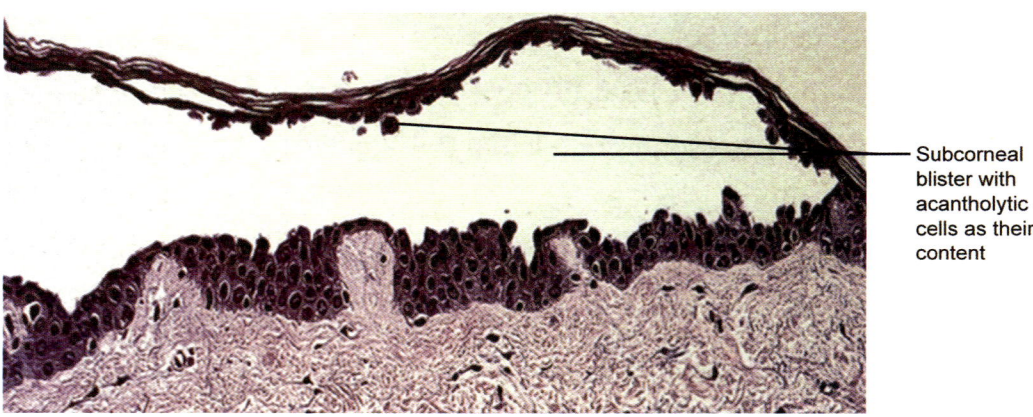

- Subcorneal blister with acantholytic cells as their content

Fig. 21.12: Pemphigus foliaceus

- Blister cavity can show neutrophils as their contents

Direct Immunofluorescence (DIF)

- IgG deposits in squamous intercellular space, more pronounced in the upper epidermis

Indirect Immunofluorescence

- Autoantibodies directed against desmoglein-1

Differential diagnosis

1. *Staphylococcal scalded skin syndrome and Impetigo*
   - Immunofluorescence will help in confirming the diagnosis of pemphigus foliaceus
   - Increased acantholytic cells are seen in pemphigus foliaceus

2. *Subcorneal pustular dermatosis*
   - Produces dome-shaped subcorneal pustules
   - Bullae cavity shows sparse number of neutrophils

Pemphigus Vegetans

- Present as a verrucous plaque
- Sites—intertriginous and flexural areas

Histopathology

- Marked acanthosis, eosinophilic spongiosis with pseudoepitheliomatous hyperplasia
- Suprabasal cleft
- Contents of cleft—acantholytic cells, eosinophils (present as an eosinophilic abscess)

Direct Immunofluorescence

- IgG deposits in squamous intercellular space

Differential Diagnosis

Pyoderma Vegetans

- Intra-epithelial and sub-epithelial microabscesses containing neutrophils and eosinophils

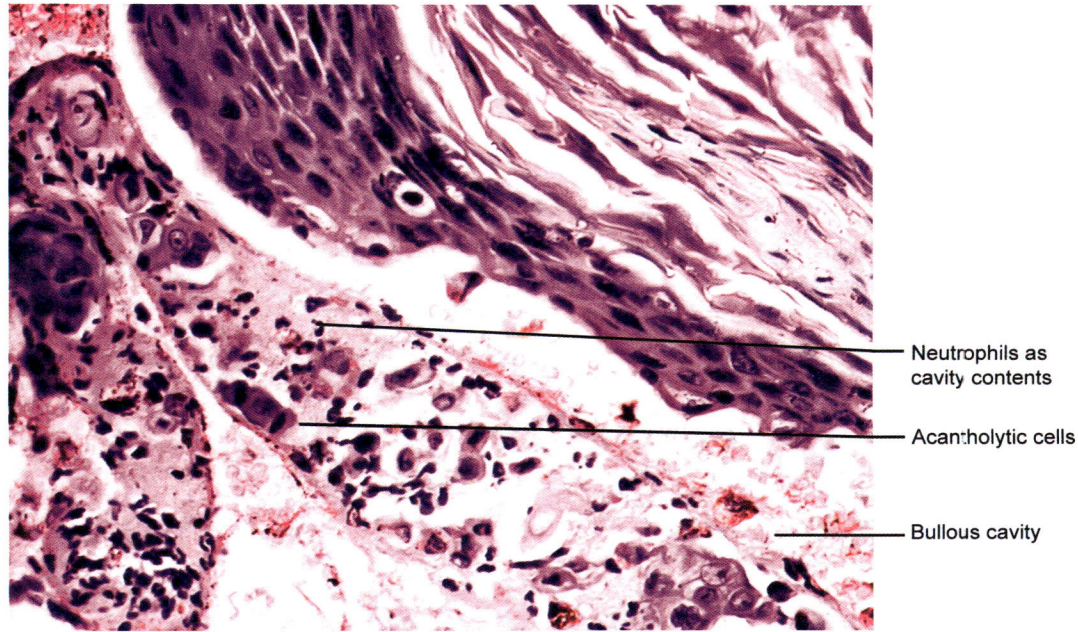

Neutrophils as
cavity contents

Acantholytic cells

Bullous cavity

Fig. 21.13: Pemphigus foliaceus with subcorneal bullae

- Focal acantholysis can be seen
- Direct immunofluorescence is negative

Paraneoplastic Pemphigus

- Associated with non-Hodgkin lymphoma, chronic lymphocytic leukemia, Castleman disease, thymoma
- Present as oropharyngeal ulceration and erosions
- Autoimmune basis—IgG autoantibodies against desmoplakins and desmogleins
- Poor prognosis

Histopathology

- Suprabasal blister with acantholytic cells and necrotic keratinocytes (pemphigus vulgaris like change)
- Basal cell vacuolar change with lichenoid lympho-cytic infiltrate (lichen planus like pattern)

Direct Immunofluorescence

- IgG deposits in squamous intercellular space and basement membrane

Indirect Immunofluorescence

- Autoantibodies directed against desmoglein 1, 3 and plakins

IgA pemphigus

- Presents as pruritic, flaccid pustules with an erythe-matous base
- Age group—affects middle age and elderly patients

- **Sites**—axilla, groin, trunk, proximal extremities, lower abdomen
- **Pathogenesis**—IgA auto-antibodies directed against desmocollin-1
- **Two types**—intraepidermal neutrophilic type and subcorneal pustular dermatosis type

Histopathology

- Intraepidermal neutrophilic type: Suprabasal pustule with neutrophils as its content
- Subcorneal pustular dermatosis type: Subcorneal pustule with neutrophils as its content

Direct Immunofluorescence

- IgA deposits in the squamous intercellular space

Indirect Immunofluorescence

- Autoantibodies directed against desmocollin-1, desmoglein-1 and 3

Pemphigus Erythematosus (PE)

- Presents as an erythematous plaque and patch
- Most commonly affects the malar area (lupus erythematosus like lesion)
- Can also present as erythematous, scaly crusted plaque over seborrheic areas like scalp, chest wall (Fig. 21.14)

Histopathology

- Resembles pemphigus foliaceus
- Subcorneal bullae with separation of stratum corneum and granular layer

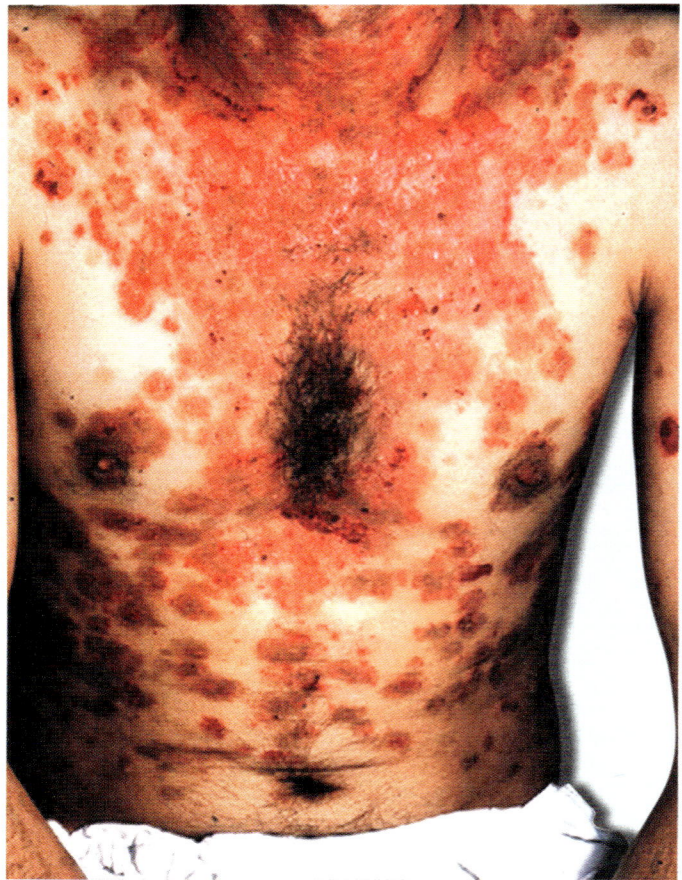

Fig. 21.14: Pemphigus erythematosus: Erythematous patches over the trunk

- Subcorneal blister can show acantholytic keratinocytes with neutrophils as their contents

Direct Immunofluorescence
- IgG deposits in the squamous intercellular space

Drug-induced Pemphigus
- Causative agents include drugs like penicillamine and captopril

Histopathology
- Sub-corneal acantholysis
- Eosinophilic spongiosis, parakeratosis
- Dermis shows eosinophils

BULLOUS PEMPHIGOID (BP)

INTRODUCTION
- Patient presents with large tense bullae
- Affects predominantly elderly individuals

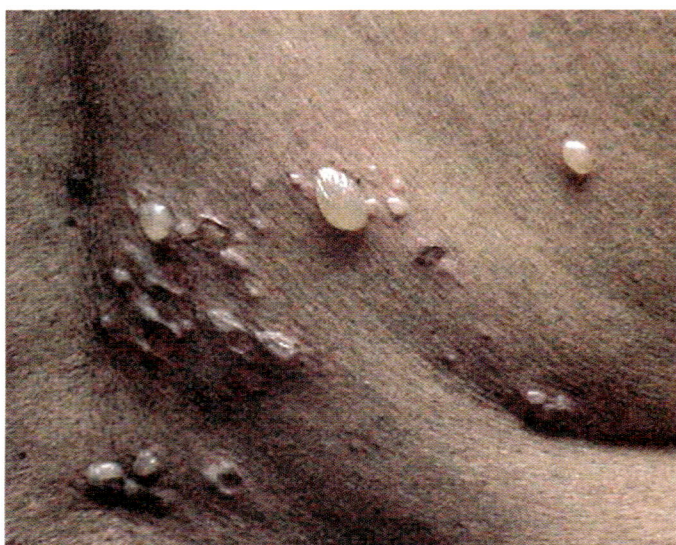

Fig. 21.15: Bullous pemphigoid. Tense bulla on an erythematous, non-inflammatory base. Eventually the bullae rupture, leaving moist erosions and crusts that resolve without scarring

- Pemphigoid antibodies are directed against BPAg-1 and BPAg-2 proteins
- Sites—trunk, extremities, intertriginous areas and oral mucosa (Fig. 21.15)

HISTOPATHOLOGY (Figs 21.16 and 21.17)

Pre-bullous Phase
- Eosinophilic spongiosis
- Presence of eosinophils around the dermoepidermal junction and in the dermis
- Dermal edema

Bullous-phase
- Cell poor bullous pemphigoid—sub-epidermal bulla with a few inflammatory cells as their contents
- Cell rich bullous pemphigoid—sub-epidermal bulla with eosinophils (dermal papillae eosinophilic microabscesses) and a few neutrophils as their contents
- Superficial and deep dermis show perivascular and interstitial eosinophilic, neutrophilic and lymphocytic infiltrate

IMMUNOFLUORESCENCE
- **Direct immunofluorescence (DIF)**—linear deposition of IgG and/or C3 at the dermoepidermal junction (DEJ) or basement membrane zone
- **Salt-split skin immunofluorescence**—IgG antibodies are present on the epidermal roof (blister roof)

DIFFERENTIAL DIAGNOSIS

Epidermolysis Bullosa Acquisita

- Subepidermal blister with sparse infiltrate of neutrophils, eosinophils and lymphocytes
- Direct Immunofluorescence—linear IgG deposits at dermoepidermal junction
- Salt-split skin immunofluorescence—IgG antibodies bind to the dermal floor
- Indirect immunofluorescence—shows antibodies in the serum against type VII collagen

Dermatitis Herpetiformis

- Subepidermal blister with dermal papillae containing neutrophilic microabscesses
- Direct immunofluorescence—IgA deposits in dermal papillae or dermo-epidermal junction

Porphyria Cutanea Tarda

- Subepidermal blister
- PAS positive hyaline material is seen in walls of the blood vessels in upper dermis

Bullous Systemic Lupus Erythematosus
(Figs 21.18 and 21.19)

- Epidermal necrolysis
- Subepidermal blister

- Blister cavity contains neutrophils and fibrinous material
- Neutrophilic abscesses in the papillary dermis
- Edema of upper dermis
- Direct immunofluorescence—linear or granular deposits of IgG and C3 at dermoepidermal junction

DERMATITIS HERPETIFORMIS

INTRODUCTION

- Autoimmune disorder, also called Duhring disease
- Associated with gluten-sensitive enteropathy, with an increased risk of lymphoma
- Patients show increased frequency of HLA-DQ-2 and DQ-8 positivity
- Presents as pruritic papulovesicular lesions (Fig. 21.20)
- Sites—symmetric involvement of elbows, knees, scalp, buttocks and scapula

LABORATORY TESTS

- IgA anti-endomysium and anti-tissue transglutaminase antibodies are detected in the serum of patients
  Site of the biopsy—early blister with perivesicular skin

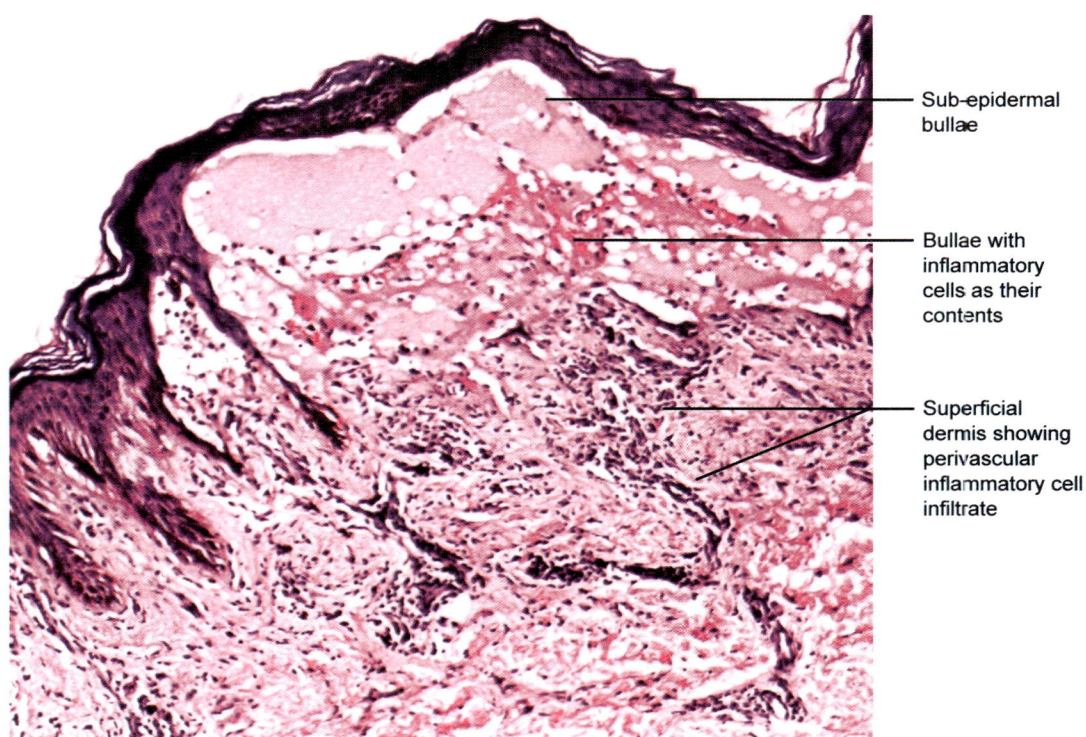

Sub-epidermal bullae

Bullae with inflammatory cells as their contents

Superficial dermis showing perivascular inflammatory cell infiltrate

Fig. 21.16: Bullous pemphigoid

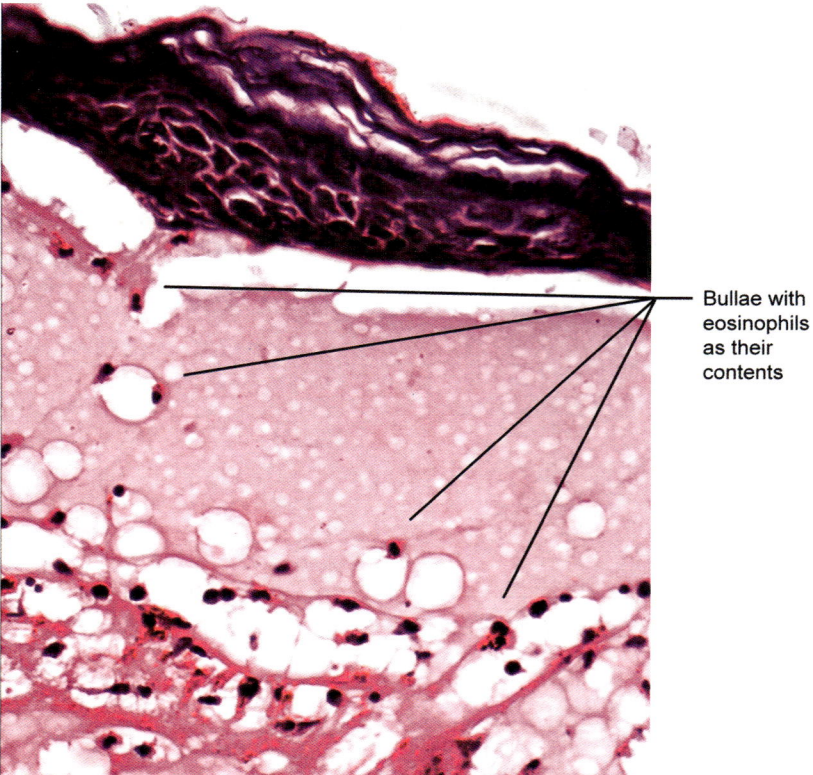

Bullae with eosinophils as their contents

Fig. 21.17: Bullous pemphigoid

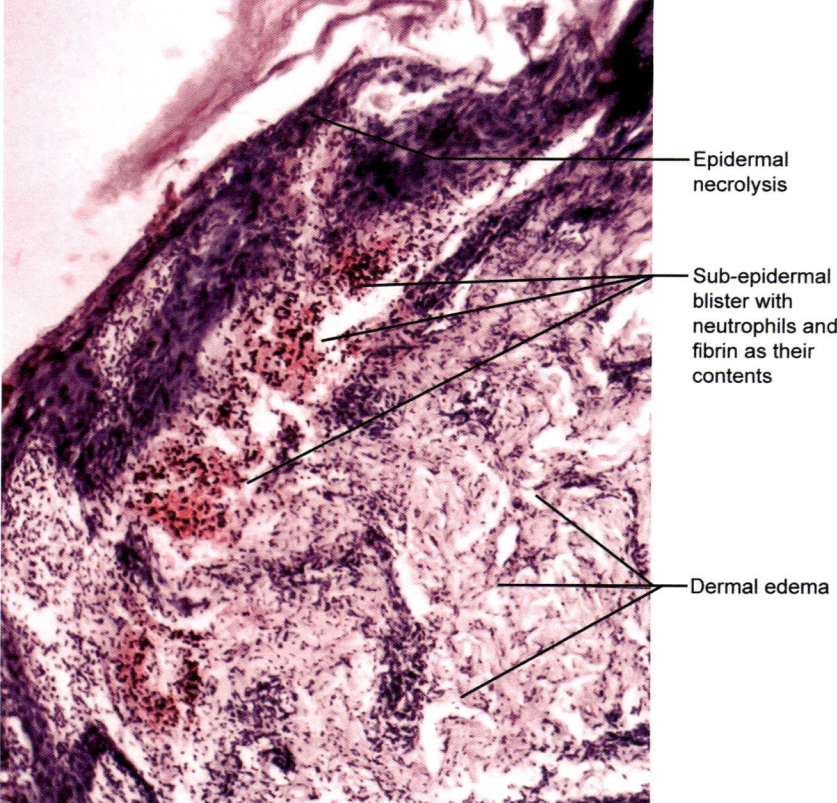

Epidermal necrolysis

Sub-epidermal blister with neutrophils and fibrin as their contents

Dermal edema

Fig. 21.18: Bullous SLE

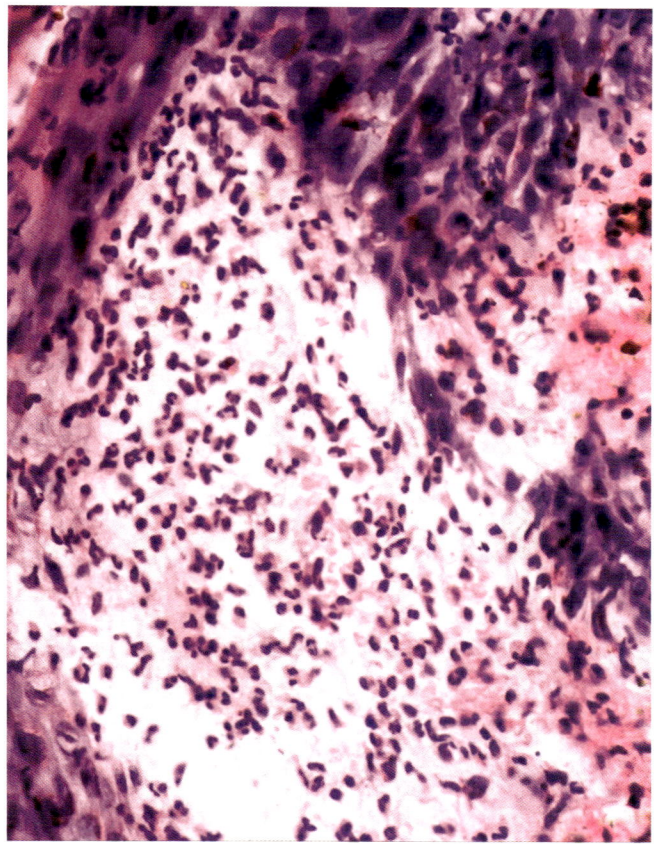

Fig. 21.19: Bullous SLE. Papillary dermal neutrophilic micro-abscesses

HISTOPATHOLOGY (Fig. 21.21)

- Subepidermal blister with numerous neutrophils
- Dermal papillary microabscesses

- Superficial perivascular mixed inflammatory cell infiltrate

DIRECT IMMUNOFLUORESCENCE

- Granular IgA deposits along the dermoepidermal junction and in papillary dermis

DIFFERENTIAL DIAGNOSIS

Bullous Pemphigoid

- Subepidermal bullae with eosinophils and neutrophils as its contents
- Direct immunofluorescence—linear deposition of IgG and/or C3 at the dermo-epidermal junction (DEJ) or basement membrane zone

Linear IgA Dermatosis (Fig. 21.22)

- Subepidermal blister with neutrophils as their contents
- Direct immunofluorescence—IgA in linear pattern along the basement membrane zone

Bullous Lupus Erythematosus

- Subepidermal blister with neutrophils
- Direct immunofluorescence—linear or granular deposition of C3 or IgG at dermoepidermal junction

Epidermolysis Bullosa Acquisita

- Subepidermal blister with sparse infiltrate of neutrophils, eosinophils and lymphocytes
- Direct immunofluorescence—linear IgG deposits at dermoepidermal junction
- Indirect immunofluorescence—shows antibodies in serum against type VII collagen

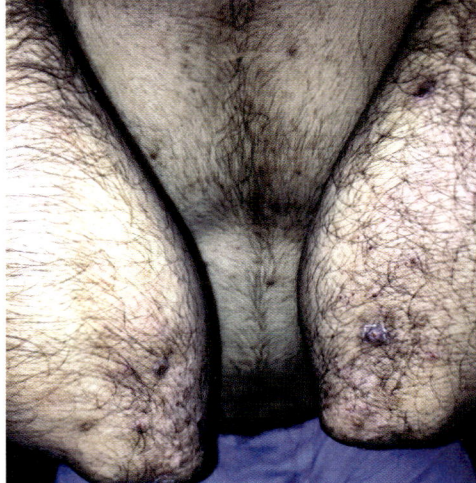
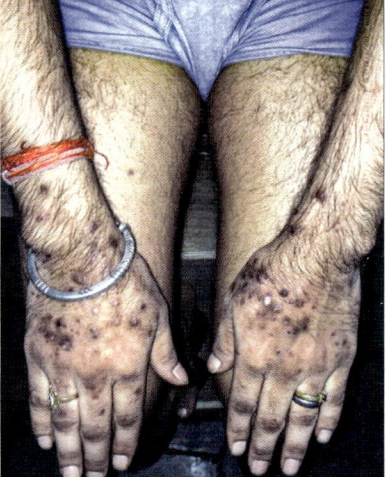

Fig. 21.20: Dermatitis herpetiformis. Multiple intensely pruritic papules and vesicles that occur in groups ("herpetiform arrangement")

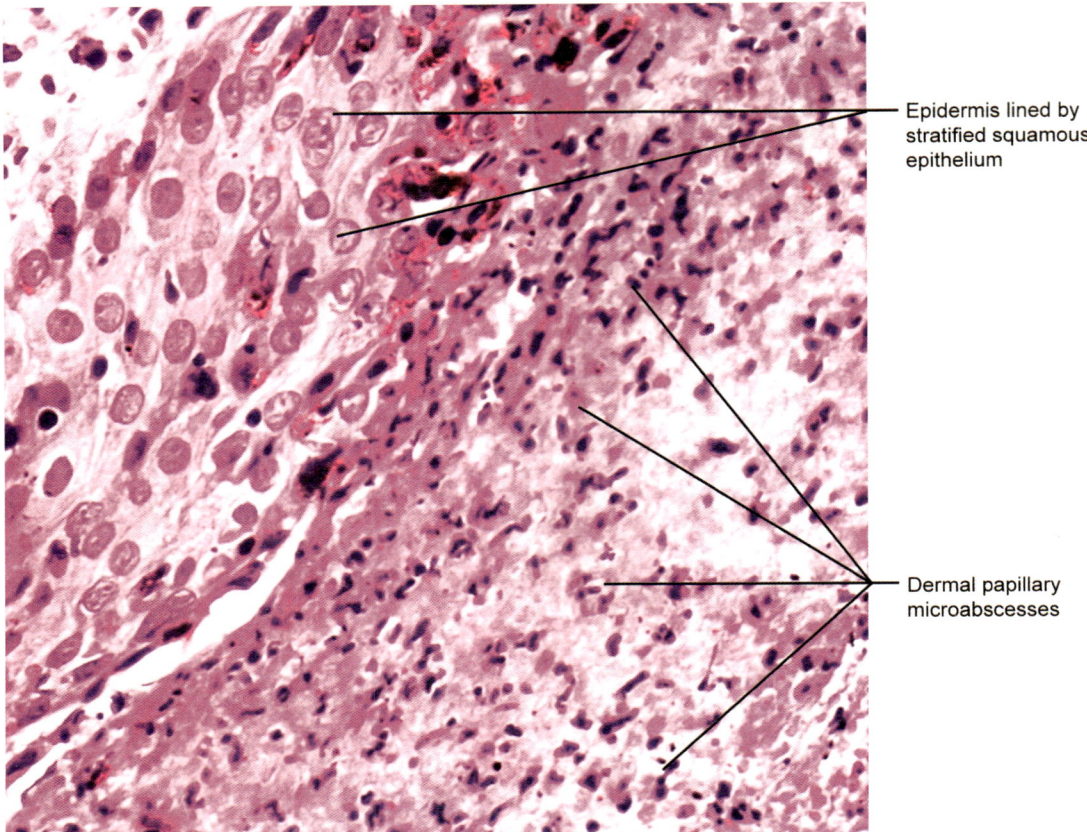

Epidermis lined by stratified squamous epithelium

Dermal papillary microabscesses

Fig. 21.21: Dermatitis herpetiformis

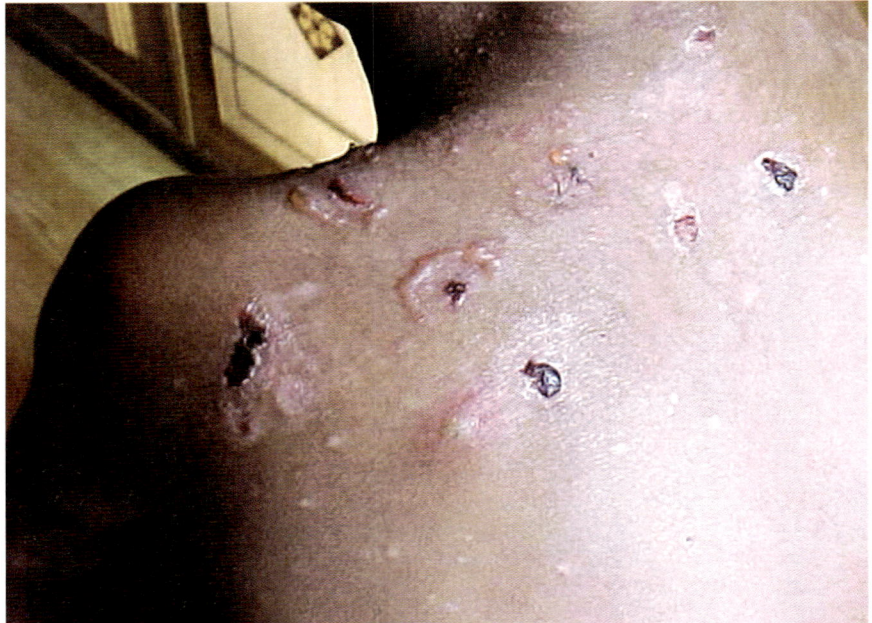

Fig. 21.22: Linear IgA bullous dermatosis. Bullae on site of inflamed skin with new blisters at the periphery of resolving lesions, resulting in an archiform or annular appearance

EPIDERMOLYSIS BULLOSA ACQUISITA

INTRODUCTION

- Presents as cutaneous vesicles and bullae
- Sites—hands, feet, elbows, knees
- Pathogenesis—antibodies against type VII collagen at the dermal–epidermal junction

HISTOPATHOLOGY (Figs 21.23 and 21.24)

- Subepidermal bullae with inflammatory cell infiltrate composed of neutrophils and eosinophils
- Superficial dermis shows perivascular and interstitial aggregates of neutrophils and eosinophils

IMMUNOFLUORESCENCE

- Direct immunofluorescence—linear IgG deposits at the dermoepidermal junction
- Salt-split skin immunofluorescence—IgG antibodies bind to the dermal floor
- Indirect immunofluorescence—antibodies in the serum against type VII collagen

DIFFERENTIAL DIAGNOSIS

Bullous Pemphigoid

- Subepidermal bullae with eosinophils and neutrophils as its contents

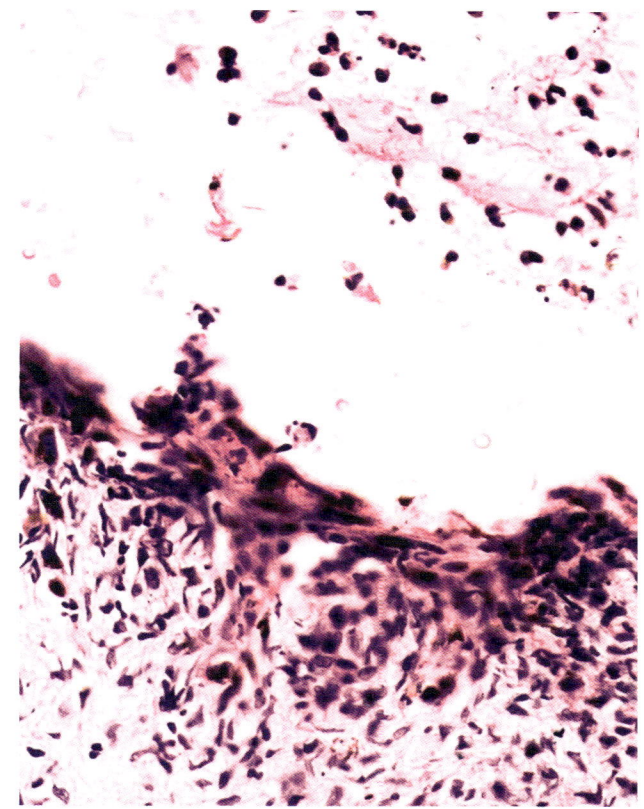

Fig. 21.24: Epidermolysis bullosa acquisita. Blister with sparse neutrophils and eosinophils as its ccntents

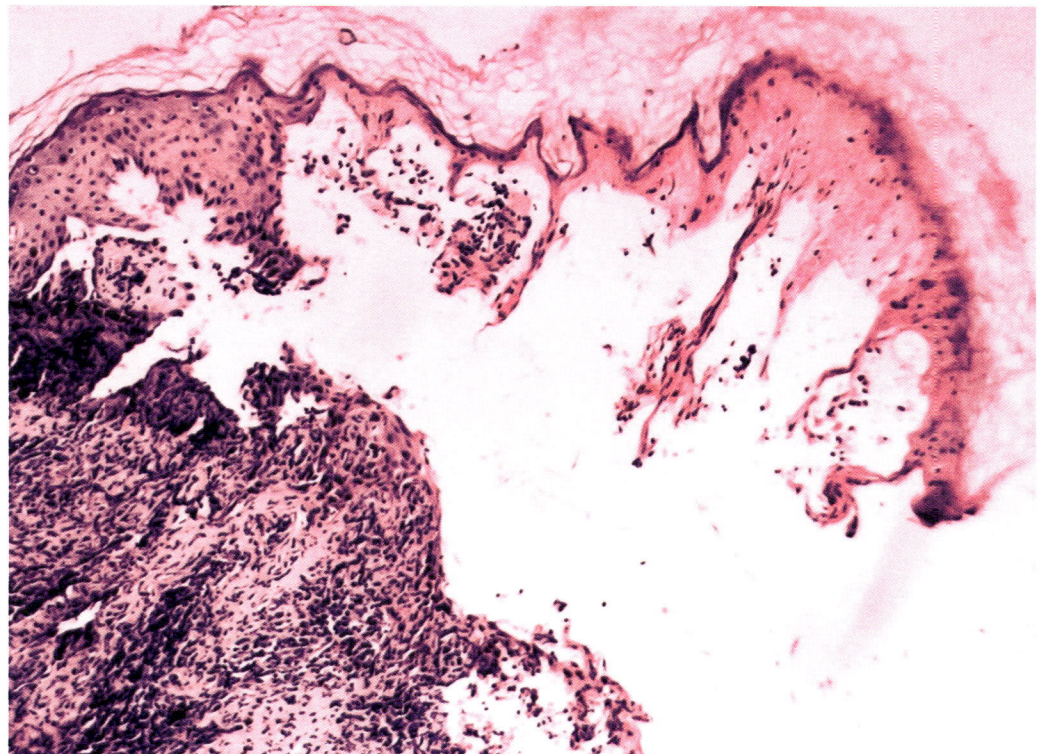

Fig. 21.23: Epidermolysis bullosa acquisita. Subepidermal blister with contents

- Direct immunofluorescence—linear deposition of IgG and/or C3 at the dermoepidermal junction (DEJ) or basement membrane zone
- Salt-split skin immunofluorescence—IgG deposits bind to epidermal roof

Cicatricial Pemphigoid
- Subepidermal blister with neutrophils, lymphocytes and histiocytes as their contents
- Blister can extend down the adnexal structures
- Hallmark—lamellar fibrosis beneath the epidermis

Linear IgA Dermatosis
- Subepidermal blister with neutrophils as their contents
- Direct immunofluorescence—IgA in linear pattern along the basement membrane zone

Bullous Systemic Lupus Erythematosus
- Subepidermal blister with neutrophils
- Direct immunofluorescence—linear or granular deposits of C3 or IgG at dermoepidermal junction

Porphyria Cutanea Tarda (PCT)
- Subepidermal blister
- PAS positive hyaline material in the walls of blood vessels in upper dermis

PORPHYRIA CUTANEA TARDA

INTRODUCTION
- Presents as vesicles and bullae with erosions and ulcers
- Site—sun-exposed areas (hands, arms, ears and face)

HISTOPATHOLOGY
- Cell poor subepidermal bullae
- Festooning—retained dermal papillae that extends into the blister lumen
- Superficial dermis shows eosinophilic PAS positive material around small blood vessels
- Caterpillar bodies—Type IV collagen positive basement membrane fragments in the stratum spinosum

DIFFERENTIAL DIAGNOSIS

Toxic Epidermal Necrolysis
- Blister with epidermis showing necrosis

Bullous Pemphigoid
- Subepidermal blister with eosinophils and neutrophils in the dermis

Epidermolysis Bullosa Acquisita
- Subepidermal bullae with sparse inflammatory cell infiltrate

Bullous Lupus Erythematosus
- Subepidermal bullae with papillary dermal neutrophilic microabscesses

SUBCORNEAL PUSTULAR DERMATOSIS

INTRODUCTION
- Presents as pustules, which can show pus accumulation
- Affects most commonly females
- Age group—fourth to fifth decade
- Sites—trunk, intertriginous areas, flexor areas of extremities

HISTOPATHOLOGY (Figs 21.25 and 21.26)
- Subcorneal vesicle filled with neutrophils and occasional eosinophils
- Pustules rest above the epidermis
- Epidermis shows minimal spongiosis
- Dermal papillae shows perivascular inflammation with neutrophils and occasional eosinophils

DIFFERENTIAL DIAGNOSIS

Pustular Psoriasis
- Spongiotic epidermis with Munro's microabscesses
- Spongiform pustules are seen

Acute Generalized Exanthematous Pustulosis
- Spongiosis and acanthosis of epidermis
- Subcorneal neutrophilic pustules

Pemphigus Foliaceous
- Subcorneal bullae with separation of stratum corneum and granular layer
- Subcorneal blister can show acantholytic keratinocytes or dyskeratotic granular keratinocytes
- Blister cavity shows neutrophils as their contents

Bullous Impetigo
- Subcorneal bulla with neutrophils as its contents
- Acantholytic cells in superficial epidermis
- Gram stain can demonstrate bacterial colonies

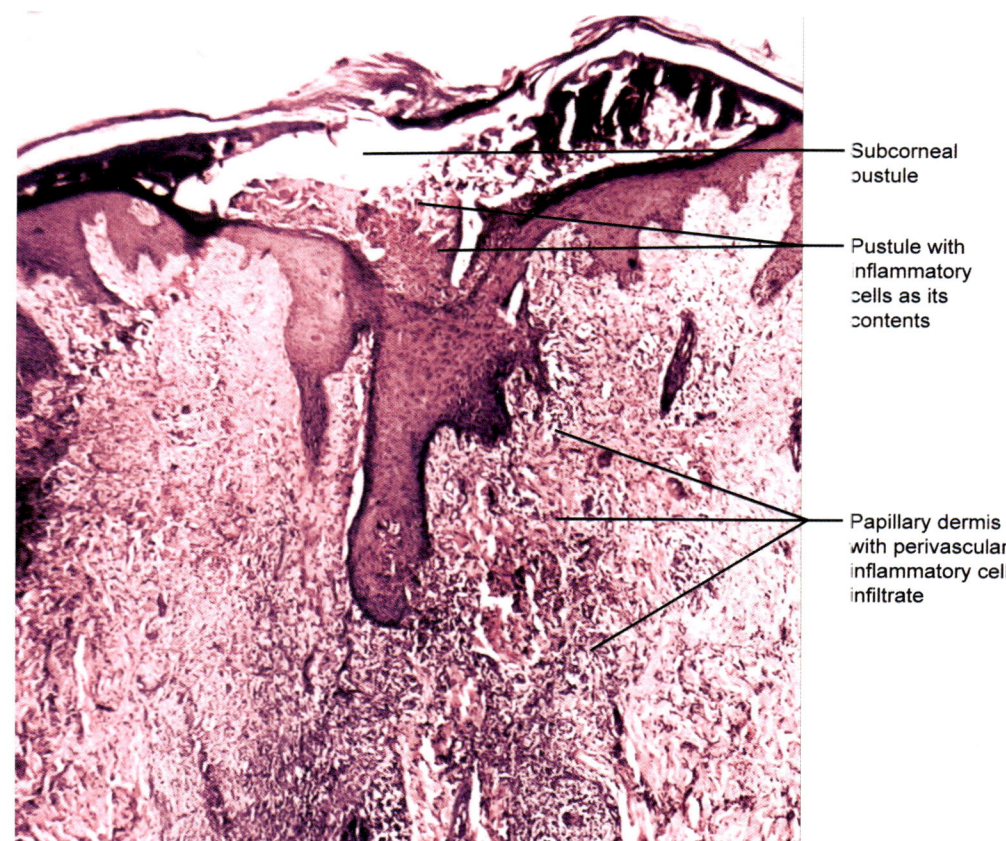

Subcorneal pustule

Pustule with inflammatory cells as its contents

Papillary dermis with perivascular inflammatory cell infiltrate

Fig. 21.25: Subcorneal pustular dermatosis

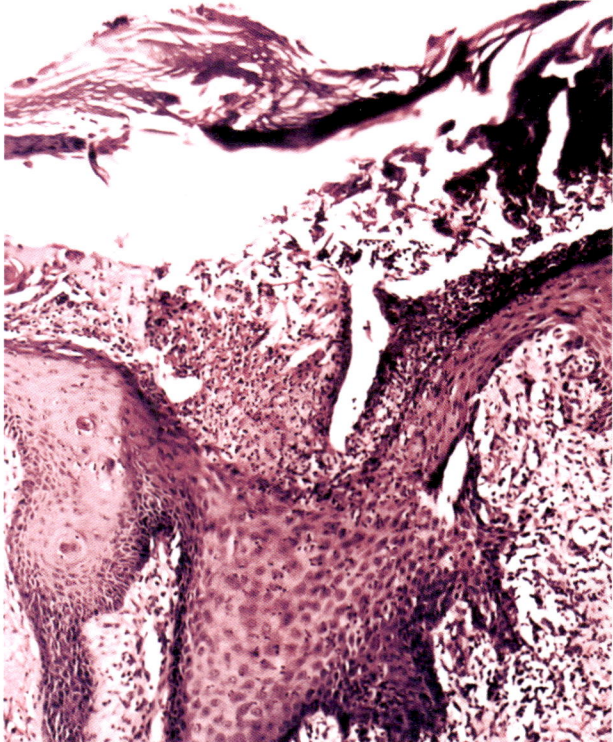

Fig. 21.26: Subcorneal pustular dermatosis with neutrophils as pustule contents

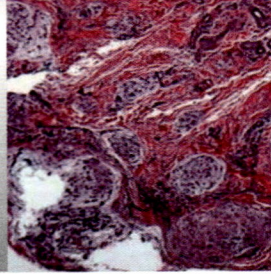

Borreliosis/Lyme Disease

INTRODUCTION

- Tick borne infection (Ixodes species tick)
- Causative organism—*Borrelia burgdorferi*

CUTANEOUS MANIFESTATIONS OF LYME DISEASE

Erythema Chronicum Migrans

- Presents as solitary or multiple erythematous papules
- Histopathology—superficial and deep perivascular, perineural and perieccrine infiltrate of lymphocytes, plasma cells, eosinophils and macrophages
- Warthin starry stain can detect spirochete

Differential Diagnosis

1. *Urticaria*
   - Dermal edema
   - Perivascular infiltrate of neutrophils, eosinophils and in chronic cases, lymphocytes are seen

2. *Erythema multiforme*
   - Epidermis—shows necrotic keratinocytes
   - Basal cell layer vacuolization, lymphocytic infiltrate along the dermoepidermal junction

3. *Drug reaction*
   - Perivascular lymphocytic and eosinophilic infiltrate
   - Absence of plasma cells

4. *Erythema annulare centrifugum*
   - Subepidermal bullae
   - Epidermis shows mild spongiosis and parakeratosis
   - Perivascular lymphohistiocytic infiltrate

Acrodermatitis Chronica Atrophicans

- Presents as diffuse or localized erythema
- Sites—upper and lower extremities, especially around joints

Histopathology

- Paraorthokeratotic epidermis showing acanthosis or atrophy
- Dermis shows perivascular, perineural, perifollicular and perieccrine infiltrate of lymphocytes and histiocytes
- Destruction of vessel walls and collagen can be seen
- Late stages—epidermal atrophy and dermal sclerosis

Differential Diagnosis

1. *Morphea*
   - Dermis shows thickened, dense, closely packed, hypocellular collagen bundles

2. *Lichen sclerosus et atrophicus*
   - Tri-layered appearance of epidermis
   - Superficial dermis shows edema and deep dermis shows homogenization of collagen

Lymphocytoma Cutis (Pseudo-Lymphoma)

- Presents as firm nodules and plaques
- Sites—earlobes, nipples and areola

Histopathology

Epidermis—spongiosis

Dermis

- Perivascular, perineural, and perieccrine infiltrate of lymphocytes
- Granulomatous vasculitis with luminal thrombosis
- Dermis shows dense mixed inflammatory cell infiltrate
- Lymphoid follicles with germinal centers can be seen

Ancillary tests

- Immunohistochemistry
- Polymerase chain reaction
- Serologic testing—enzyme-linked immunosorbent assay (ELISA) or immunofluorescence assay (IFA) followed by Western blot

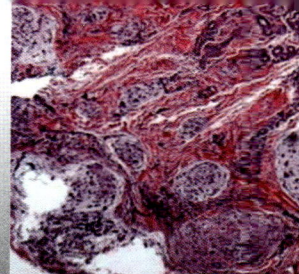

Urticaria

INTRODUCTION

- Presents as raised, pruritic, erythematous papules (Fig. 23.1)
- Lesions appear abruptly and are transient
- Predisposing factors—soluble antigens in food and drugs, snake venom, contact allergens, autoimmune conditions

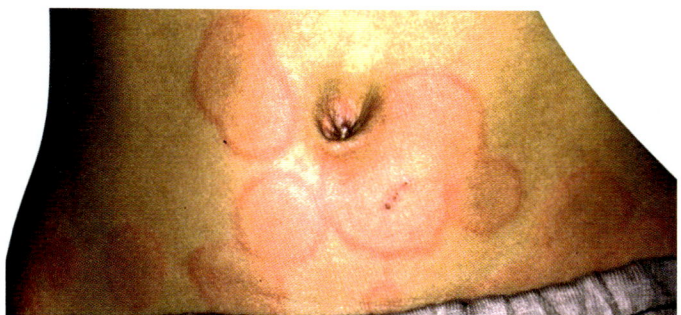

Fig. 23.1: Urticaria. Circumscribed, raised, erythematous plaques with central pallor

- Chronic urticaria—disease persisting for more than 6 weeks
- Etiology—histamine release brought about by mast cell and eosinophilic degranulation
- Dermatographism—sharply localized wheal and surrounding flare on stroking of the skin

HISTOPATHOLOGY (Figs 23.2 and 23.3)

- Early lesions—dermal edema, dilated vessels with neutrophils in their lumen
- Perivascular and interstitial neutrophils can also be seen
- As lesions age, dermis shows perivascular and interstitial mixed inflammatory cell infiltrate comprising of eosinophils, neutrophils and lymphocytes

TYPES

Angioedema

- Swelling of the skin, mucus membranes

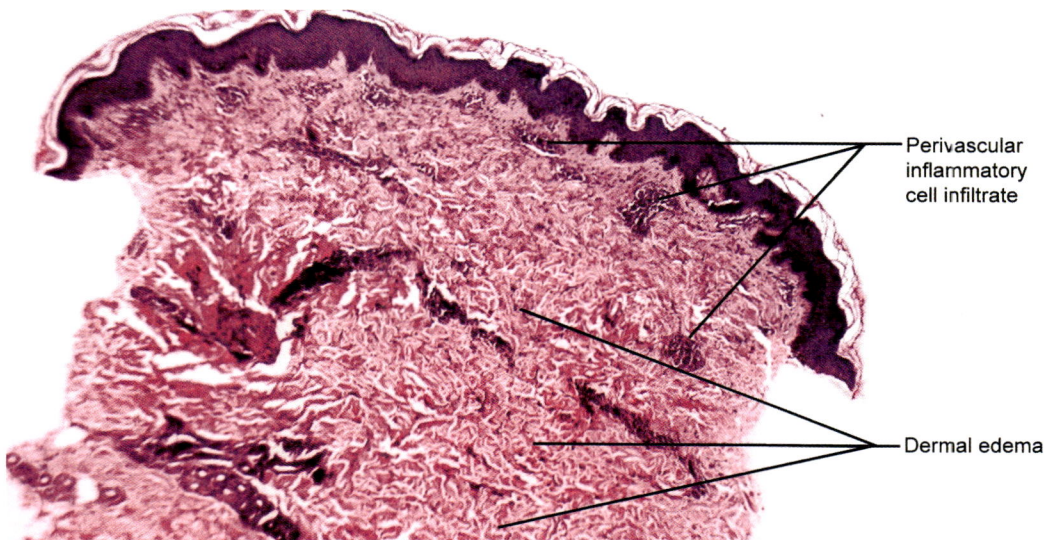

Perivascular inflammatory cell infiltrate

Dermal edema

Fig. 23.2: Urticaria

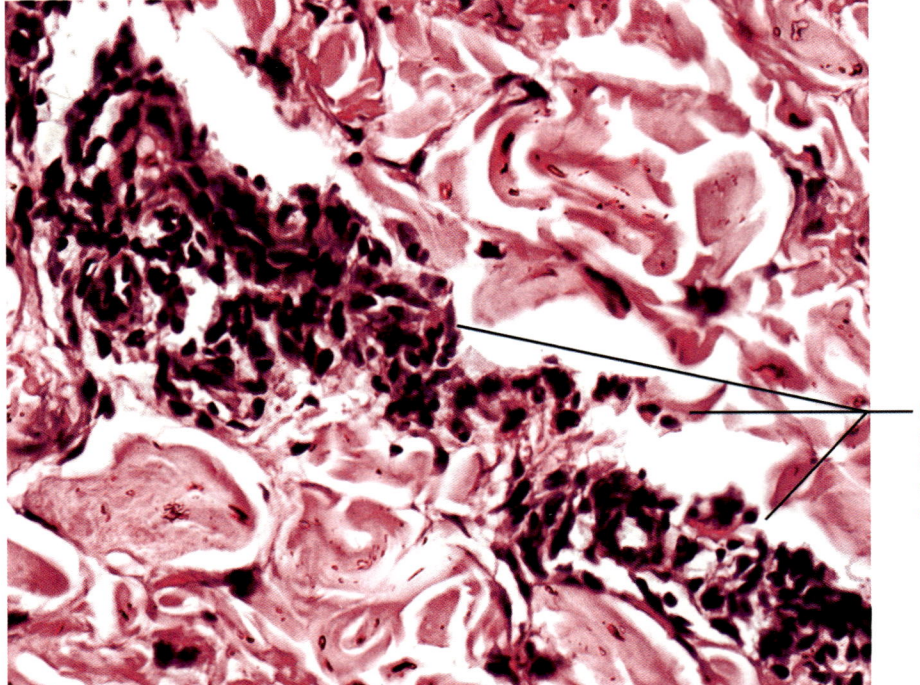

Perivascular chronic inflammatory cell infiltrate comprising of lymphocytes and eosinophils

Fig. 23.3: Urticaria

- Involvement of subcutaneous or submucosal tissues of lips, eyelids and genital area
- Hereditary angioedema—due to deficiency of C1-esterase inhibitor (C1-INH)

Histopathology

- Inflammatory infiltrate and edema, that extends to the subcutaneous tissue
- In hereditary angioedema, there occurs subcutaneous and mucosal edema without inflammatory infiltrate

Urticarial Vasculitis

- Urticarial lesions associated with arthralgia, abdominal pain, glomerulonephritis

Histopathology

- Dermis shows features of leukocytoclastic vasculitis and erythrocyte extravasation

Drug-induced Urticaria

- Causative agent—Penicillin, NSAIDs and sulfonamides

Contact Urticaria

- Due to allergies (hypersensitivity reactions) and irritants (non-immunologically mediated)

Papular Urticaria

- More common in young children
- Lesions persist for longer duration
- Can result from hypersensitivity reaction to insect bites

Histopathology (Fig. 23.4)

- Perivascular dense lymphocytic and eosinophilic infiltrate

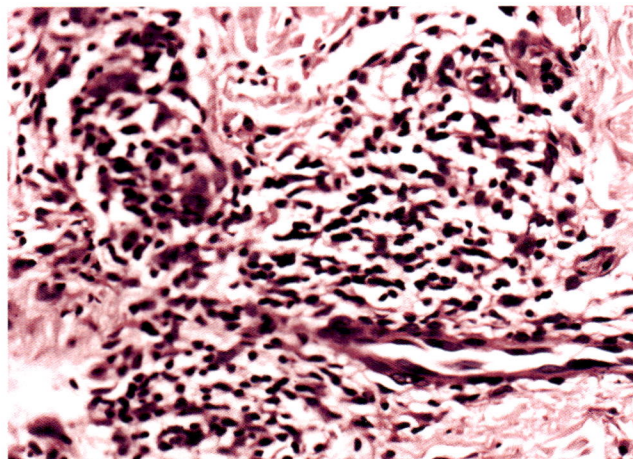

Fig. 23.4: Papular urticaria. Dermis shows dense perivascular lymphocytic and eosinophilic infiltrate

DIFFERENTIAL DIAGNOSIS

Drug Eruptions

- Perivascular lymphocytic infiltrate with eosinophils
- Absence of neutrophils in the vessel wall lumina

Acute Febrile Neutrophilic Dermatosis

- Diffuse band-like infiltrate of neutrophils in upper and mid-dermis, which can extend into the subcutis

Erythema Annulare Centrifugum

- Epidermis shows mild spongiosis and parakeratosis
- Perivascular lymphohistiocytic infiltrate

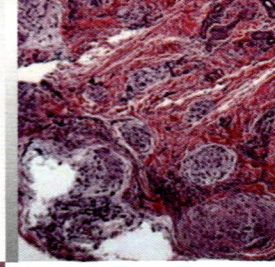

Acute Febrile Neutrophilic Dermatosis

INTRODUCTION

- Also called Sweet's syndrome
- Characterized by abrupt onset of fever, leucocytosis and raised, painful, erythematous nodules or plaques
- Sites—face and extremities
- Predominantly affects females
- Etiology—result of hypersensitivity reaction

HISTOPATHOLOGY (Figs 24.1 and 24.2)

- Normal epidermis
- Dermis shows a dense band-like perivascular neutrophilic infiltrate, which can extend into the subcutis
- Upper dermal edema, endothelial cell swelling and erythrocyte extravasation are seen

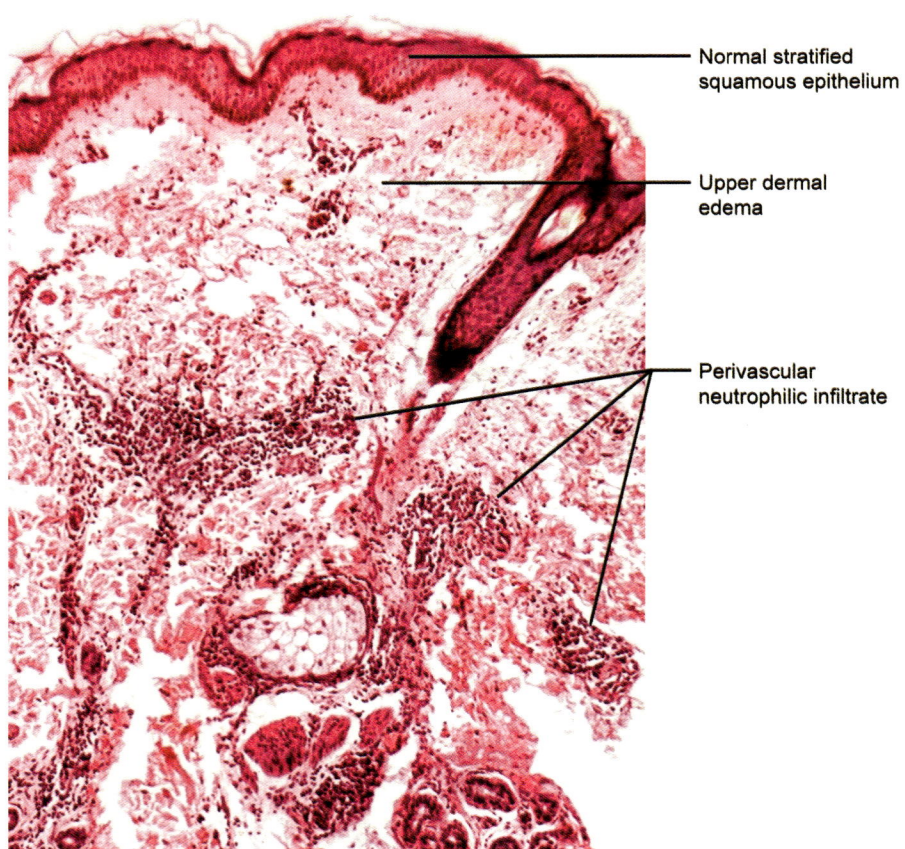

Normal stratified squamous epithelium

Upper dermal edema

Perivascular neutrophilic infiltrate

Fig. 24.1: Sweet's syndrome

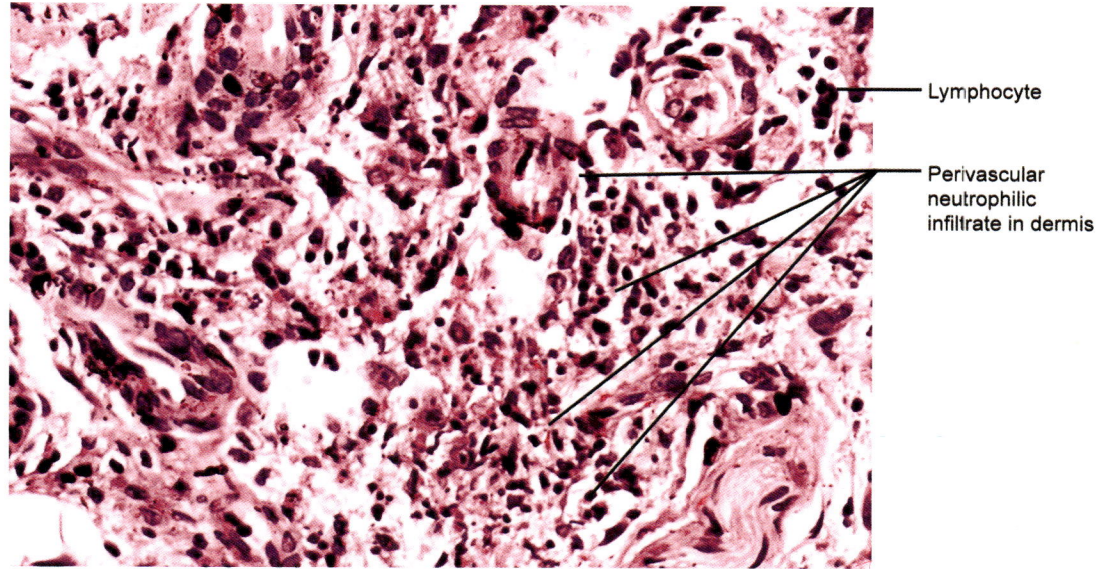

Lymphocyte

Perivascular neutrophilic infiltrate in dermis

Fig. 24.2: Sweet's syndrome

- As lesions age, perivascular lymphocytes and histiocytes predominate
- Subepidermal blister formation can also be seen

DIFFERENTIAL DIAGNOSIS

Pyoderma Gangrenosum
- Dermis shows necrotizing suppurative inflammation
- Perivascular lymphocytic infiltrate
- Leukocytoclastic vasculitis can be seen

Urticaria
- Dermal edema, dilated vessels with perivascular and interstitial infiltrate of lymphocytes, neutrophils and eosinophils

Erysipelas
- Superficial dermal edema
- Dermis shows neutrophilic infiltrate, which extends into the subcutaneous fat
- Perivascular neutrophilic infiltrate

Eosinophilic Cellulitis (Wells Syndrome)
- Diffuse dermal infiltrate of perivascular and interstitial infiltrate of eosinophils
- Absence of vasculitis

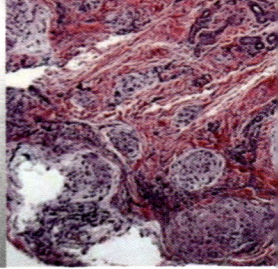

Eosinophilic Cellulitis

INTRODUCTION

- Inflammatory dermatosis
- Presents as persistent or recurrent plaques with erythematous border
- Sites—trunk and extremities

HISTOPATHOLOGY

- Normal epidermis with upper dermis showing edema
- Perivascular and interstitial infiltrate of eosinophils
- Flame figures—brightly eosinophilic damaged collagen fibers
- Subcutis shows necrotizing granulomas

DIFFERENTIAL DIAGNOSIS

Acute Febrile Neutrophilic Dermatosis

- Diffuse dermal infiltrate of neutrophils

Urticaria

- Dermal edema, dilated vessels with perivascular and interstitial infiltrate of lymphocytes, neutrophils and eosinophils

Urticarial Vasculitis

- Urticarial lesions associated with arthralgia, abdominal pain, glomerulonephritis
- Leukocytoclastic vasculitis of small vessels

Hypereosinophilic Syndrome

- Increased number of eosinophils in peripheral blood
- Superficial and deep perivascular infiltrate of eosinophils

Drug Reaction

- Superficial perivascular lymphocytic infiltrate admixed with eosinophils

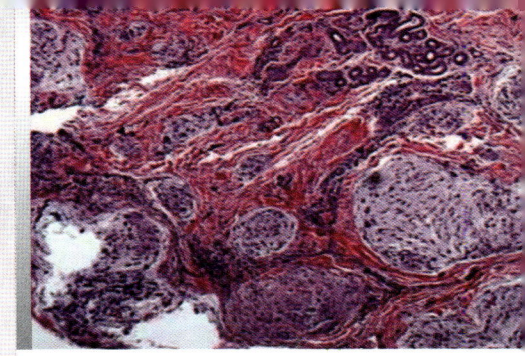

Connective Tissue Diseases

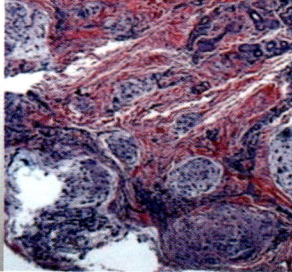

Morphea

INTRODUCTION

- Commonest form of scleroderma
- Lesions are localized to the skin and subcutaneous tissues
- Antibodies to *Borrelia burgdorferi* have been found in serum of these patients, suggesting an infective etiology

LESIONS CAN BE CLASSIFIED INTO THE FOLLOWING TYPES

Plaque Type

- Most common manifestation of morphea
- Round or oval to irregular lesions with violaceous border, that shows induration
- Most common site—trunk

Linear Type (Fig. 26.1)

- Most common subtype in children
- Site—extremities and scalp
- *En coup de sabre* variant—induration of anterior portion of the scalp and forehead

Segmental Type

- Localized to one side of the face and can result in one-sided facial atrophy

Generalized Type

- Most commonly affects children
- Any of the patterns described above can be seen
- Pan-sclerotic morphea—disability and significant morbidity in form of muscle atrophy, joint contractures and non-healing ulcers can occur

HISTOPATHOLOGY (Figs 26.2 and 26.3)

- Adequate amount of subcutaneous tissue should be there in biopsy for diagnosis

Early Lesion

- Interstitial lymphoplasmacytic infiltrate among deep dermal collagen bundles
- Lymphoplasmacytic infiltrate surround the eccrine ducts in the deeper dermis with resultant loss of adipose tissue around these ducts

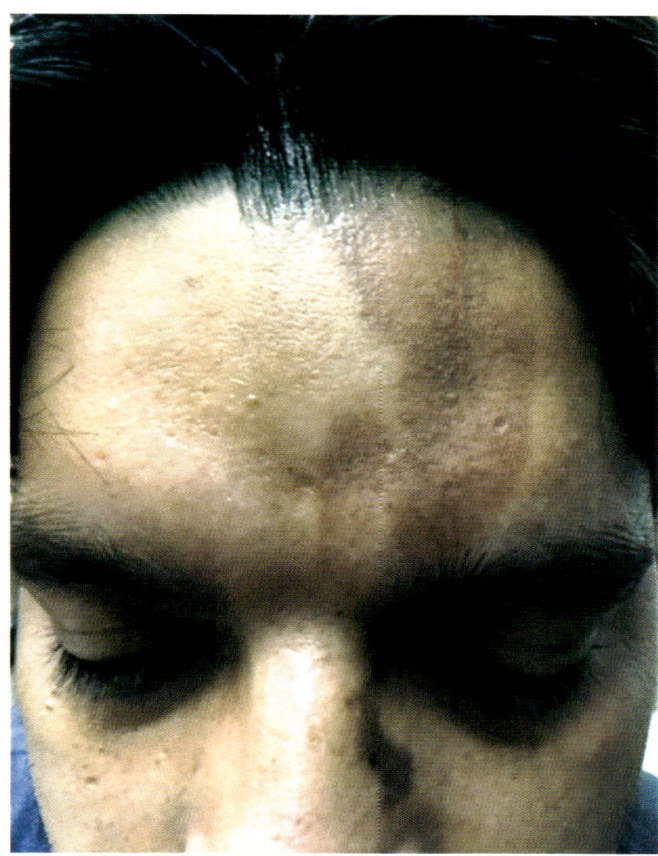

Fig. 26.1: Linear morphea (*En coup de sabre*). Hyperpigmented atrophic plaques resembling the cut of a sword

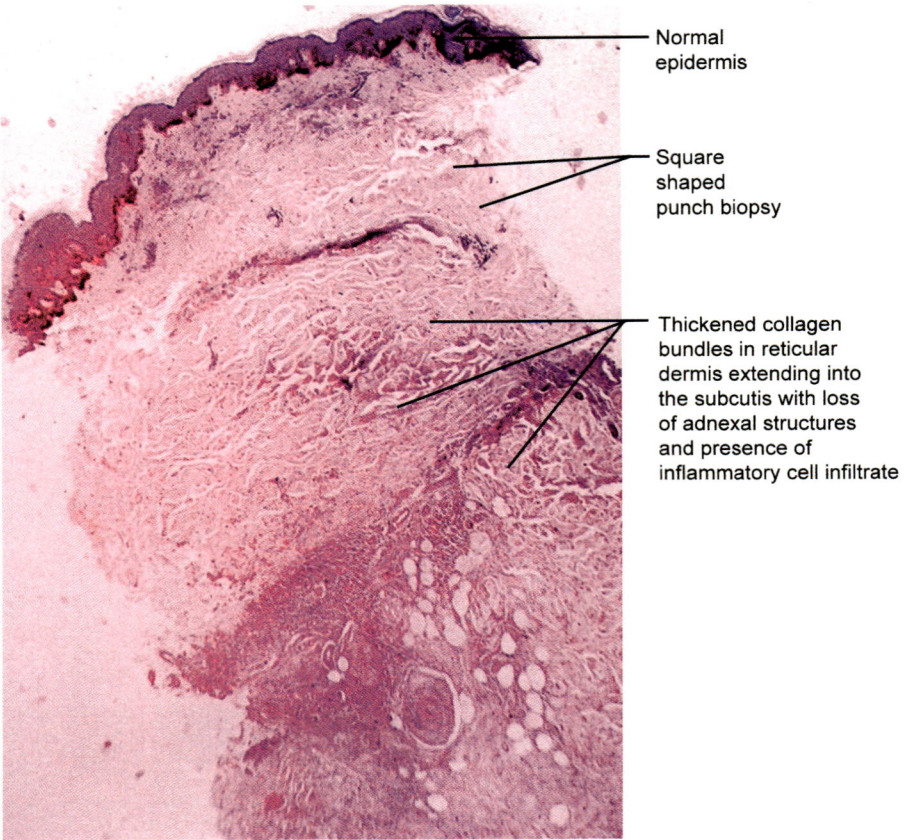

Normal epidermis

Square shaped punch biopsy

Thickened collagen bundles in reticular dermis extending into the subcutis with loss of adnexal structures and presence of inflammatory cell infiltrate

Fig. 26.2: Morphea

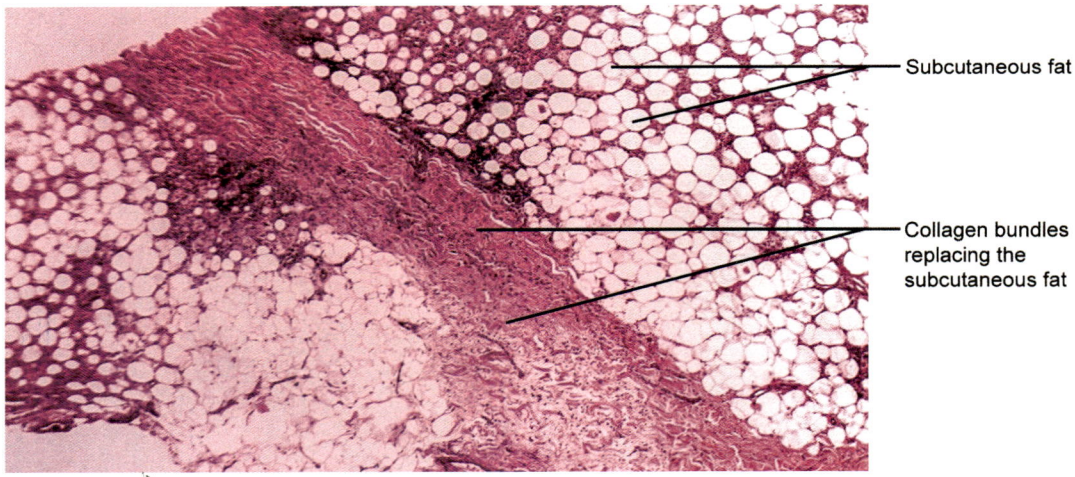

Subcutaneous fat

Collagen bundles replacing the subcutaneous fat

Fig. 26.3: Morphea

- As the lesions progress, subcutaneous fat shows newly formed collagen and inflammatory cell infiltrate

Established Lesion
- Epidermis is normal
- Square appearance of punch biopsy

- Reticular dermis—thickened, dense, closely packed collagen bundles
- Atrophy of eccrine glands, which if present, is seen in the upper dermis (as newly formed thick, collagen bundles replace the subcutaneous fat)
- Sparse inflammation at the dermal subcutaneous interface

DIFFERENTIAL DIAGNOSIS

	Morphea	Lichen sclerosus et atrophicus
1. Epidermis	Normal	Thinning of the rete ridges
2. Follicular plugging	Absent	Present
3. Hydropic degeneration	Absent	Present
4. Subepidermal bullae	Absent	Can be seen
5. Dermis	Homogenized collagen	Marked edema
6. Subcutaneous inflammation	Present	Absent
7. Subcutaneous fibrosis	Present	Absent

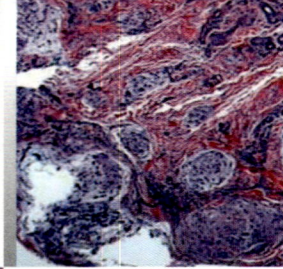

Scleroderma

INTRODUCTION

Two forms:

1. Circumscribed scleroderma (morphea)
2. Systemic scleroderma (progressive systemic sclerosis)

Systemic Scleroderma can be localized or systemic:

1. Localized scleroderma or CREST syndrome

- Calcinosis, Raynaud phenomenon, esophageal dysfunction, sclerodactyly (skin thickening distal to metacarpophalangeal joints) and telangiectasia
- Skin thickening distal to elbows and knees
- Associated with anti-centromere autoantibody

2. Systemic scleroderma

- Generalized skin involvement, which becomes hard with development of flexion contractures
- Skin thickening proximal to the elbows or knees
- Associated with anti-topoisomerase-1 auto-antibody

HISTOPATHOLOGY (Figs 27.1 and 27.2)

Early Lesion

- Superficial and deep perivascular, periadnexal and perineural lymphoplasmacytic infiltrate
- Thick collagen bundles

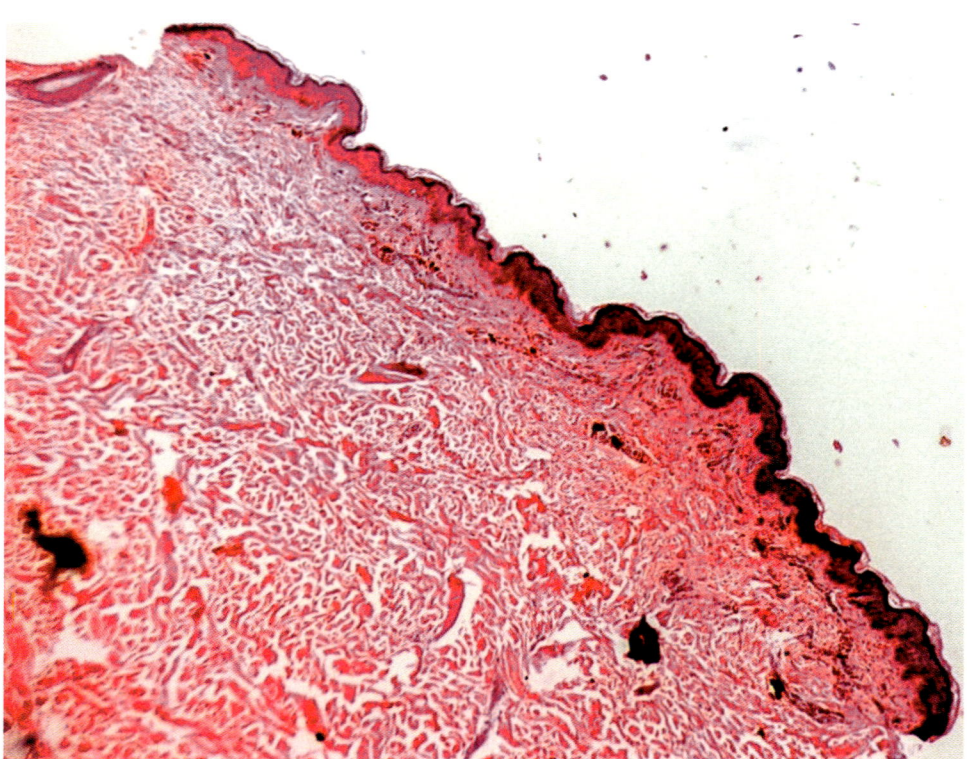

Fig. 27.1: Scleroderma. Thickened collagen bundles in dermis

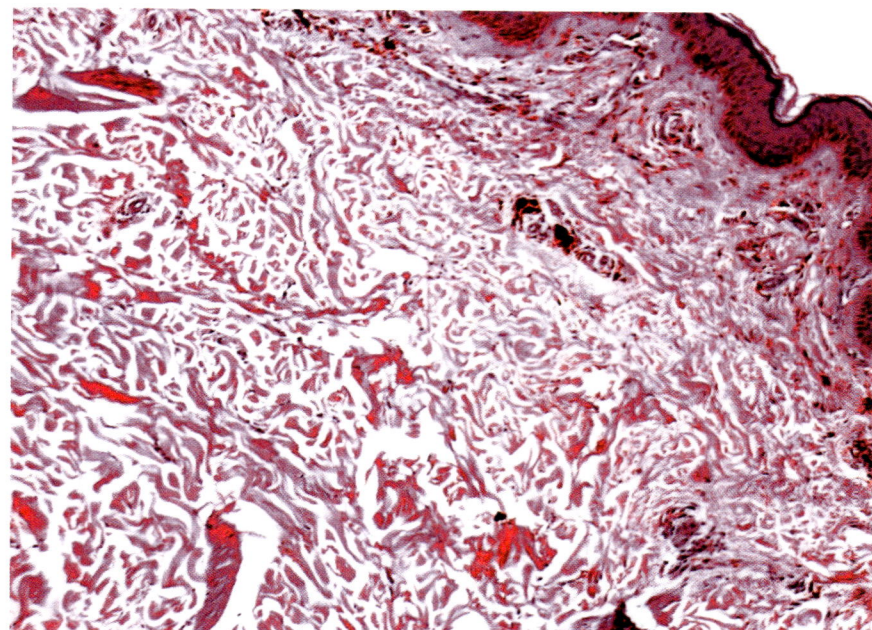

Fig. 27.2: Scleroderma. Thick collagen bundles, paucity of blood vessels and adnexal structures in the dermis

Developed Lesion

- Thick collagen bundles, that extend into the subcutis
- Paucity of dermal blood vessels, with thickening and hyalinization of their walls
- Thick, coarse elastic fibers parallel to collagen bands, which can be highlighted on Van Gieson stain

DIFFERENTIAL DIAGNOSIS

Scleredema

- Thickened dermal collagen, with infiltrate of mucin in the deeper dermis

- Absence of prominent inflammatory cell infiltrate

Scleromyxedema

- Dermis shows prominent mucin deposition
- Proliferation of irregularly arranged fibroblasts

Lichen Sclerosus et Atrophicus

- Tri-layered or striped appearance of the epidermis
- Basal cell layer vacuolization
- Superficial dermal edema and deep dermis show homogenization of collagen

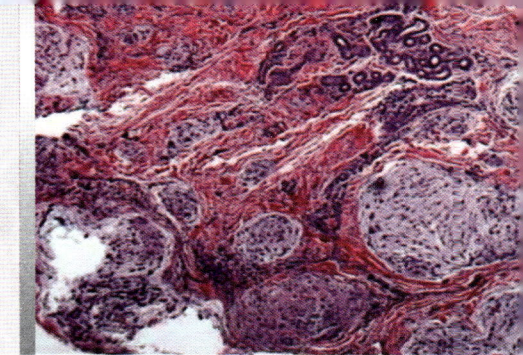

Panniculitis

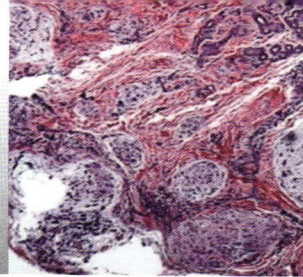

Erythema Nodosum

INTRODUCTION

- Most common type of panniculitis
- Presents as tender, bilateral, symmetrical, erythematous nodules or plaques (Fig. 28.1)
- Size of nodules—1–5 cm
- Causes—drug induced, infections (bacterial, fungal, protozoal and viral), leukemia, Hodgkin disease, non-Hodgkin lymphoma, autoimmune diseases
- Most common cause in children—Streptococcal infection
- Most common site—anterior surface of lower legs

HISTOPATHOLOGY (Figs 28.2 and 28.3)

- Subcutis shows thickened septa
- Septal and paraseptal regions show neutrophilic aggregates
- Later stages show mixed inflammatory cell infiltrate comprising of lymphocytes, macrophages, giant cells with septal fibrosis
- **Miescher's radial granulomas**—aggregates of macrophages and neutrophils around small blood vessels

- Vascular damage—vessel wall shows mixed neutrophilic and macrophage infiltrate
- Later lesions show widening of the septa, granulomas and multinucleated giant cells
- **Erythema nodosum migrans (chronic form)**—characterized by numerous large epithelioid histiocytic granulomas and lipogranulomas

DIFFERENTIAL DIAGNOSIS

Erythema Induratum

- Vasculitis and fat necrosis are commonly seen

Nodular Vasculitis

- Vessel wall shows lymphocytic infiltrate with fibrous thickening and obliteration of vascular lumens

Ruptured Epidermoid Cyst

- Cysts in deep dermis, associated with inflammation that extends into the subcutaneous fat

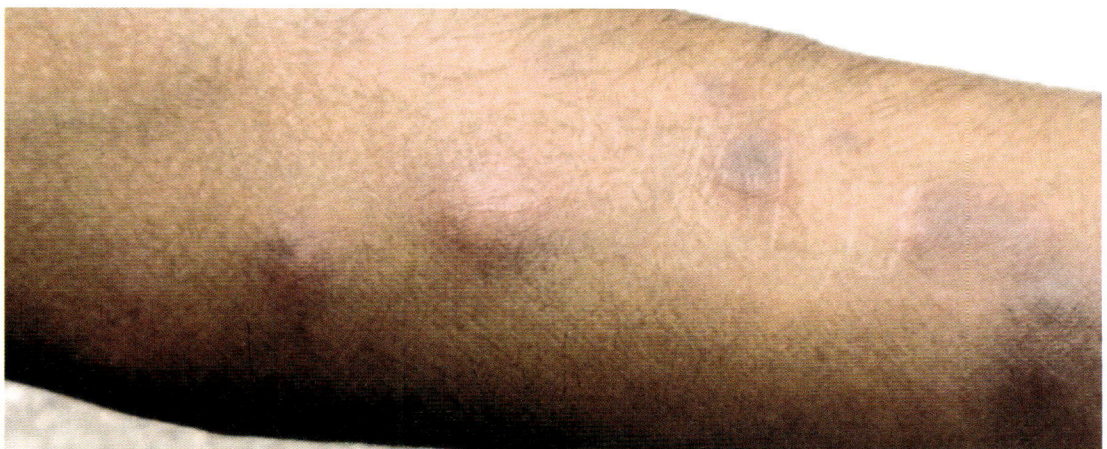

Fig. 28.1: Erythema Nodosum. Erythematosus, tender, non-ulcerated, immobile nodules with healed lesions showing secondary bruising

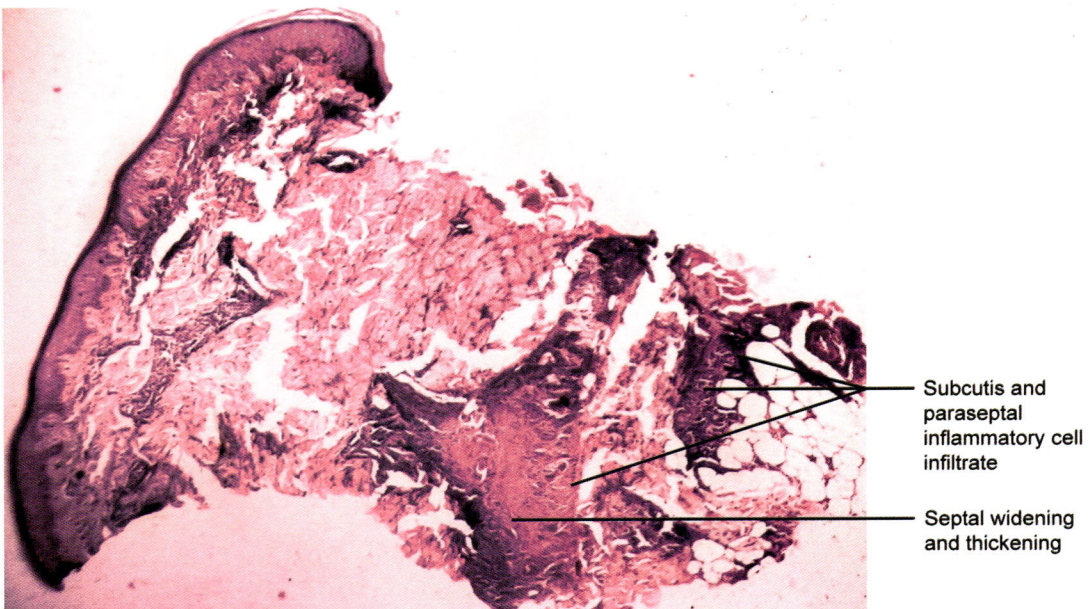

Subcutis and
paraseptal
inflammatory cell
infiltrate

Septal widening
and thickening

Fig. 28.2: Erythema nodosum

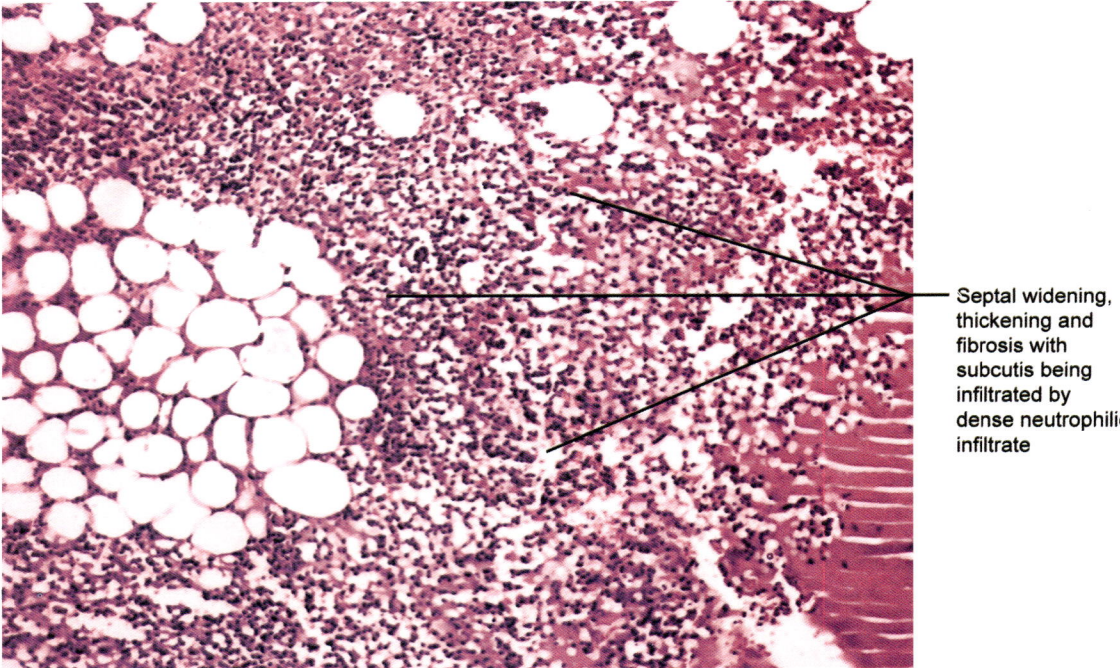

Septal widening,
thickening and
fibrosis with
subcutis being
infiltrated by
dense neutrophilic
infiltrate

Fig. 28.3: Erythema nodosum

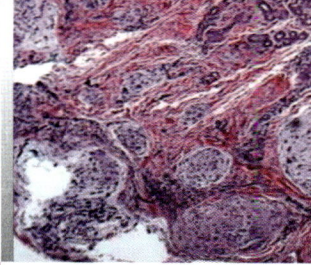

Lupus Panniculitis

INTRODUCTION

- Seen in patients with chronic discoid lupus erythematosus or systemic lupus erythematosus
- Sites—trunk and extremities, scalp, face
- Presents as erythematous plaques and ulcerated nodules

HISTOPATHOLOGY (Figs 29.1 to 29.3)

- Epidermal and dermal changes of lupus erythematosus can be seen
- Lymphocytic infiltration of the fat lobules and septa
- Lymphoid follicles with germinal center formation can occur
- Lymphocytic vasculitis—concentric lymphocytic infiltrate surrounding the blood vessels
- Mucin deposition between collagen bundles in dermis

DIFFERENTIAL DIAGNOSIS

Weber–Christian Disease

- Disease is localized to fat lobules
- Absence of mucin deposits and perivascular lymphocytic infiltrate

Subcutaneous Panniculitis-like T-cell Lymphoma

- Presence of atypical lymphocytes within fat
- Absence of other histopathological features of lupus panniculitis

Erythema Induratum

- Lobular or septo-lobular granulomatous panniculitis
- Absence of mucin in dermis

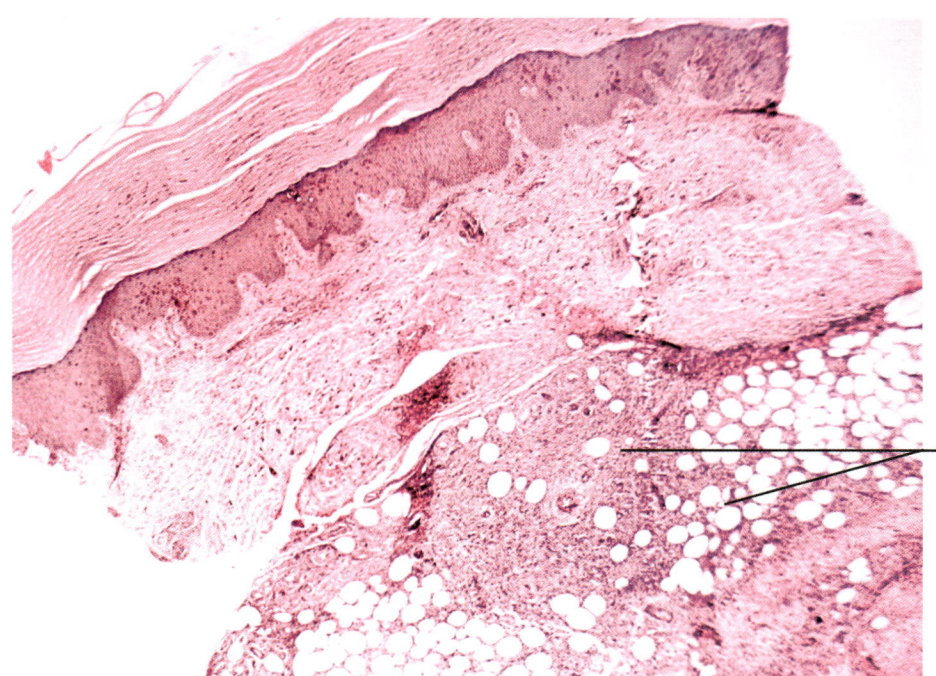

Septal thickening, widening and infiltration of subcutis by lymphoid cells

Fig. 29.1: Lupus panniculitis

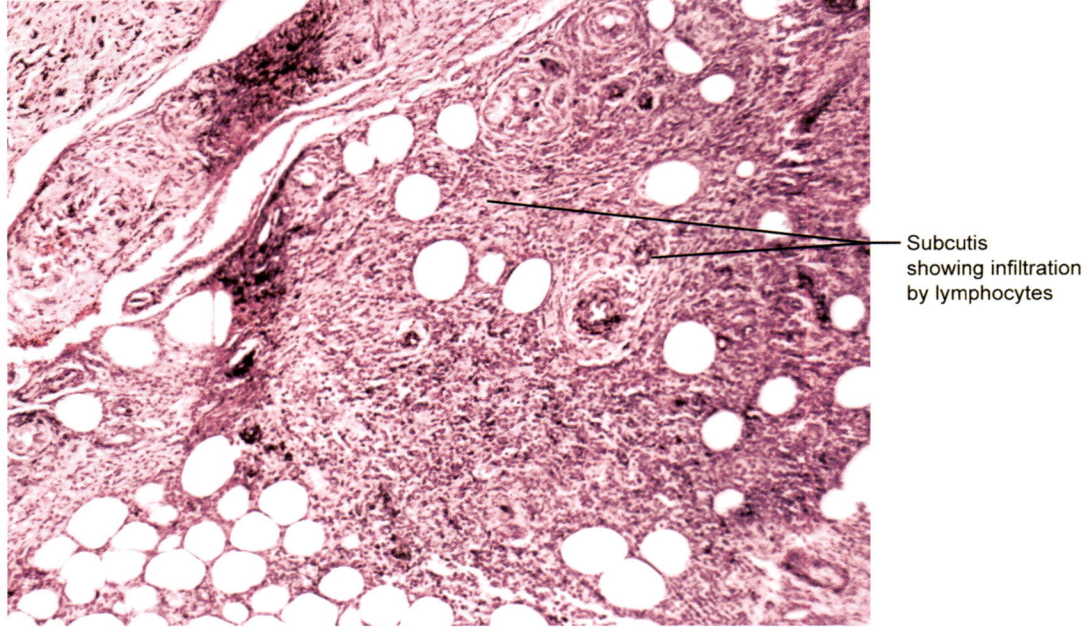

Subcutis
showing infiltration
by lymphocytes

Fig. 29.2: Lupus panniculitis

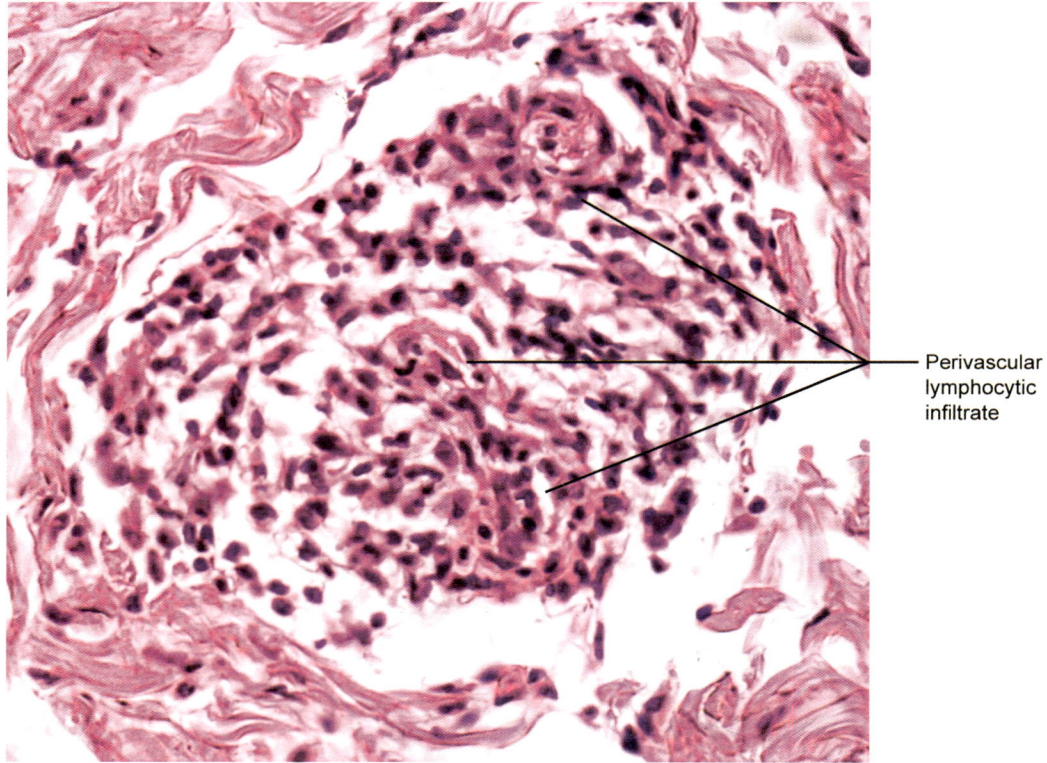

Perivascular
lymphocytic
infiltrate

Fig. 29.3: Lupus panniculitis

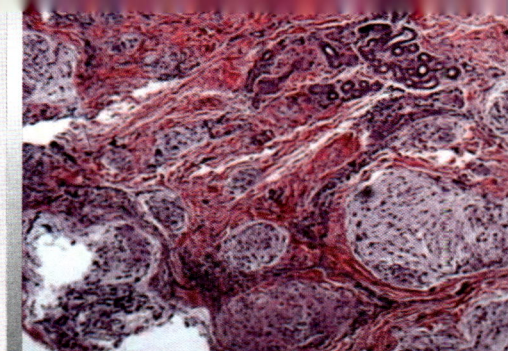

Granulomatous Inflammatory Disorders

Part 5

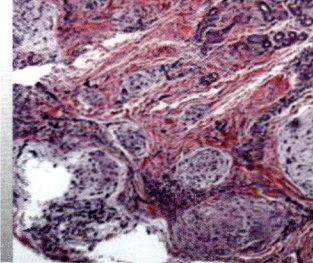

Foreign Body Granuloma

INTRODUCTION

- Granulomatous inflammation in response to a foreign body
- Most common cause of foreign body granulomatous inflammatory reaction—rupture of epidermoid or trichilemmal cyst
- Other commonly encountered cutaneous foreign bodies—wood, paraffin, lead, tattoos, silica, talc, suture material
- Presents as firm, skin colored to reddish—brown nodule

HISTOPATHOLOGY (Fig. 30.1)

- Epidermis is normal

- Dermis shows granulomas comprising of histiocytes, multinucleated foreign body giant cells and a diffuse mixed inflammatory cell infiltrate surrounding the foreign body

DIFFERENTIAL DIAGNOSIS

Sarcoidosis

- Non-caseating granulomas comprising of epithelioid histiocytes with multinucleated giant cells
- Absence of foreign body and inflammatory cells

Deep Fungal Infection

- Pseudoepitheliomatous hyperplasia
- Fungal organisms can be highlighted by PAS stain

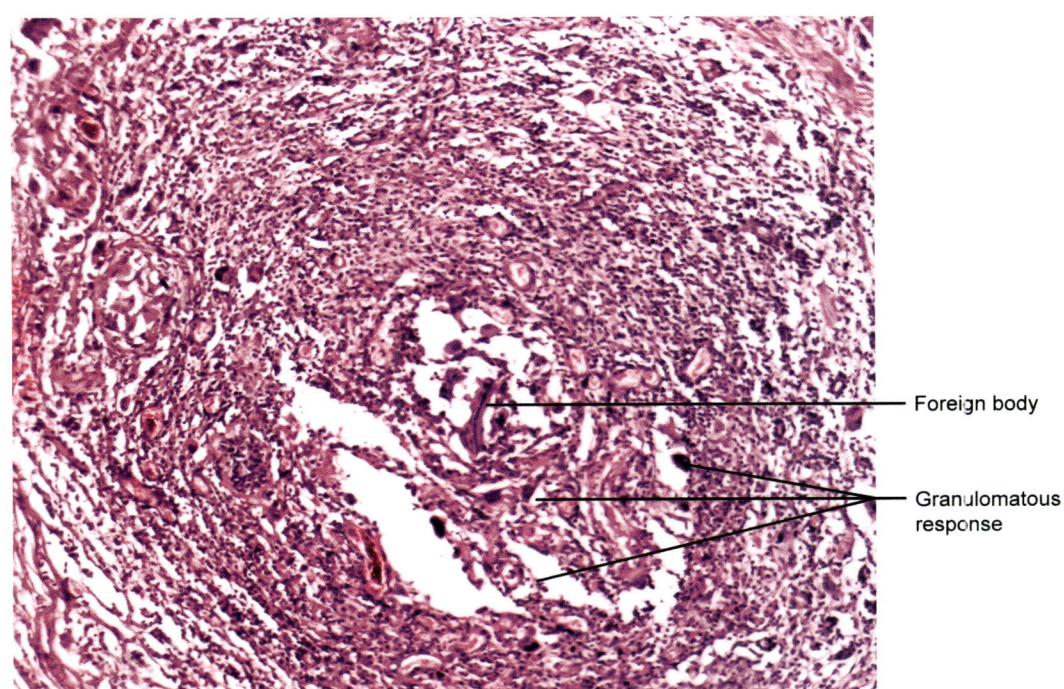

Fig. 30.1: Foreign body granuloma

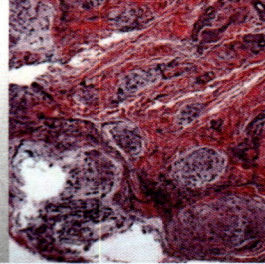

Granuloma Annulare

INTRODUCTION

- Idiopathic granulomatous skin disorder
- Presentation—multiple, skin colored, small papules, arranged in an annular pattern (Fig. 31.1)
- Age group—more common in children and young adults
- Females are more commonly affected than males
- Site—arms, hands, legs and feet
- Forms—localized, generalized, subcutaneous and deep
- Spontaneous regression can occur
- Associations—diabetes mellitus, HIV/AIDS

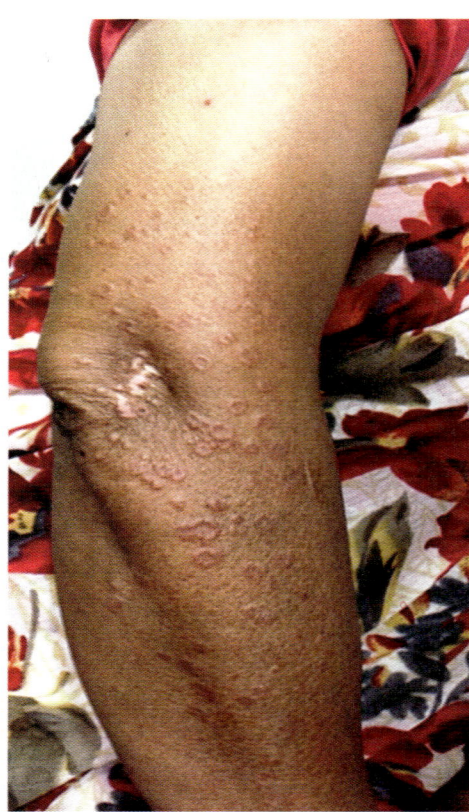

Fig. 31.1: Granuloma annulare. Widespread erythematous annular plaques with rope-like border and central clearing

HISTOPATHOLOGY (Figs 31.2 to 31.5)

- Areas of collagen destruction can be seen in the dermis
- These areas are surrounded by a peripheral rim of histiocytes and lymphocytes
- Granulomas can be seen surrounding these areas of collagen destruction
- Necrobiotic areas show increased mucin which can be demonstrated by colloidal iron or alcian blue
- Histiocytes are present either in (a) interstitial pattern or (b) palisading pattern
- Interstitial pattern—histiocytes and perivascular lymphocytes are seen interspersed between the collagen bundles
- Palisading pattern—histiocytes surround central mucin

DIFFERENTIAL DIAGNOSIS

Necrobiosis Lipoidica

- Focal dermal involvement, usually upper dermis
- Linear array of histiocytes, that are horizontally arranged
- Dermal sclerosis and thickened subcutaneous septa
- Increased number of giant cells, thickened blood vessel walls
- Extensive deposition of lipids in the dermis
- Mucin deposition is not prominent
- Plasma cells make a component of inflammatory cell component, which are rare in granuloma annulare

Xanthomas

- Can be confused with granuloma annulare (interstitial pattern)
- Presence of foamy histiocytes
- Absence of mucin and perivascular lymphocytic infiltrate

Mycosis Fungoides

- Epidermotropism of atypical lymphocytes (lymphocytes arranged throughout the dermo-epidermal junction) is seen
- These atypical lymphocytes have cereberiform nuclei

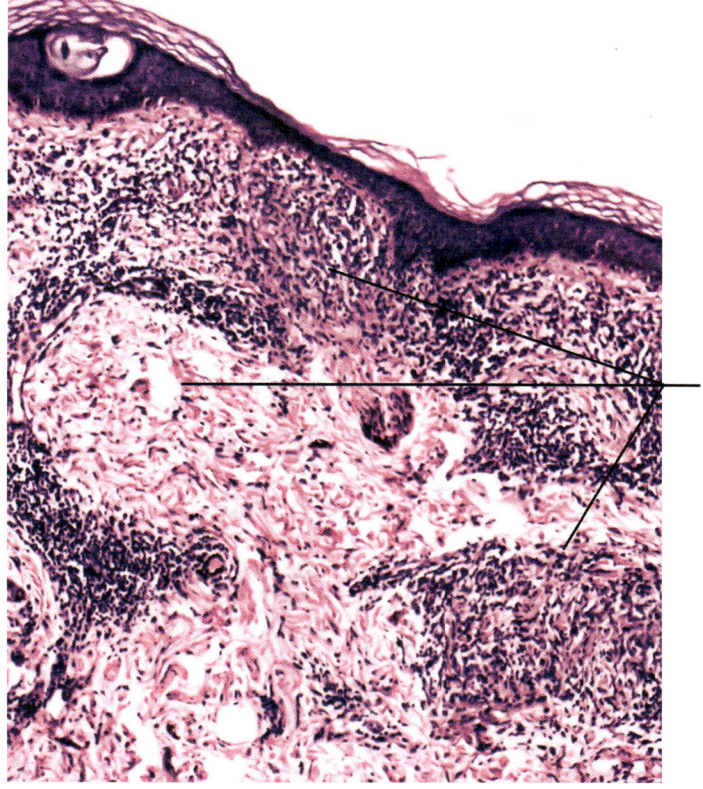

Dermis with degenerated collagen bundles, histiocytes and inflammatory cell infiltrate

Fig. 31.2: Granuloma annulare

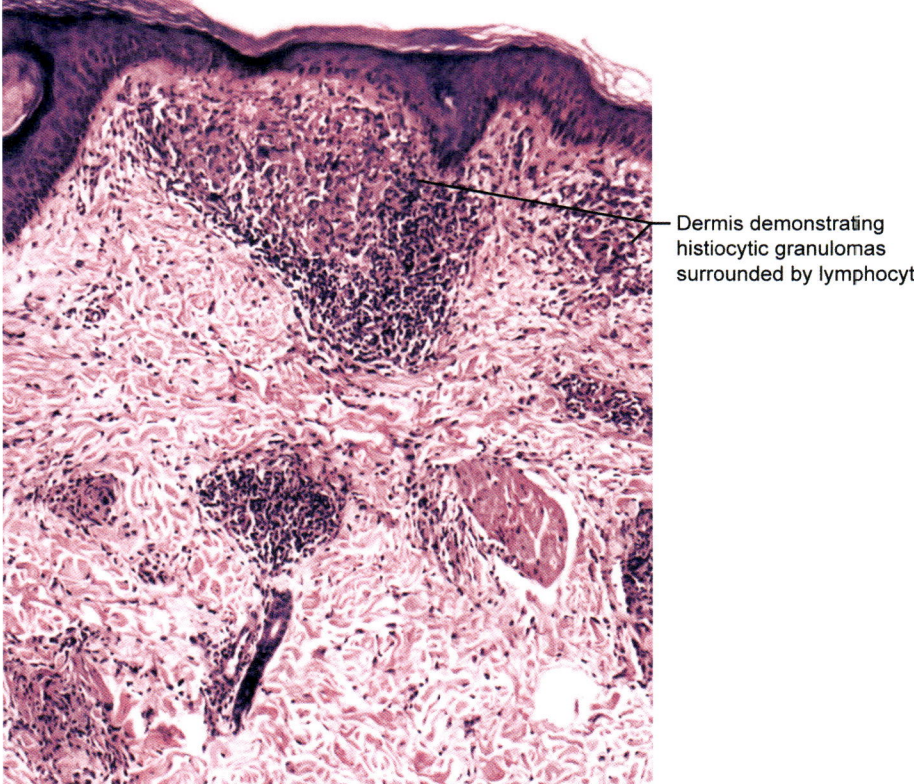

Dermis demonstrating histiocytic granulomas surrounded by lymphocytes

Fig. 31.3: Granuloma annulare

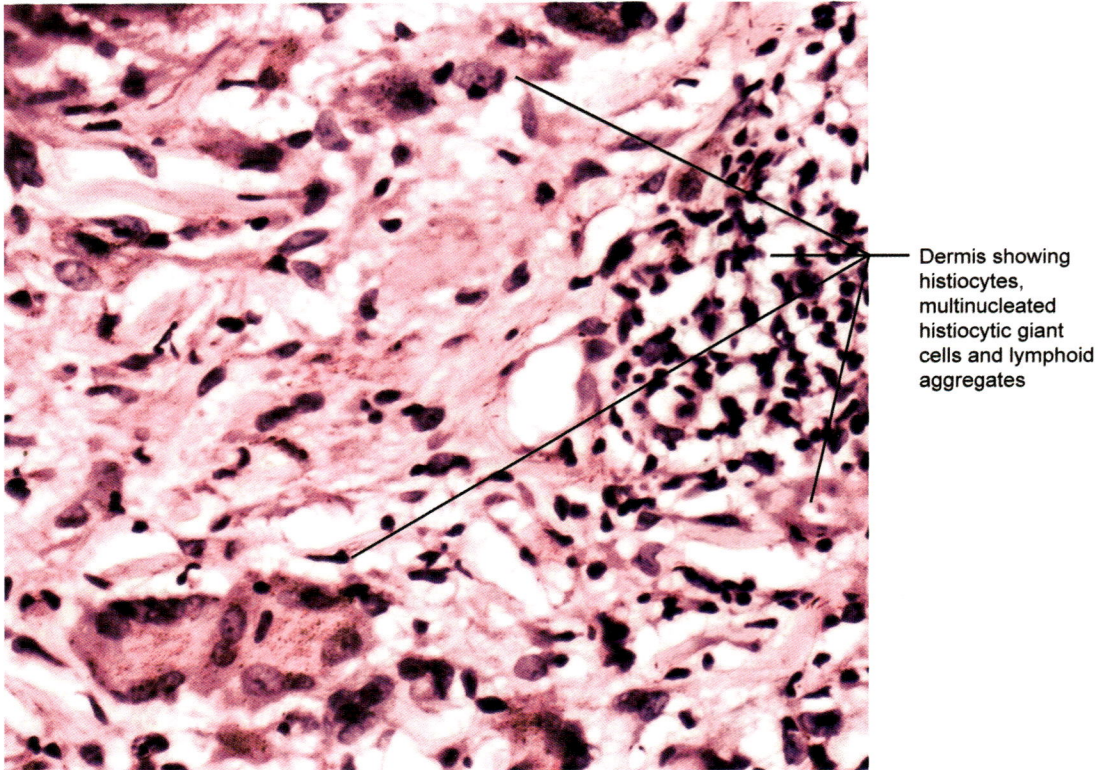

Dermis showing histiocytes, multinucleated histiocytic giant cells and lymphoid aggregates

Fig. 31.4: Granuloma annulare

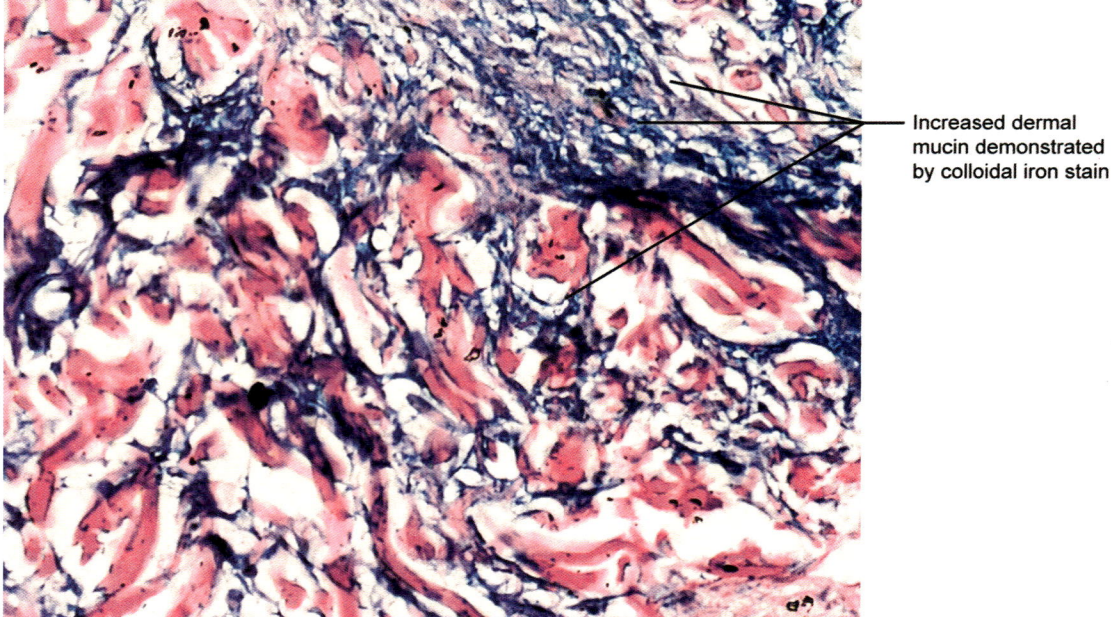

Increased dermal mucin demonstrated by colloidal iron stain

Fig. 31.5: Granuloma annulare

Rheumatoid Nodule

- Fibrinoid degeneration of collagen, surrounded by palisaded histiocytes
- Absence of mucin
- Foreign body giant cell reaction
- Stroma shows proliferation of blood vessels with perivascular fibrosis

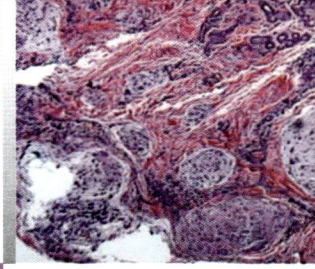

Leishmaniasis

INTRODUCTION

- Causative organism—parasitic protozoa of genus Leishmania
- Transmitted to humans by the bite of infected female sand-fly
- Two forms——promastigote (flagellated form) in sand-fly and amastigote (non-flagellated form) in humans
- Transformation to amastigotes occurs in histiocytes in humans and is favored by low pH and lysosomal enzymes

- Site: Face, neck, scalp, arms, extremities
- Lesion starts as an erythematous papule, which can transform into a nodule and plaque and can show spontaneous regression

HISTOPATHOLOGY (Figs 32.1 and 32.2)

- Epidermis—hyperkeratosis, parakeratosis, epidermal atrophy or hyperplasia
- Dermis—diffuse infiltrate of histiocytes, lymphocytes, plasma cells and occasional eosinophils
- Cytoplasm of histiocytes contains round to oval bodies, with basophilic nucleus and a rod-shaped

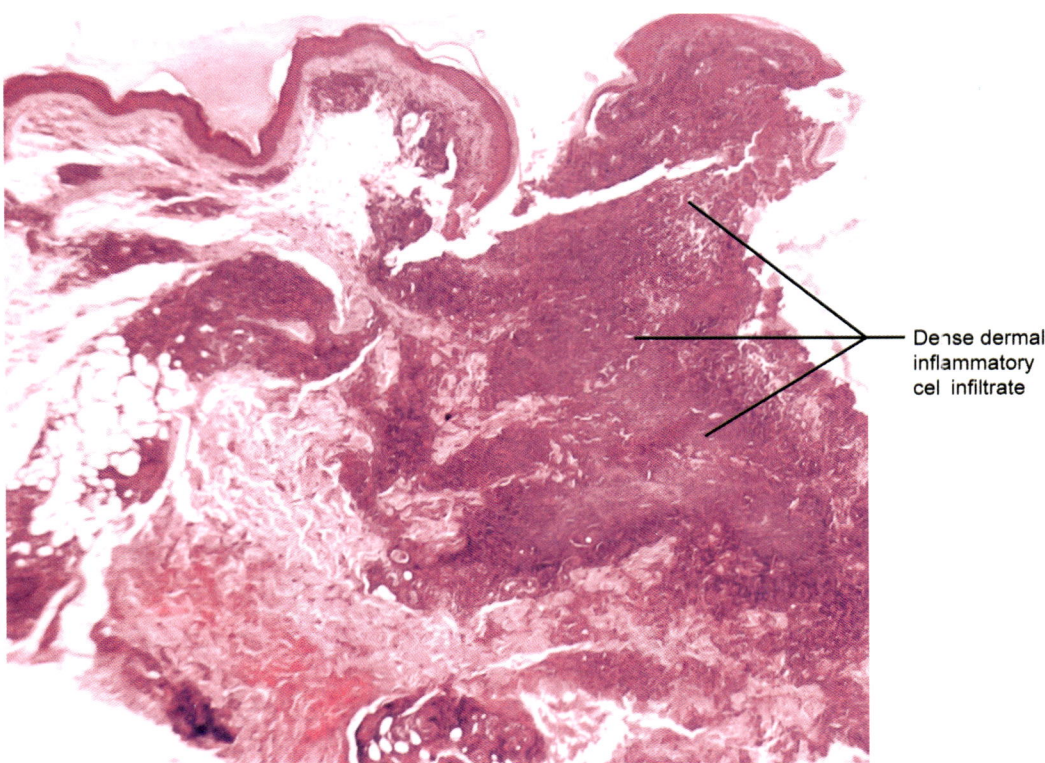

Dense dermal inflammatory cell infiltrate

Fig. 32.1: Leishmaniasis

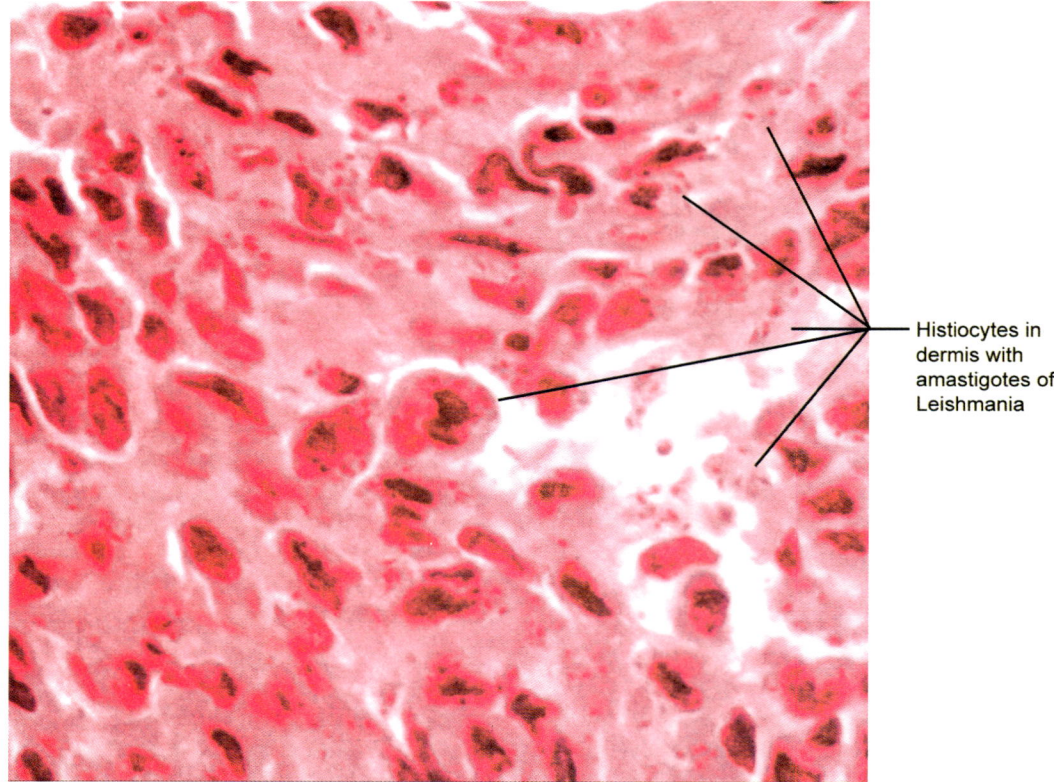

Histiocytes in dermis with amastigotes of Leishmania

Fig. 32.2: Leishmaniasis

eccentrically located kinetoplast (Leishman-Donovan bodies or LD bodies)
- They lack capsule, which helps in differentiating them from histoplasma capsulatum
- Identification of nucleus and kinetoplast is diagnostic
- LD bodies stain red or dark blue with Giemsa stain

Ancillary Tests and Special Stains
- Polymerase chain reaction (PCR)—most sensitive test for detection of DNA in tissues
- Giemsa stain on a tissue biopsy can highlight the organism

Visceral Leishmaniasis/Kala Azar
- Causative agent—*Leishmania donovani*
- Systemic disease characterized by fever, lymphadenopathy, hepatosplenomegaly, ascitis and pancytopenia
- Diffuse darkening of the skin, face, hands and feet
- On histopathological examination, numerous intracytoplasmic LD bodies are seen within the histiocytes

DIFFERENTIAL DIAGNOSIS

Histoplasmosis
- Capsulated organisms/spores with surrounding halo and absence of kinetoplast
- Organism stains with PAS and GMS (LD bodies does not stain with both)

Cryptococcus
- Round capsulated organism with peripheral capsular halo
- Capsule stains with methylene blue, alcian blue or mucicarmine
- Capsule shows negative staining with India ink preparation

Rhinoscleroma
- Numerous Mikulicz cells (foamy macrophages) with organisms inside them
- Numerous plasma cells with Russell bodies

Lupus Vulgaris
- Tuberculoid granulomas with necrosis
- Ziehl-Neelsen stain demonstrates acid-fast bacilli

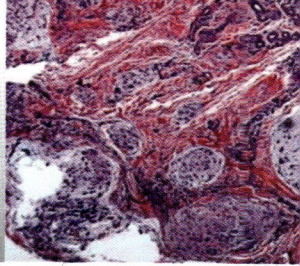

Leprosy

Chapter

33

INTRODUCTION

- Also known as Hansen's disease
- Causative agent—Mycobacterium leprae (acid-fast, gram-positive bacteria)
- Site—acral skin, peripheral nerves, eyes, ears, nose, mucous membranes, testes
- Mode of transmission: Inhalation of bacilli
- *Age:* Bimodal distribution with peaks at 10–14 years and 35–44 years
- *Presentation:* Hypoesthetic cutaneous lesions, enlarged peripheral nerves
- *Classification based upon number of lesions and number of bacilli:* Pauci-bacillary or Multi-bacillary

RIDLEY-JOPLING CLASSIFICATION

Categorizes leprosy into 5 major forms

Tuberculoid Leprosy (TT)

- Most common type in India
- Localized form with asymmetric distribution of anesthetic plaques

- Sites—trunk and limbs
- Lepromin test is positive

Histopathology

- Dermis shows non-caseating epithelioid histiocytic granulomas (perineural, periadnexal and peri-vascular) comprising of epithelioid histiocytes, lymphocytes and Langhans giant cells
- Epidermal involvement by granulomas is commonly seen
- Bacilli are difficult to demonstrate by Fite stain

Borderline Leprosy

- Includes borderline tuberculoid (BT), mid-borderline (BB) and borderline lepromatous (BL)

Borderline Tuberculoid (BT) Leprosy

- Lesions are larger and more in number than tuberculoid leprosy (TT) (Fig. 33.1)

Histopathology (Figs 33.2 to 33.4)

- Presence of subepidermal grenz zone

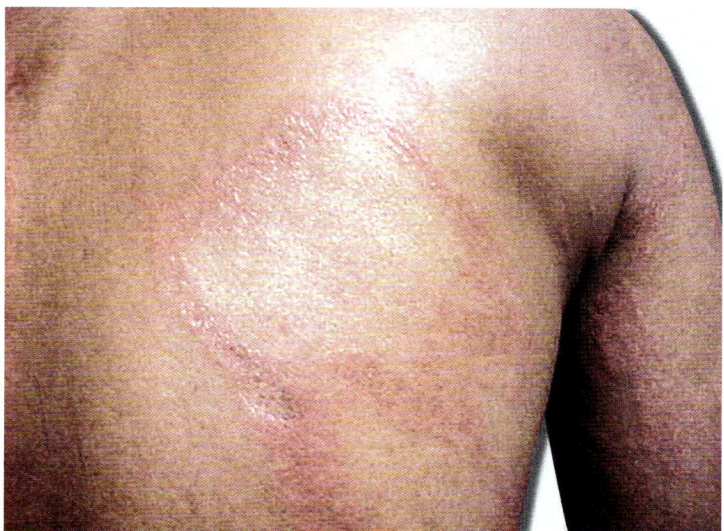

Fig. 33.1: Borderline tuberculoid leprosy. Erythematous annular plaque with satellite lesions

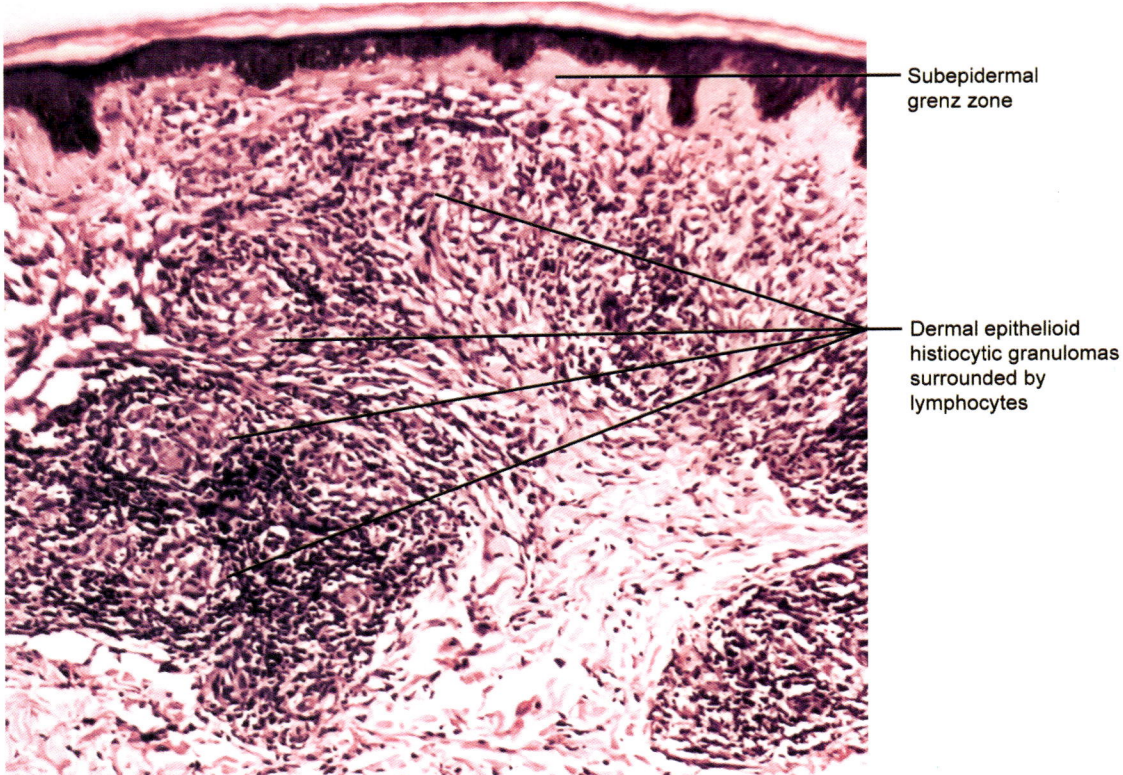

Subepidermal grenz zone

Dermal epithelioid histiocytic granulomas surrounded by lymphocytes

Fig. 33.2: Borderline tuberculoid (BT) leprosy with type 1 reaction

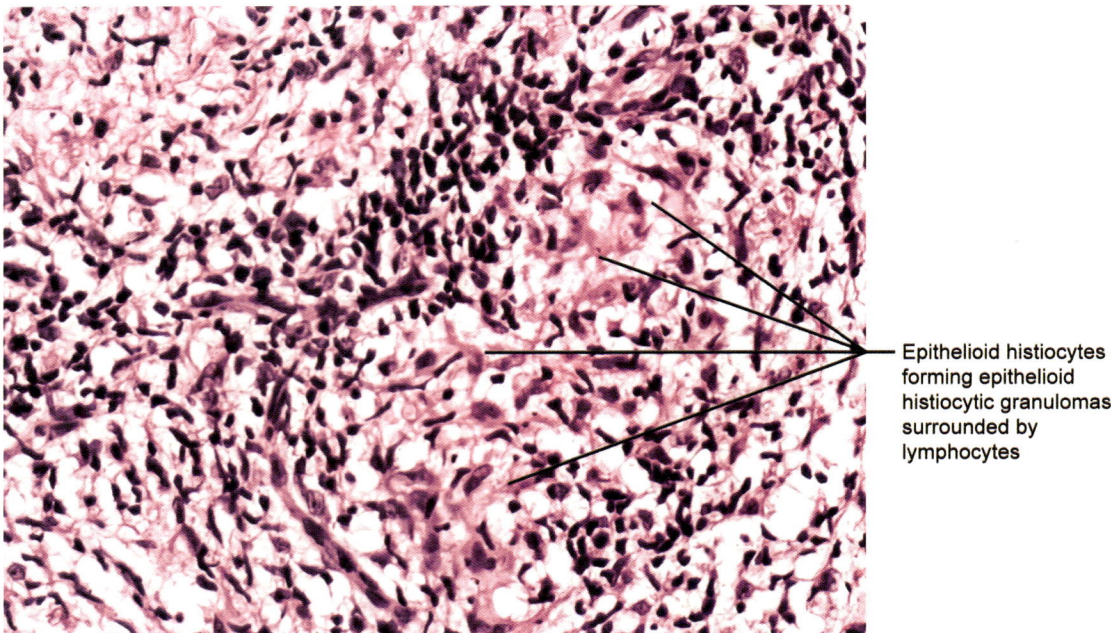

Epithelioid histiocytes forming epithelioid histiocytic granulomas surrounded by lymphocytes

Fig. 33.3: Borderline tuberculoid leprosy with type 1 lepra reaction

- Dermis demonstrate epithelioid histiocytic granulomas
- Bacilli though difficult to identify, can be demonstrated

Borderline Leprosy (BB)

- Erythematous annular patches with ill-defined margins (Fig. 33.5)

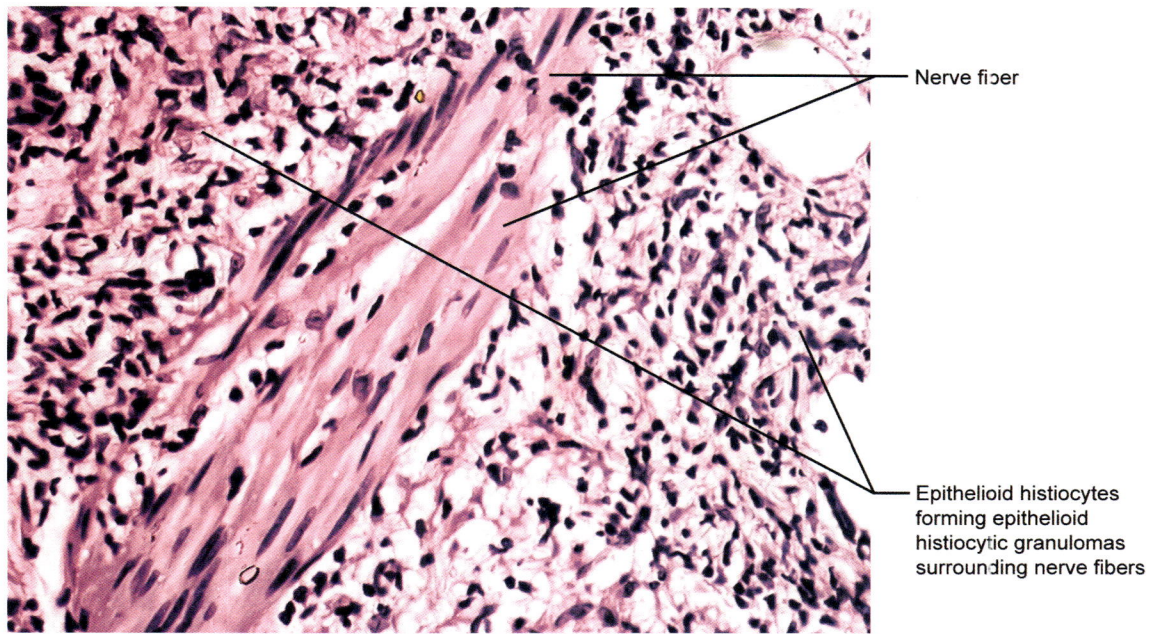

Nerve fiber

Epithelioid histiocytes forming epithelioid histiocytic granulomas surrounding nerve fibers

Fig. 33.4: Borderline tuberculoid leprosy with type 1 lepra reaction

Histopathology
- Epithelioid histiocytic aggregates without well-defined epithelioid histiocytic granulomas
- Bacilli can be demonstrated by Fite stain

Borderline Lepromatous (BL)
- Numerous ill-defined lesions with selective anesthesia of the lesions

Histopathology
- Presence of subepidermal grenz zone
- Presence of small aggregates of macrophages without epithelioid histiocytes
- Bacilli are easily demonstrable by Fite stain

Lepromatous Leprosy (LL)
- Symmetrical, widely distributed erythematous macules, papules and nodules (Fig. 33.6)
- Involvement of upper respiratory tract, oropharynx, kidneys, liver, spleen, bones, and testes can occur
- Leonine facies – facial involvement by leprosy
- Saddle nose deformity due to nasal septal destruction or perforation
- Nerve lesions can result in claw hand and foot drop

Histopathology (Figs 33.7 and 33.8)
- Presence of grenz zone
- Dermis shows diffuse infiltrate of foamy macrophages (Lepra cells or Virchow cells)
- Globi—organisms in clusters within the macrophages
- Bacilli can be demonstrated in nerves, vascular endothelium, Schwann cells or sweat glands

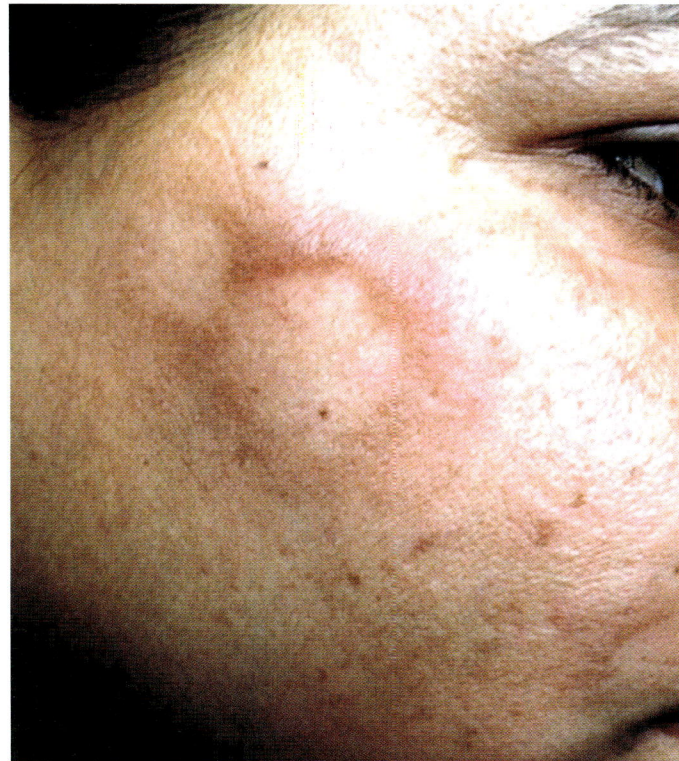

Fig. 33.5: Borderline borderline leprosy. Erythematous annular plaque with punched out lesion

Indeterminate Leprosy (IL)
- Single or multiple hypopigmented macules with or without loss of sensations

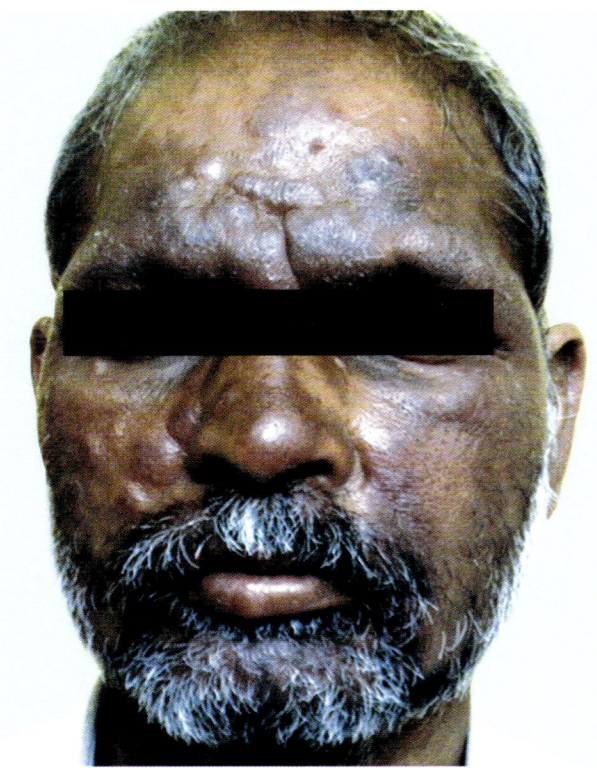

Fig. 33.6: Lepromatous leprosy. Multiple erythematous to hyperpigmented plaques and nodules, with loss of eyebrows

- Most commonly affects limbs
- Lesions can heal spontaneously or can develop into determinate types

Histopathology
- Superficial and deep dermal perivascular, peri-adnexal and/or perineural lymphohistiocytic infiltrate
- Rarely, bacilli (in small numbers) can be seen near nerves

Histioid Leprosy (HL)
- Rare variant of lepromatous leprosy
- Characterized by cutaneous or subcutaneous nodules and plaques

Histopathology (Figs 33.9 to 33.10)
- Grenz zone is present
- Well-circumscribed lesion comprising of spindle shaped cells/histiocytes
- Histiocytes contain numerous cytoplasmic acid-fast bacilli, which are longer than usual acid-fast lepra bacilli
- Interspersed foamy macrophages may be seen

LEPRA REACTIONS

Type I Lepra Reaction
- Example of Type IV hypersensitivity reactions
- Affect patients of borderline leprosy
- Associated with shift towards tuberculoid (upgrading) or Lepromatous pole (downgrading reaction)

Histopathology
1. *Type 1 upgrading/ reversal reaction*
   – Edema, clusters of epithelioid cells, increased lymphocytes, giant cells

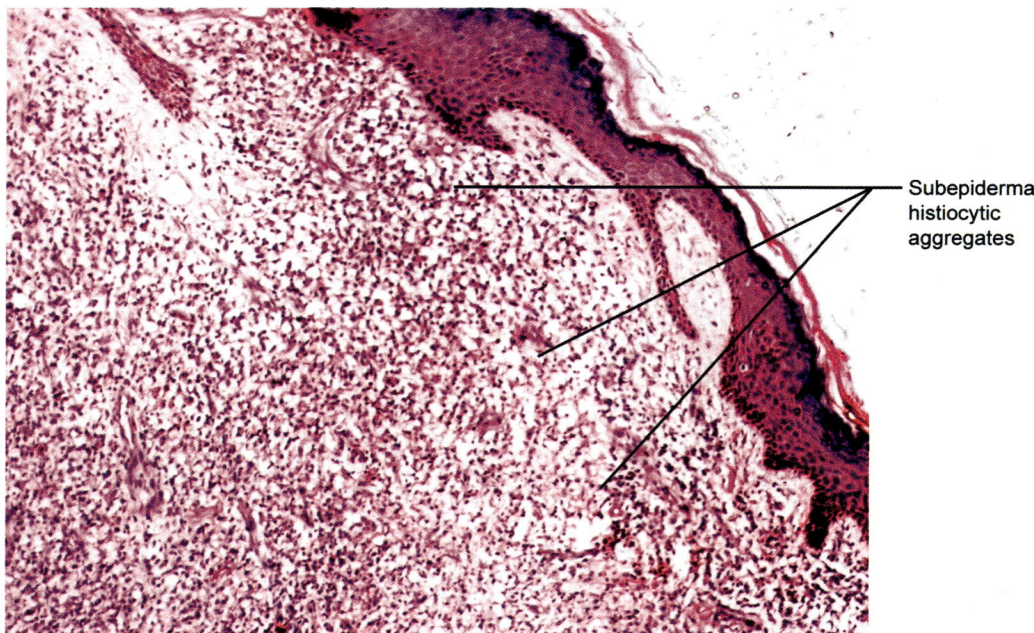

Subepidermal histiocytic aggregates

Fig. 33.7: Lepromatous leprosy

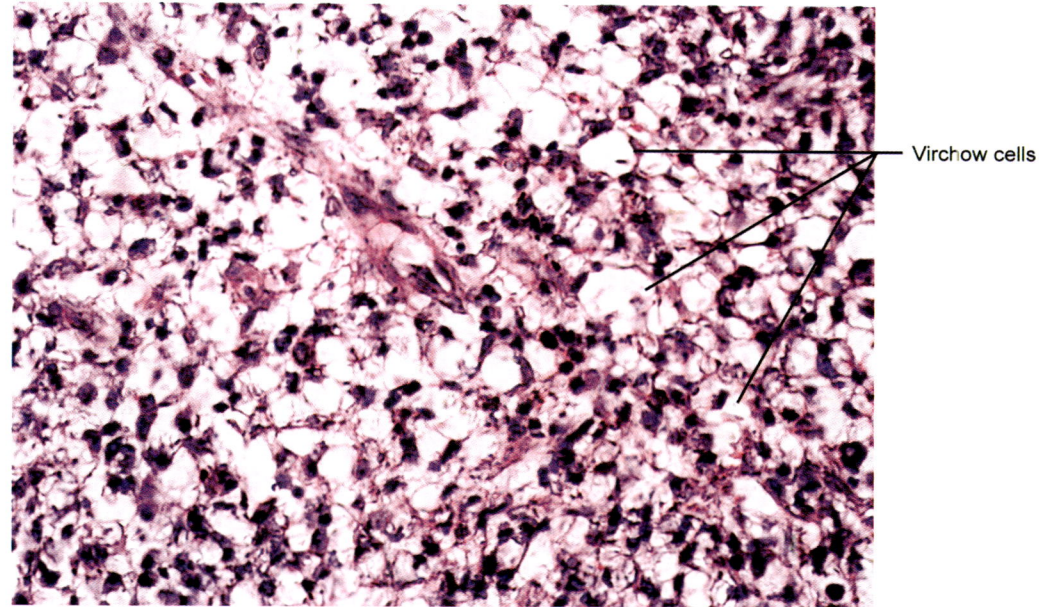

Fig. 33.8: Lepromatous leprosy

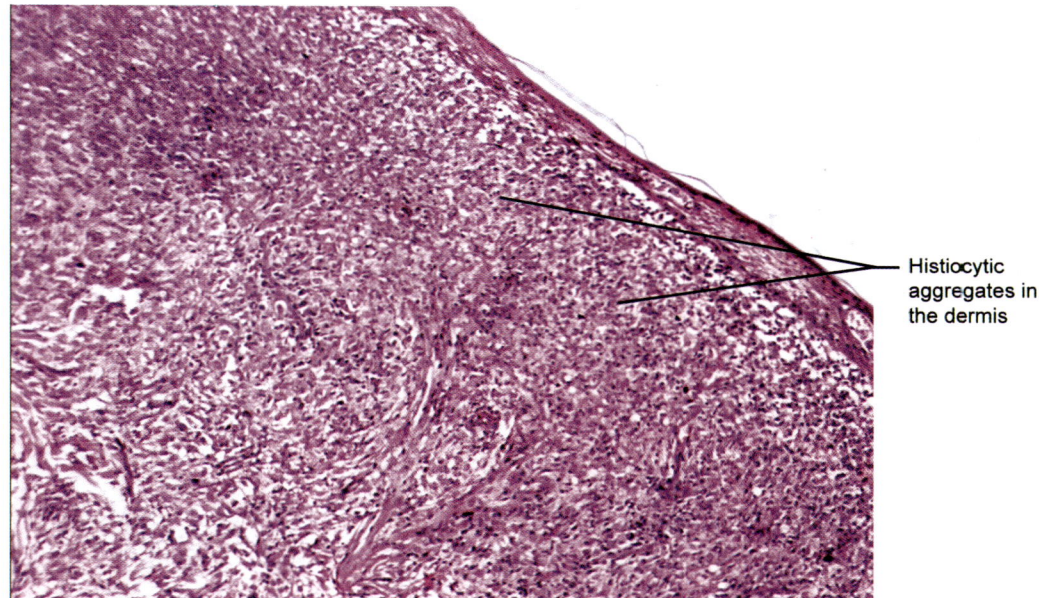

Fig. 33.9: Histioid leprosy

2. *Type I downgrading reaction*
   – Decreased lymphocytes and epithelioid cells
   – Increased number of macrophages, containing bacilli

Type II Lepra Reaction

- Also known as erythema nodosum leprosum (ENL)
- Cause—due to immune complex mediated vasculitis
- Seen in lepromatous leprosy (LL) following initiation of the treatment

- Presents as painful, erythematous cutaneous nodules involving the extremities

Histopathology

- Papillary dermis shows edema
- Dermis shows neutrophilic and lymphocytic infiltrate with macrophages containing bacilli
- Macrophages can be seen extending up to the subcutaneous fat
- Septal and lobular panniculitis can be seen
- Vasculitis is often present

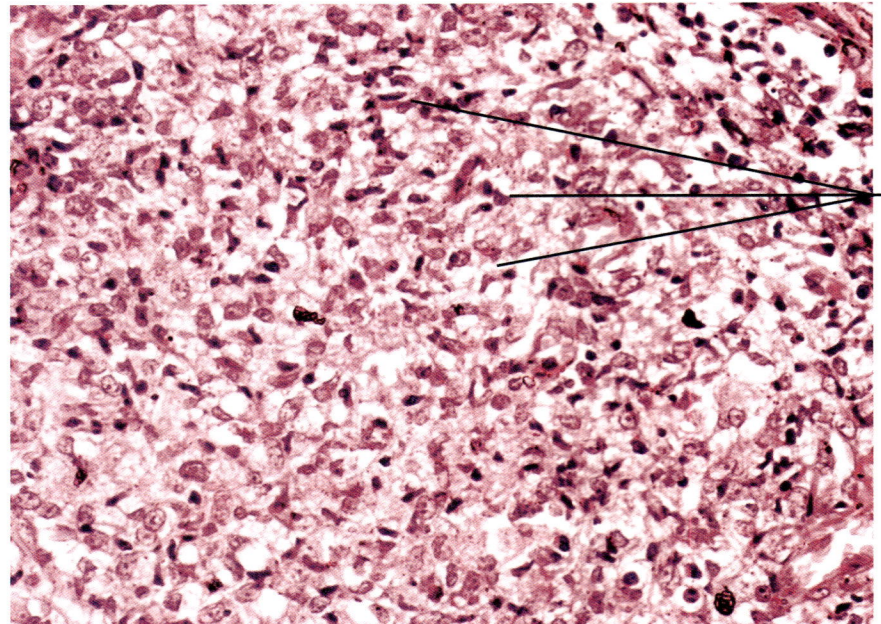

Spindle shaped cells/ histiocytes within the dermis

Fig. 33.10: Histioid leprosy

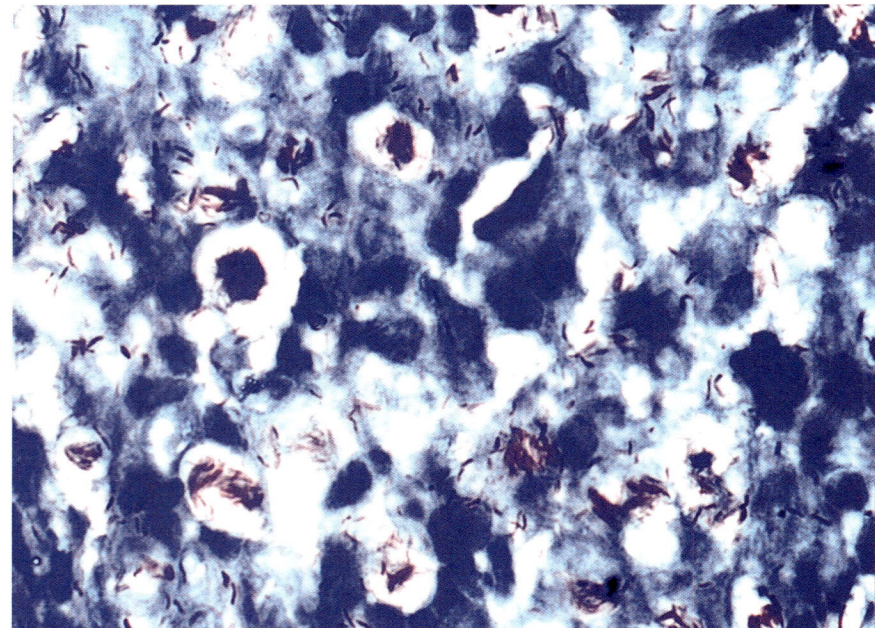

Fig. 33.11: Fite stain demonstrating numerous acid-fast bacilli within macrophages

Lucio's Phenomenon
- Patients present as nodules or ulcers on extremities
- Seen in lepromatous leprosy (LL) patients

Histopathology
- Vasculitis of the vessel wall in upper and mid-dermis
- Epidermal and dermal necrosis can be seen
- Vessel wall shows endothelial cell swelling
- Endothelial cells and macrophages show numerous bacilli

Ancillary Tests
- Polymerase chain reaction
- Special stains—modified Ziehl-Neelsen (Fite-Faraco) stain which stains organisms bright red (Fig. 33.11)

Bacillary Index (BI)

0 : No bacilli visualized
1 : 1 to 10 bacilli in 10 to 100 high power fields (hpf)
2 : 1 to 10 bacilli in 1 to 10 hpf
3 : 1 to 10 bacilli per hpf
4 : 10 to 100 bacilli per hpf
5 : 100 to 1000 bacilli per hpf
6 : > 1000 bacilli per hpf

Differential Diagnosis

1. ***Tuberculoid leprosy (TT) has to be differentiated from***
   – Tuberculosis, atypical mycobacterial infections, histoplasmosis, cat-scratch disease, syphilis and other infectious granulomatous diseases
2. ***Lepromatous leprosy has to be differentiated from***
   – Xanthomas, rhinoscleroma, malakoplakia, leishmaniasis, atypical mycobacterial infections
3. ***Histioid leprosy has to be differentiated from***
   – Fibrohistiocytoma

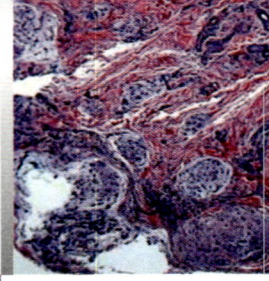

Mycobacterial Infections

CUTANEOUS TUBERCULOSIS

Infection of the skin by *Mycobacterium tuberculosis* can occur by three routes
1. **Direct inoculation**—e.g. primary chancre, tuberculosis verrucosa cutis
2. **Hematogenous spread**—e.g. lupus vulgaris, miliary tuberculosis
3. **Spread by direct extension**—e.g. scrofuloderma

Primary Cutaneous Tuberculosis

* Rare
* Causes—direct inoculation, needle stick injury
* Manifests as tuberculous chancre (crust covered ulcer)

Histopathology (Fig. 34.1)

* Dermis shows neutrophils, lymphocytes, plasma cells
* Over the course of disease, caseous necrosis, epithelioid histiocytic granulomas and Langhans multinucleated giant cells are seen

Tuberculosis Verrucosa Cutis

* Presents as a verrucous plaque with fissures and discharging pus (Fig. 34.2)
* Sites—hands, knees, buttocks, thighs

Histopathology

* Acanthotic, hyperkeratotic stratified squamous epithelium
* Upper dermis—abscess formation
* Mid-dermis—tuberculoid granulomas with necrosis
* Tubercle bacilli can be demonstrated by Ziehl-Neelsen stain

Lupus Vulgaris

* Site—head and neck
* Presents as red-brown patch to nodule, which can undergo atrophic change
* Characteristic feature—new lesions develop over the areas of atrophy

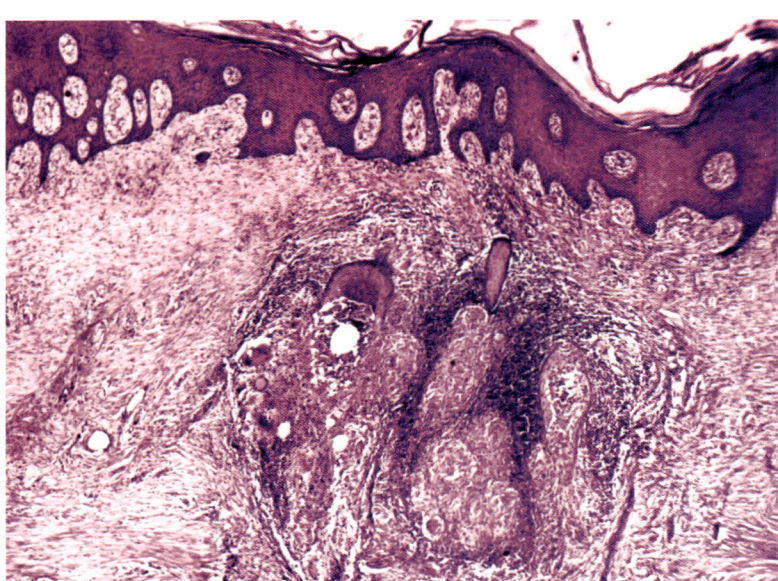

Fig. 34.1: Cutaneous tuberculosis. Confluent caseating epithelioid histiocytic granulomas in dermis

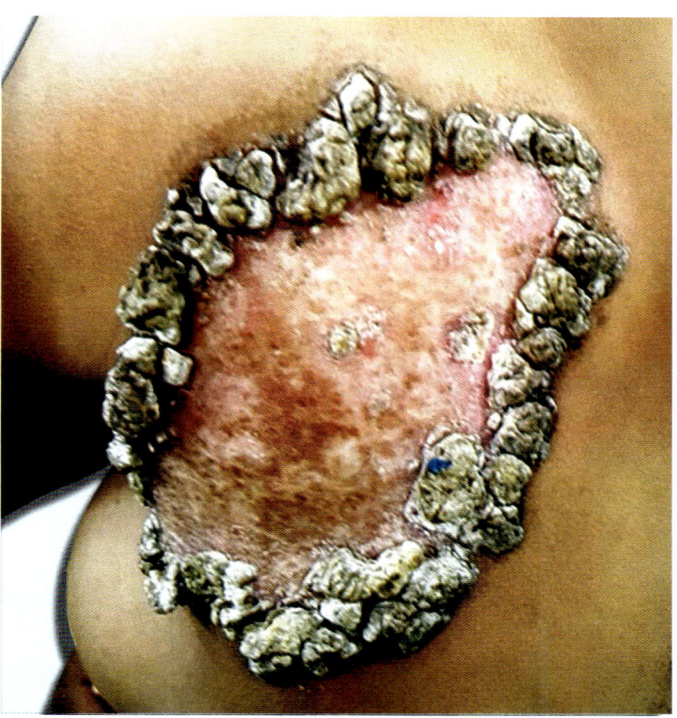

Fig. 34.2: Tuberculosis verrucosa cutis. Painless, violaceous, indurated warty plaques growing via peripheral extension with central clearing and atrophy

- Rarely, squamous cell carcinoma can develop at margins of the ulcer
- Cause—due to reactivation of primary tuberculosis

Histopathology (Figs 34.3 and 34.4)

- Epidermis—can show atrophy or features of acanthosis, hyperkeratosis and papillomatosis
- Dermis—shows confluent epithelioid histiocytic granulomas with or without caseous necrosis and dense infiltrate of lymphocytes

Miliary Tuberculosis

- Presents as erythematous papules and pustules measuring 2–5 mm in diameter

Scrofuloderma (Figs 34.5 and 34.6)

- Tuberculous involvement of skin resulting from the direct extension from an underlying focus of tuberculosis in a bone or lymph node

TUBERCULIDS

Lichen Scrofulosorum

- Presents as yellow-brown follicular papules
- Size—0.5–3.0 mm in diameter
- Most common site—trunk

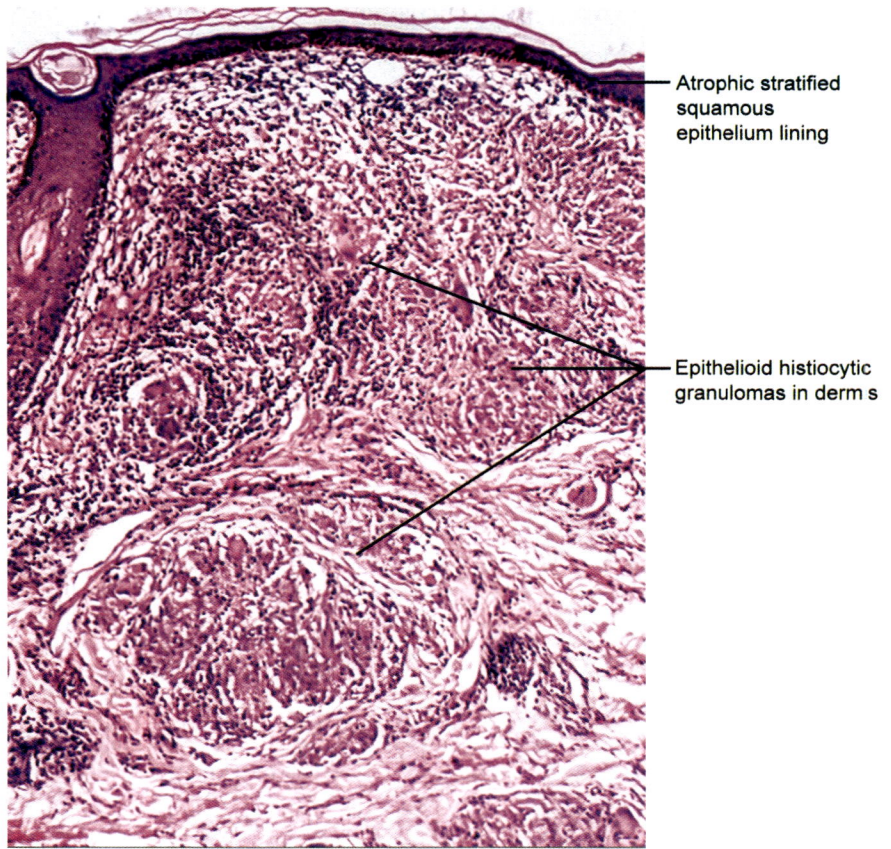

Atrophic stratified squamous epithelium lining

Epithelioid histiocytic granulomas in derm s

Fig. 34.3: Lupus vulgaris

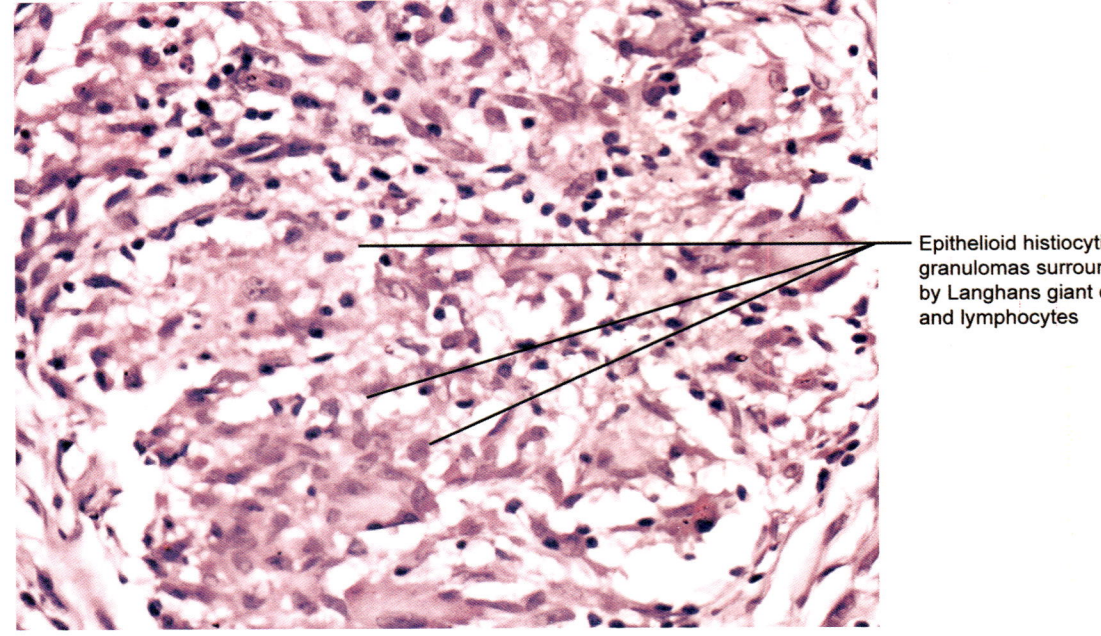

Epithelioid histiocytic granulomas surrounded by Langhans giant cells and lymphocytes

Fig. 34.4: Lupus vulgaris

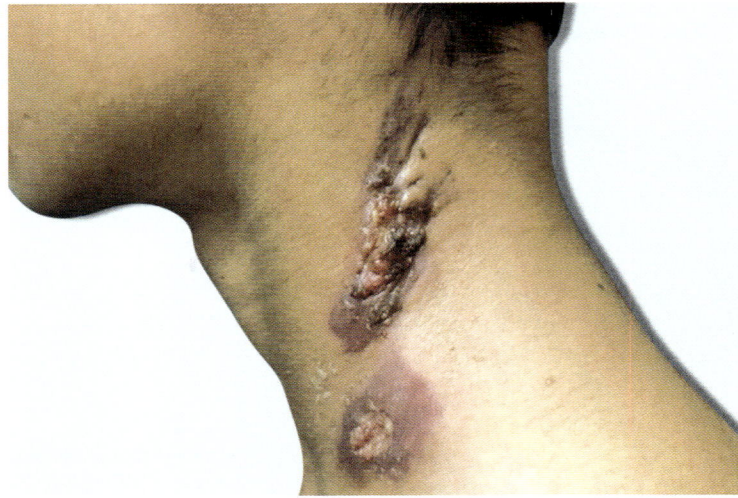

Fig. 34.5: Scrofuloderma. Firm, painless, red-brown nodules that overly foci of tuberculous infection. Nodules enlarge and form ulcers and sinus tracts that drain watery, purulent material

- Occurs due to hematogenous spread of acid-fast bacilli to the skin

Histopathology

- Superficial dermal epithelioid histiocytic granulomas, seen in close proximity to the hair follicles/sweat glands
- Absence of caseous necrosis and tubercle bacilli

GRANULOMATOUS ROSACEA

- Associated with HIV infection
- Most common sites—cheeks, chin, nose, forehead
- Early lesions show perivascular lymphocytic infiltrate
- Older lesions show tuberculoid granuloma comprising of epithelioid histiocytes and Langhans giant cells (Figs 34.7 and 34.8)

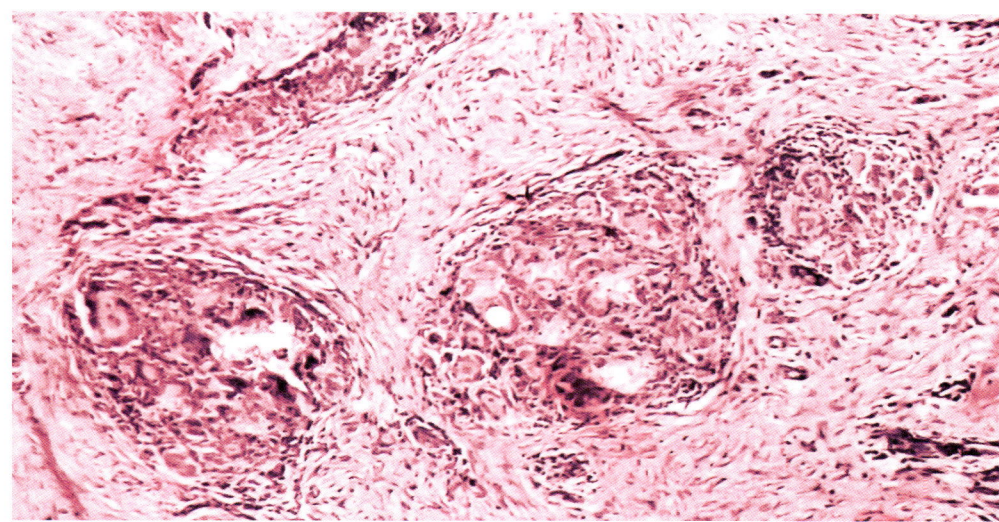

Fig. 34.6: Scrofuloderma. Dermal epithelioid histiocytic granulomas with surrounding Langhans giant cells

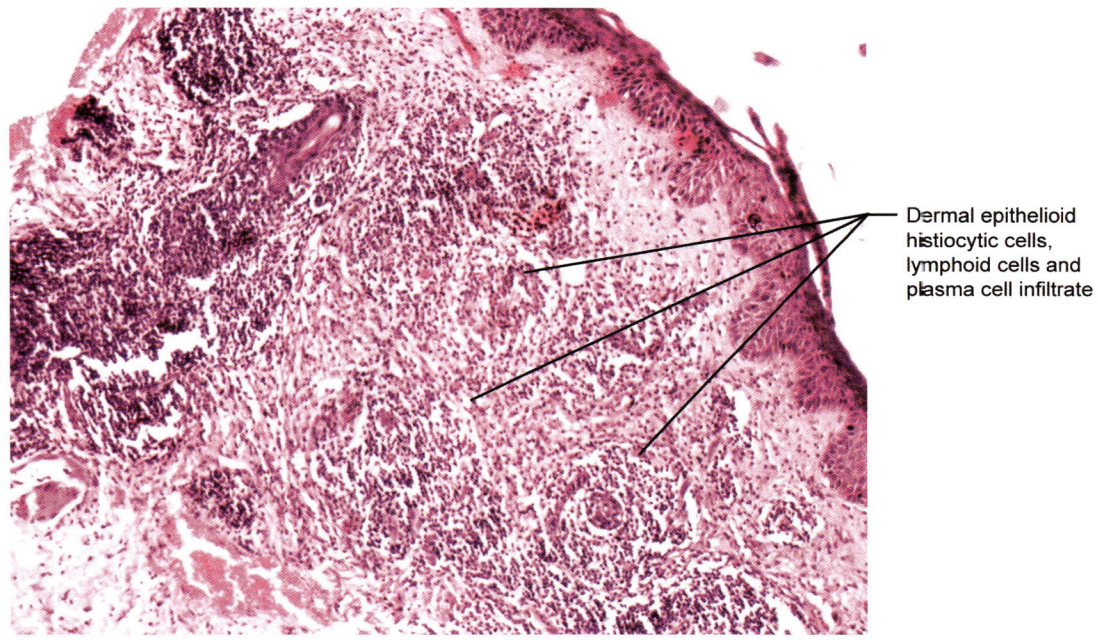

Dermal epithelioid histiocytic cells, lymphoid cells and plasma cell infiltrate

Fig. 34.7: Granulomatous rosacea

- Perifollicular arrangement of epithelioid histiocytic granulomas are also seen

NON-TUBERCULAR MYCOBACTERIUM

Examples

1. *Mycobacterium avium-intracellulare*
   - Most commonly affects immunocompromised individuals
   - Presents as cutaneous papules and nodules

Histopathology

a. Granulomas and mixed inflammatory cell infiltrate or
b. Macrophages containing large number of bacilli without necrosis

2. *Mycobacterium marinum*
   - Exposure to bacilli occurs in the swimming pools or aquariums
   - Sites – fingers, knees, elbows, feet

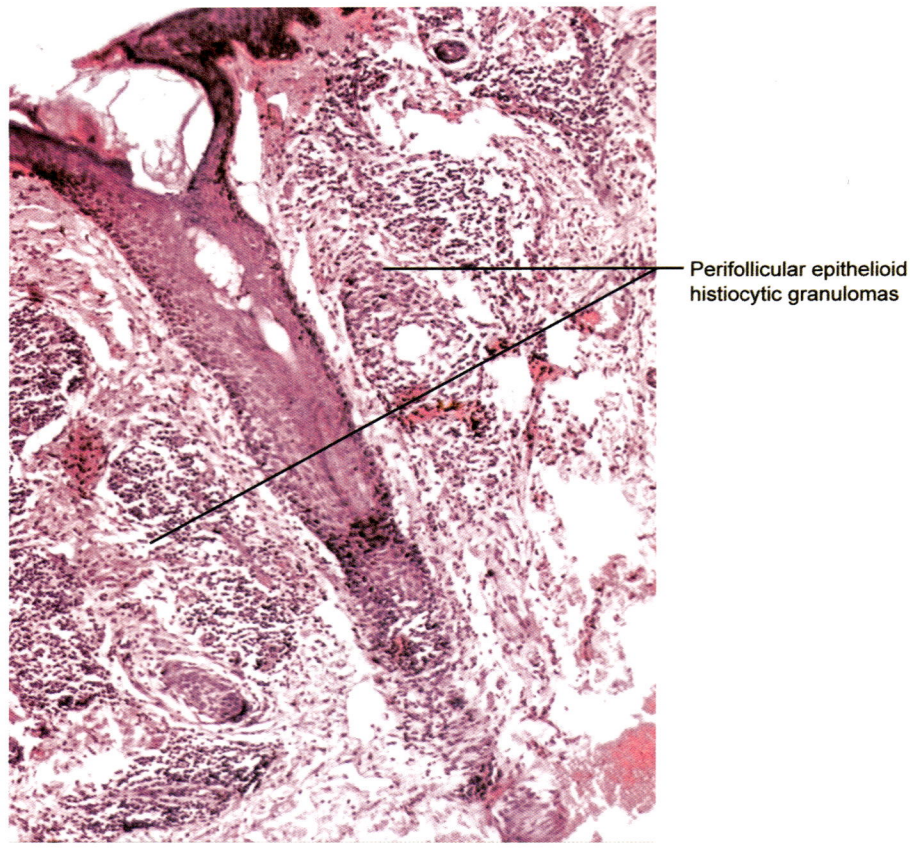

Perifollicular epithelioid histiocytic granulomas

Fig. 34.8: Granulomatous rosacea

Histopathology
a. Pseudoepitheliomatous epidermal hyperplasia
b. Inflammatory cell infiltrate in upper dermis
c. Few small epithelioid histiocytic granulomas

3. *Mycobacterium ulcerans (Buruli ulcer)*
   – Most commonly affects children and young adults
   – Presents as papules or pustules or painless ulcers over the extremities

Histopathology
   – Extensive coagulative necrosis of dermal collagen and subcutaneous fat
   – Extensive fat necrosis
   – Ziehl-Neelsen stain shows clumps of acid-fast bacilli within fat necrosis

DIFFERENTIAL DIAGNOSIS

Leprosy (Tuberculoid)
• Well-formed granulomas with multinucleated histiocytic giant cells surrounded by lymphocytes
• Fite-stain for acid-fast bacilli—positive

Fungal Infection
• Pseudo-epitheliomatous hyperplasia
• Fungal organisms can be demonstrated by GMS or PAS stain

Sarcoidosis
• Naked granulomas with sparse lymphocytic infiltrate
• Absence of caseous necrosis

Foreign Body Granuloma
• Foreign body giant cell reaction surrounding the foreign material
• Absence of caseous necrosis

LUPUS MILIARIS DISSEMINATUS FACIEI
• Presents as yellow brown papules
• Sites—face, eyebrow, eyelids
• Presents as papular lesions over the face, which can progress to scar
• Age group—adolescents and young adults
• **Histopathology**—dermis shows necrosis surrounded by epithelioid cell granulomas (Figs 34.9 and 34.10)

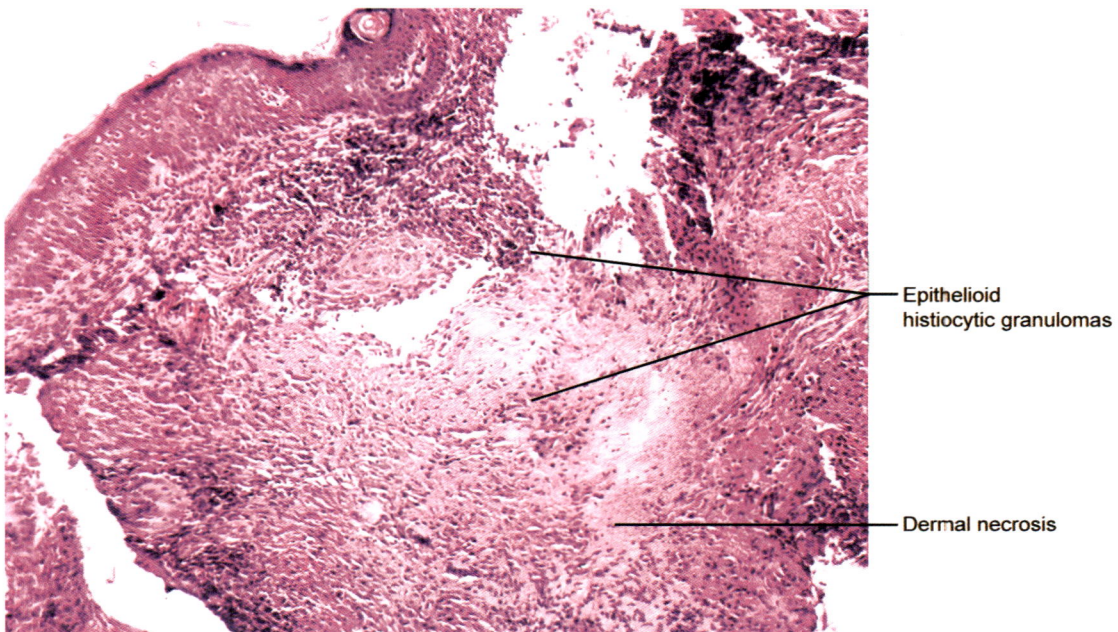

Epithelioid histiocytic granulomas

Dermal necrosis

Fig. 34.9: Lupus miliaris

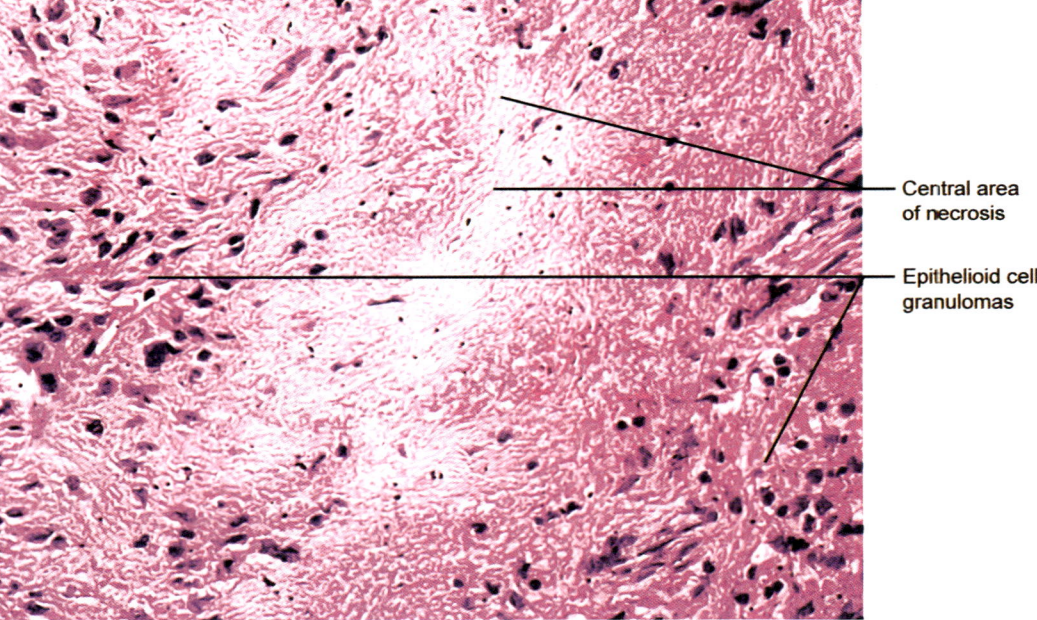

Central area of necrosis

Epithelioid cell granulomas

Fig. 34.10: Lupus miliaris

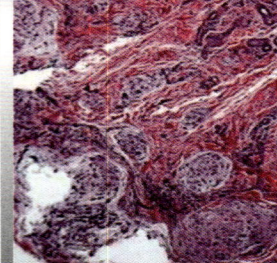

Necrobiosis Lipoidica

INTRODUCTION

- Most commonly affects diabetic patients
- Presents as yellow brown patches or plaques
- Sites—lower extremities/shins (most common), ankles, calf, thigh

HISTOPATHOLOGY (Figs 35.1 and 35.2)

- Epidermis—thinned out, normal or thickened
- Mid-dermis and deep dermis show granulomas, degenerated collagen (necrobiosis), and sclerosis
- Histiocytes and giant cells (Langhans, Touton and foreign body type) are commonly found
- Palisades of histiocytes around the degenerated collagen
- Absence of mucin

- Perivascular lymphocytic infiltrate
- Blood vessel wall thickening with endothelial cell proliferation is seen in mid-dermis and deep dermis

DIFFERENTIAL DIAGNOSIS

Granuloma Annulare

- Dermis shows degenerated collagen bundles and mucin
- Colloidal iron or alcian blue is used to demonstrate mucin

Mycobacterium Infection

- Granulomas with caseation necrosis, multinucleated giant cells, lymphocytic infiltrate
- Mycobacterium can be demonstrated by Ziehl-Neelsen stain

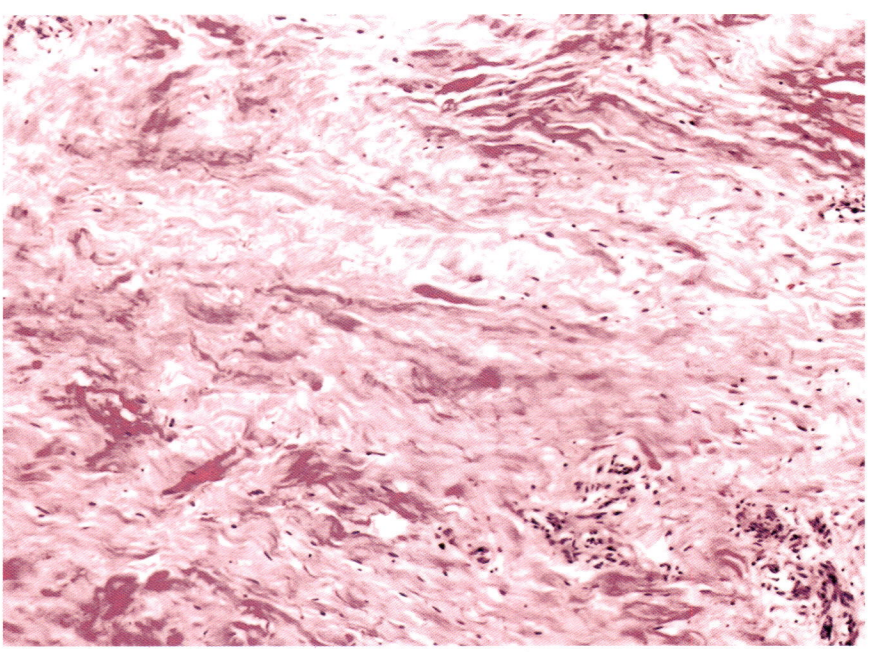

Fig. 35.1: Degenerated collagen in necrobiosis lipoidica

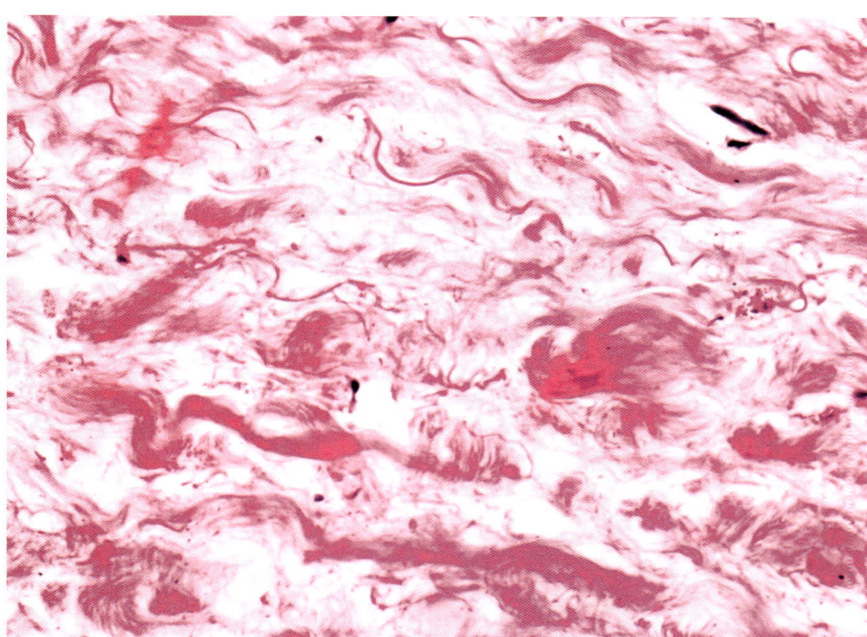

Fig. 35.2: Necrobiosis lipoidica. Degenerated collagen bundles

Necrobiotic Xanthogranuloma

- Dense inflammation with foamy histiocytes
- Extensive inflammation of subcutis
- Granulomatous inflammation of the vessel wall with thrombosis

Sarcoidosis

- Epithelioid histiocytic aggregates (can also be seen in necrobiosis lipoidica)
- Absence of collagen degradation

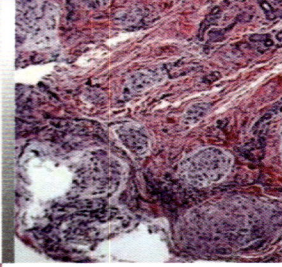

Sarcoidosis

INTRODUCTION

- Systemic granulomatous disease
- Cutaneous involvement—lesions present as red-brown papules, nodules and plaques
- Sites—most commonly affects lungs, lymph nodes, liver, spleen, eyes and skin
- Lupus pernio—when plaques or papules are situated on nose, cheeks and ears

HISTOPATHOLOGY (Figs 36.1 to 36.4)

- Epidermis is normal
- Well-circumscribed, nodular aggregates of epithelioid histiocytes in the dermis forming noncaseating granulomas (which are scattered throughout the dermis)
- Sparse or no lymphocytes seen at the periphery of epithelioid cell granulomas (naked granuloma)

- Epithelioid histiocytes can extend into the subcutaneous tissue
- Multi-nucleated giant cells (Langhan's type) are seen admixed with epithelioid histiocytic aggregates
- Asteroid bodies: Star-shaped eosinophilic inclusions with radiating spikes, seen in multi-nucleated giant cells (Fig. 36.4)
- Schaumann bodies: Concentric calcium complexes, within giant cells
- Lupus pernio: Associated with dense lymphocytic infiltrate

DIFFERENTIAL DIAGNOSIS

Foreign Body Granuloma

- Foreign body material is seen
- Granulomas with foreign body type giant cells

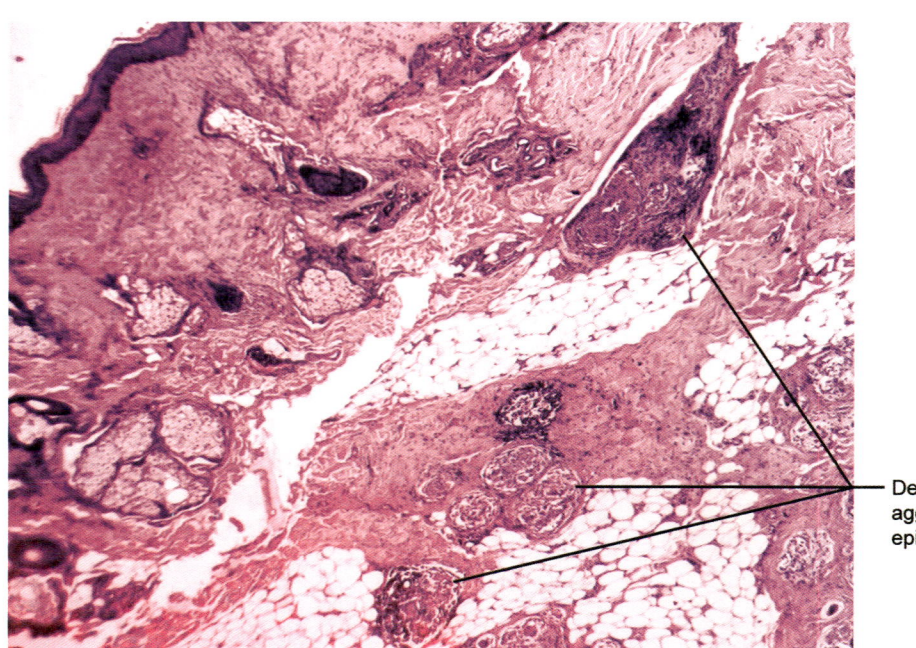

Dermis with nodular aggregates of epithelioid histiocytes

Fig. 36.1: Sarcoidosis

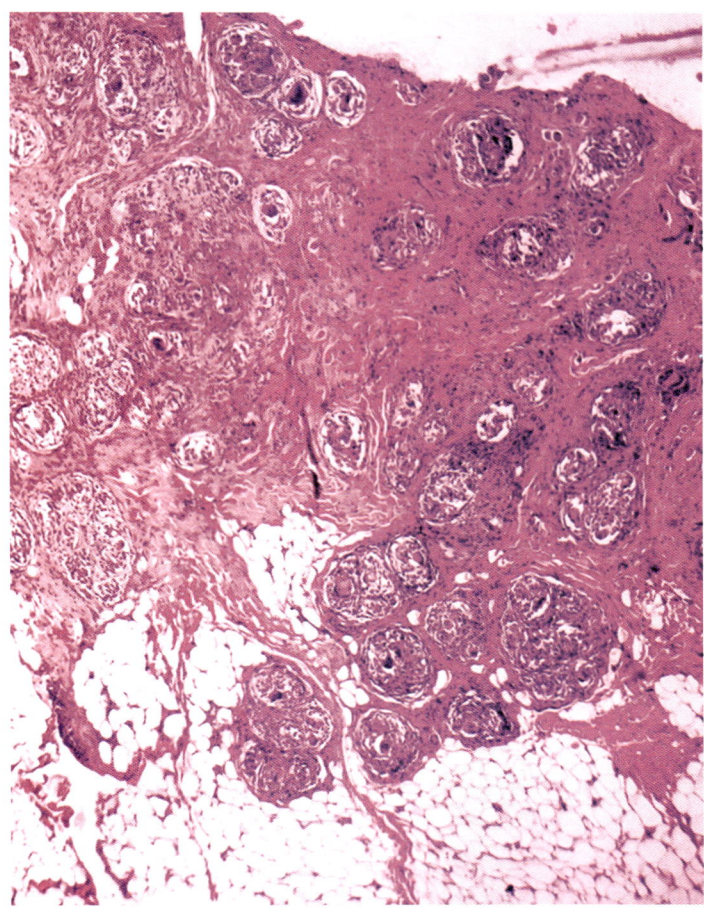

Fig. 36.2: Numerous epithelioid histiocytic granulomas in dermis and subcutis

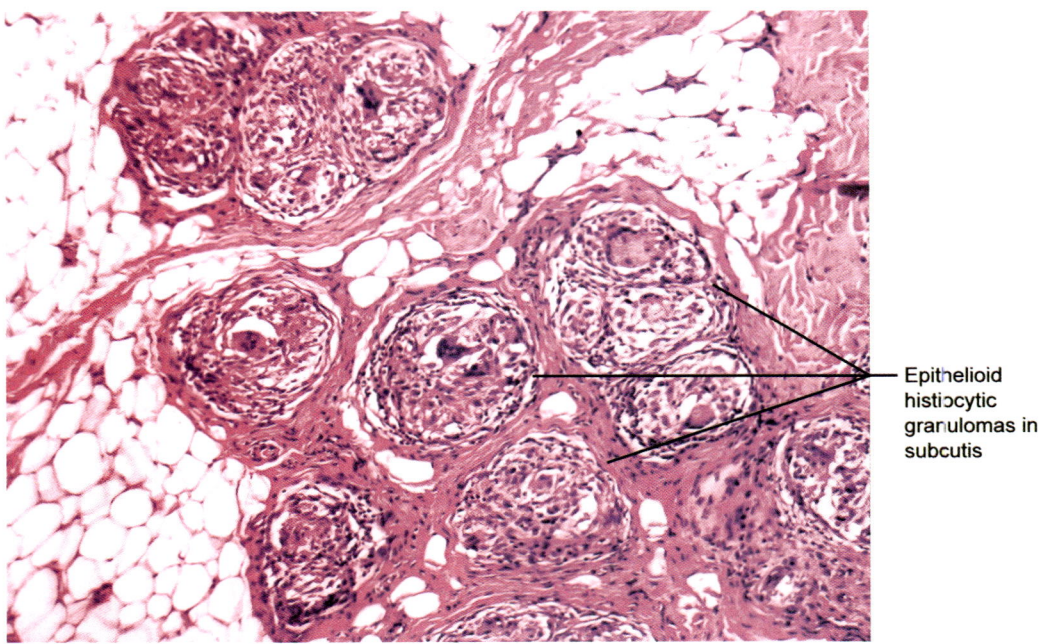

Epithelioid histiocytic granulomas in subcutis

Fig. 36.3: Sarcoidosis

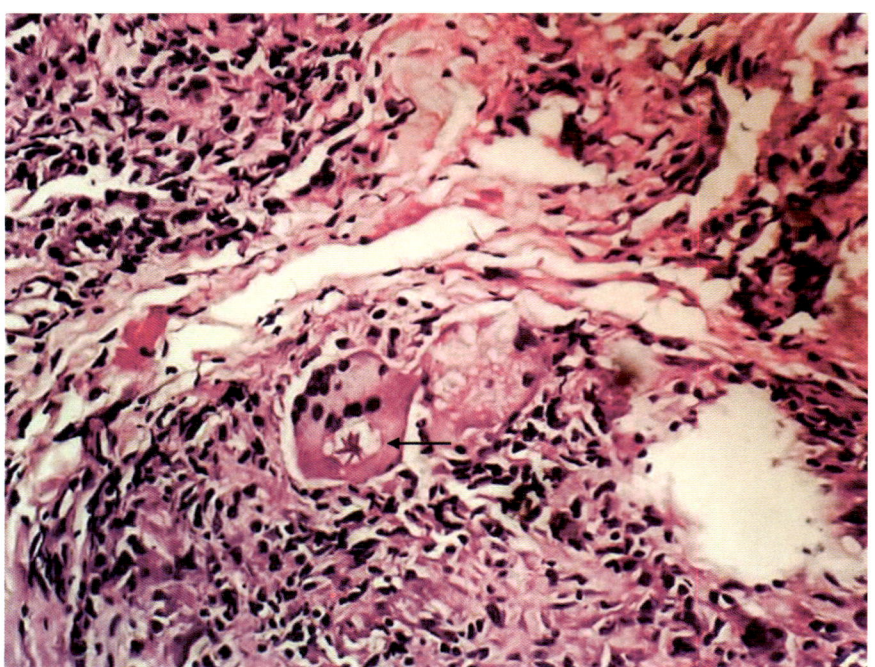

Fig. 36.4: Asteroid body seen in multinucleated giant cell (arrow)

Cutaneous Tuberculosis

- Caseating granulomas with central necrosis
- AFB stain demonstrates mycobacterium bacilli

Tuberculoid Leprosy

- Epithelioid histiocytic granulomas surrounding the nerve fibers
- Granulomas show small areas of central necrosis

Lupus Vulgaris

- Epidermis—acanthotic, ulcerated with pseudo-epitheliomatous hyperplasia
- Marked inflammatory cell reaction around and in between the granulomas
- Granulomas and infiltrate are located close to the epidermis

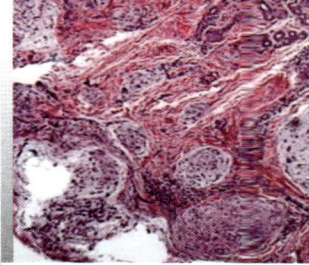

Syphilis

INTRODUCTION

- Sexually transmitted disease
- Causative organism: *Treponema pallidum*
- Three stages: Primary, secondary and tertiary

STAGE I/PRIMARY SYPHILIS

- Hard, painless, indurated papule, nodule or plaque (chancre) containing organisms (Fig. 37.1)
- Sites—genitals, perianal skin
- Serous exudates from the ulcer contain numerous treponemes

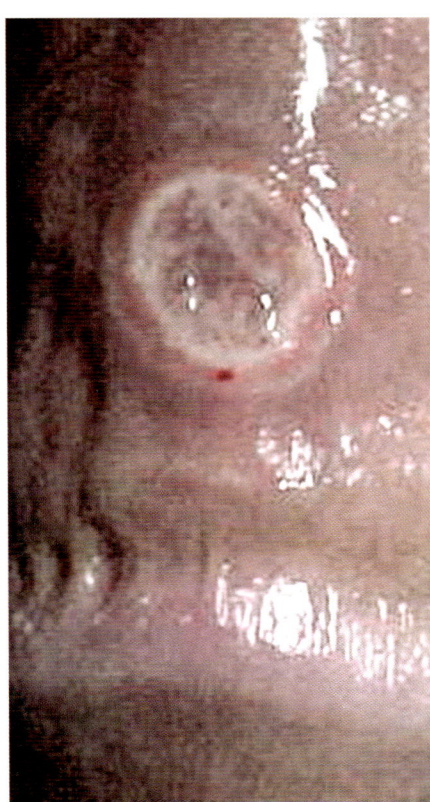

Fig. 37.1: Syphilis (primary chancre). Ulcer with raised indurated margin and a nonexudative base

Histopathology

- Epidermis—acanthosis, spongiosis, exocytosis of lymphocytes and neutrophils, ulceration
- Dermis—edema with dense, perivascular lympho-histiocytic infiltrate
- Endarteritis obliterans—endothelial cell swelling and hyperplasia, lymphohistiocytic infiltrate with luminal attenuation
- Warthin-Starry silver stain can highlight the organism

STAGE II/SECONDARY SYPHILIS

- Develops 4–8 weeks after chancre development
- Due to hematogenous spread of the organism
- Lesions present as brown-red macules, papules and nodules (Fig. 37.2)
- Verrucous lesions seen in anogenital area (Condylomata lata)

Histopathology (Fig. 37.3)

- Epidermis—orthohyperparakeratotic psoriasiform epidermal hyperplasia, spongiosis, basal cell layer vacuolation, interface lymphocytic dermatitis
- Dermis—marked papillary dermal edema, perivascular-periadnexal lymphohistiocytic and plasma cell infiltrate

STAGE III/TERTIARY SYPHILIS

Can present as:
- Lesions confined to the skin or
- Gummatous lesions—involving the skin, bone and liver or
- Systemic involvement—cardiovascular and neurological disorders

Histopathology (Figs 37.4 and 37.5)

- **Lesions confined to the skin**—shows epithelioid histiocytic granulomas in dermis and multinucleated giant cells

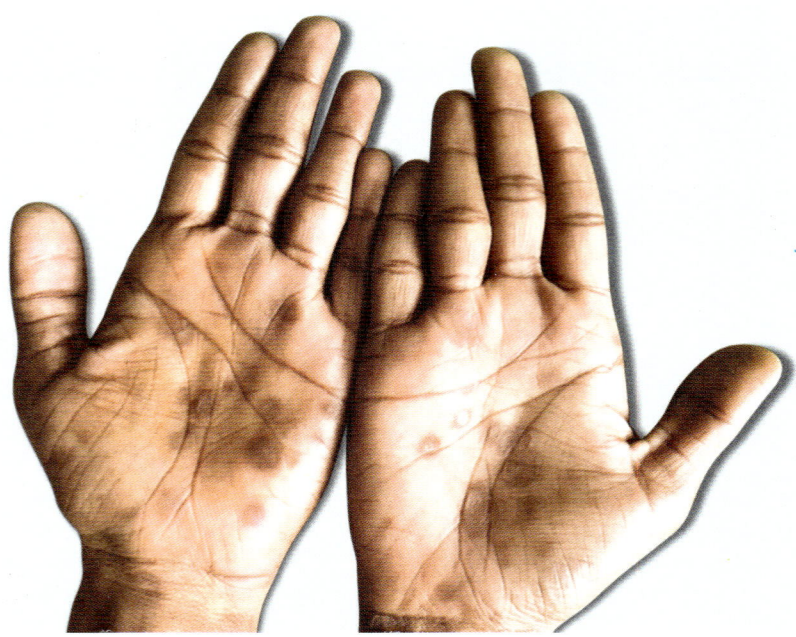

Fig. 37.2: Secondary syphilis. Symmetrical macular or papular eruption. Individual lesions are discrete, copper-red or reddish-brown

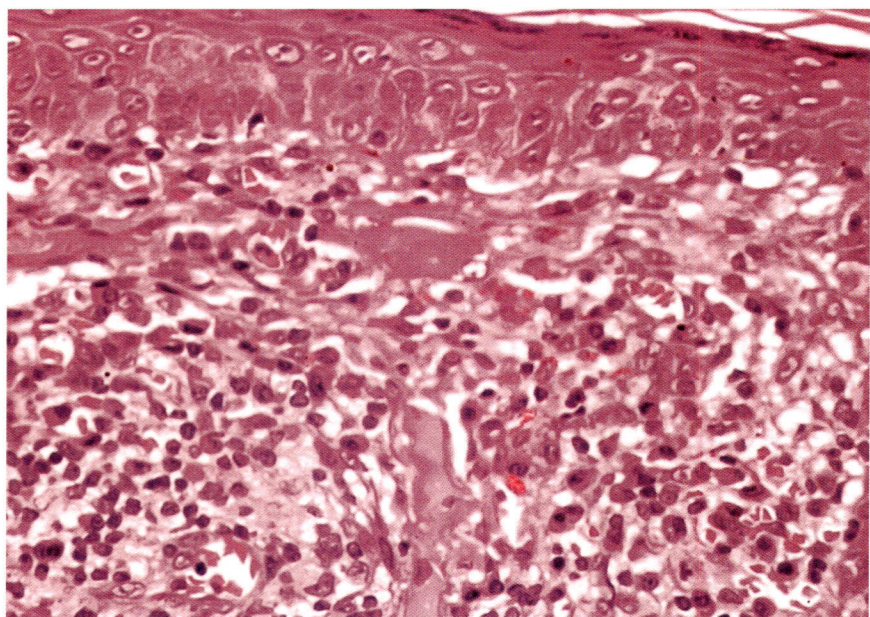

Fig. 37.3: Secondary syphilis. Dermis shows dense perivascular lymphoplasmacytic infiltrate

- **Gummatous lesions**—granulomatous inflammation with central zones of necrosis and endarteritis obliterans in cutaneous lesions
- **Systemic involvement**
  - *Cardiovascular syphilis*—arterial fibrosis, with neovascularization
  - *Meningeal syphilis*—endarteritis obliterans of the meningeal vessels

ANCILLARY TESTS

Immunohistochemistry
- Most sensitive test for diagnosis of *Treponema pallidum* infection
- Polyclonal antibody directed against *T. pallidum* for identifying the organism
- Spirochetes can be found in epidermis, upper dermis and around blood vessels

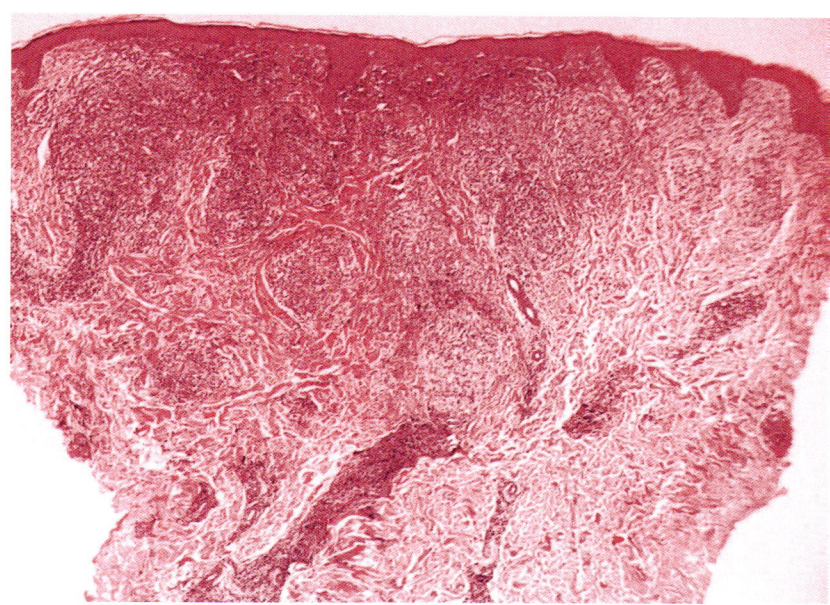

Fig. 37.4: Tertiary syphilis. Confluent epithelioid histiocytic granulomas in dermis

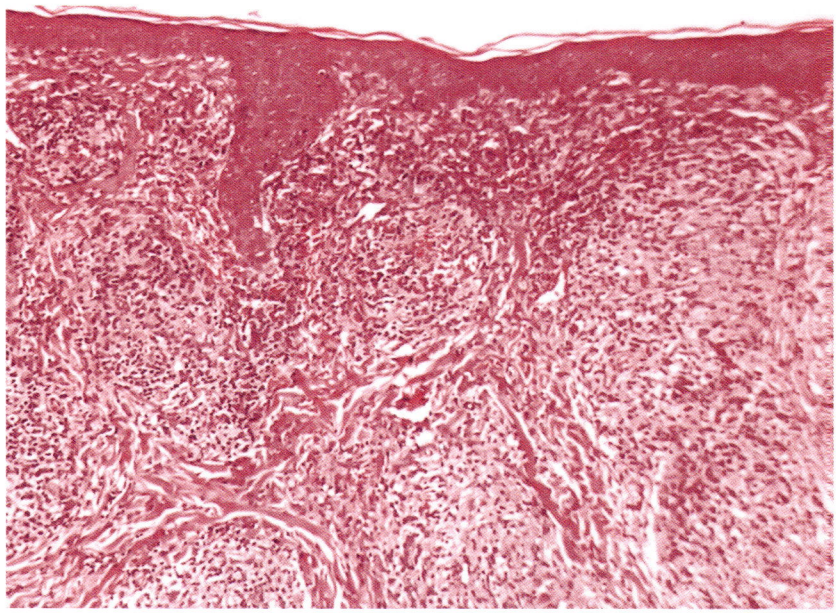

Fig. 37.5: Tertiary syphilis with dermal granulomas

DIFFERENTIAL DIAGNOSIS

Lichen Planus

- Compact orthokeratosis, acanthosis, hypergranulosis, saw-toothed rete-ridges
- Lichenoid interface dermatitis with basal cell layer vacuolization and colloid bodies

Psoriasis

- Psoriasiform hyperplasia often with neutrophils in stratum corneum

Pityriasis Lichenoides

- Perivascular lymphocytic infiltrate in the mid-dermis without plasma cells
- Apoptotic keratinocytes, exocytosis of lymphocytes and erythrocytes

Acrodermatitis Chronica Atrophicans

- Atrophic epidermis
- Numerous dilated blood vessels with perivascular plasma cell infiltrate

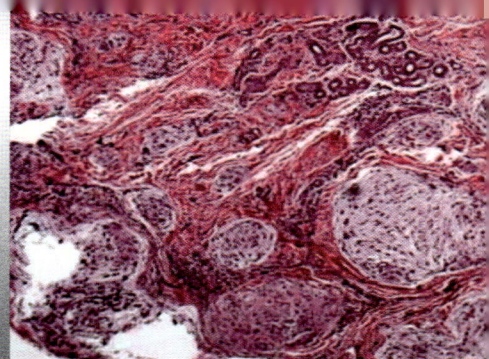

Degenerating Diseases, Perforating Disorders and Metabolic Diseases Affecting Skin

Part 6

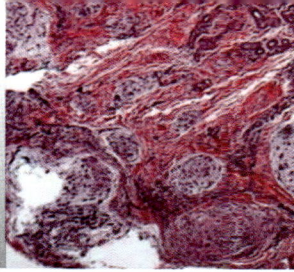

Acanthosis Nigricans

INTRODUCTION

- Presents as symmetrical, velvety, pigmented plaques
- Sites—axillae, lips, oral mucosa, neck, face, palms, sole, and knuckles
- Associated with carcinomas (gastrointestinal tract, kidney, liver, lung, bladder), endocrine disorders (hyper-insulinemia, obesity), genetic disorders (Down's syndrome) and drugs (corticosteroids, niacin, OCPs)

HISTOPATHOLOGY (Figs 38.1 and 38.2)

- Acanthosis, papillomatosis and hyperkeratosis

- Papillomatosis produces intervening valleys
- Hyperpigmentation of the basal layer

DIFFERENTIAL DIAGNOSIS

Linear Epidermal Nevi

- Marked acanthosis
- Orthokeratotic stratum corneum
- Rudimentary pilosebaceous units

Hypertrophic Type of Seborrheic Keratosis

- Marked acanthosis
- Presence of horn cysts and pseudohorn cysts

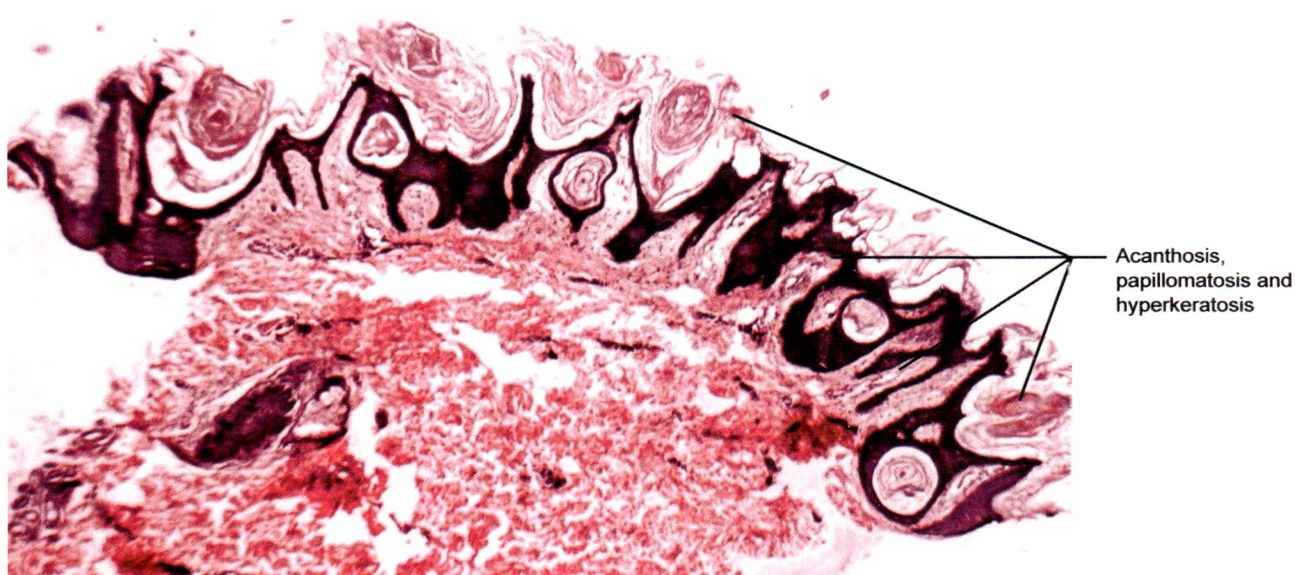

Acanthosis, papillomatosis and hyperkeratosis

Fig. 38.1: Acanthosis nigricans

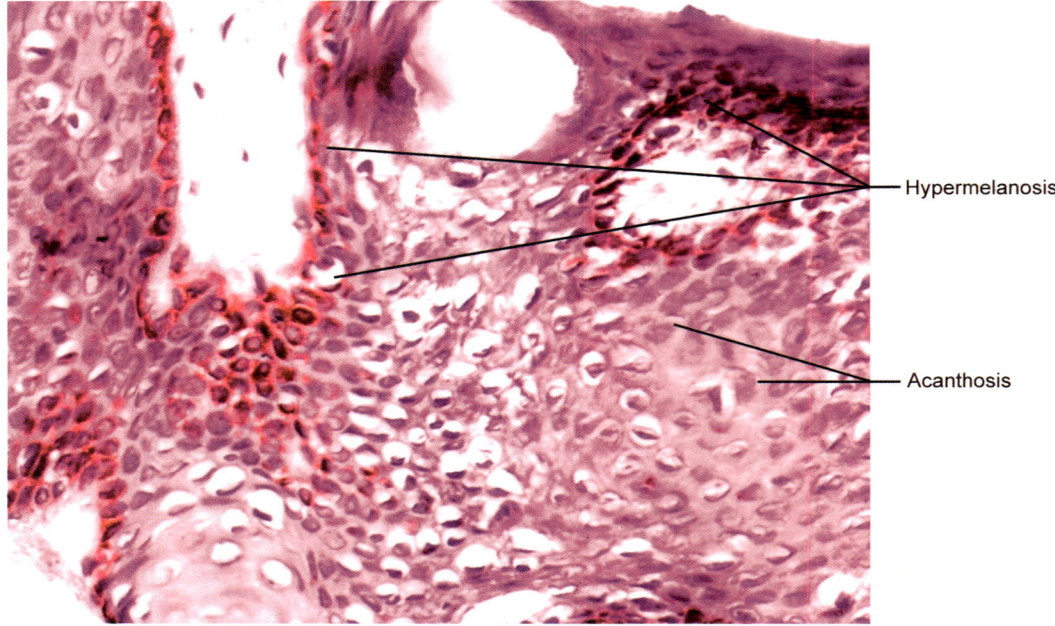

Fig. 38.2: Acanthosis nigricans

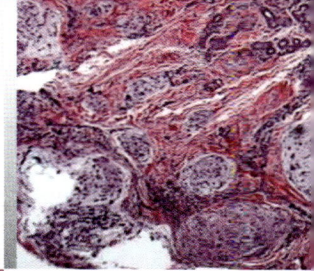

Calcinosis Cutis

INTRODUCTION

- Idiopathic deposition of calcium salts

PRESENTATION

Can present as:
1. Solitary nodule on head (ear)
2. Single or multiple lesions over the scrotum
3. Deposits on periarticular soft tissue over joints (Tumoral calcinosis)
4. Small nodules in the genital area, thighs, knees
5. Deposits seen in dystrophic and metastatic calcification
6. Calcification of the vessel wall of the dermis and subcutis (Calciphylaxis)
7. Calcification arising in trichilemmal cysts, pilomatricoma, epidermal inclusion cysts, trichoepithelioma

HISTOPATHOLOGY (Figs 39.1 to 39.3)

- Small to large subcutaneous calcium deposits
- In calciphylaxis, calcification is seen in the vessel walls

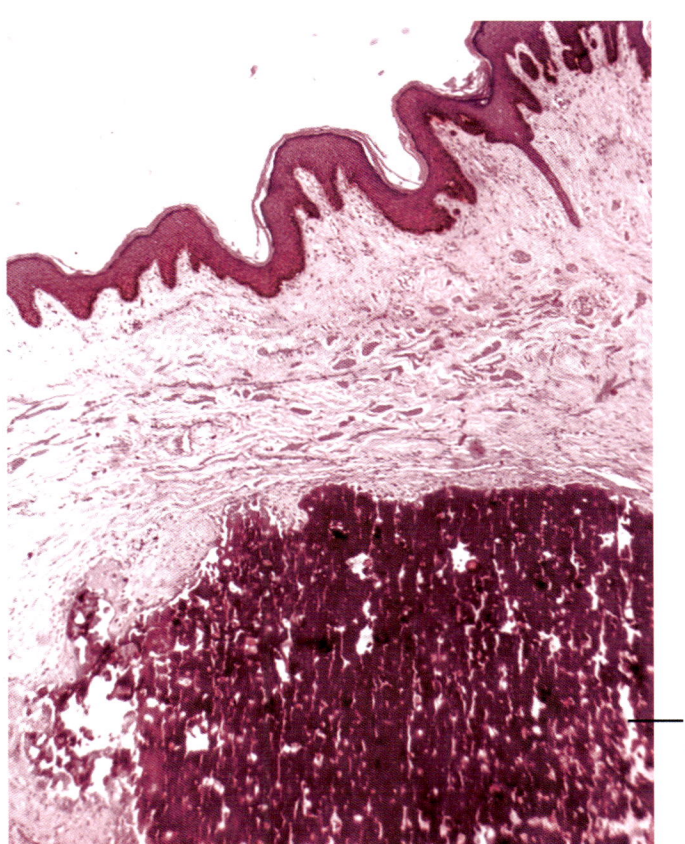

—— Dermal calcium deposits

Fig. 39.1: Calcinosis cutis

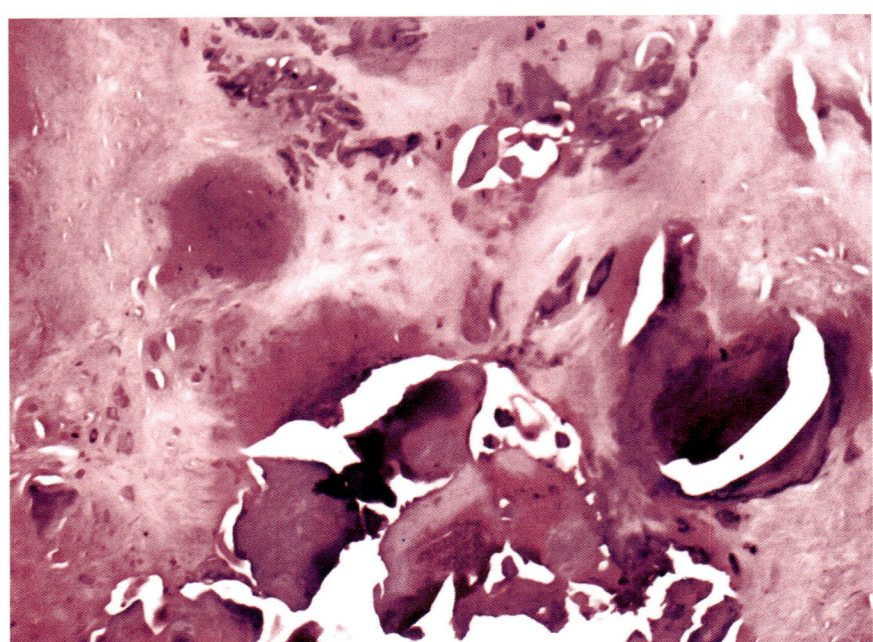

Fig. 39.2: Calcinosis cutis

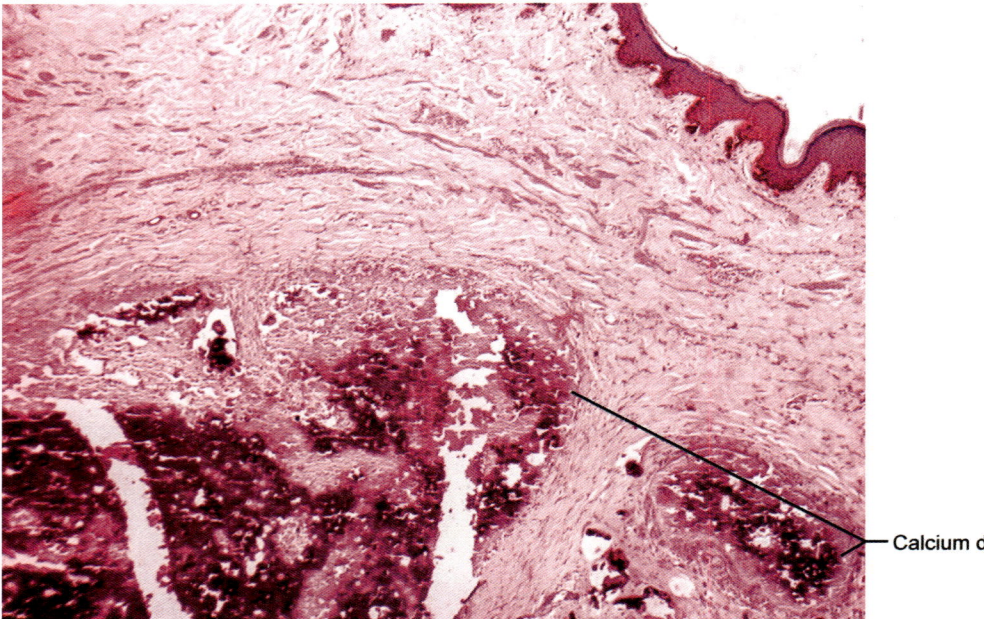

Calcium deposits

Fig. 39.3: Idiopathic scrotal calcinosis cutis

- On hematoxylin and eosin stain, calcium deposits appear deeply basophilic/deep blue

- On von Kossa silver stain, these calcium salts appear black in color

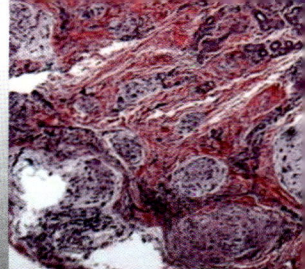

Chondrodermatitis Nodularis Helicis

INTRODUCTION

- Presents as a single, tender, erythematous nodule on the upper part of ear
- Age group—affects male above 40 years of age
- Cause—attempt at trans-epidermal elimination of the dermal collagen (perforating dermatosis)

HISTOPATHOLOGY

- Central epidermis shows a defect with surrounding epidermis showing features of acanthosis, hyperkeratosis and parakeratosis
- Underneath the defect, dermis shows fibrinoid degeneration of the collagen
- Fibrous thickening of the perichondrium, present directly underneath the degenerated collagen
- Surrounding dermis shows small blood vessel proliferation and dilatation with sparse lymphocytic infiltrate

DIFFERENTIAL DIAGNOSIS

Relapsing Polychondritis

- Neutrophilic destruction of cartilage
- Cartilage is replaced by fibrous tissue

Elastotic Nodule

- Clumps of elastic tissue in the dermis
- Absence of ulceration and cartilage damage

Gouty Tophus

- Dermal aggregates of crystals

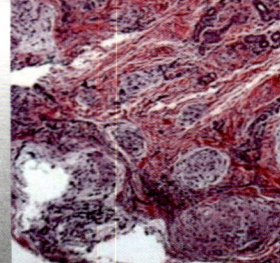

Cutis Laxa (Elastolysis)

INTRODUCTION

- Characterized by loose pendulous skin
- Pathogenesis—fibulin-5 gene mutations has recently been described
- Patterns of inheritance—autosomal dominant, autosomal recessive and X-linked recessive
- Individuals show premature aging

HISTOPATHOLOGY (Figs 41.1 and 41.2)

- Papillary dermis shows reduced elastic fibers
- Preserved dermal elastic fibers show variation in diameter, fragmentation with irregular borders
- Chronic inflammatory cell infiltrate can be seen
- van Gieson stain can demonstrate elastin loss or its reduction in affected portions

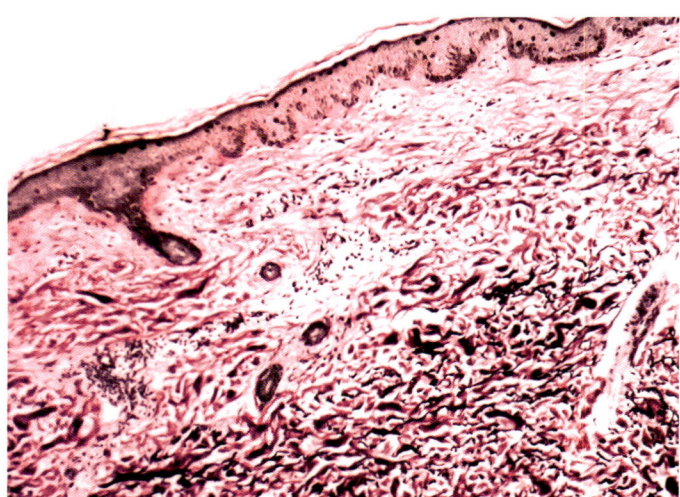

Fig. 41.1: Cutis laxa. Elastin fibers in the upper dermis appear to be completely absent on H&E stain

Fig. 41.2: Cutis laxa. Verhoeff van Gieson stain demonstrates loss of elastin fibers in the upper dermis. Deeper dermis shows waviness along with fragmentation of elastic fibers

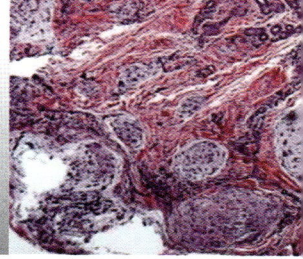

Elastosis Perforans Serpiginosa (EPS)

INTRODUCTION

- Also called perforating elastosis
- Demonstrates trans-epidermal elimination
- Most commonly affects males
- Age group—second decade
- Sites—head and neck, upper extremities
- Presents as small papules which can coalesce or are arranged in a serpiginous fashion
- Associated with penicillamine intake

HISTOPATHOLOGY (Figs 42.1 to 42.3)

- Acanthotic epidermis
- Epidermis demonstrates transepidermal channel
- Through this transepidermal channel, fragmented brightly, eosinophilic elastic fibers and basophilic nuclear debris are eliminated

DIFFERENTIAL DIAGNOSIS

Kyrle's Disease and Perforating Folliculitis

- Both of these disorders show transepidermal elimination of basophilic degenerated material
- However, unlike elastosis perforans serpiginosa, both of these disorders do not show marked increase in elastic tissue

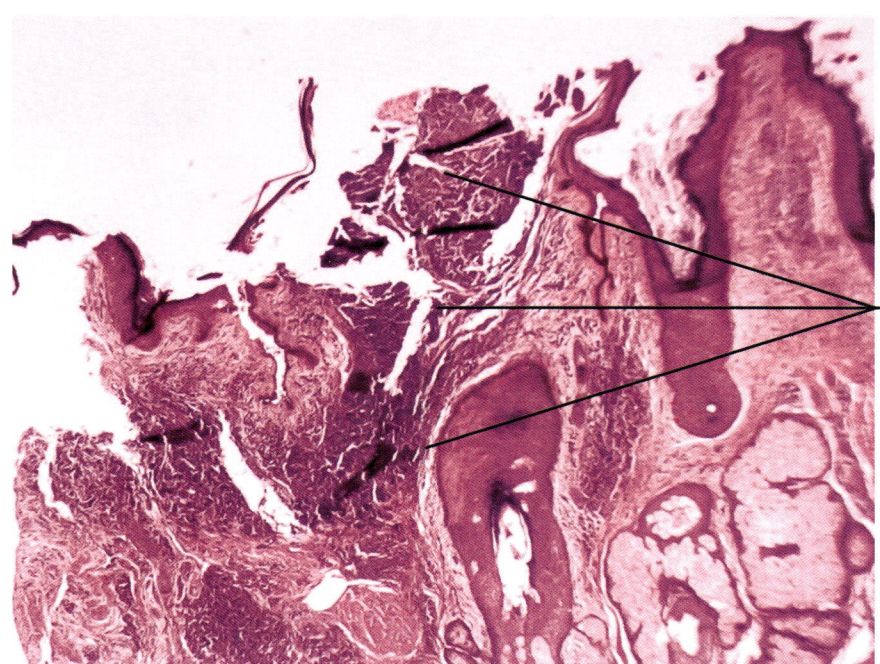

Transepidermal channel showing elimination of degenerated material

Fig. 42.1: Elastosis perforans serpiginosa

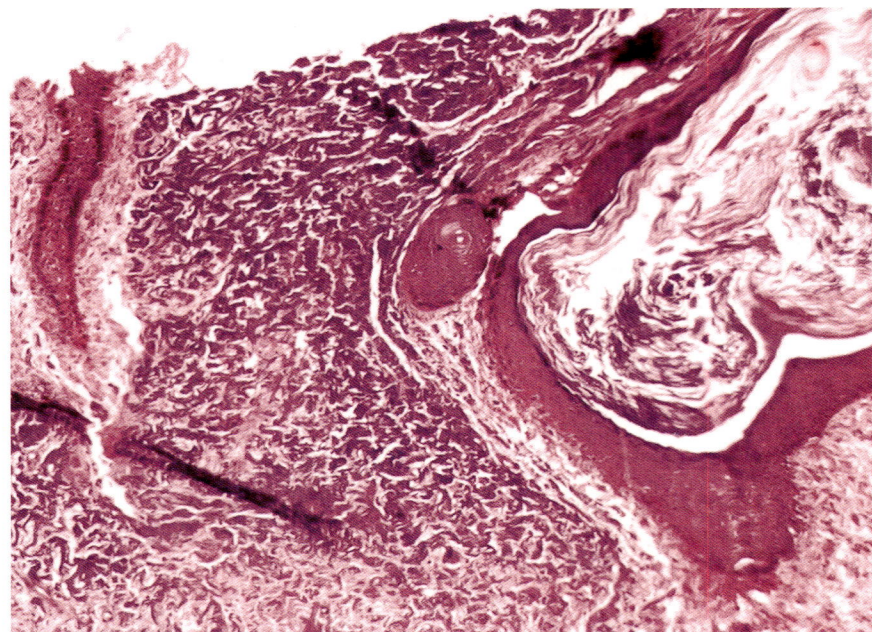

Fig. 42.2: Trans-epidermal elimination in elastosis perforans serpiginosa

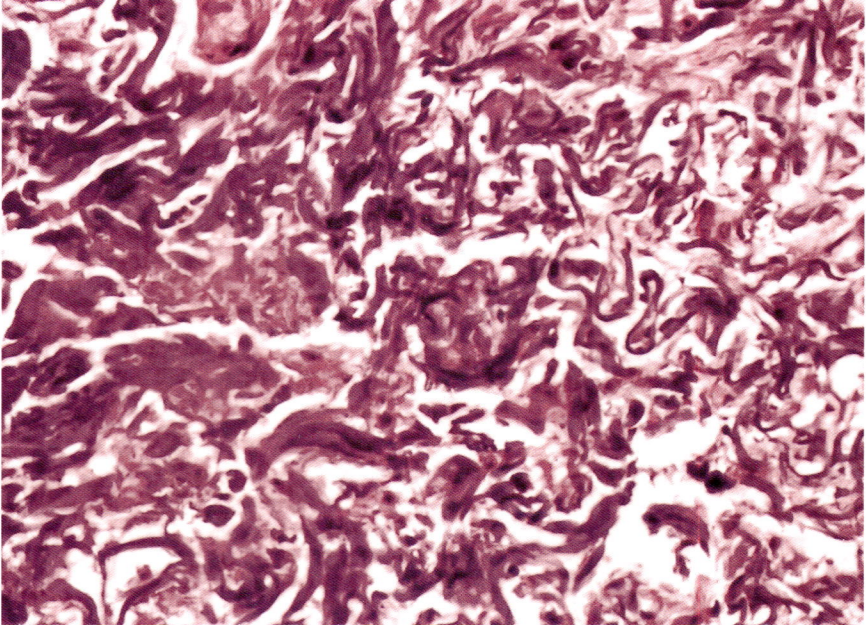

Fig. 42.3: Elastic fibers form a major content in elastosis perforans serpiginosa

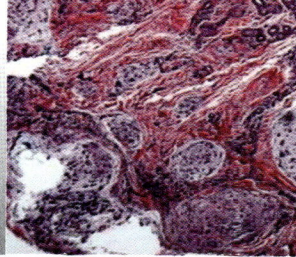

Kyrle's Disease

INTRODUCTION

- Presents as hyperkeratotic papule with a central plug
- Sites—lower limbs, upper limbs, head and neck
- Seen in patients with chronic renal failure, liver diseases, congestive heart failure, diabetes mellitus

HISTOPATHOLOGY (Figs 43.1 and 43.2)

- Epidermis can be normal, atrophic or acanthotic

- Keratotic plug is seen in epidermis, or in dermis and when seen in latter, often a connection of dermal keratotic plug with overlying epidermis can be well appreciated
- Keratotic plug shows basophilic cellular debris and focal area of parakeratosis
- Collagen is not demonstrated with Masson's trichrome

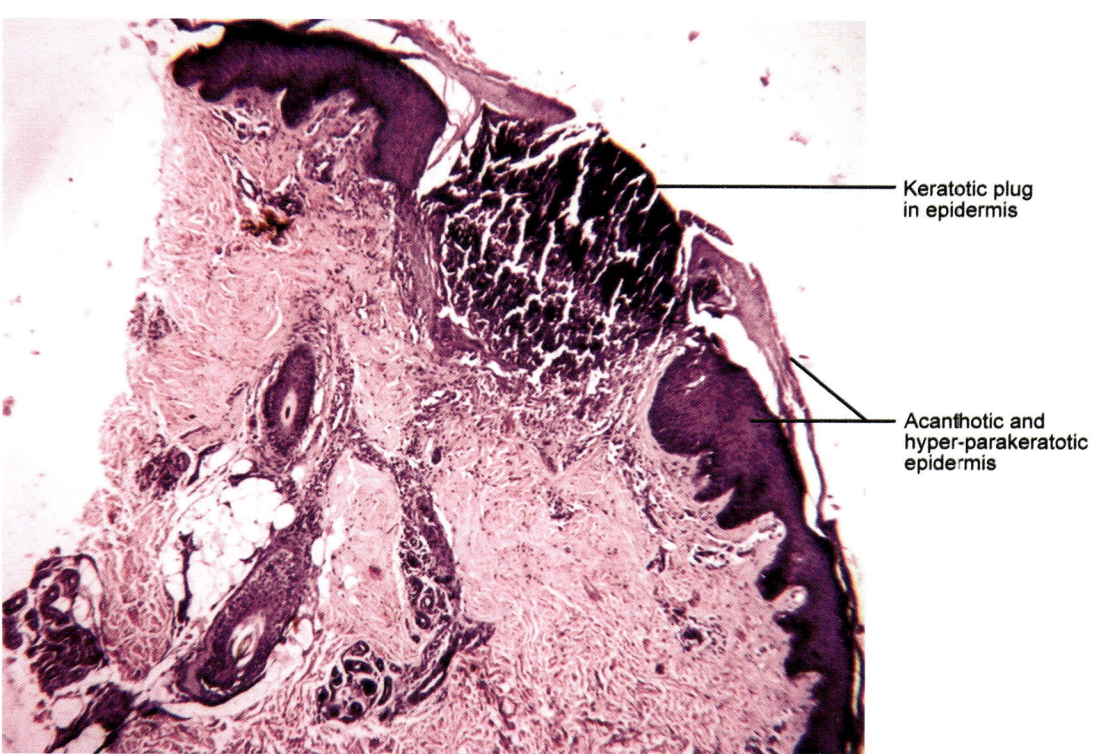

Keratotic plug in epidermis

Acanthotic and hyper-parakeratotic epidermis

Fig. 43.1: Kyrle's disease

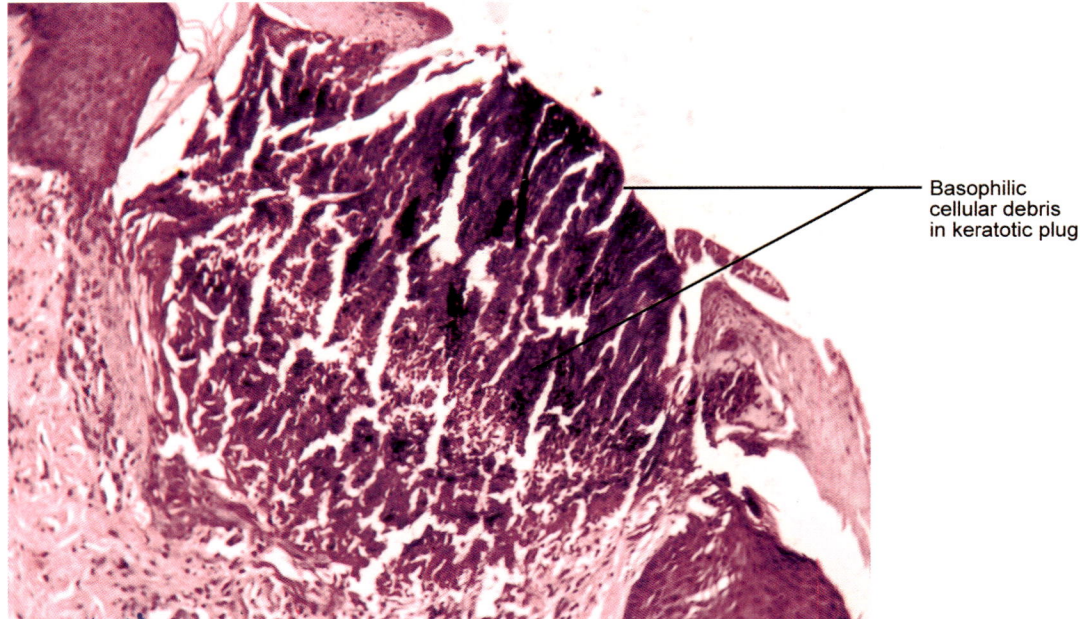

Basophilic
cellular debris
in keratotic plug

Fig. 43.2: Kyrle's disease

DIFFERENTIAL DIAGNOSIS

1. Acquired perforating collagenosis
2. Perforating folliculitis
3. Elastosis perforans serpiginosa
4. Granuloma annulare
5. Pseudoxanthoma elasticum

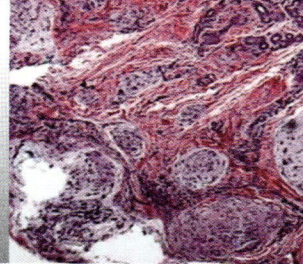

Macular Amyloidosis

INTRODUCTION

- Presents as pruritic macules or hyperpigmented patches
- Sites—trunk, inter-scapular region, upper back

HISTOPATHOLOGY (Figs 44.1 and 44.2)

- Papillary dermis shows small globular deposits of amyloid
- Amyloid is difficult to detect on H & E stains and can be easily missed out

- Amyloid can be demonstrated by Congo red stain or crystal violet dye
- Direct immunofluorescence—amyloid fluoresce positively for IgM and C3

DIFFERENTIAL DIAGNOSIS

Lichen Amyloidosis (Fig. 44.3)

- Presents as pruritic papules
- Sites—lower extremities
- Hyperkeratosis, epidermal hyperplasia along with papillary dermal amyloid deposits

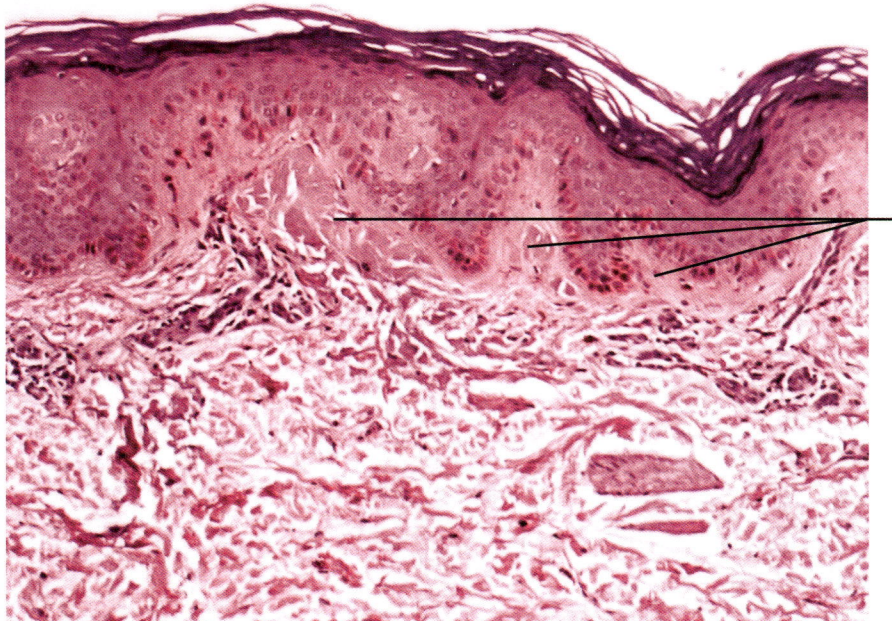

Amyloid deposits beneath the epidermis

Fig. 44.1: Macular amyloidosis

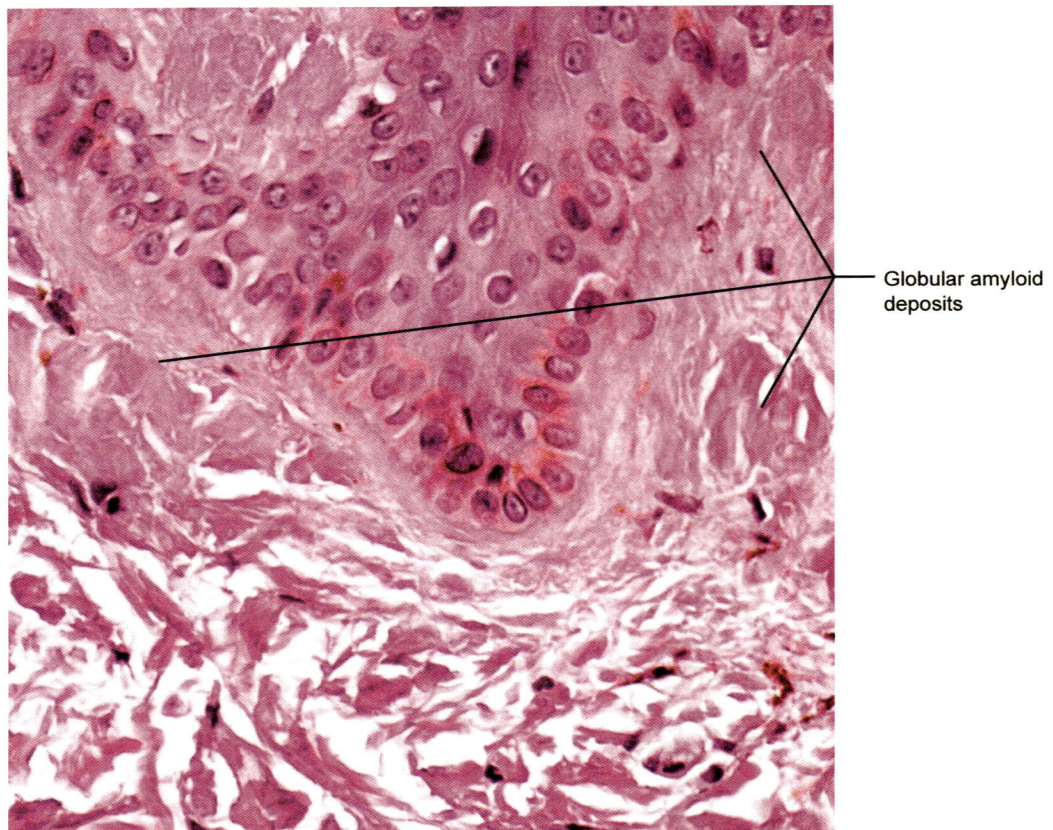

Globular amyloid deposits

Fig. 44.2: Macular amyloidosis

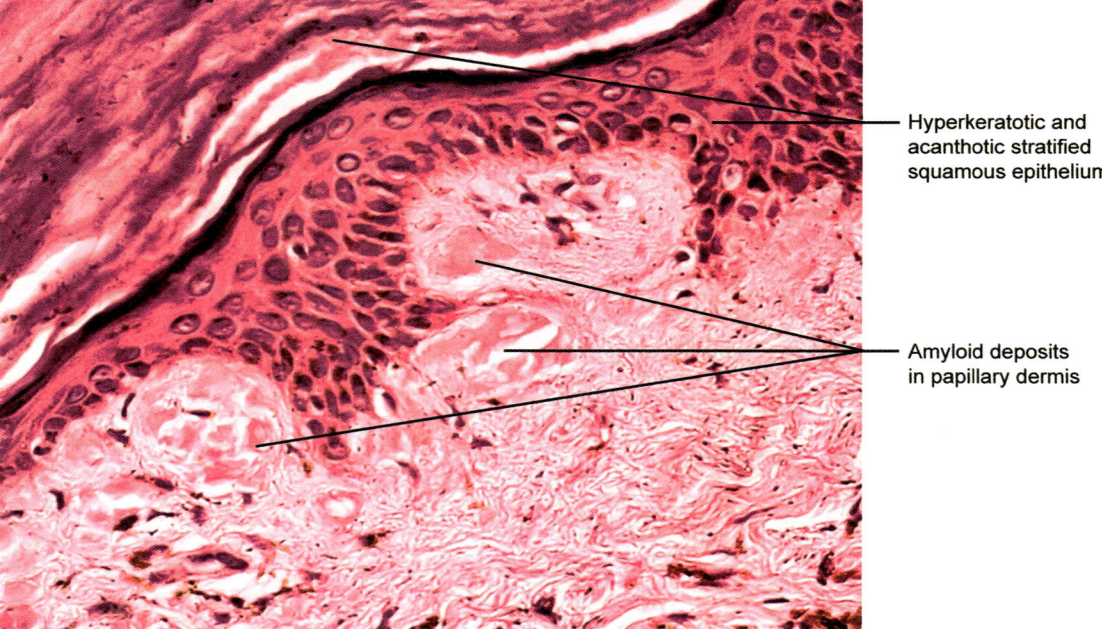

Hyperkeratotic and acanthotic stratified squamous epithelium

Amyloid deposits in papillary dermis

Fig. 44.3: Lichen amyloidosis

Pseudoxanthoma Elasticum

INTRODUCTION

- Inherited disorder characterized by calcification of elastic fibers in the dermis, retina and blood vessels
- Age group—second to third decade
- Etiology—mutations in ABCC6 (ATP binding cassette family C member-6) gene, which encodes MRP-6 (multidrug resistance-associated protein 6)
- Sites—neck, axillae and groin

- Presents as yellow coalescing papules (Fig. 45.1)
- Arterial involvement—gastric, coronary and large peripheral arteries

HISTOPATHOLOGY (Figs 45.2 and 45.3)

- Epidermis appears normal
- Mid-dermis and deep dermis show short, swollen, curled, frayed, elastic fibers

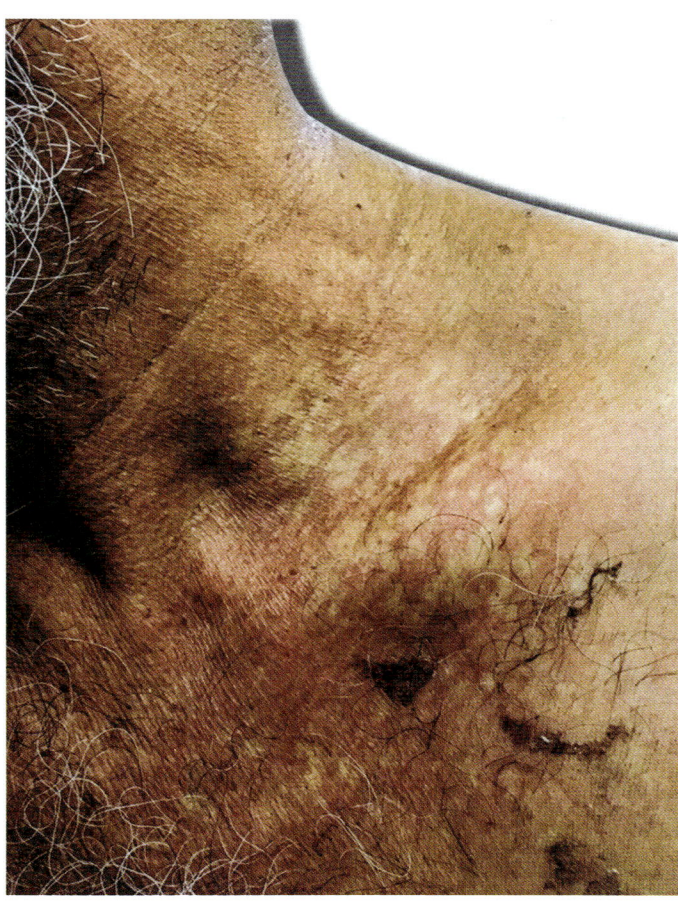

Fig. 45.1: Pseudoxanthoma elasticum. 2–5 mm yellow to orange papules with normal surrounding skin

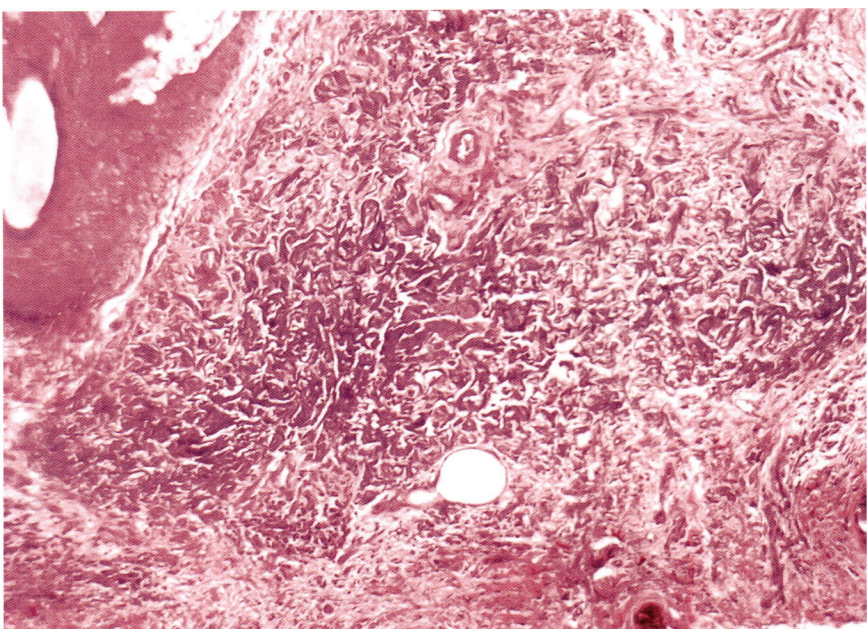

Fig. 45.2: Pseudoxanthoma elasticum. Dermis shows swollen and degenerated basophilic elastic fibers

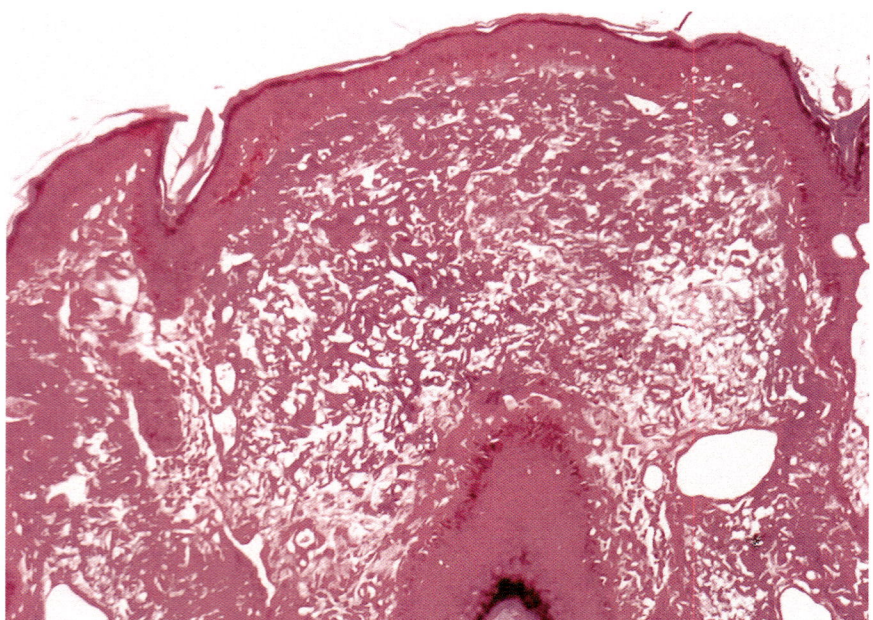

Fig. 45.3: Pseudoxanthoma elasticum. Basophilic degenerated collagen fibers in the dermis

- Elastic fibers appears basophilic with H&E stain, black with Orcein and Verhoeff's stain and calcium deposition can be highlighted by von Kossa stain

DIFFERENTIAL DIAGNOSIS

Solar/Actinic Elastosis

- Accumulation of irregularly thickened elastic fibers in the upper one-third (superficial) of dermis
- Presents as dense masses without calcification

Elastosis Perforans Serpiginosa

- Trans-epidermal elimination of elastic fibers, degenerated epithelial cells, inflammatory debris through hyperplastic epidermis
- van Gieson stain can highlight elastic fibers undergoing trans-epidermal elimination

Calcinosis Cutis

- Calcium deposits in dermis, which stains deep-blue on hematoxylin and eosin stain

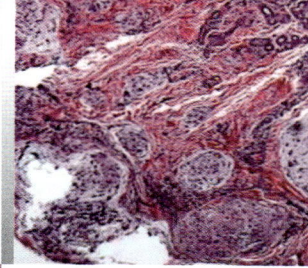

Reactive Perforating Collagenosis

- A rare disorder characterized by trans-epidermal elimination of altered collagen through the epidermis
- In children, it presents as recurrent umbilicated papules, on extremities (palms and soles) with keratotic plugs in the center
- Lesions can regress by themselves, but recurrence is common
- In adults (acquired perforating collagenosis), association with diabetes and chronic renal failure is seen

- Other triggering factors include minor trauma, arthropod bites, scratching, scabies

HISTOPATHOLOGY (Figs 46.1 and 46.2)

- Epidermis is filled with parakeratotic keratin plug comprising of degenerated collagen fibers and inflammatory debris
- Through the epidermis, collagen fibers are extruded in vertical orientation

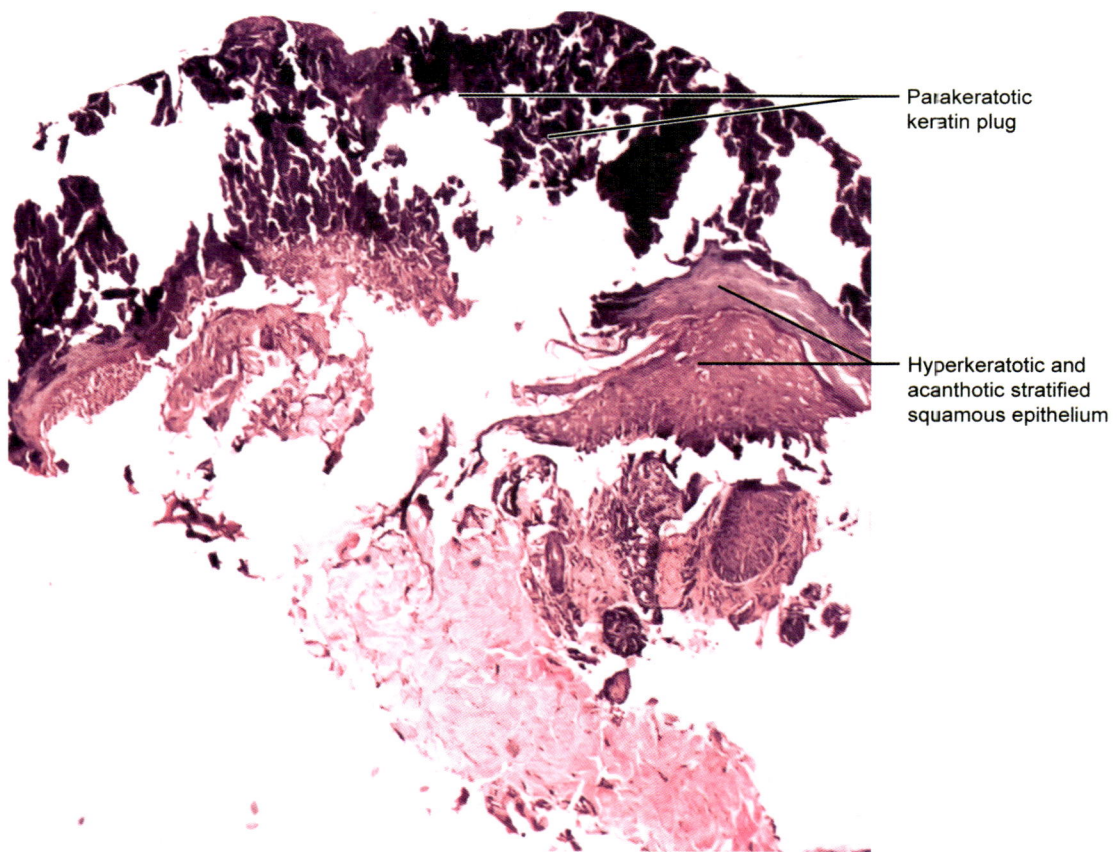

Parakeratotic keratin plug

Hyperkeratotic and acanthotic stratified squamous epithelium

Fig. 46.1: Reactive perforating collagenosis

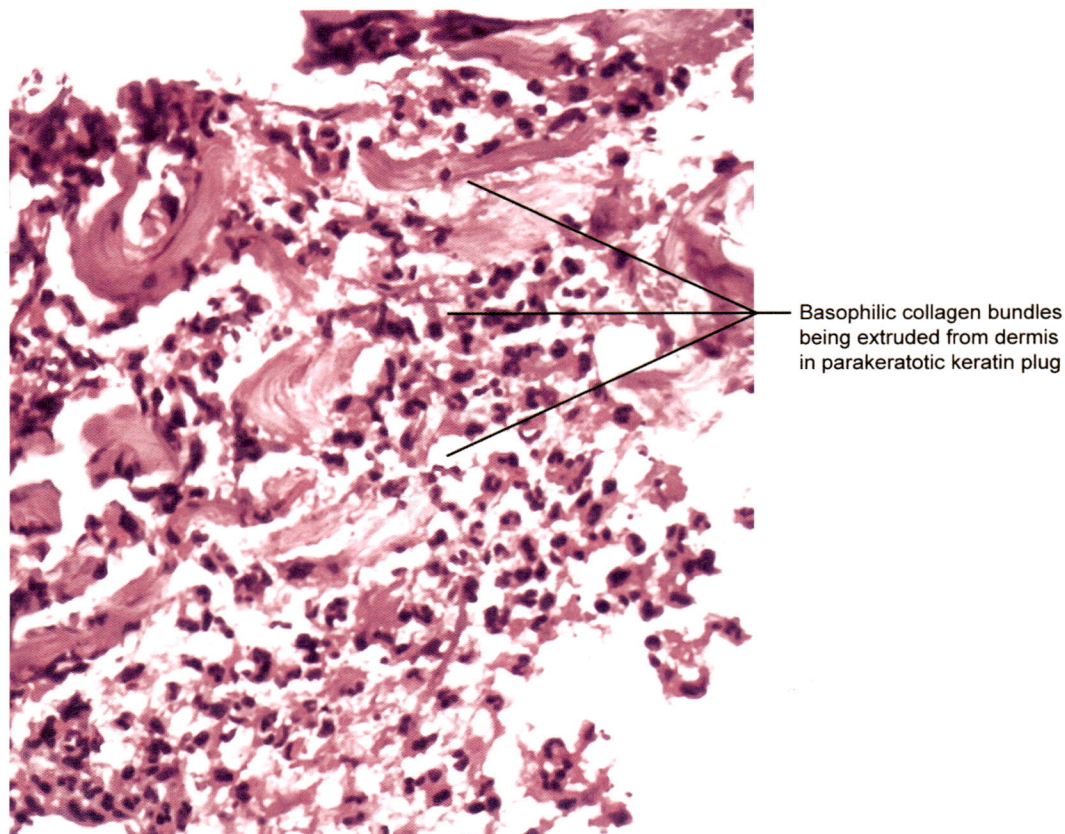

Basophilic collagen bundles being extruded from dermis in parakeratotic keratin plug

Fig. 46.2: Reactive perforating collagenosis

DIFFERENTIAL DIAGNOSIS

Elastosis Perforans Serpiginosa

- Presents as keratotic papules with atrophy and desquamation in center
- Lesions are arranged in a serpiginous fashion

Perforating Folliculitis

- Presents as isolated papules, with white keratotic plugs in the center

Kyrle's Disease

- Presents as hyperkeratotic papule with a central keratotic plug

Xanthoma

INTRODUCTION

- Localized collection of lipid-laden macrophages
- Cause—elevated serum lipid levels (LDL and VLDL)
- Associations—hereditary lipoproteinemias

VARIANTS

- Xanthelasma
- Eruptive xanthoma
- Tuberous xanthoma
- Tendinous xanthoma
- Planar xanthoma
- Plexiform xanthomas
- Verruciform xanthoma

Xanthelasma

- Most common form of xanthoma
- Presents as yellowish plaques on eyelids (Fig. 47.1)
- Sites—eyelids and periorbital skin

Histopathology

- Thinned-out epidermis
- Superficially located foam cells (in lobules), muscle fibers and blood vessels

Eruptive Xanthoma

- Sudden onset of multiple, small, red-yellow papules
- Sites—gluteal region, thighs, extensor surfaces of arms and legs

Histopathology

- Early lesions show non-foamy cells, lymphocytes, macrophages and neutrophils
- Well-formed lesions show foamy cells

Tuberous Xanthoma

- Firm, yellow, subcutaneous nodules and plaques
- Sites—elbow, knee, fingers, buttocks
- Association with familial hyper-lipoproteinemia is seen

Histopathology (Figs 47.2 and 47.3)

- Large aggregates of foam cells throughout the dermis
- Lipid within the foam cells can be demonstrated by oil-red O stain

Tendinous Xanthomas

- Predisposing factor—elevated LDL levels

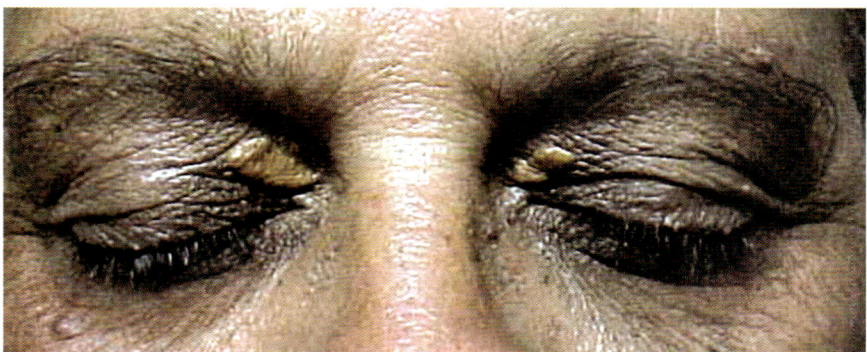

Fig. 47.1: Xanthelasma. Cholesterol-filled, soft, yellow plaques, on the medial aspect of eyelids

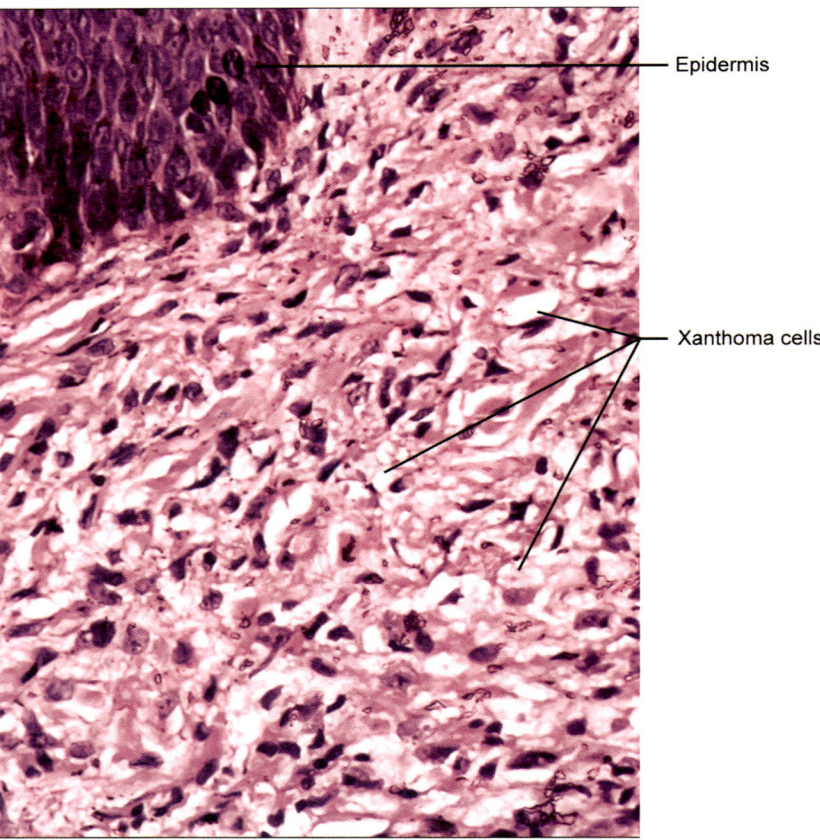

Fig. 47.2: Xanthoma

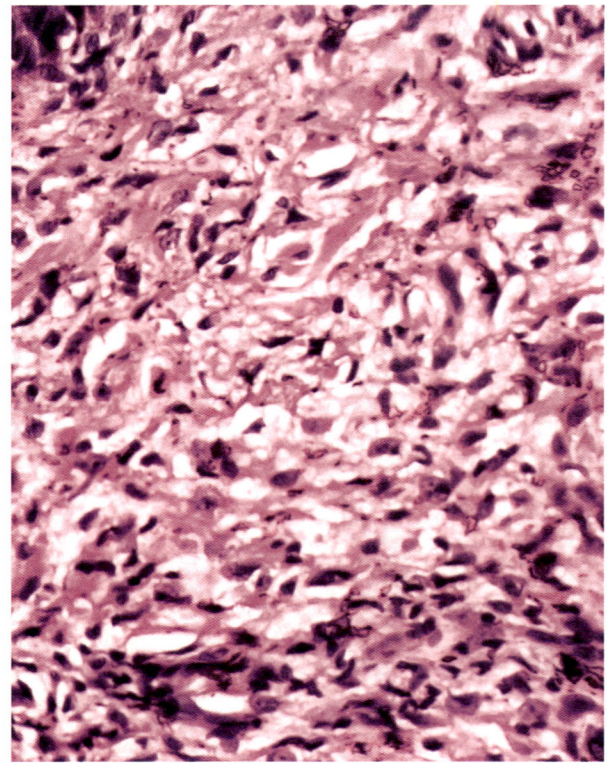

Fig. 47.3: Xanthoma. Numerous xanthoma cells in dermis

- Sites—Achilles tendon, extensor tendons of hands and feet
- Lesions are firm to hard, flesh colored nodules

Histopathology
- Presence of foam cells and cholesterol clefts

Planar Xanthomas
- Seen on skin folds, palm creases

Histopathology
- Thickened epidermis with hyperkeratosis
- Dermis—numerous foamy macrophages with their peripherally displaced nuclei

Plexiform Xanthoma
- Presents as solitary lesions

Histopathology
- Tumors are located in the dermis and subcutis
- Plexiform arrangement of epithelioid and xanthomatous cells are seen

Verruciform Xanthoma
- Solitary, flat, plaques
- Sites—oral cavity, genital skin

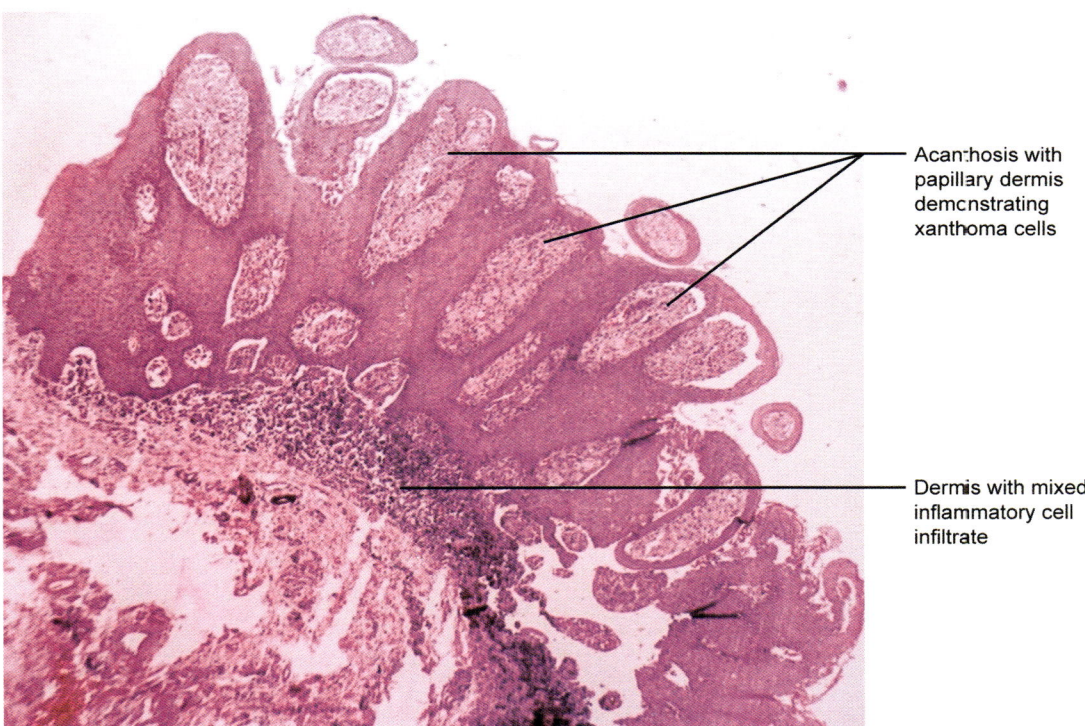

Acanthosis with papillary dermis demonstrating xanthoma cells

Dermis with mixed inflammatory cell infiltrate

Fig. 47.4: Verruciform xanthoma

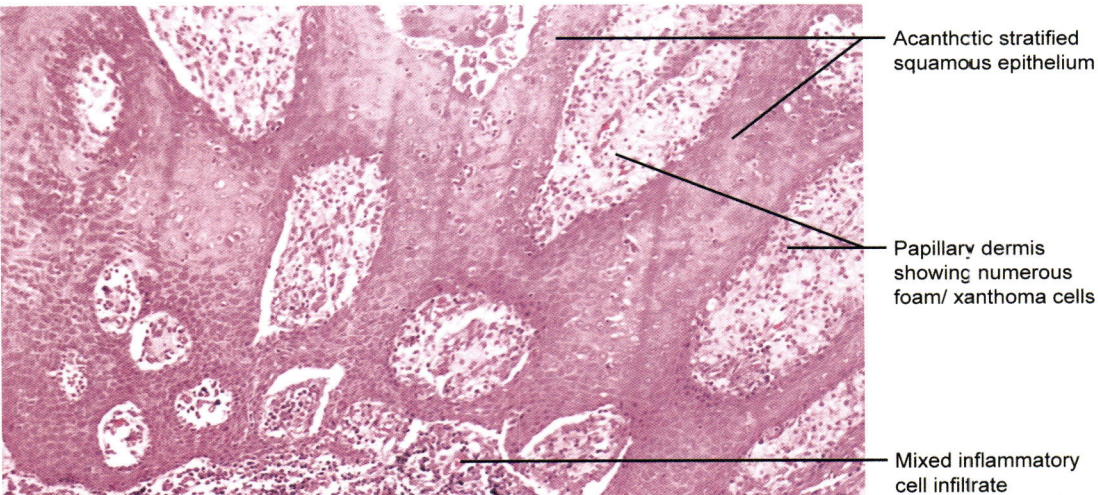

Acanthotic stratified squamous epithelium

Papillary dermis showing numerous foam/ xanthoma cells

Mixed inflammatory cell infiltrate

Fig. 47.5: Verruciform xanthomas

- Seen in immunocompromised patients, i.e. HIV patients

Histopathology (Figs 47.4 to 47.6)

- Acanthosis, hyperkeratosis, focal parakeratosis
- Papillary dermis shows numerous large xanthoma cells
- Lymphocytes, plasma cells, neutrophils and eosinophils are seen in between and underneath these xanthoma cells

- Foam cells demonstrate CD68 positivity

DIFFERENTIAL DIAGNOSIS

Granuloma Annulare

- Dermis shows degenerated collagen bundles and mucin
- Palisading of macrophages/histiocytes around the degenerated collagen bundles
- Foam cells are absent

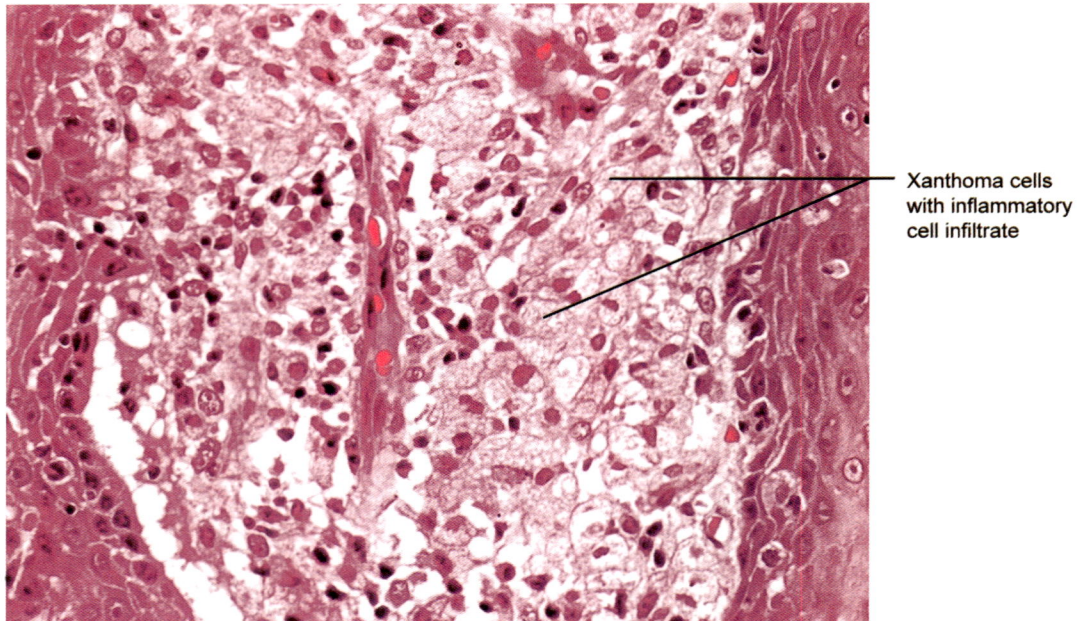

Xanthoma cells
with inflammatory
cell infiltrate

Fig. 47.6: Verruciform xanthomas

Granular Cell Tumor

- Cells with granular cytoplasm, demonstrating S-100 positivity
- Foam cells are absent

Juvenile Xanthogranuloma

- Foam cells with Touton giant cells
- Mixed inflammatory cell infiltrate comprising of macrophages, eosinophils and lymphocytes

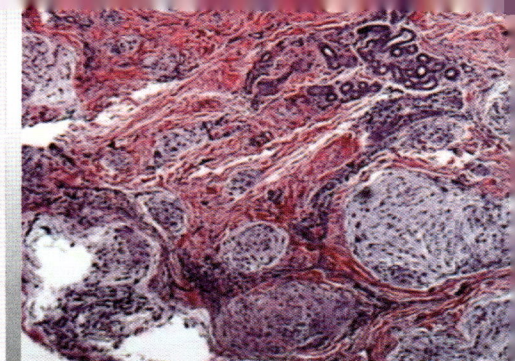

Vascular Disorders Affecting Dermis

Part 7

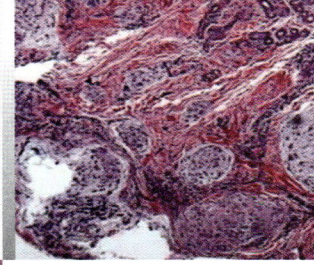

Granuloma Faciale

INTRODUCTION

- Presents as small vessel leukocytoclastic vasculitis
- Clinical presentation—presents as plaques or nodules
- Most common site—face
- Most commonly affects elderly males

HISTOPATHOLOGY (Figs 48.1 and 48.2)

- Dermis shows polymorphous inflammatory cell infiltrate comprising of lymphocytes, eosinophils, plasma cells and neutrophils
- Dermal inflammatory cell infiltrate separated from the epidermis by grenz zone
- Neutrophils can surround the vessels, and can show fragmentation (leukocytoclasis)

- At later stages, dermal capillaries show concentric fibrosis

DIFFERENTIAL DIAGNOSIS

Sweet Syndrome

- Monomorphic inflammatory cell infiltrate, comprising of neutrophils
- Vessel wall may show features of leukocytoclasis (fragmented nuclei of neutrophils in the vessel wall)
- Extensive vessel wall involvement is not seen

Erythema Elevatum Diutinum

- Dermis shows more neutrophils than eosinophils
- Early lesions—perivascular neutrophils with leucocytoclasis

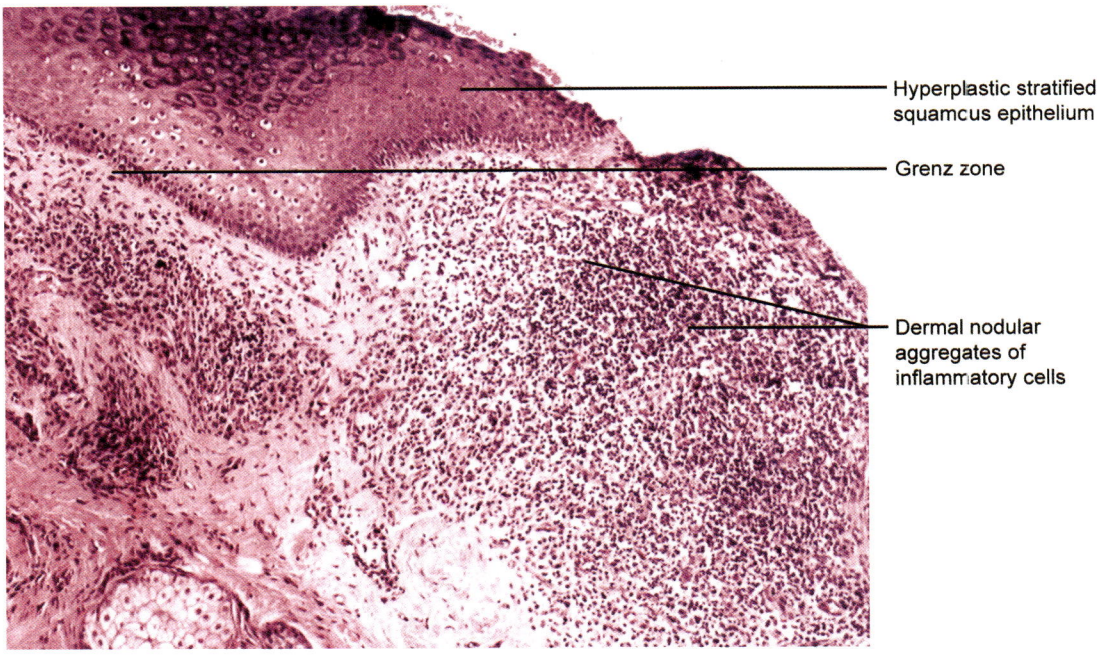

Hyperplastic stratified squamcus epithelium

Grenz zone

Dermal nodular aggregates of inflammatory cells

Fig. 48.1: Granuloma faciale

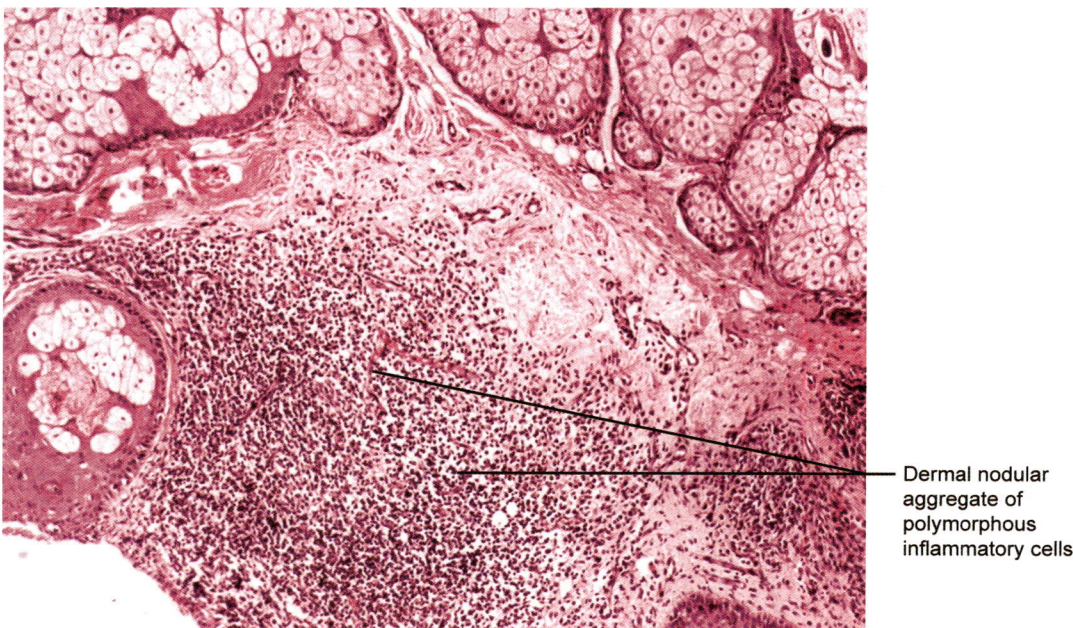

Fig. 48.2: Granuloma faciale

- Late lesions—fibrinoid material in the capillary lumen, with "onion skinning" fibrosis around the vessel wall

Leukocytoclastic Vasculitis

- Leucocytoclasis
- Less dense inflammatory cell infiltrate
- Extravasation of erythrocytes is more prominent

ERYTHEMA ELEVATUM DIUTINUM

INTRODUCTION

- Presents as red-brown to yellow, nodules, papules or plaques
- Sites—symmetrical involvement of extensor surface of the extremities

HISTOPATHOLOGY

Early Lesion

- Perivascular neutrophils with leukocytoclasis
- Fibrin deposits around the small dermal blood vessels

Established Lesion

- Capillary proliferation with neutrophilic infiltrate

- Capillaries may show fibrinoid material within their lumen
- Onion-skin fibrosis around the vessels occurs late in course of disease

DIFFERENTIAL DIAGNOSIS

Granuloma Faciale

- Presence of grenz zone, due to sparing of the superficial papillary dermis
- Facial involvement is more common
- Presence of eosinophils and plasma cells in addition to neutrophils

Sweet Syndrome

- Perivascular neutrophilic infiltrate
- Features of vasculitis can be seen, though they are uncommon
- Extensive vessel wall involvement is not seen

Behçet's Disease

- Can present as oral ulcers, genital ulcers, uveitis, synovitis and vasculitis
- Neutrophilic vascular reaction
- Features of leukocytoclastic vasculitis can occur
- Dense dermal neutrophilic microabscesses can be seen

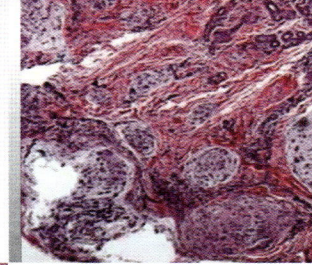

Leukocytoclastic Vasculitis

INTRODUCTION

- Clinical presentation—palpable purpura (Fig. 49.1)
- Most common site—shins

CAUSES

1. Infections (meningococcal)
2. Autoimmune disorders
3. Antibody mediated disorders (ANCA mediated – Wegener's granulomatosis, microscopic polyangiitis, Churg-Strauss syndrome)
4. Immune complex mediated disorders (Henoch-Schönlein purpura, urticarial vasculitis, cryoglobulinemia)
5. Carcinomas

HISTOPATHOLOGY (Figs 49.2 to 49.4)

- Affected vessel includes dermal post-capillary venules
- Perivascular neutrophilic infiltrate, resulting in destruction of the vessel wall

- Due to fragmentation of nuclei (leukocytoclasis), term leukocytoclastic vasculitis is used
- Fibrinoid degeneration (fibrinoid necrosis)—endothelial cell swelling, fibrin deposition around the vessel walls, giving it a smudgy appearance
- Erythrocyte extravasation from the vessel wall in dermis is seen
- As the lesions progress, neutrophils are replaced by mononuclear cells

DIFFERENTIAL DIAGNOSIS

Sweet's Syndrome (Acute Febrile Neutrophilic Dermatoses) (Fig. 49.5)

- Tender plaques or nodules on face, extremities
- Dense perivascular neutrophilic infiltrate in the upper and mid-dermis
- Vessel wall may show features of leukocytoclasis (fragmented nuclei of neutrophils, within vessel wall)
- Extensive vessel wall involvement is not seen
- Absence of fibrinoid vascular change

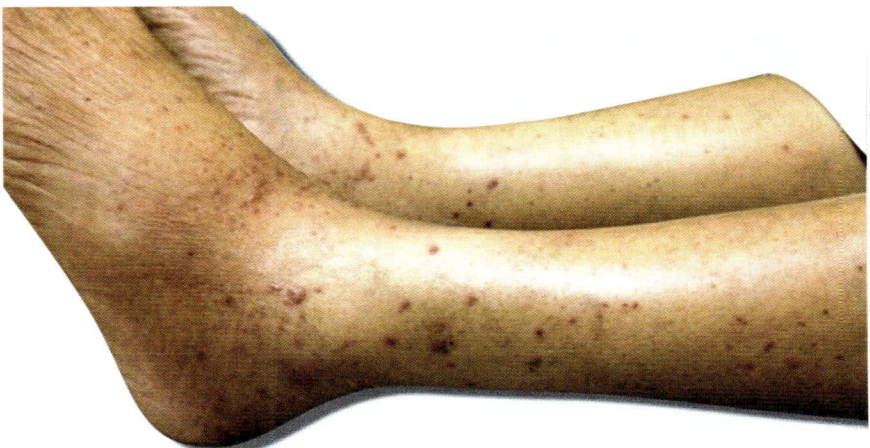

Fig. 49.1: Leukocytoclastic vasculitis. Palpable purpura and non-blanching petechiae

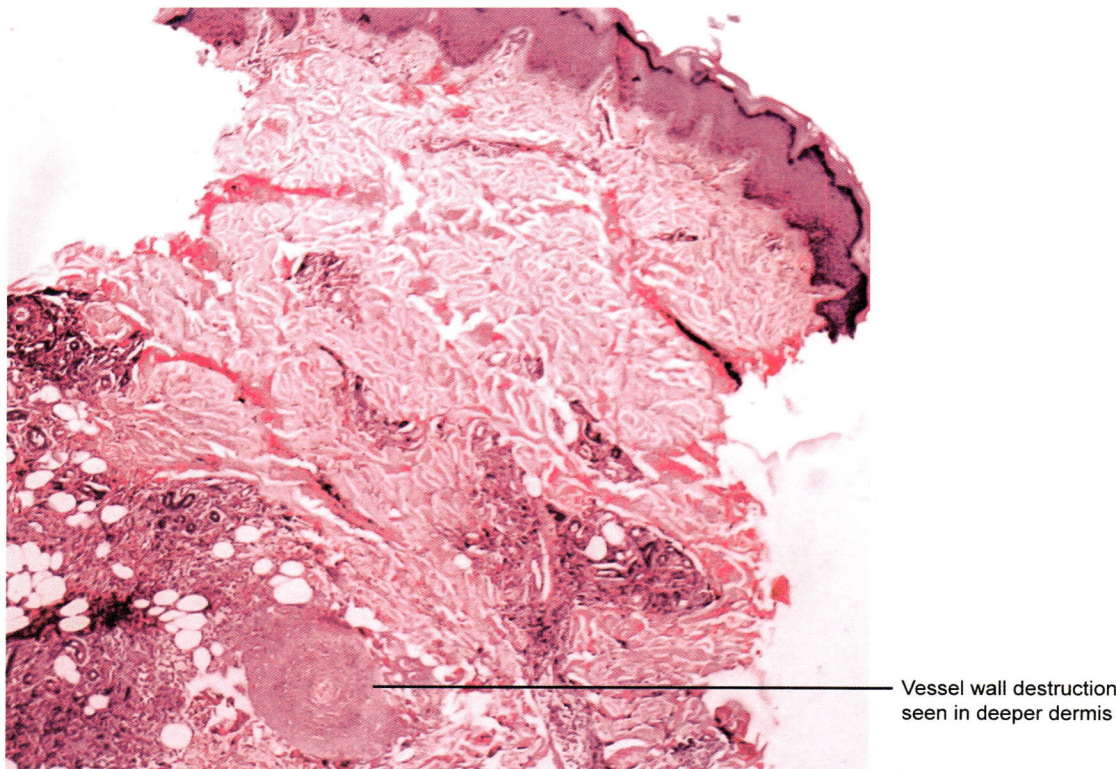

Vessel wall destruction seen in deeper dermis

Fig. 49.2: Vasculitis

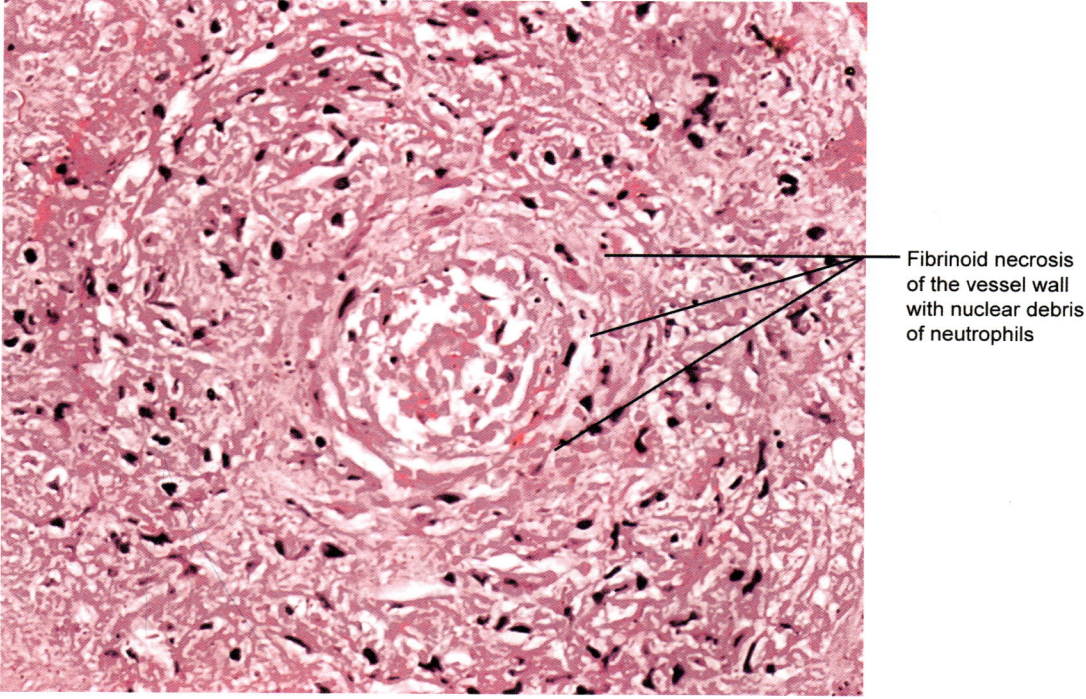

Fibrinoid necrosis of the vessel wall with nuclear debris of neutrophils

Fig. 49.3: Leukocytoclastic vasculitis

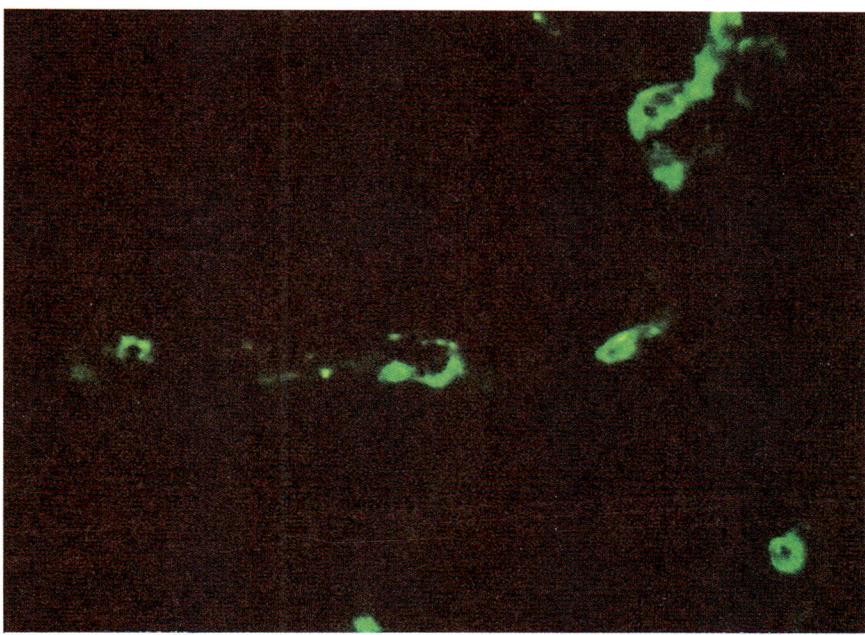

Fig. 49.4: Direct immunofluorescence demonstrating IgA deposits in vessel walls of patient suffering from Henoch-Schönlein purpura (IgA vasculitis)

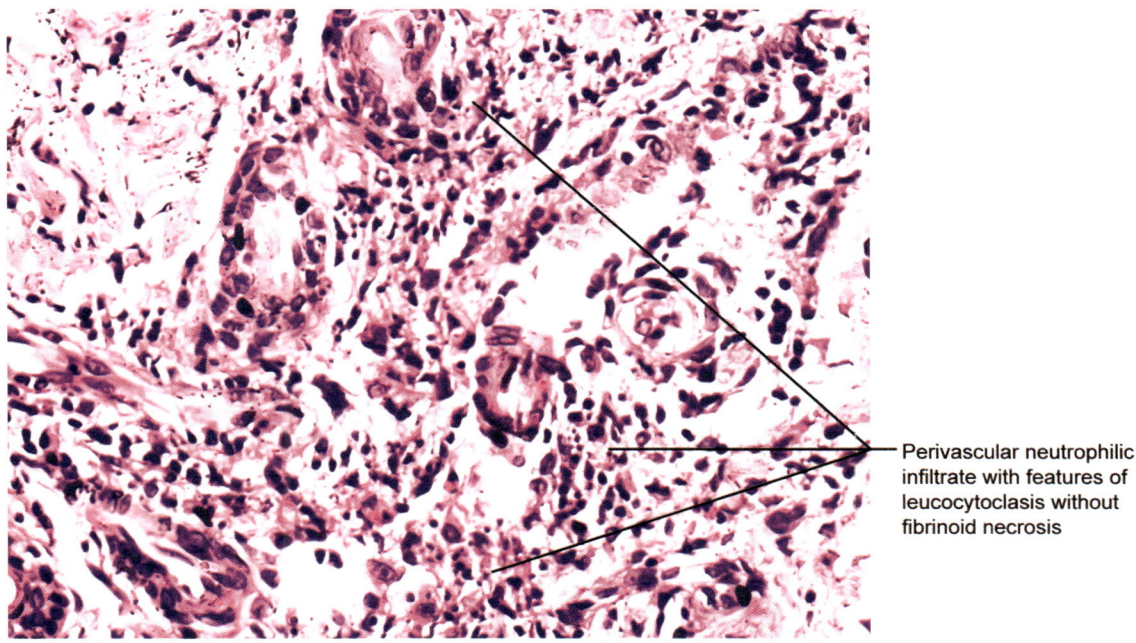

Perivascular neutrophilic infiltrate with features of leucocytoclasis without fibrinoid necrosis

Fig. 49.5: Sweet syndrome

Lymphocytic Vasculitis (Figs 49.6 and 49.7)

- Perivascular lymphocytic infiltrate with lymphocytes in the vessel wall
- Absence of leukocytoclasis

Livedoid Vasculitis (Atrophie Blanche)

- Epidermal necrosis with underlying vasculopathy
- Fibrinoid material within the vessel wall or vessel lumen

- In late stages, dermal vessel wall shows hyalinization and thickening of the intima

Granuloma Faciale

- Polymorphous inflammatory cell infiltrate in the upper dermis, which is separated from the epidermis by grenz zone
- Neutrophils surround the vessels and can show fragmentation (neutrophilic vascular reaction)

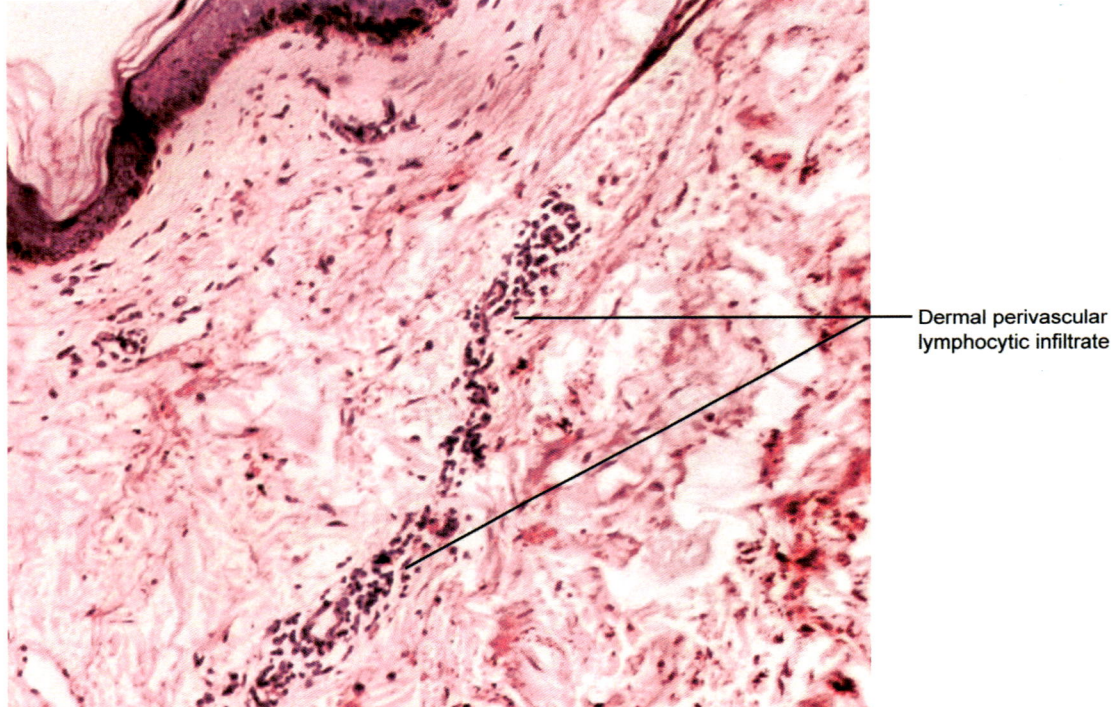

Dermal perivascular
lymphocytic infiltrate

Fig. 49.6: Lymphocytic vasculitis

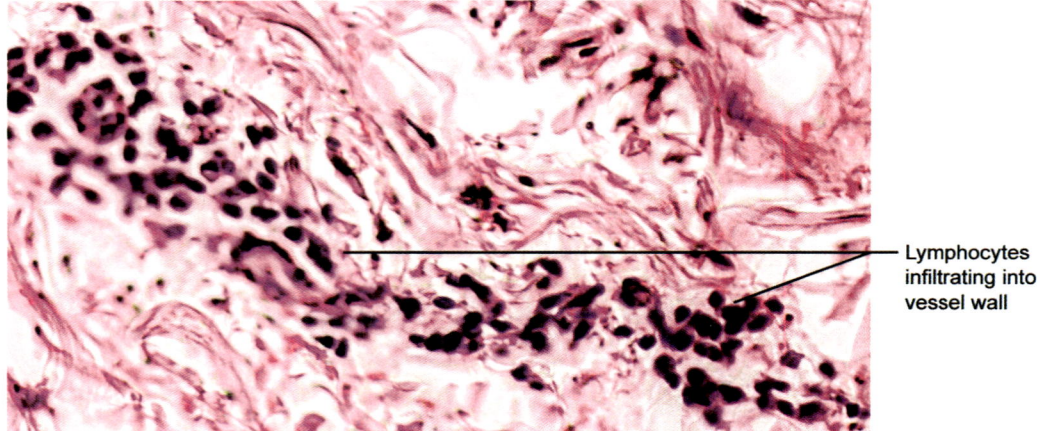

Lymphocytes
infiltrating into
vessel wall

Fig. 49.7: Lymphocytic vasculitis

Erythema Elevatum Diutinum (EED)

- Early lesions—perivascular neutrophils with leuco-cytoclasis
- Late lesions—fibrinoid material in the capillary lumen, with "onion skinning" fibrosis around the vessels

Cryoglobulinemia

- Amorphous material is deposited throughout the vessel wall and in its lumen
- Features of leukocytoclastic vasculitis are uncommon, but can be seen

Polyarteritis Nodosa

- Early stage—necrotizing leukocytoclastic vasculitis in the dermal vessels
- Late stage—intimal proliferation and thrombosis with resultant occlusion of vessel wall

Wegener's Granulomatosis

- Leukocytoclastic small vessel vasculitis with granulomatous inflammation
- Granulomas comprise necrobiotic collagen, necrotic debris with neutrophils

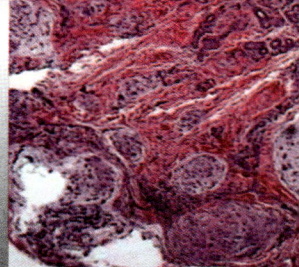

Polyarteritis Nodosa

INTRODUCTION

- Vasculitis of medium and/or small-sized blood vessels
- Cutaneous involvement—presents as tender subcutaneous nodules or ulcerations
- Age group—fourth to sixth decade
- Most commonly affects males
- Site—lower extremities

- Predisposing factor—Group A beta hemolytic streptococci, hepatitis B infection
- Most common cause of death—renal involvement

HISTOPATHOLOGY (Fig. 50.1)

Early Lesion

- Degeneration of the arterial wall with deposition of fibrinoid material

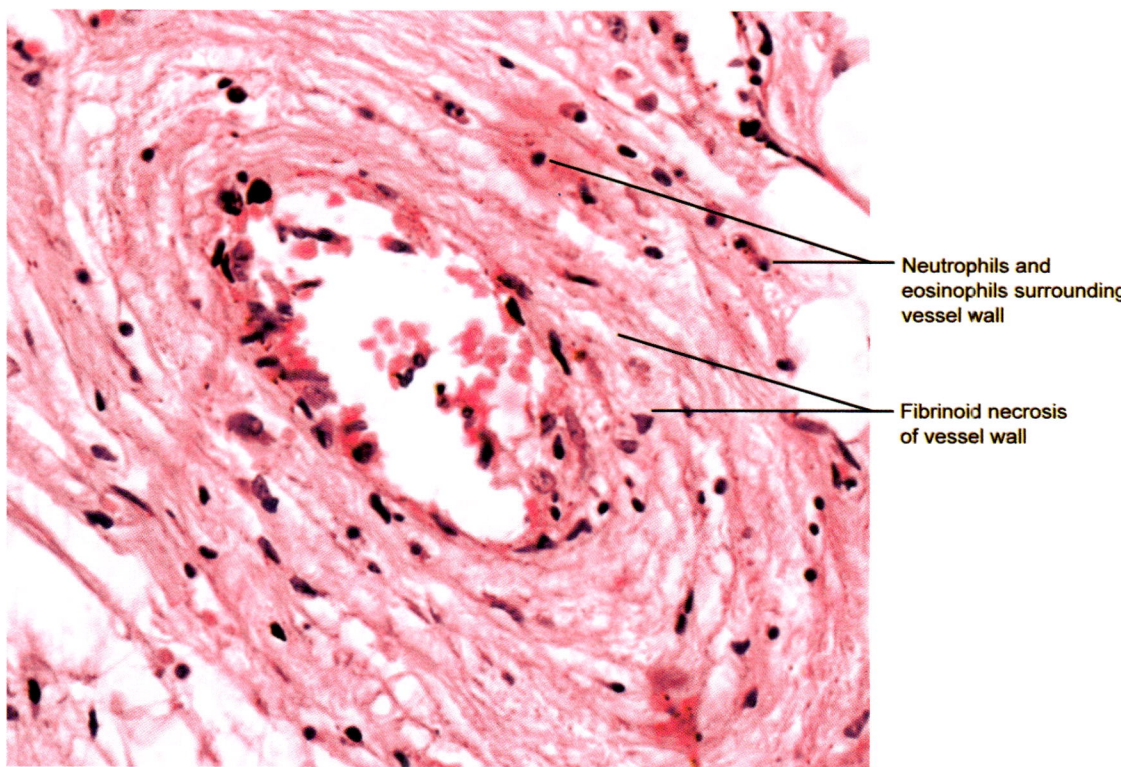

Neutrophils and eosinophils surrounding vessel wall

Fibrinoid necrosis of vessel wall

Fig. 50.1: Vasculitis

- Presence of neutrophils and eosinophils surrounding the vessel wall with leucocytoclasis

Late Lesion
- Intimal proliferation and thrombosis with occlusion of the vessel wall
- Intimal fibrosis of the vessel wall

Direct Immunofluorescence
- Shows IgM and C3 deposits in affected arterial walls

DIFFERENTIAL DIAGNOSIS

Nodular Vasculitis
- Leukocytoclastic vasculitis of subcutaneous vessels
- Inflammation extend into the fat lobules

Cryoglobulinemia
- Leukocytoclastic vasculitis

- Fibrin plug/thrombi within the vessel wall lumen, demonstrated by PAS

Microscopic Polyangiitis
- Neutrophilic vasculitis affecting capillaries, venules or arterioles (small blood vessels)
- Serology—positive p-ANCA (perinuclear anti-neutrophilic cytoplasmic antibody)

Granulomatosis with Polyangiitis (Wegener's Granulomatosis)
- Necrotizing/ leukocytoclastic small vessel vasculitis
- Granulomatous inflammation
- Serology—positive c-ANCA (cytoplasmic anti-neutrophilic cytoplasmic antibody)

Churg-Strauss Syndrome
- Necrotizing granulomatous vasculitis
- With accompanying eosinophilia and asthma

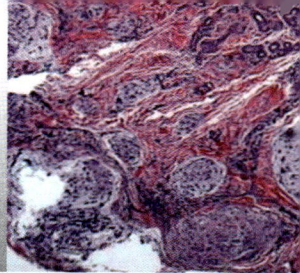

Cryoglobulinemia

INTRODUCTION

- Presents as superficial painful ulcers, purpura, urticaria or gangrene
- Most common site—ankles
- Predisposing factor—cold

THREE TYPES

Type I

- Monoclonal IgG or IgM cryoglobulins
- Associated with lymphoproliferative disorders, leukemia, myeloma, Waldenstrom's macroglobulinemia

Type II

- Monoclonal and polyclonal cryoglobulins
- Idiopathic forms are termed essential mixed cryoglobulinemia

Type III

- Polyclonal cryoglobulins
- Associated with SLE, Sjögren syndrome, rheumatoid arthritis, hepatitis C
- Idiopathic forms are termed essential mixed cryoglobulinemia

HISTOPATHOLOGY

Type I

- Dermal vessels show eosinophilic material deposited throughout the vessel wall and in its vascular lumen, which can be highlighted by PAS stain

- Inflammation is absent
- RBCs extravasation into the dermis

Type II and III

- Leukocytoclastic vasculitis with dense inflammation and resultant vessel wall damage
- Exocytosis of RBCs

DIRECT IMMUNOFLUORESCENCE

- Dense granular IgM, IgG and C3 deposits within the vessel walls

DIFFERENTIAL DIAGNOSIS

Disseminated Intravascular Coagulation

- Widespread fibrin thrombi in the capillaries and venules
- Features of ischemic damage to the tissues

Livedo Vasculopathy (Atrophie Blanche)

- Epidermal necrosis with underlying vasculopathy
- Fibrinoid material within the vessel wall or in vessel lumen
- In late stages, dermal vessel walls show hyalinization and intimal thickening

Leukocytoclastic Vasculitis and Polyarteritis Nodosa

- Damage to the small and medium-sized blood vessels
- Perivascular neutrophilic infiltrate
- Leukocytoclasis and fibrinoid necrosis of the vessel wall
- Erythrocyte extravasation into dermis

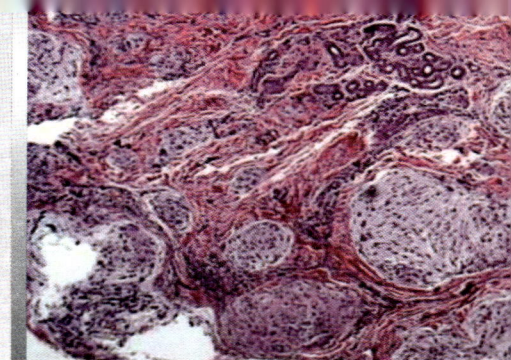

Inflammatory Disorders of Adnexal Structures

Part

8

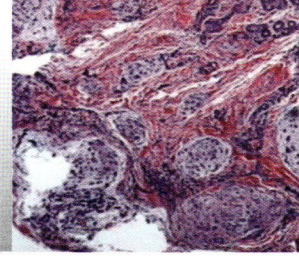

Chapter

Alopecia Areata

52

INTRODUCTION

- Autoimmune disorder
- Results in non-scarring hair loss
- Mediated by T-cells (CD8+ and CD4+), which induce premature anagen arrest and involution
- Diffuse infiltration of CD1a+ Langerhans cell around the hair bulb
- Presents as oval or circular patches of hair loss
- Most common site—scalp (Fig. 52.1)

HISTOPATHOLOGY

- Anagen follicles show peribulbar lymphocytic infiltrate (swarm of bees)
- Inflammatory cell destruction leads to conversion of anagen follicles to catagen follicles, as a result catagen and telogen follicles predominate
- This same cycle repeats and when the follicle re-enters anagen phase from telogen phase, they come under lymphocyte attack
- Chronic cases show miniaturized hair follicle and peribulbar fibrosis
- Conclusion—catagen and telogen hair with a miniaturized hair follicle are signs of alopecia areata

DIFFERENTIAL DIAGNOSIS

Tinea Capitis

- Perifollicular inflammation
- Fungal hyphae in stratum corneum, outside and within the hair follicles

Telogen Effluvium

- Presents with sudden increase in hair loss
- Anagen hair is decreased and telogen hair number is increased
- Absence of significant inflammation or miniaturization

Androgenetic Alopecia

- Diminution or miniaturization of hair follicles is a hallmark feature

- Patterned alopecia with a family history of baldness
- Absence of peribulbar or perivascular inflammation
- Absence of fibrosis

Trichotillomania

- Dilated hair follicles with fragments of hair shafts, which also contain melanin
- Peribulbar or perivascular inflammation is absent

Inflammatory Scarring Alopecia

- Dense peri-follicular infiltrate
- Infiltrate is also present at the dermo-epidermal junction
- In late stages, follicles are replaced by fibrosis

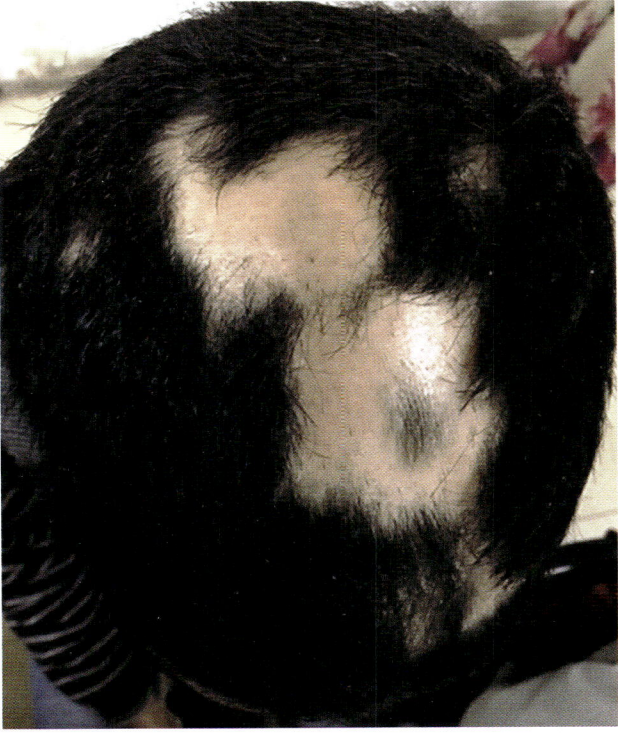

Fig. 52.1: Alopecia areata. Smooth, circular areas of complete hair loss

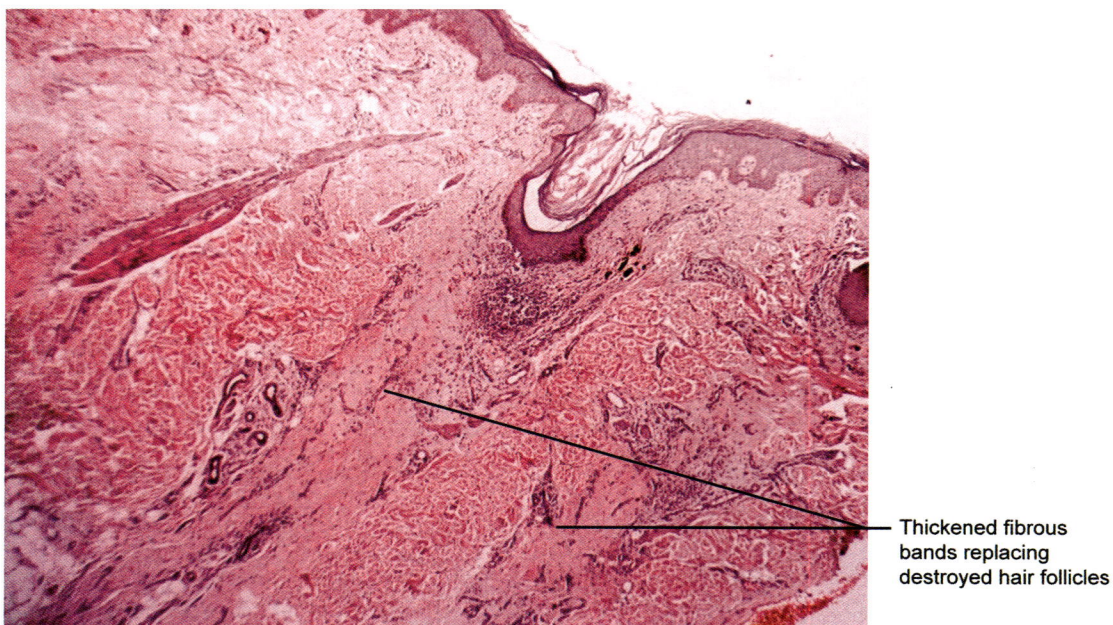

Fig. 52.2: Alopecia (scarring)

Thickened fibrous bands replacing destroyed hair follicles

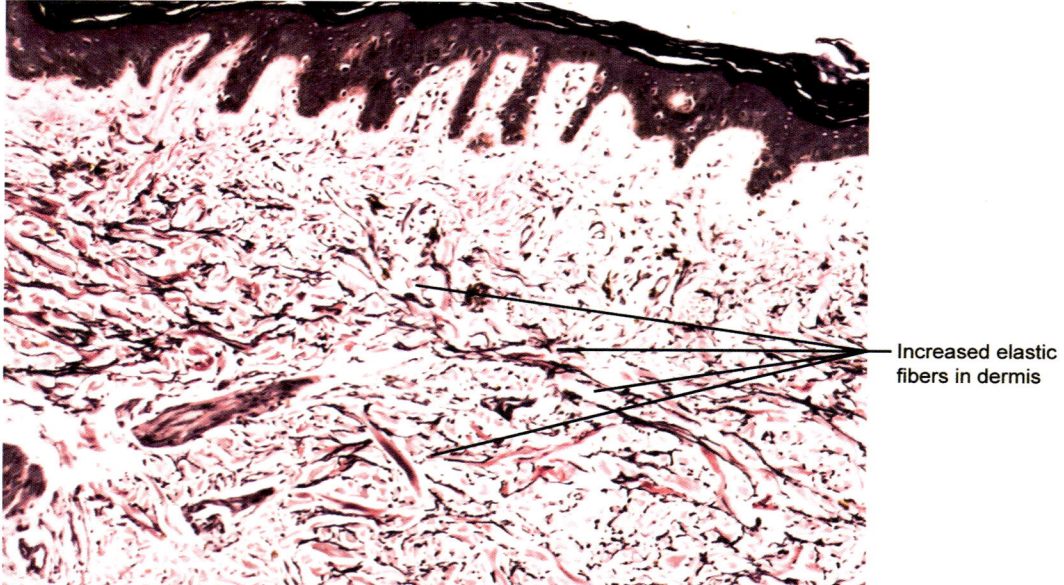

Fig. 52.3: Verhoeff-van Gieson stain in scarring alopecia

Increased elastic fibers in dermis

Idiopathic Scarring Alopecia (Pseudopelade)
(Figs 52.2 and 52.3)

- Characterized by patchy hair loss
- Preceding history of folliculitis, lichen planus, lupus erythematosus should be absent
- Replacement of hair follicles and sebaceous glands by bands of fibrous tissue
- These fibrous bands contain elastic fibers
- Verhoeff-van Gieson stain demonstrates increased elastic fibers amongst these fibrous bands

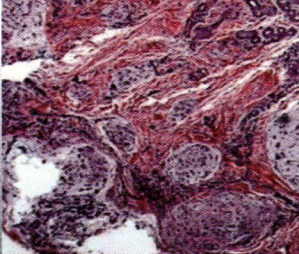

Folliculitis

INTRODUCTION

- Infectious inflammation of the hair follicle
- Presents as erythematous papules or pustules
- Sites—trunk, buttocks and extremities (Fig. 53.1)

HISTOPATHOLOGY (Figs 53.2 and 53.3)

- Intrafollicular and perifollicular infiltrate of neutrophils, eosinophils and plasma cells
- Spongiosis with follicular epithelial destruction
- Foreign body granulomatous reaction around the ruptured hair follicle
- Acute folliculitis—intrafollicular abscess or suppuration
- Chronic folliculitis—perifollicular fibrosis
- Staphylococcal folliculitis (furuncle)—gram-positive cocci can be identified within the follicular lumen

ANCILLARY STUDIES

- Bacterial colonies can be demonstrated by Gram stain
- Fungal organisms can be demonstrated by PAS or GMS stains

DIFFERENTIAL DIAGNOSIS

Rosacea

- Inflammatory disorder which affects nose, cheek, glabella and chin
- Presents as papules and pustules
- Dilatation of upper and mid-dermal vessels
- Perivascular and perifollicular mixed inflammatory cell infiltrate comprising of lymphocytes, histiocytes and neutrophils

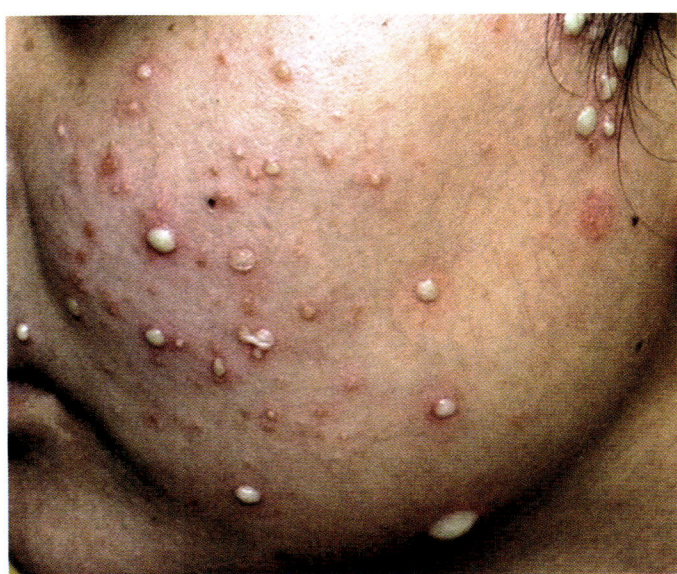

Fig. 53.1: Folliculitis. Follicular pustules and erythematous papules on hair-bearing area

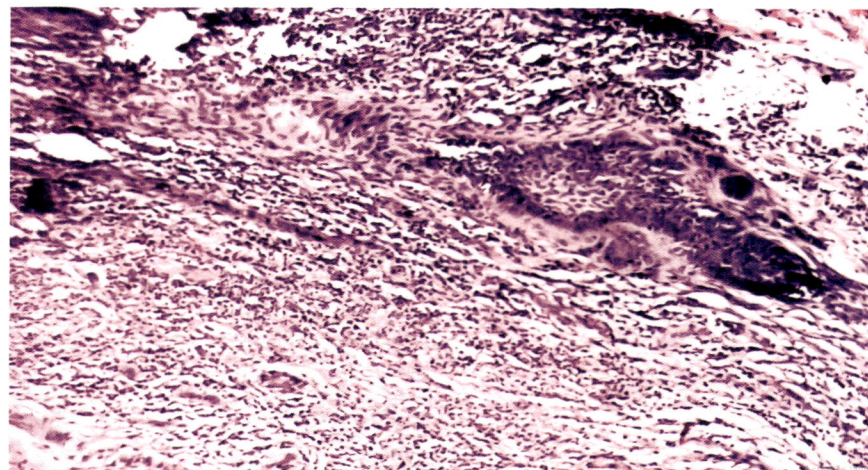

Fig. 53.2: Folliculitis. Dense neutrophilic infiltrate surrounding the follicles. Follicular destruction is also evident

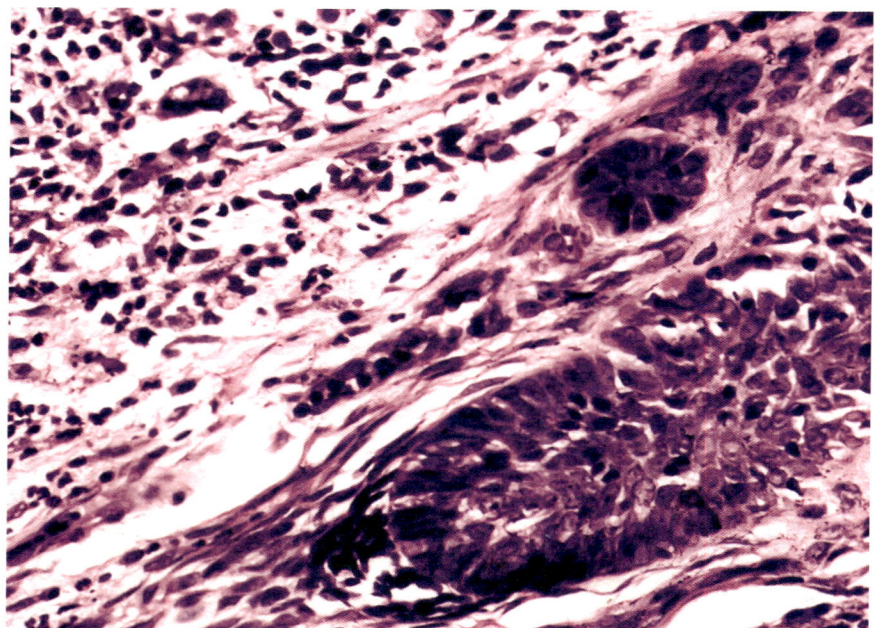

Fig. 53.3: Folliculitis. Perifollicular and intrafollicular inflammatory cell infiltrate with follicular destruction

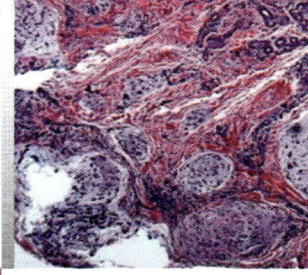

Folliculitis Decalvans

INTRODUCTION

- Inflammatory scarring alopecia
- Causative agent—*Staphylococcus aureus*
- Most common site—scalp
- Age: Young to middle-aged adults
- Presents as single or multiple plaques of alopecia with painful follicular pustules, crusts and papules

HISTOPATHOLOGY (Figs 54.1 and 54.2)

Early-stage Disease

- Dilation of the upper segment of hair follicle
- Perifollicular neutrophilic aggregates
- Gram stain can be used to highlight bacterial colonies

Late-stage Disease

- Perifollicular lymphoplasmacytic infiltrate

- Scarring and follicular loss
- Peri-follicular concentric fibrosis

DIFFERENTIAL DIAGNOSIS

Follicular Lichen Planus (Lichen Planopilaris)

- Hypergranulosis of the follicular epithelium
- Perifollicular lymphocytic infiltrate with interface change
- Late stage—hourglass appearance (perifollicular fibrosis with loss of hair follicles and adnexal structures)

Central Centrifugal Cicatricial Alopecia

- Eccentric thinning of the follicular epithelium
- Perifollicular lymphoplasmacytic infiltrate and concentric fibrosis
- Dermal follicular scarring

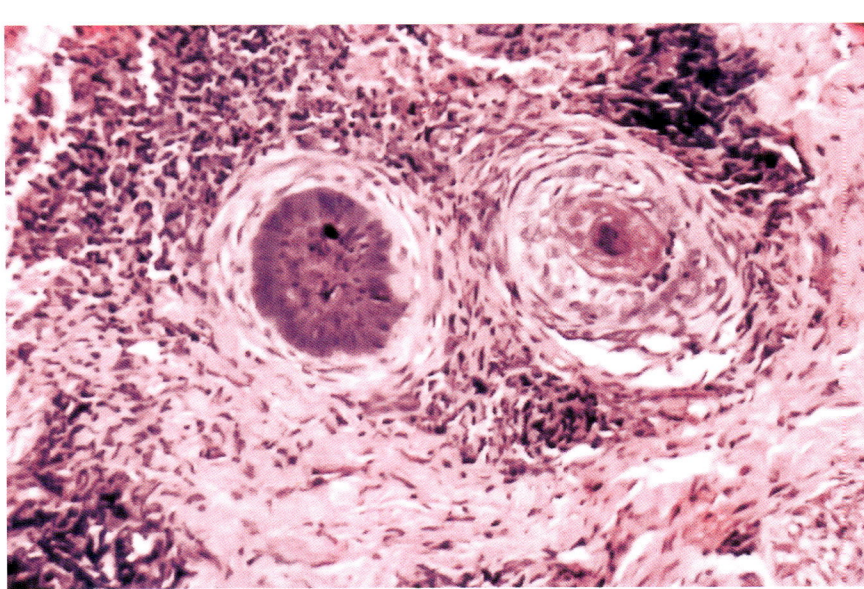

Fig. 54.1: Folliculitis decalvans. Interstitial and perifollicular concentric fibrosis with dense neutrophilic and lymphocytic infiltrate

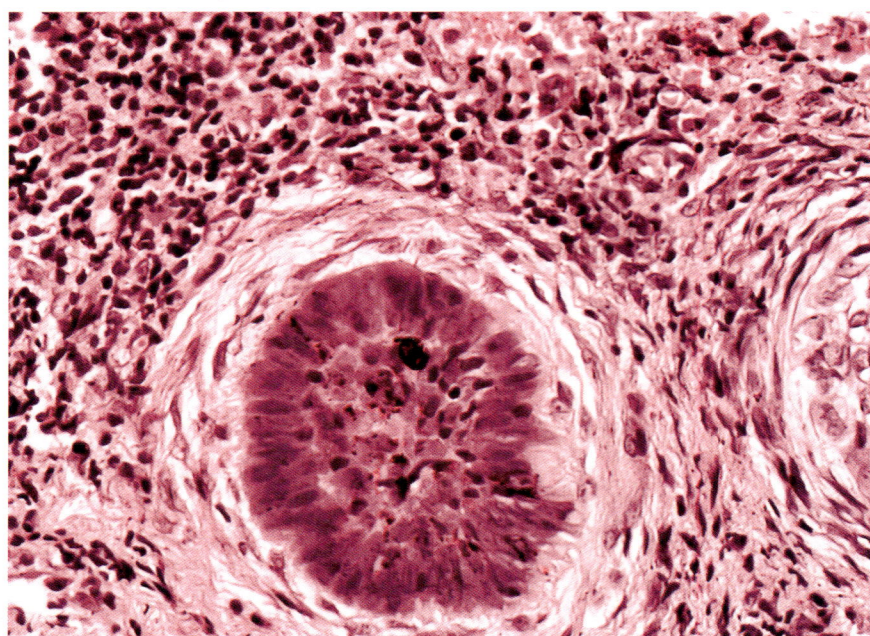

Fig. 54.2: Folliculitis decalvans. Perifollicular concentric fibrosis with predominant interstitial lymphocytic infiltrate

Lupus Erythematosus

- Perifollicular lymphocytic infiltrate with interface changes
- Perivascular lymphocytic infiltrate
- Mucin deposits between bands of collagen
- Late stage—hair follicle loss with perifollicular fibrosis

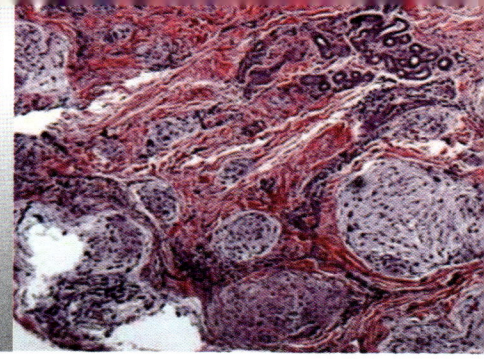

Drug Reactions

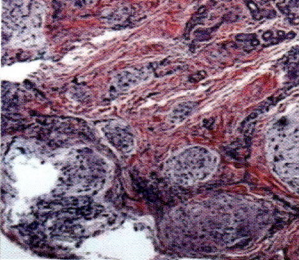

Drug Reactions

FIXED DRUG ERUPTION

INTRODUCTION

- Presents as edematous and erythematous patches following intake of a drug
- History of repeated similar episodes in past can be found
- Sites—lips, genitalia, proximal extremity, lower back (Fig. 55.1)

HISTOPATHOLOGY

- Hydropic degeneration of the basal cell layer
- Lichenoid inflammatory cell infiltrate
- Epidermis shows presence of necrotic keratinocytes (colloid bodies or civatte bodies)
- Upper dermis shows pigment incontinence with melanophages
- Bullous variant—subepidermal clefting is seen

DIFFERENTIAL DIAGNOSIS

Graft Versus Host Reaction

- Interface dermatitis with apoptotic keratinocytes
- Vacuolar degeneration along the dermal-epidermal junction
- Fibrosis of the papillary dermis

Erythema Multiforme

- Orthokeratotic stratum corneum
- Necrotic keratinocytes which can progress to full thickness epidermal necrosis

TOXIC EPIDERMAL NECROLYSIS

- Patient presents with diffuse erythematous rash (Fig. 55.2)
- Drugs being implicated as etiological agents includes sulfonamides, phenytoin, NSAIDs, steroids

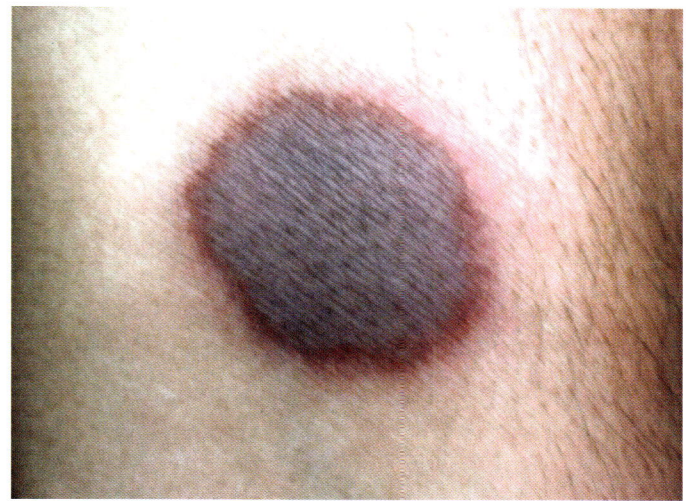

Fig. 55.1: Fixed drug eruption. Well-demarcated, round to oval, reddish-brown macule

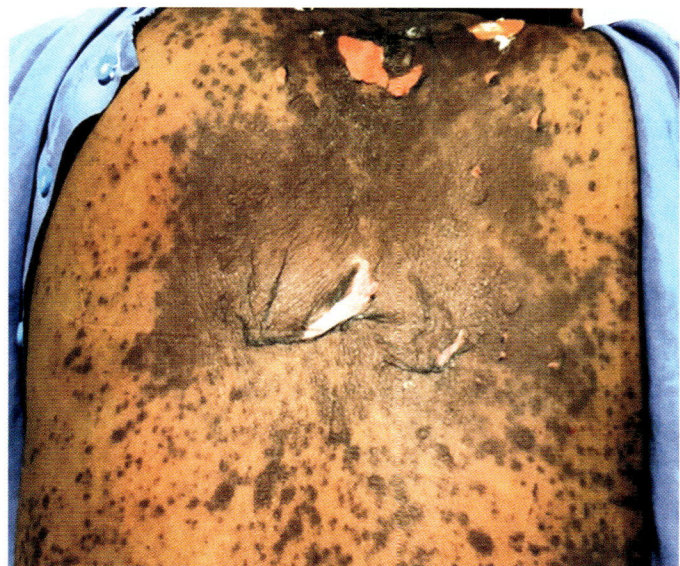

Fig. 55.2: Stevens-Johnson syndrome. Ill-defined, coalescing, erythematous to hyperpigmented macules with purpuric centers along with peeling of skin

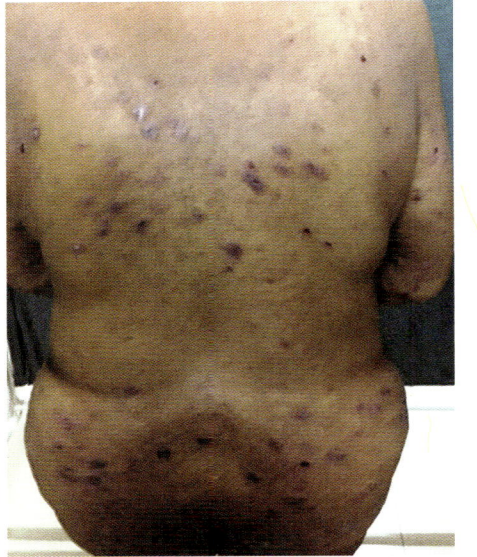

Fig. 55.3: Lichenoid drug eruption. Symmetric eruption of flat-topped, erythematous or violaceous papules

HISTOPATHOLOGY

- Widespread keratinocyte necrosis
- Subepidermal blister can be seen
- Dermal infiltrate of lymphocytes and eosinophils

LICHENOID DRUG ERUPTION (LDE)

INTRODUCTION

- Presents as erythematous macules, papules or plaques (Fig. 55.3)
- Sites—trunk and limbs
- Shares feature with lichen planus

HISTOPATHOLOGY

- Hyperparakeratotic stratified squamous epithelium with saw-toothed appearance of rete-ridges
- Basal cell vacuolization, interface dermatitis with a band-like infiltrate of lymphocytes
- Superficial and deep dermis show perivascular lymphocytic and eosinophilic infiltrate

DIFFERENTIAL DIAGNOSIS

Lichen Planus

- Wedge-shaped hypergranulosis with absence of parakeratosis

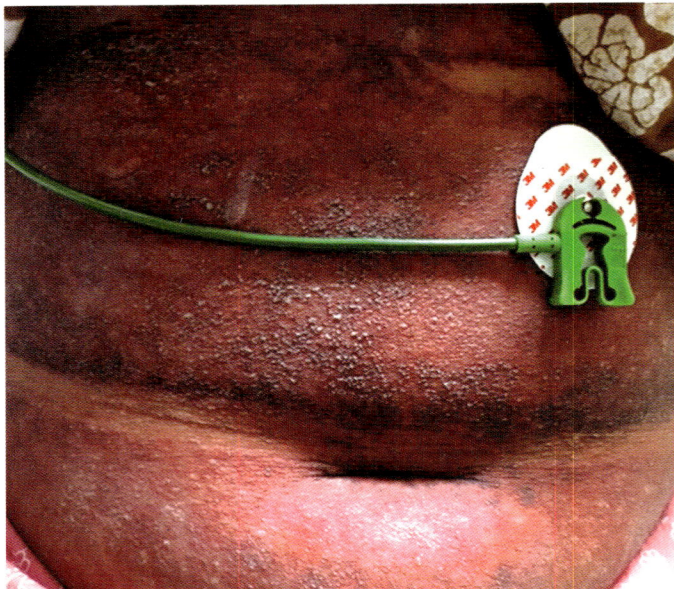

Fig. 55.4: Acute generalized exanthematous pustulosis. Numerous sterile, pin-head sized pustules on a background of erythema

- Absence of perivascular eosinophils in upper and mid-dermis
- Presence of melanophages in papillary dermis

MACULOPAPULAR DRUG REACTION

INTRODUCTION

- Maculopapular rash following ingestion of drug (Fig. 55.4)
- Most commonly affects older individuals

HISTOPATHOLOGY

- Keratinocyte necrosis at the dermo-epidermal junction
- Basal cell layer vacuolization
- Superficial dermis—perivascular and interstitial infiltrate comprising of lymphocytes and eosinophils

DIFFERENTIAL DIAGNOSIS

Urticaria

- Absence of interface change or necrotic keratinocytes
- Presence of dermal edema

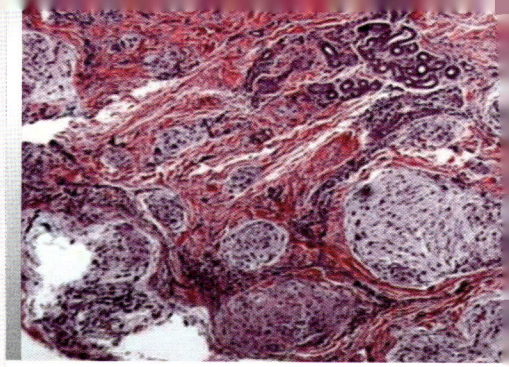

Pigmentary Disorders of Skin

Part

10

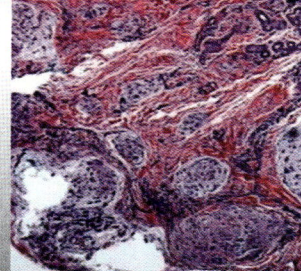

Vitiligo

INTRODUCTION

- Acquired disorder, that occurs due to the destruction of melanocytes
- Characterized by depigmented macules
- Sites—face, axillae, groin, genitalia, knees and elbows
- Associated autoimmune disorders include Hashimoto's thyroiditis, pernicious anemia, hyperthyroidism, Addison's disease, alopecia areata, pemphigus vulgaris, Crohn's disease

HISTOPATHOLOGY (Figs 56.1 and 56.2)

- Epidermis shows loss of melanin pigment and absence of melanocytes
- Edge of the lesion can show increased melanin pigment and melanocytes with an occasional lymphocyte
- Upper dermis can show perivascular lymphocytic infiltrate

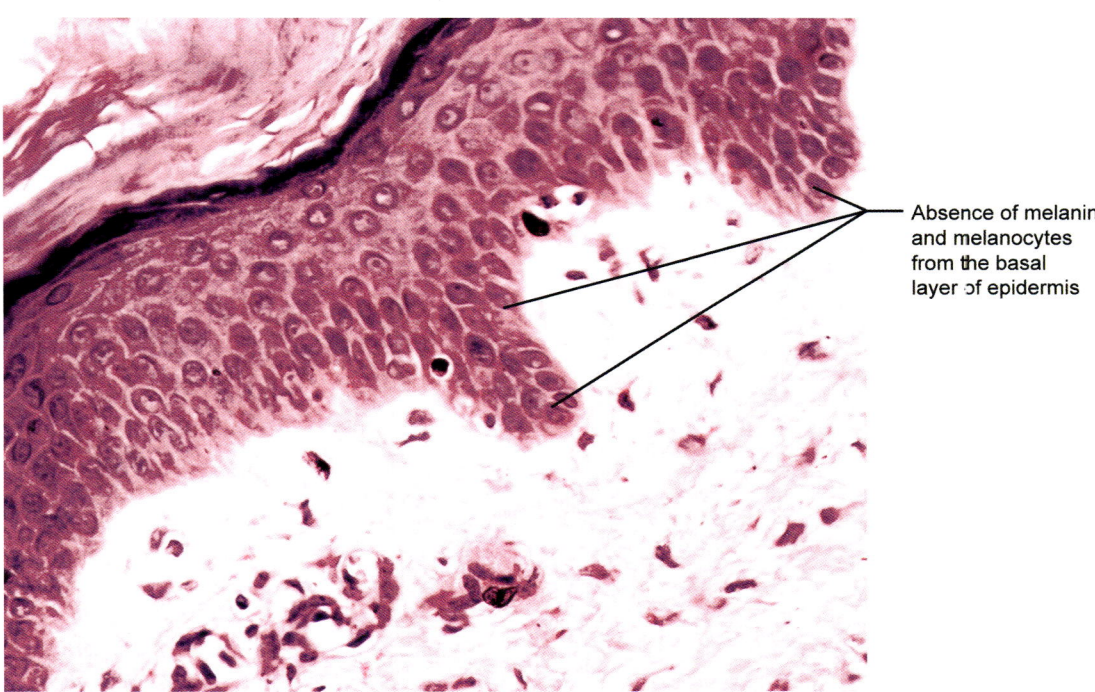

Absence of melanin and melanocytes from the basal layer of epidermis

Fig. 56.1: Vitiligo

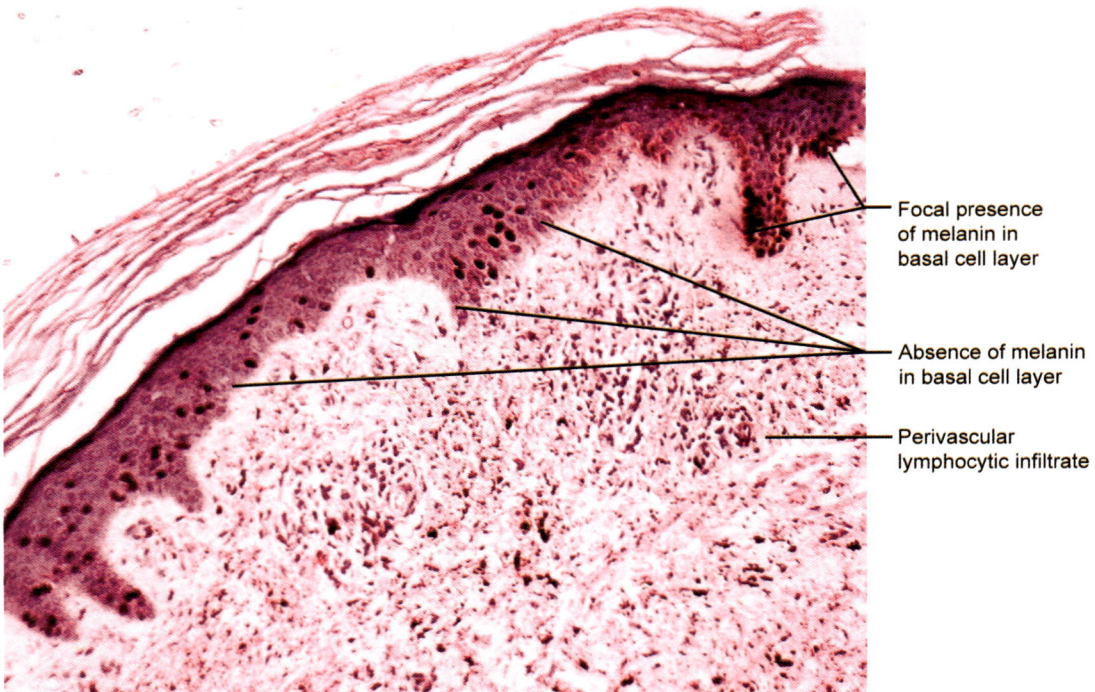

Focal presence of melanin in basal cell layer

Absence of melanin in basal cell layer

Perivascular lymphocytic infiltrate

Fig. 56.2: Vitiligo

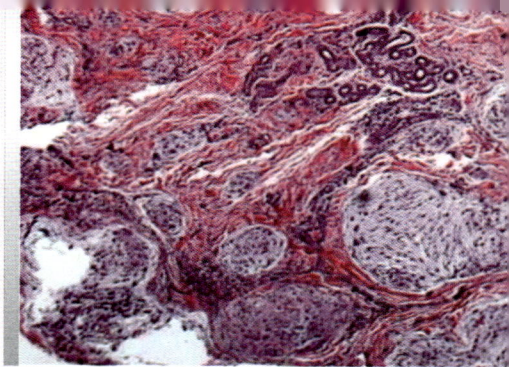

Cysts Affecting Skin

Part 11

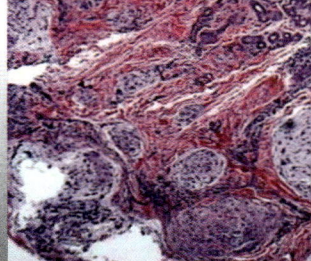

Dermoid Cyst

INTRODUCTION

- Presents as asymptomatic subcutaneous cystic mass at birth
- Site—midline neck
- Size—1–4 cm in diameter

HISTOPATHOLOGY (Fig. 57.1)

- Cyst is lined by stratified squamous epithelium
- Cyst wall can show pilosebaceous units, hair follicles, eccrine and apocrine glands, sebaceous glands, smooth muscle, cartilage, areas of calcification
- Cyst wall rupture can result in foreign body granulomatous reaction

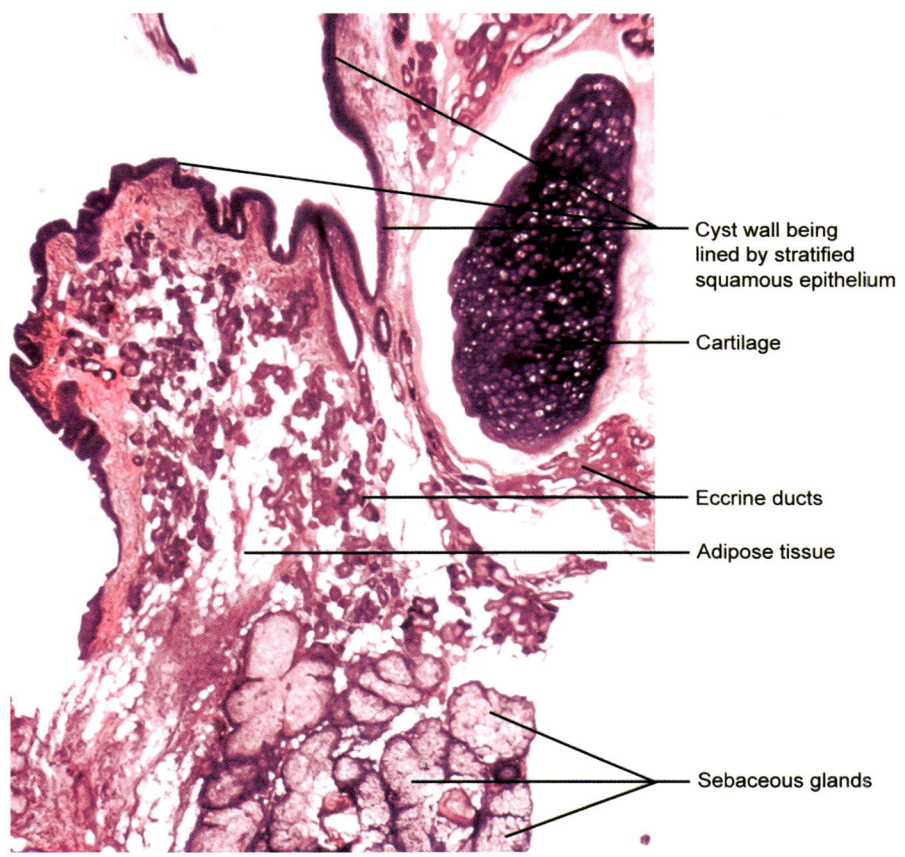

Cyst wall being lined by stratified squamous epithelium

Cartilage

Eccrine ducts

Adipose tissue

Sebaceous glands

Fig. 57.1: Dermoid cyst

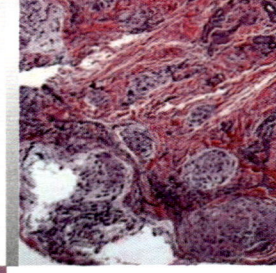

Epidermoid/Epidermal Cyst

INTRODUCTION

- Uni-locular cysts
- Site—face, neck and trunk
- Size—can measure up to 5 cm
- Dome-shaped lesions with smooth surface and can show a dot-like punctum (Fig. 58.1)
- Etiology—develops due to damage of pilosebaceous unit or following trauma

HISTOPATHOLOGY (Figs 58.2 and 58.3)

- Cyst lined by stratified squamous epithelium with the presence of granular layer
- Contents of the cyst—laminated keratin
- Ruptured cyst results in a foreign body reaction with multinucleated giant cells
- Hybrid cyst—a cyst showing features of epithelial and trichilemmal keratinization

- Malignant transformation can be seen rarely

DIFFERENTIAL DIAGNOSIS

Trichilemmal Cyst

- Absence of granular layer
- Abrupt trichilemmal keratinization

Eruptive Vellus Hair Cyst

- Cyst wall is lined by thin stratified squamous epithelium with presence of granular layer
- Laminated keratin with numerous small hair shafts make its contents

Steatocystoma

- Epithelial cyst with cuticle lining and sebaceous glands within the cyst wall

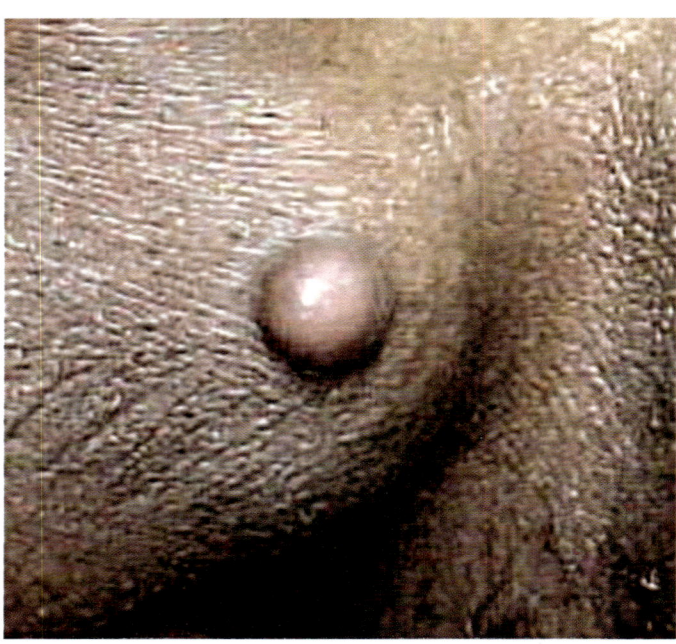

Fig. 58.1: Epidermoid cyst. Skin-colored nodule with a central punctum

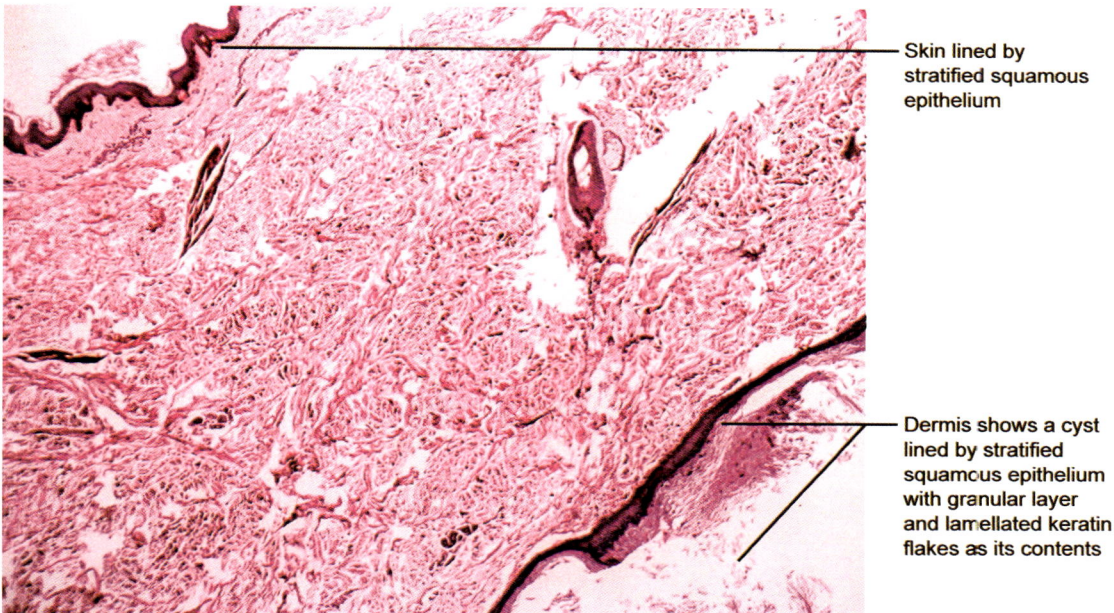

Skin lined by stratified squamous epithelium

Dermis shows a cyst lined by stratified squamous epithelium with granular layer and lamellated keratin flakes as its contents

Fig. 58.2: Epidermal inclusion cyst

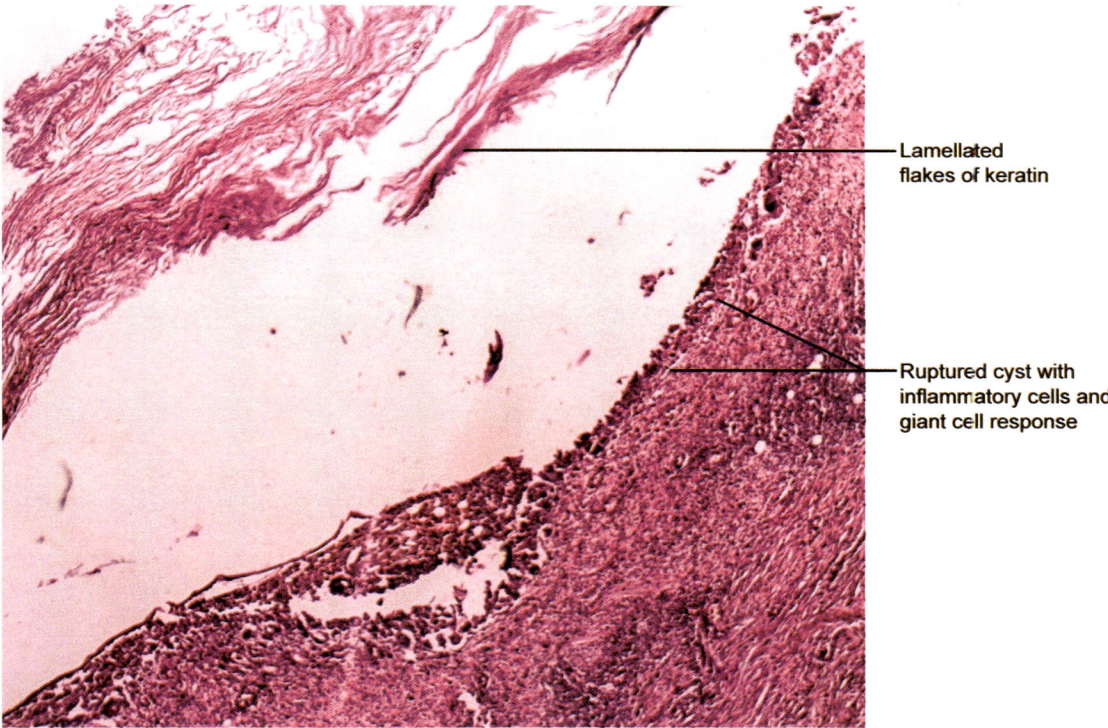

Lamellated flakes of keratin

Ruptured cyst with inflammatory cells and giant cell response

Fig. 58.3: Epidermal inclusion cyst

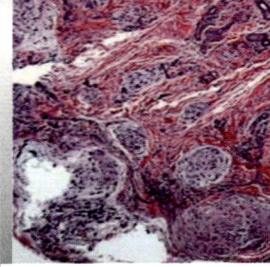

Eruptive Vellus Hair Cyst

INTRODUCTION

- Presents as multiple, asymptomatic papules measuring between 1 and 4 mm
- Site—chest wall, axilla, face, neck and extremities
- Age group—children or young adults
- Can undergo spontaneous regression

HISTOPATHOLOGY (Figs 59.1 and 59.2)

- Deep dermis show cysts, which are lined by stratified squamous epithelium
- Lumen of the cysts contains keratin and vellus hair shafts (refractile)

- Dual cysts/hybrid cysts can occur together—i.e. vellus hair cyst and steatocystoma
- Rupture of the cyst wall can result in foreign body granulomatous reaction
- Transepidermal elimination of the cyst contents can occur due to a connecting pore at the skin surface which can result in spontaneous resolution

DIFFERENTIAL DIAGNOSIS

Steatocystoma

- Cyst lined by squamous epithelium with sebaceous glands in its wall

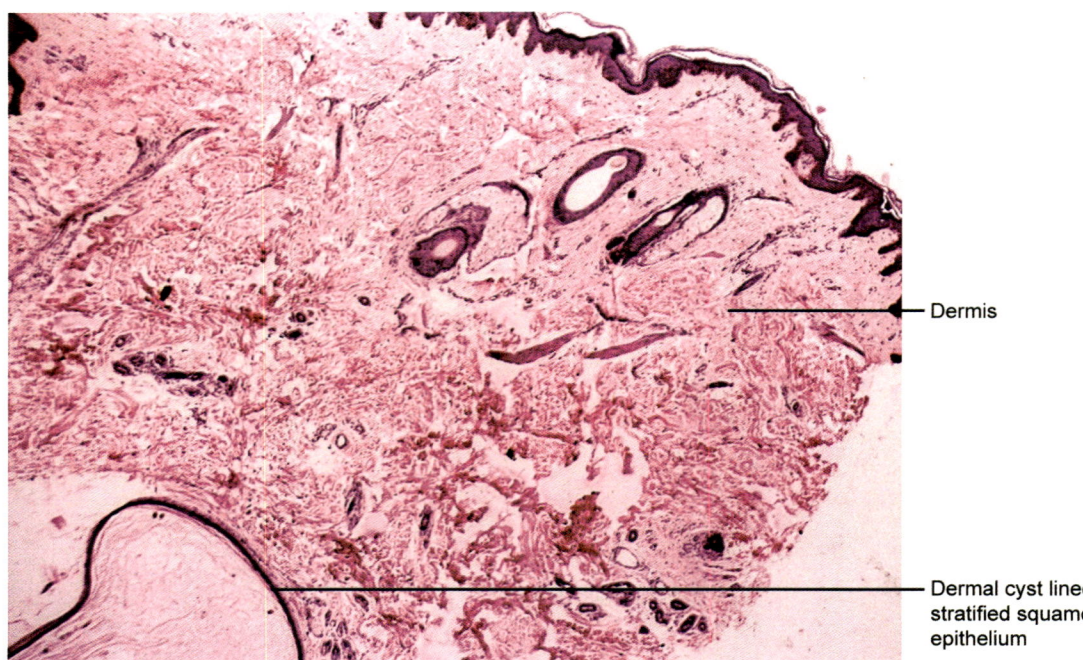

Fig. 59.1: Vellus hair cyst

Dermis

Dermal cyst lined by stratified squamous epithelium

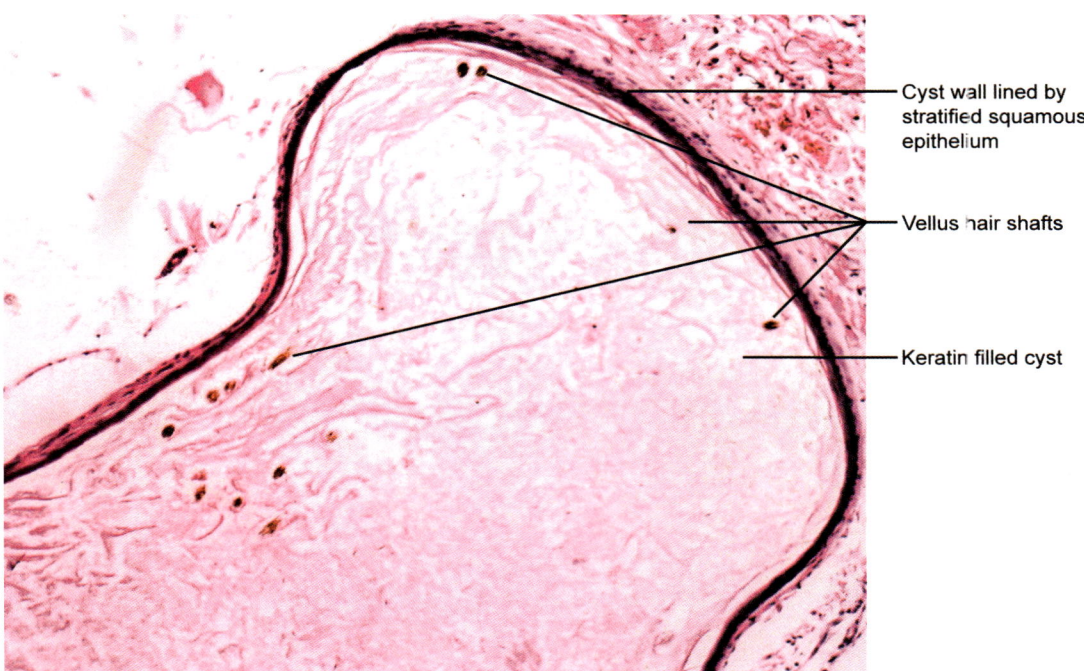

Cyst wall lined by
stratified squamous
epithelium

Vellus hair shafts

Keratin filled cyst

Fig. 59.2: Vellus hair cyst

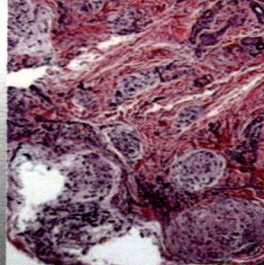

Digital Mucous Cyst

INTRODUCTION

- Presents as a solitary, dome-shaped, round to oval papule or nodule
- Site: Dorsal aspect of interphalangeal joint and distal phalanx of the digits

HISTOPATHOLOGY

- Cyst wall is devoid of lining epithelium
- Subepidermal cystic space with mucin collection
- Mucin can also be demonstrated by colloidal iron and alcian blue stain

DIFFERENTIAL DIAGNOSIS

Ganglion

- Lakes of mucin with presence of synovial cells
- Pseudo-capsule surrounds the mucin

Epidermoid Cyst

- Lined by stratified squamous epithelium with preserved granular layer
- Devoid of mucin

Myxoid Neurothekeoma

- Proliferation of basaloid tumor cells within mucin pool
- Tumor cells show S-100 positivity

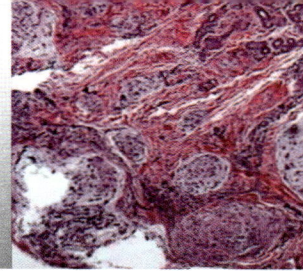

Steatocystoma

INTRODUCTION

- Presents as small, round, cystic, asymptomatic nodules measuring from few mm to 3 cm in diameter (Fig. 61.1)
- Steatocystoma simplex—solitary lesions, seen on axillae, face, neck, chest
- Steatocystoma multiplex—multiple lesions, seen most commonly on trunk

HISTOPATHOLOGY (Fig. 61.2)

- Cyst comprising of multilayered squamous epithelial lining
- Inner lining of cyst wall contains homogeneous eosinophilic horny layer (cuticle) without granular layer
- Characteristic feature is presence of sebaceous glands within the cyst wall

DIFFERENTIAL DIAGNOSIS

Eruptive Vellus Hair Cyst

- Cyst wall lined by stratified squamous epithelium with presence of granular layer
- Laminated keratin with numerous small hair shafts

Epidermoid Cyst

- Cyst lined by stratified squamous epithelium with preserved granular layer
- Cyst is filled with laminated keratin
- Lacks sebaceous glands, follicular structures and vellus hairs

Trichilemmal Cyst

- Cyst lined by stratified squamous epithelium that undergoes trichilemmal keratinization
- Absence of the granular layer
- Calcification can be seen

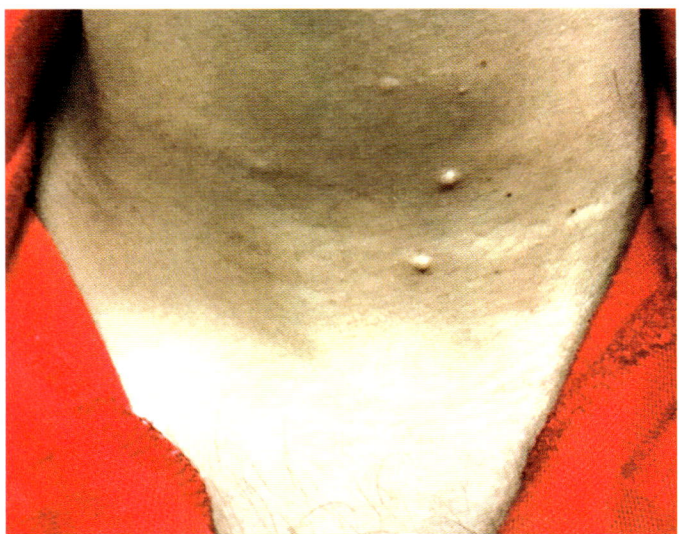

Fig. 61.1: Steatocystoma. Multiple, dermal, sebum-containing cysts

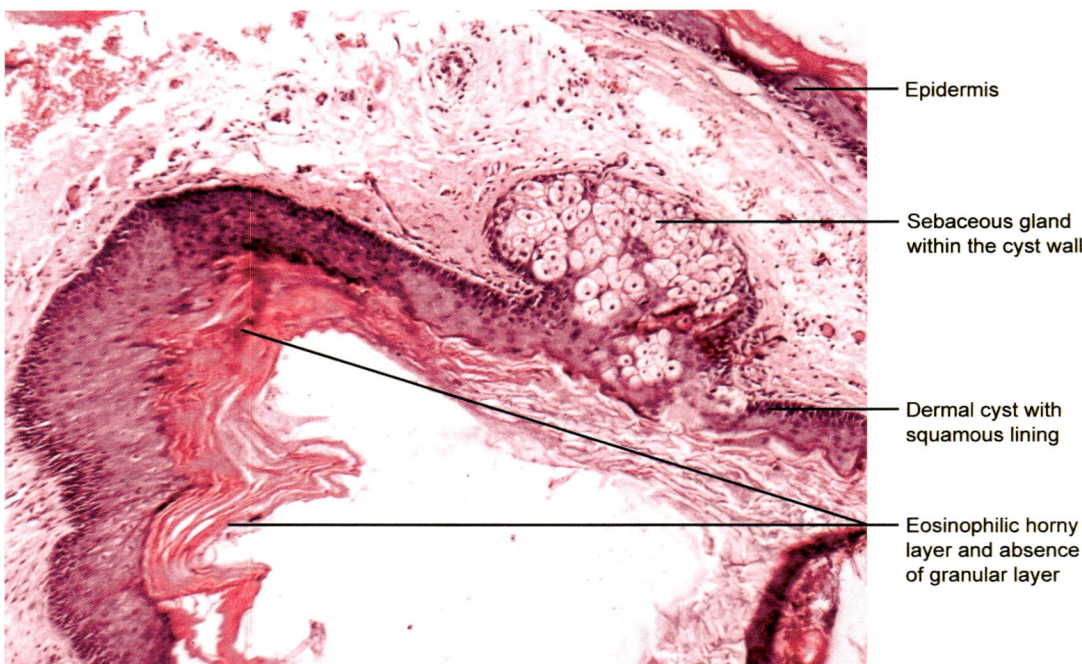

Epidermis

Sebaceous gland within the cyst wall

Dermal cyst with squamous lining

Eosinophilic horny layer and absence of granular layer

Fig. 61.2: Steatocystoma

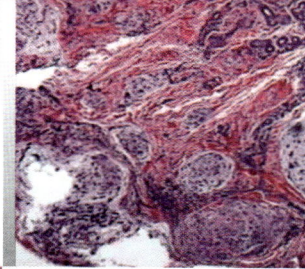

Trichilemmal Cyst (Pilar Cyst)

INTRODUCTION

- Most common site—scalp
- Presents as asymptomatic dermal or subcutaneous nodule

HISTOPATHOLOGY (Figs 62.1 and 62.2)

- Cyst is lined by stratified squamous epithelium with absence of granular layer
- Squamous cells undergo abrupt keratinization, called trichilemmal keratinization
- Calcification can be seen
- Cyst wall rupture can show granulomatous inflammatory response

DIFFERENTIAL DIAGNOSIS

Proliferating Trichilemmal Tumor/Pilar Cyst

- Scalp is the most common site
- Tumor measures 2–10 cm in diameter

Histopathology (Figs 62.3 to 62.5)

- Lobular proliferation of nests of squamous cells
- Nests of squamous cells can show peripheral pallisading
- Epithelium in the center of lobules undergo abrupt keratinization
- Presence of squamous eddies
- Mild nuclear atypia can be seen

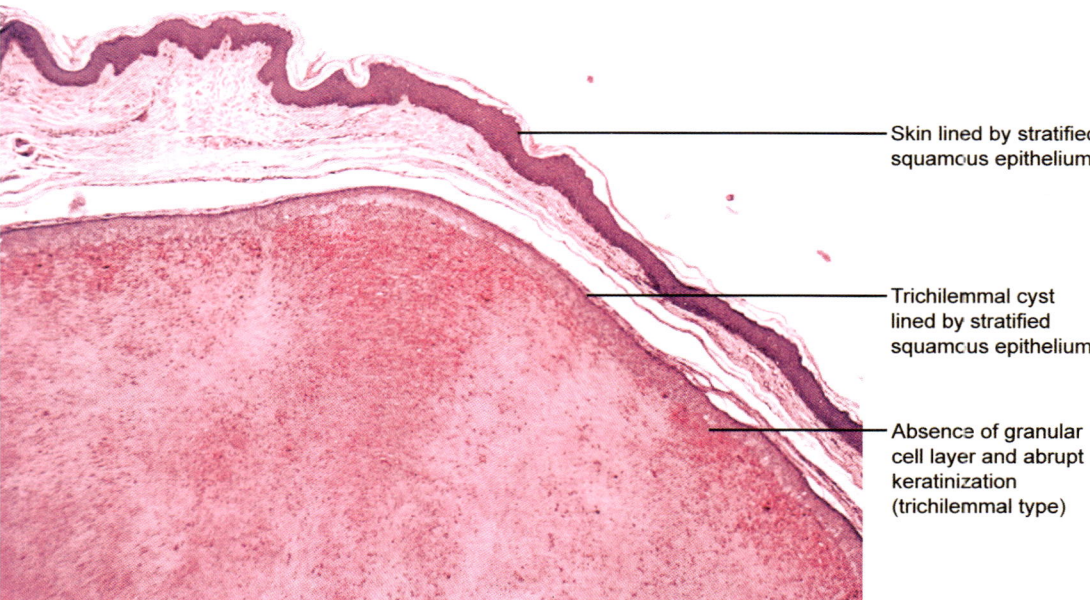

Skin lined by stratified squamous epithelium

Trichilemmal cyst lined by stratified squamous epithelium

Absence of granular cell layer and abrupt keratinization (trichilemmal type)

Fig. 62.1: Trichilemmal/pilar cyst

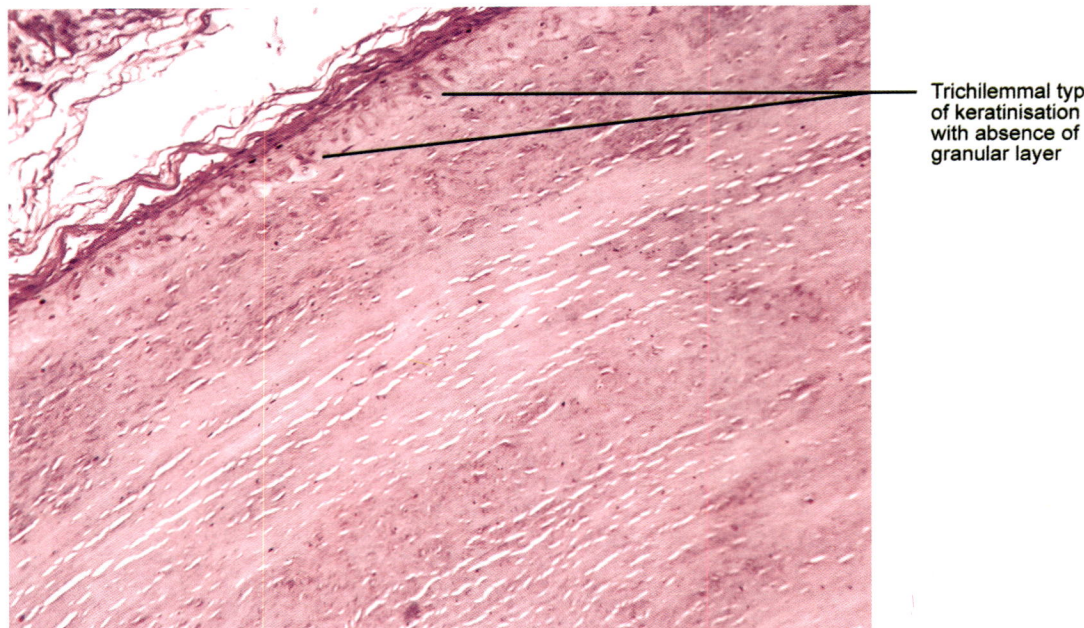

Fig. 62.2: Trichilemmal/pilar cyst

Trichilemmal type
of keratinisation
with absence of
granular layer

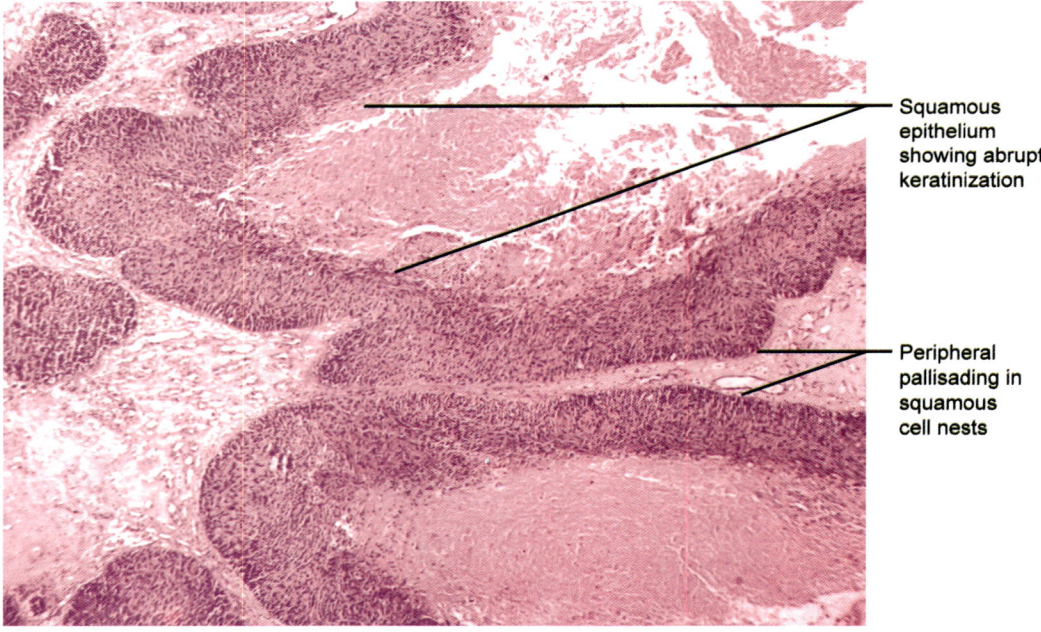

Fig. 62.3: Proliferating trichilemmal tumor

Squamous
epithelium
showing abrupt
keratinization

Peripheral
pallisading in
squamous
cell nests

Epidermal Inclusion Cyst

- Cyst lined by stratified squamous epithelium with intact granular cell layer
- Epidermal keratinization with laminated keratin
- Absence of trichilemmal keratinization

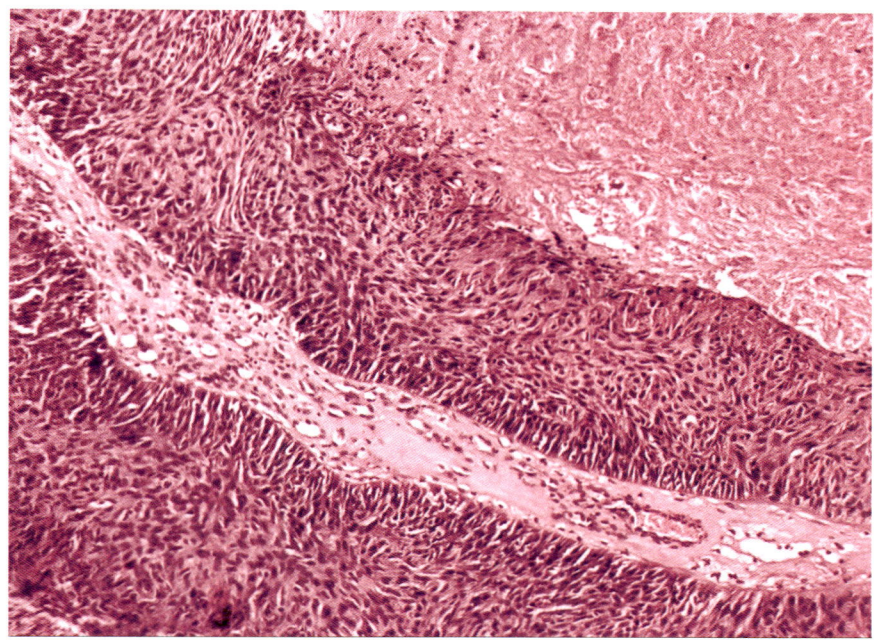

Fig. 62.4: Proliferating trichilemmal tumor. Central cavity showing abrupt type of keratinization with peripheral pallisading of squamous epithelial cells lining cyst wall

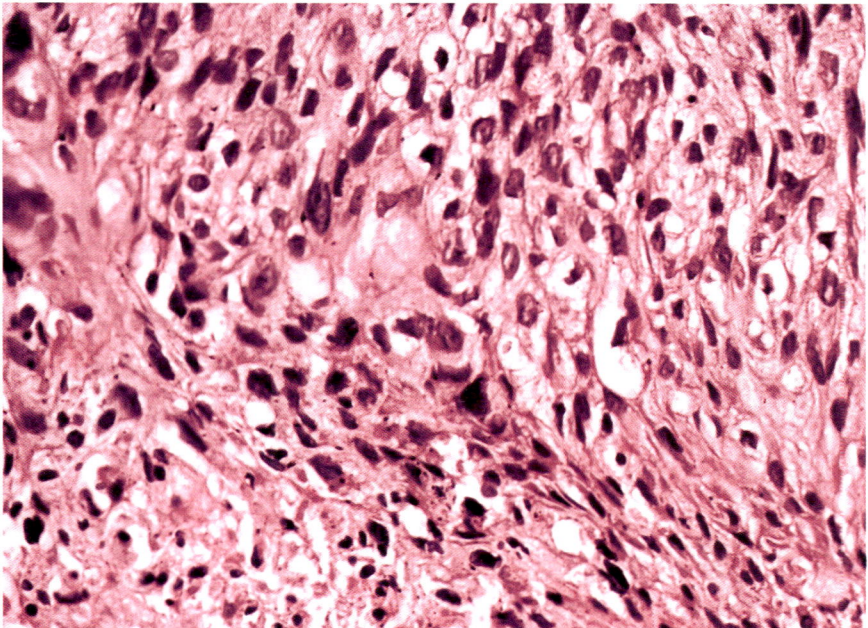

Fig. 62.5: Proliferating trichilemmal tumor. Squamous epithelial lining cells showing nuclear atypia

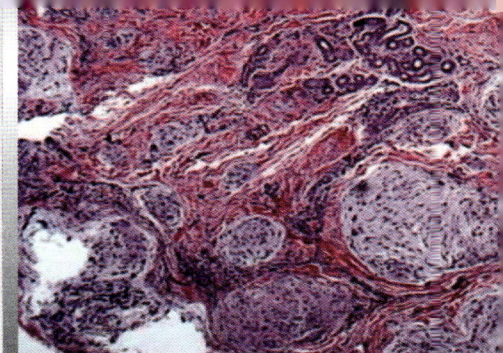

Epidermal Hamartomas and Neoplasms

Part 12

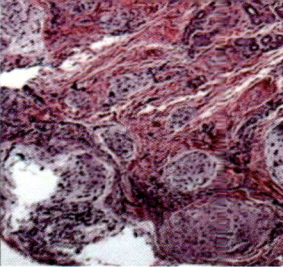

Epidermal Nevus

TWO TYPES—LOCALIZED OR SYSTEMATIZED TYPES

Localized Epidermal Nevus

- Presents as hyperkeratotic papules, arranged in a linear pattern (Fig. 63.1)
- Sites—head, trunk and extremities
- Can be present at the time of birth
- Seen in association with nevus sebaceous or syringo-cystadenoma papilliferum

Systematized Epidermal Nevus

- Presents as multiple papules in a linear configuration
- Site—trunk
- Associated with epidermal nevus syndrome

Histopathology

- Hyperkeratosis, orthokeratosis, acanthosis and papillomatosis
- Elongated rete ridges with the presence of acantholytic cells
- Epidermolytic hyperkeratosis (perinuclear vacuolization, irregularly shaped keratinocytes, acantholytic dyskeratosis and keratohyaline granules)
- Rare complications—basal cell carcinomas, squamous cell carcinomas, keratoacanthoma can arise in epidermal nevus

DIFFERENTIAL DIAGNOSIS

Seborrheic Keratosis

- Presence of pseudo-horn cysts

Verrucae Vulgaris

- Papillomatosis, parakeratosis, vacuolization of epidermal cells, elongated rete ridges

Acanthosis Nigricans

- Acanthosis, elongation of rete ridges

VARIANT

Inflammatory Linear Verrucous Epidermal Nevus (ILVEN)

- Parakeratosis, psoriasiform epithelial hyperplasia
- Superficial dermis shows perivascular lymphocytic infiltrate

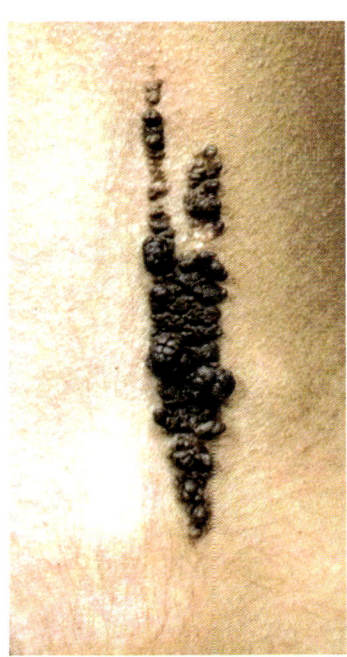

Fig. 63.1: Linear verrucous epidermal nevus. Linear patches and thin plaques consisting of coalescing skin-colored verrucous papules

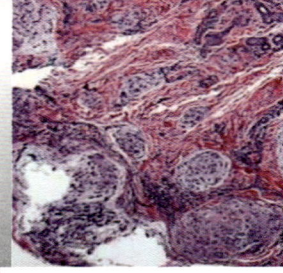

Nevus Sebaceous (Organoid Nevus)

INTRODUCTION

- Also called nevus Sebaceous of Jadassohn
- Lesion is present since birth and presents as a plaque
- As age advances, lesions become nodular
- Sites—face, forehead or scalp (Fig. 64.1)
- Size varies from 1 to 6 cm

HISTOPATHOLOGY (Figs 64.2 and 64.3)

During Childhood

- Absence of sebaceous cells
- Immature pilosebaceous units
- Hair structures with incomplete differentiation (hypoplastic hair follicles)

At Puberty

- Acanthosis, papillomatosis
- Enlarged and increased number of sebaceous glands in superficial dermis forming lobules
- Increased number of apocrine and eccrine glands in deeper dermis

ASSOCIATIONS

- Syringocystadenoma papilliferum (most frequent), trichoblastoma, pheochromocytoma, neurofibroma, meningioma

DIFFERENTIAL DIAGNOSIS

Epidermal Nevus

- Does not show increased sebaceous glands and adnexal structures in dermis

Sebaceous Hyperplasia

- Seen in elderly individuals
- Sebaceous lobules (four or more) attached to the infundibulum of each pilosebaceous unit
- Sebaceous lobules show a peripheral rim of basaloid cells

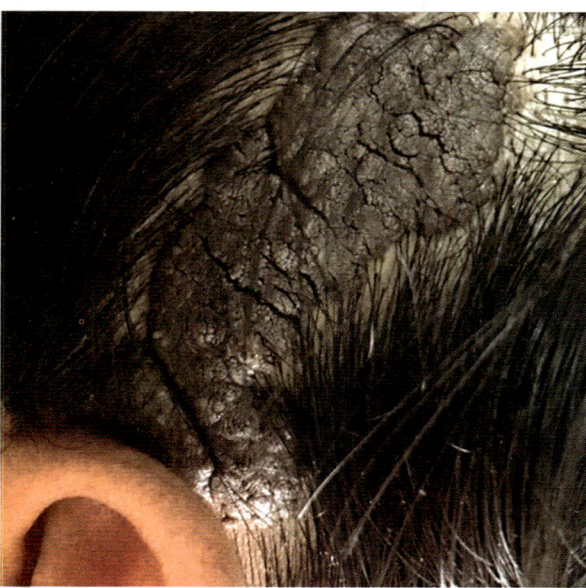

Fig. 64.1: Nevus sebaceous of Jadassohn. Well-defined localized area of alopecia showing linear plaque with cerebriform surface

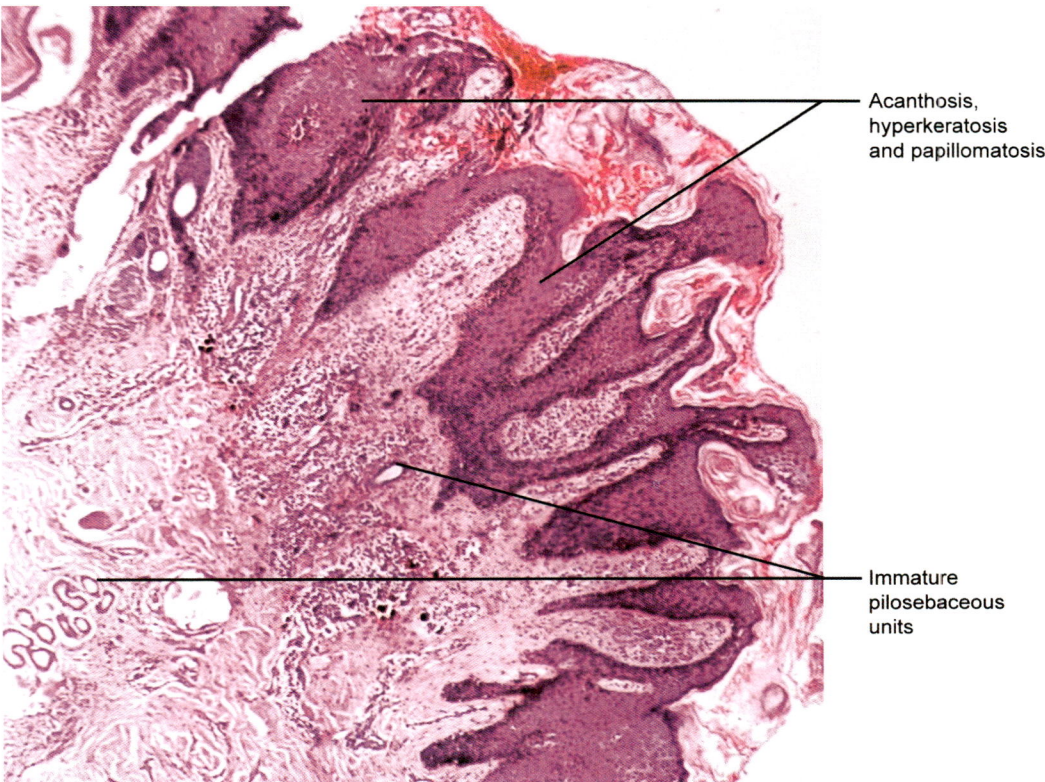

Acanthosis, hyperkeratosis and papillomatosis

Immature pilosebaceous units

Fig. 64.2: Nevus sebaceous

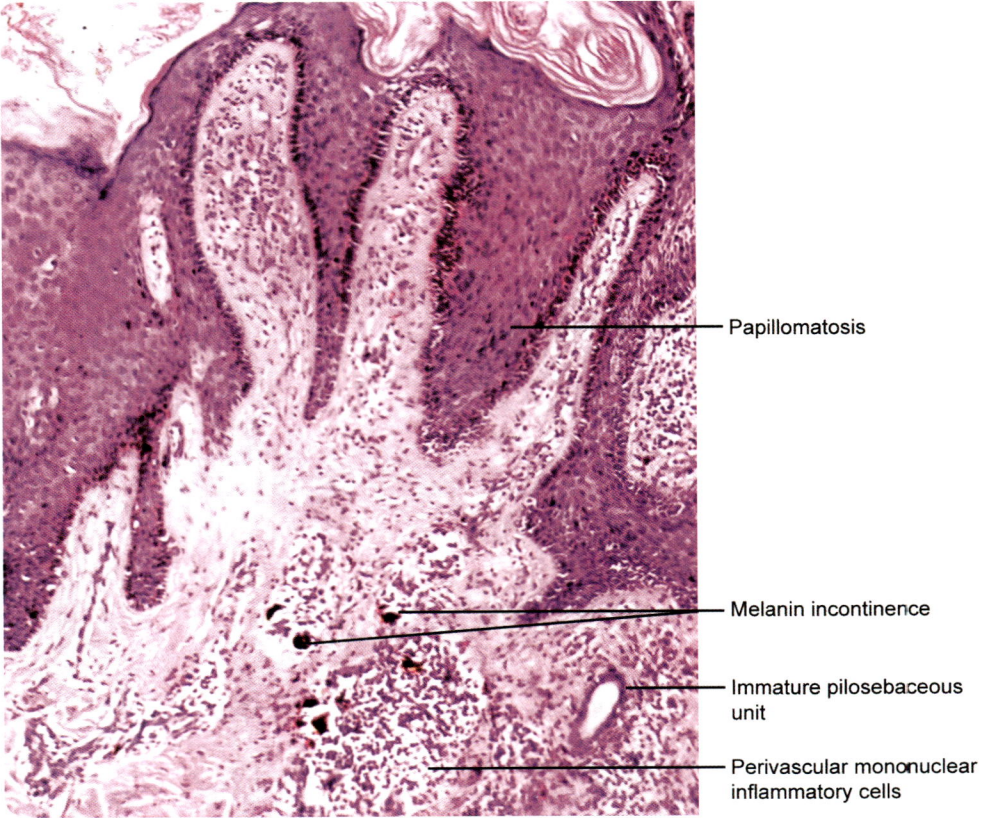

Papillomatosis

Melanin incontinence

Immature pilosebaceous unit

Perivascular mononuclear inflammatory cells

Fig. 64.3: Nevus sebaceous

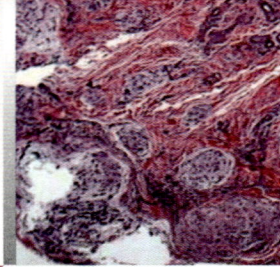

Seborrheic Keratosis

INTRODUCTION

- Commonly affects middle aged individuals
- Sites—trunk, face, extremities
- Presents as a brown, raised, plaque with keratin filled surface plug
- Size of the lesion varies from mm to less than 1 cm
- Associated with fibroblast growth factor receptor-3 (FGFR3) mutations

HISTOPATHOLOGY (Figs 65.1 and 65.2)

- Hyperkeratosis, acanthosis, papillomatosis
- Epidermis is composed of squamous cells and basaloid cells
- Lower border of tumor is arranged as a straight line
- Interspersed between these cells are numerous keratin filled cysts (horn cysts), some of which communicate with the surface (pseudo-horn cysts)

VARIANTS

Irritated Type

- Numerous, small, squamous eddies (made up of squamous cells)

Inverted Follicular Keratosis

- Endophytic verrucous proliferation with squamous eddies

Adenoid or Reticulated Pattern

- Presence of pseudo-horn cysts and rows of basaloid cells

Acanthotic Type

- Most common type
- Acanthosis, horn cysts and pseudo-horn cysts

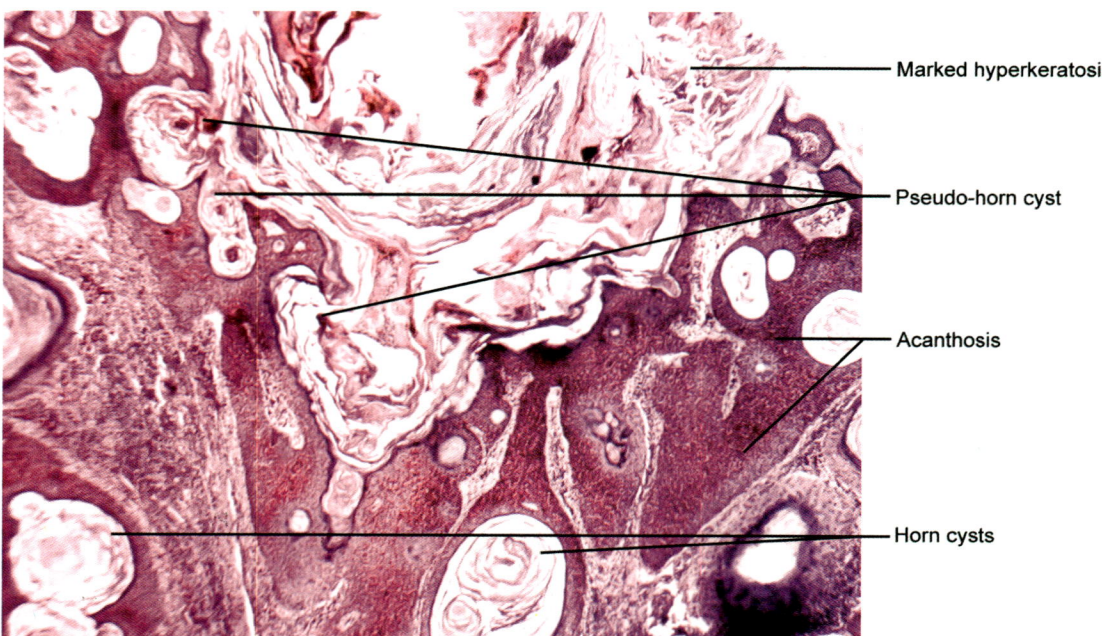

Marked hyperkeratosis

Pseudo-horn cyst

Acanthosis

Horn cysts

Fig. 65.1: Seborrheic keratosis

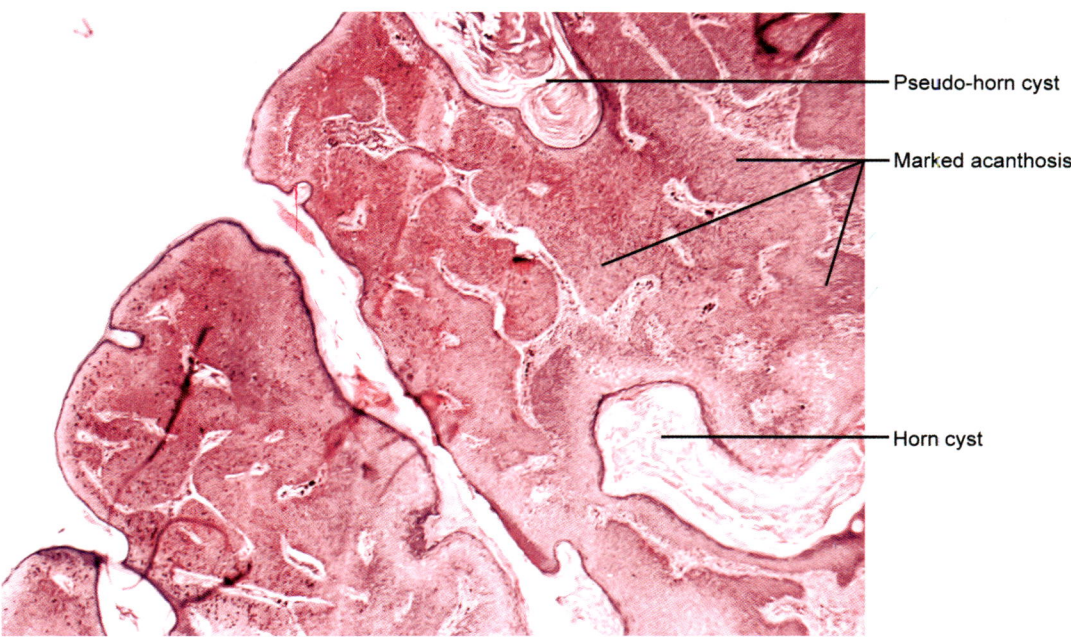

Fig. 65.2: Seborrheic keratosis

- Increased melanin pigment at the dermal-epidermal junction

Melanoacanthoma

- Marked increase in melanin, which is not only confined to dermo-epidermal junction, but are seen scattered throughout the tumor lobules

DIFFERENTIAL DIAGNOSIS

Epidermal Nevus

- Age and clinical presentation differs
- Are of localized and systematized forms
- Absence of horn cysts and pseudo-horn cysts

Verrucae Vulgaris

- Papillomatosis, parakeratosis, koilocytic atypia and elongated rete ridges

Clear Cell Acanthoma

- Epidermal cells show clear cell change
- Presence of neutrophils scattered throughout the epidermal cells (forming abscesses)

Paget Disease

- Clear tumor cells in epidermis, which show alcian blue, PAS and CK-7 positivity

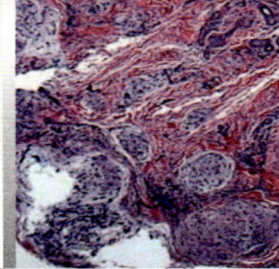

Clear Cell Acanthoma

INTRODUCTION

- Presents as a solitary dome-shaped papule or nodule, measuring 5 to 10 mm in diameter
- Most commonly affects legs

HISTOPATHOLOGY (Figs 66.1 to 66.3)

- Epidermis shows psoriasiform hyperplasia, focal acanthosis and papillomatosis
- Epidermal cells appear clear except the basal cells
- PAS stain demonstrates glycogen within these clear cells
- Epidermis shows spongiosis with presence of neutrophils forming intraepidermal abscesses

DIFFERENTIAL DIAGNOSIS

Seborrheic Keratosis

- Numerous pseudo-horn cysts

Psoriasis

- Elongated rete ridges with neutrophilic micro-abscesses in epidermis and corneal layers

Bowen Disease

- Epidermal clear cells with nuclear atypia and increased mitosis

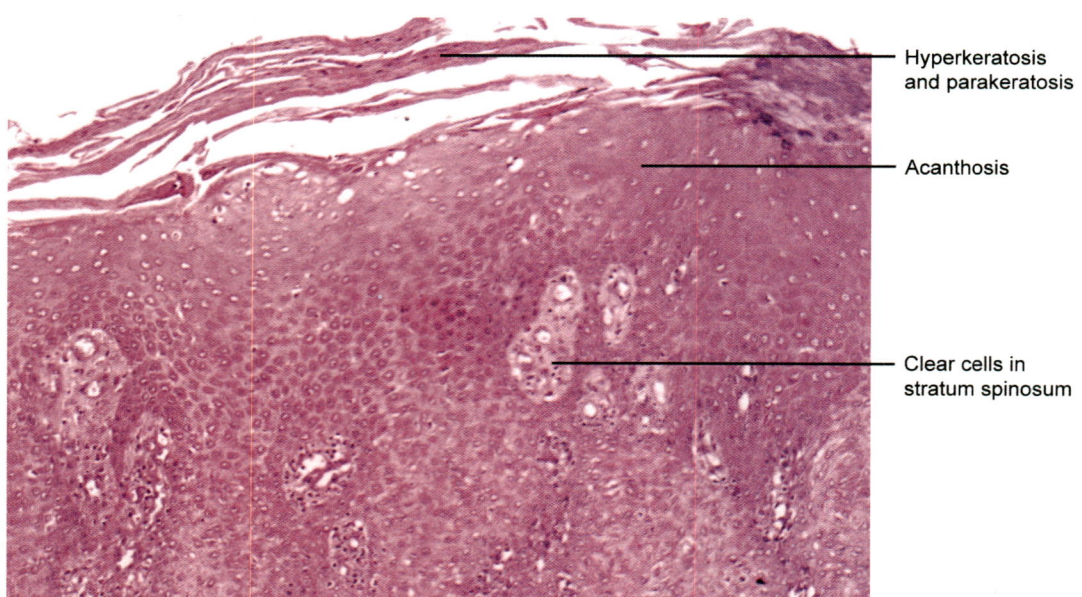

Hyperkeratosis and parakeratosis

Acanthosis

Clear cells in stratum spinosum

Fig. 66.1: Clear cell acanthoma

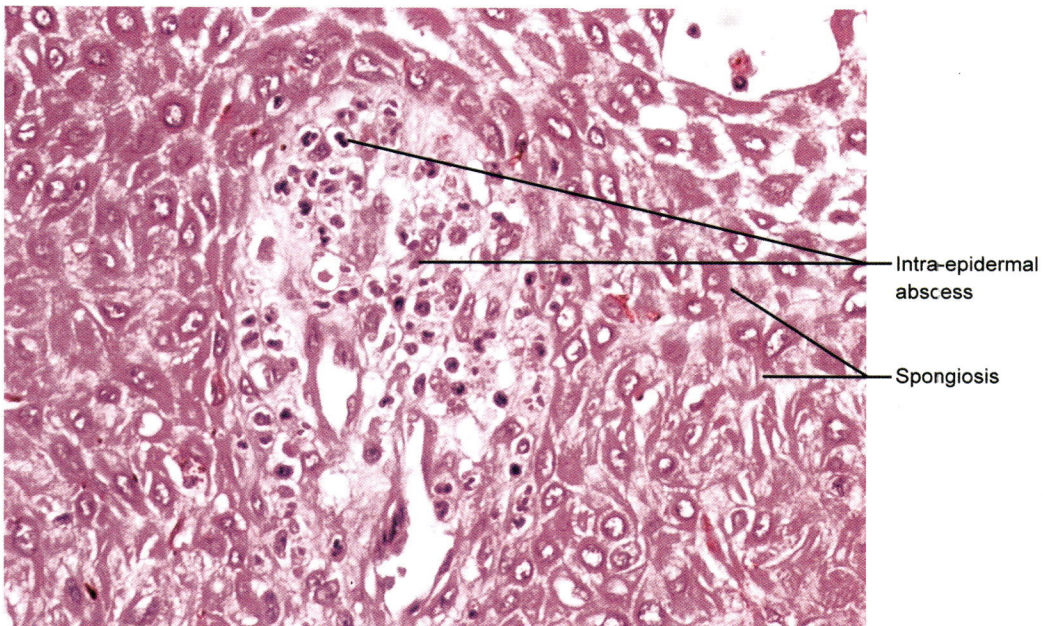

Intra-epidermal abscess

Spongiosis

Fig. 66.2: Clear cell acanthoma

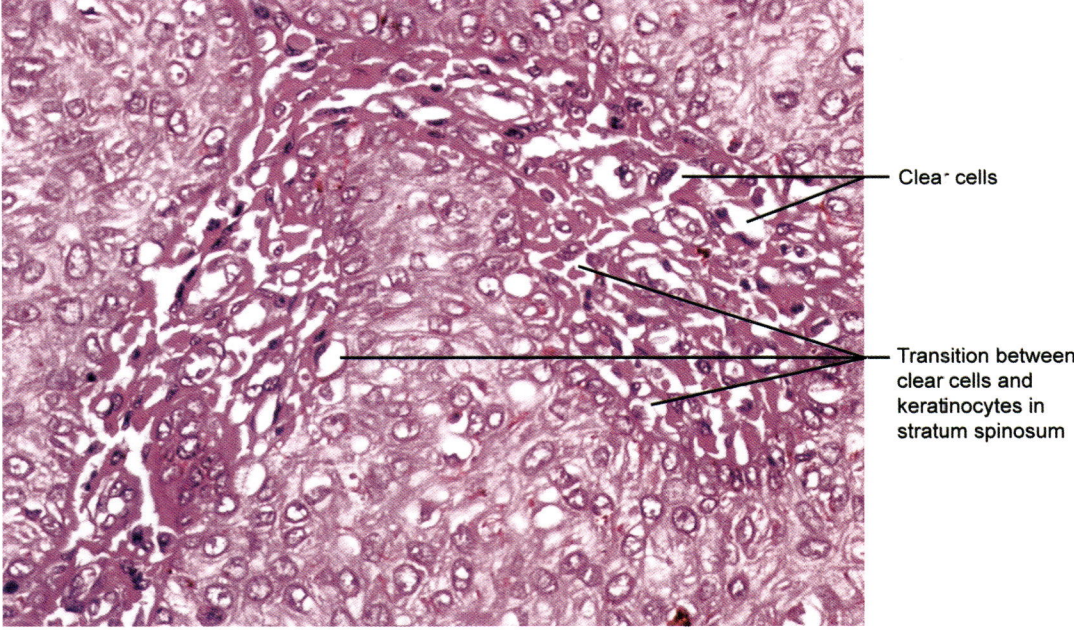

Clear cells

Transition between clear cells and keratinocytes in stratum spinosum

Fig. 66.3: Clear cell acanthoma

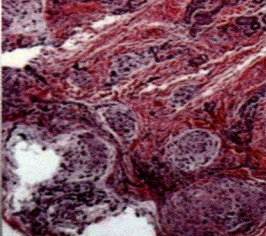

Porokeratosis

INTRODUCTION

- Due to disturbance in keratinization
- Involves face, genitalia, scalp, nails (Fig. 67.1)
- Complication—can transform into squamous cell carcinoma

FIVE TYPES

- Plaque type—porokeratosis of Mibelli (round or oval plaque with atrophic center and keratotic peripheral rim)
- Disseminated superficial actinic porokeratosis (DSAP)—most common type, affects sun-exposed areas, involves extensor surface of extremities
- Linear porokeratosis—involves a segment of body
- Porokeratosis palmaris/plantaris—seen in adolescents, present as small superficial lesions on palms and soles
- Punctate porokeratosis—affects only palms and soles, presents as numerous punctate lesions

HISTOPATHOLOGY (Figs 67.2 and 67.3)

- Epidermis shows keratin-filled invagination

- Within the center of this keratin filled invagination, arises the parakeratotic column, called cornoid lamellae
- Granular cell layer underneath the cornoid lamellae is diminished or absent
- Epidermis underneath the parakeratotic column shows irregularly arranged keratinocytes with pyknotic nuclei and can be flattened, normal or rarely acanthotic

DIFFERENTIAL DIAGNOSIS

Actinic Keratosis

- Horizontal alteration of parakeratotic and ortho-keratotic hyperkeratosis

Lupus Erythematosus

- Hyperkeratotic stratum corneum with follicular plugging
- Thickened basement membrane
- Absence of cornoid lamellae
- Perivascular and peri-adnexal lymphocytic infiltrate

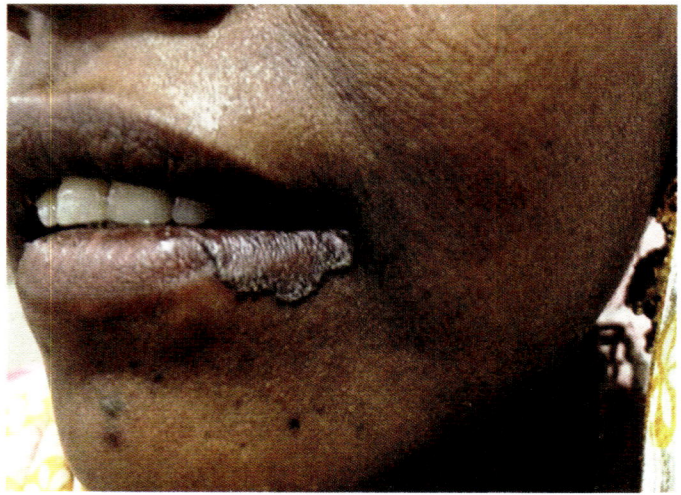

Fig. 67.1: Porokeratosis. Hyperpigmented macule with peripheral fine keratotic ridge known as cornoid lamella

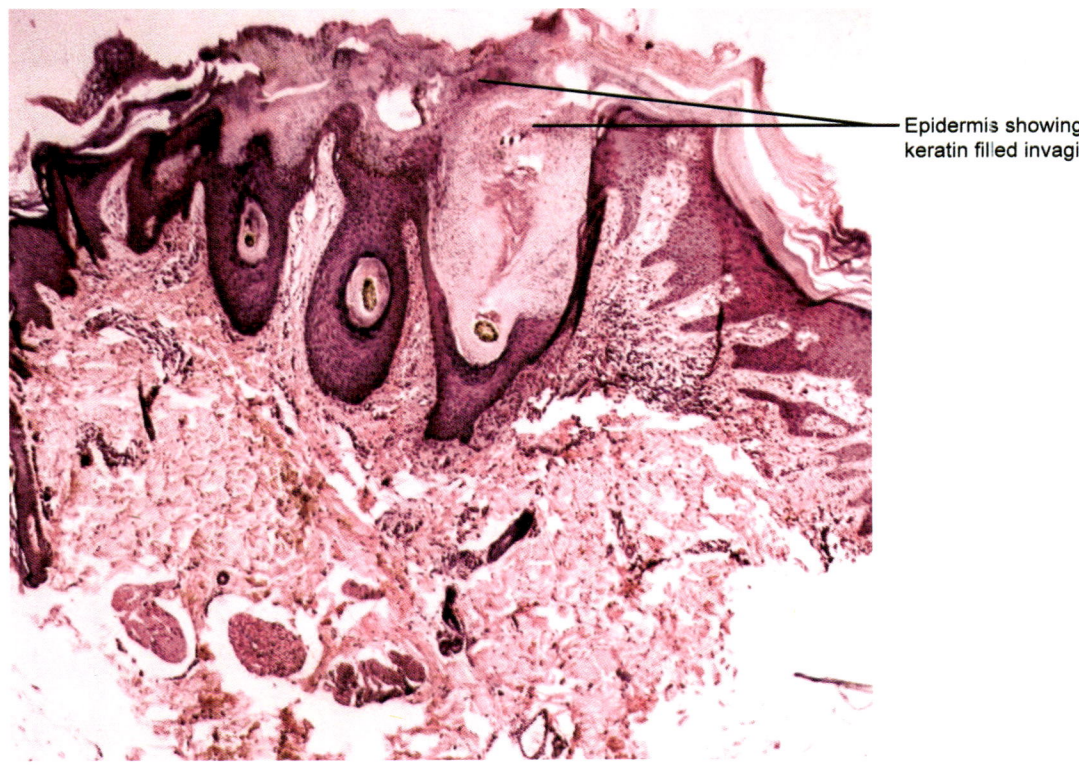

Epidermis showing
keratin filled invaginations

Fig. 67.2: Porokeratosis

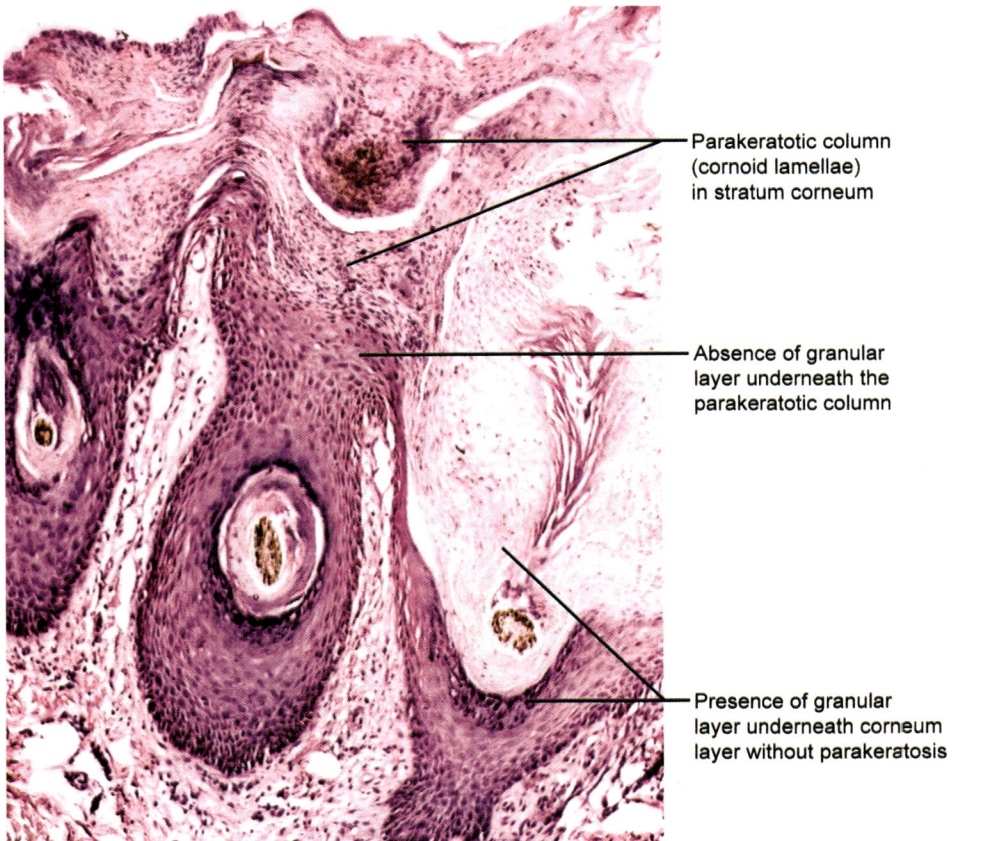

Parakeratotic column
(cornoid lamellae)
in stratum corneum

Absence of granular
layer underneath the
parakeratotic column

Presence of granular
layer underneath corneum
layer without parakeratosis

Fig. 67.3: Porokeratosis

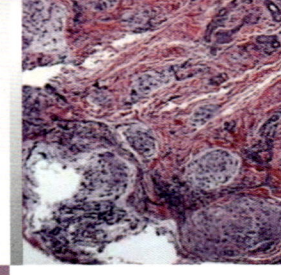

Actinic Keratosis

INTRODUCTION

- Also called solar keratosis
- Predisposing factor—sun-exposure
- Sites—face of elderly individuals
- Other sites—forearm, scalp, ears, hands
- Presents as erythematous scaly papule or plaque, measuring less than 1 cm in diameter
- Rarely, lesions can transform into squamous cell carcinoma

HISTOPATHOLOGY (Figs 68.1 and 68.2)

- Cell of origin—basal cells
- Precancerous lesions

- Also called squamous cell carcinoma *in situ*
- Malignant transformation to squamous cell carcinoma can occur
- Alternate areas of orthokeratotic and parakeratotic stratified squamous epithelium with atypical keratinocytes
- Upper dermis shows dense lymphoplasmacytic infiltrate

FIVE TYPES

Hypertrophic Type

- Acanthosis, hyperkeratosis, and papillomatosis
- Orthokeratosis with alternating parakeratosis

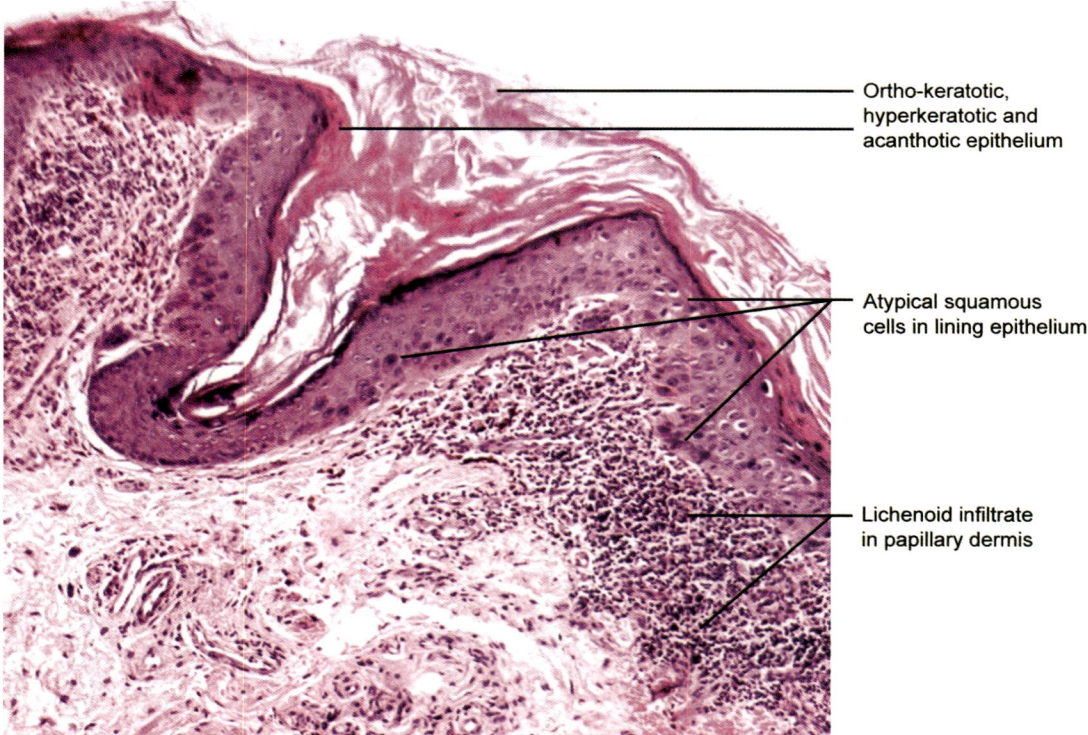

Ortho-keratotic, hyperkeratotic and acanthotic epithelium

Atypical squamous cells in lining epithelium

Lichenoid infiltrate in papillary dermis

Fig. 68.1: Actinic keratosis

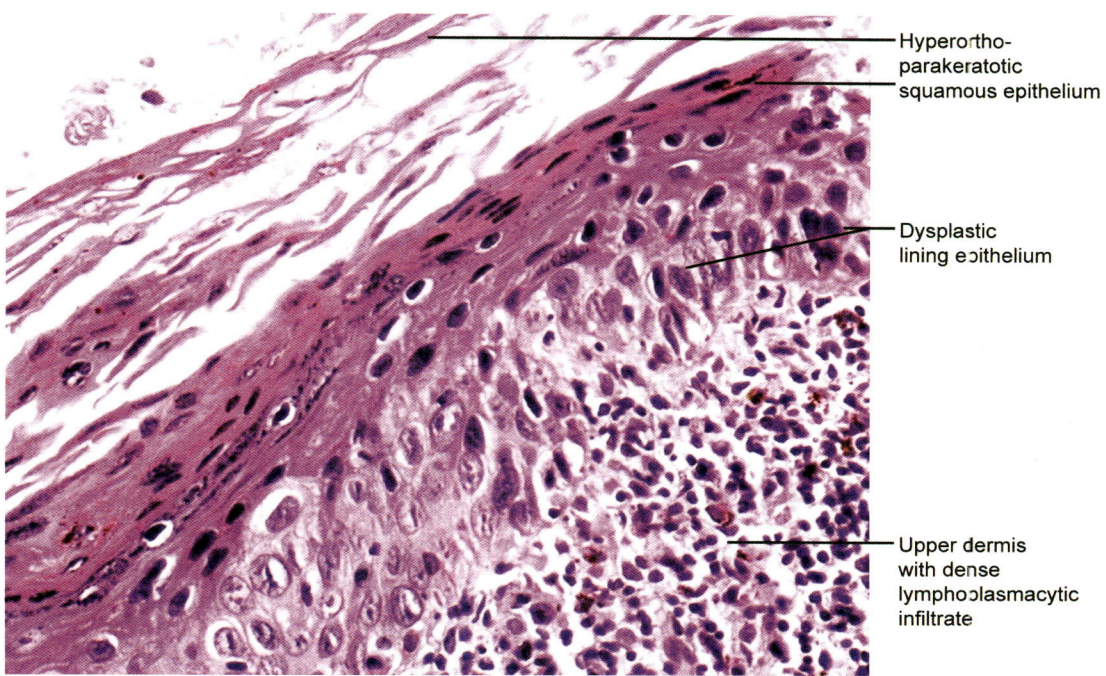

Hyperortho-
parakeratotic
squamous epithelium

Dysplastic
lining epithelium

Upper dermis
with dense
lymphoplasmacytic
infiltrate

Fig. 68.2: Actinic keratosis

- Epidermis shows atypical squamous cells, showing loss of polarity and nuclear pleomorphism
- Papillary dermis shows vertically oriented collagen bundles and dilated blood vessels
- Lichenoid actinic keratosis—variant of hypertrophic type, shows nuclear atypia, acanthosis, hyperkeratosis, basal cell vacuolization, band-like lichenoid infiltrate and civatte bodies

Atrophic Type

- Thinned out epidermis, atypical basal layer keratinocytes

Bowenoid Type (Squamous Cell Carcinoma *in situ*)

- Epidermis shows atypical squamous cells (full epithelial thickness) with marked nuclear and cytoplasmic pleomorphism and large atypical mitosis

Acantholytic Type

- Mimics basal cell carcinoma
- Hyperkeratotic epidermis, suprabasal clefts with acantholytic cells, dyskeratotic cells and atypical basal layer keratinocytes

Pigmented Type

- Increased melanin in keratinocytes of the basal cell layer with melanophages in upper dermis

DIFFERENTIAL DIAGNOSIS

Lupus Erythematosus

- Basal cell vacuolization
- Follicular plugging
- Focal peri-appendageal infiltrate

Lentigo Maligna

- Close differential of pigmented actinic keratosis
- Flattening of the epidermis
- Increased number of atypical melanocytes
- Absence of atypical basal keratinocytes

Epidermal Dysmaturation

- Epidermal changes, seen following chemotherapy
- Epidermal keratinocytes show loss of polarity, large hyperchromatic nuclei, mitotic figures and apoptotic bodies

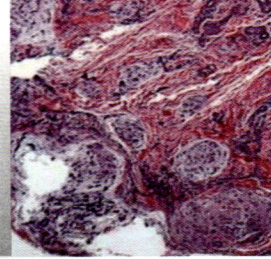

Bowen's Disease

INTRODUCTION

- Carcinoma *in situ* of skin
- Precursor lesion of squamous cell carcinoma
- Can be seen on sun-exposed and non sun-exposed areas
- Presents as a solitary erythematous scaly papule
- HPV-16 and 18 are implicated agents
- Bowenoid papulosis—associated with verrucous papules on the genitalia, resembling condyloma acuminatum, associated with HPV-16 infection

HISTOPATHOLOGY

- Parakeratotic, hyperkeratotic and acanthotic epidermis
- Elongated and thickened rete ridges
- Full thickness epidermal dysplastic changes are seen
- Squamous cells appear large with hyperchromatic nuclei and can show atypical mitosis
- Demarcation between epidermis and dermis is maintained
- Absence of invasion
- Upper dermis shows chronic inflammatory cell infiltrate
- Can progress to invasive squamous cell carcinoma

DIFFERENTIAL DIAGNOSIS/ VARIANTS

Bowenoid Papulosis (Figs 69.1 and 69.2)

- Causative agent—human papillomavirus-16 (HPV-16)

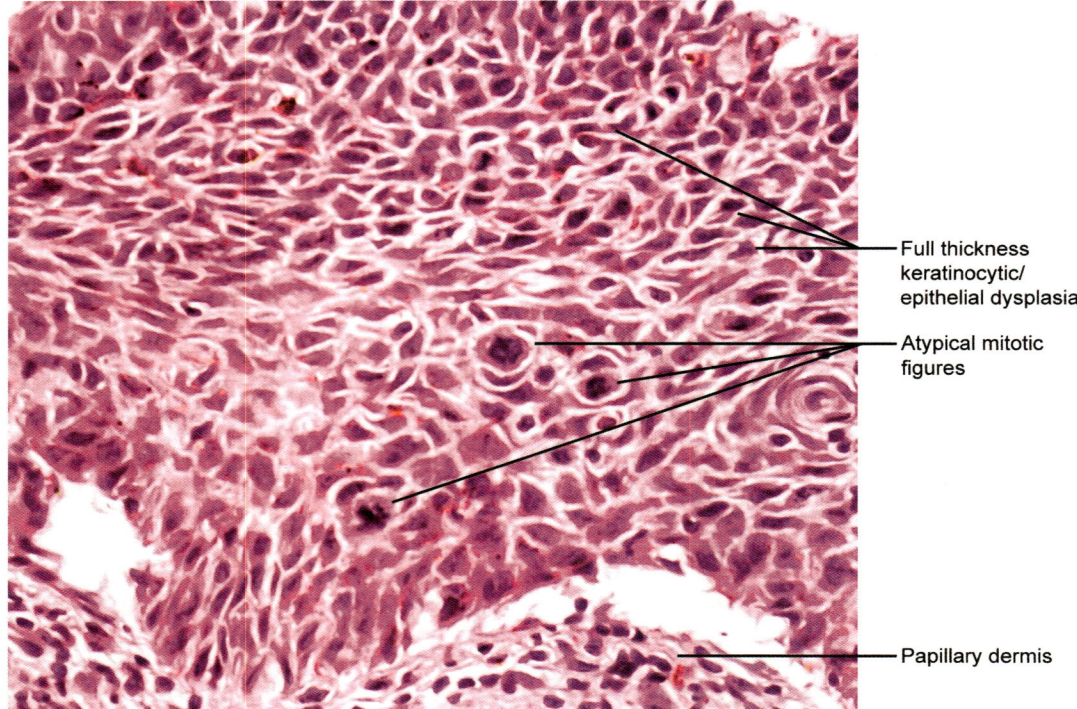

Full thickness keratinocytic/ epithelial dysplasia

Atypical mitotic figures

Papillary dermis

Fig. 69.1: Bowenoid papulosis

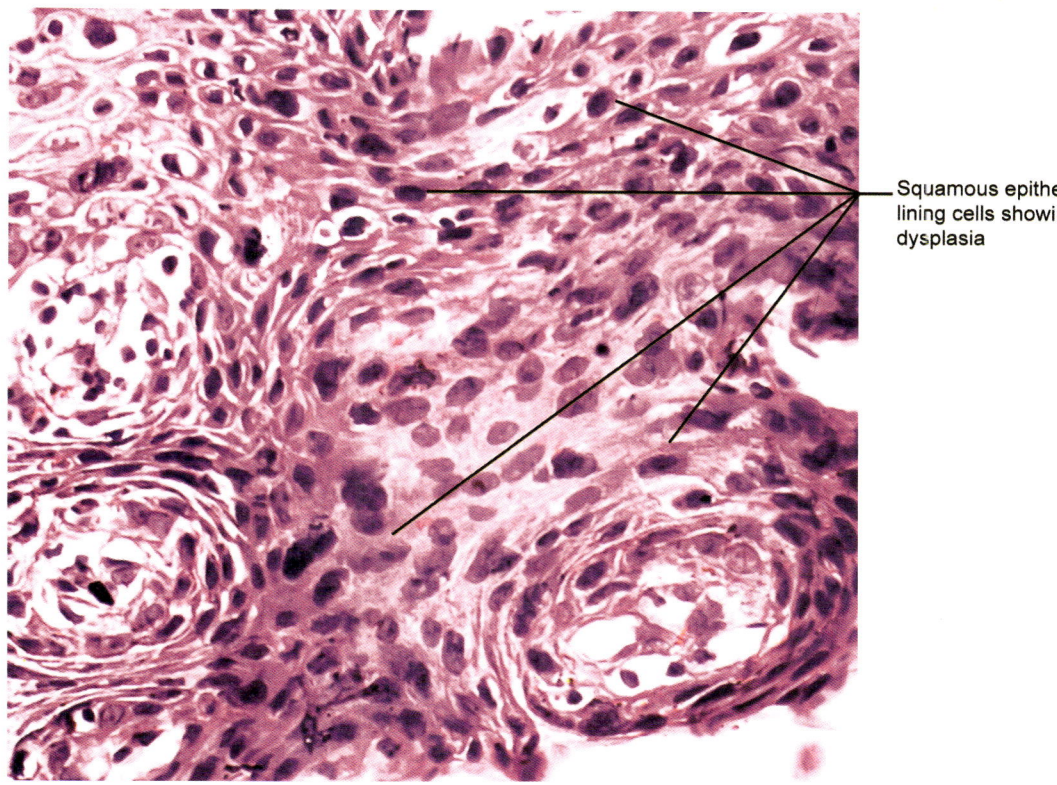

Squamous epithelial lining cells showing dysplasia

Fig. 69.2: Bowenoid papulosis

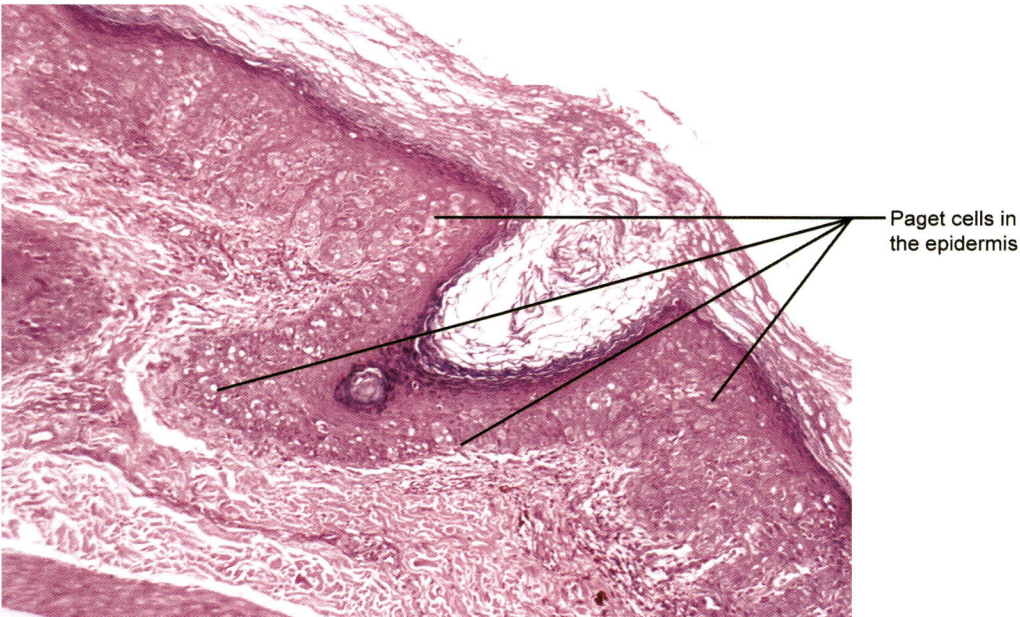

Paget cells in the epidermis

Fig. 69.3: Paget's disease (extra-mammary)

- Presents as multiple, small, verrucous papules on the genitalia of men and women
- Lesser degree of cytological atypia than Bowen's disease

- Full thickness squamous epithelial lining atypia
- Stratum corneum and granular cell layer can show basophilic rounded inclusions

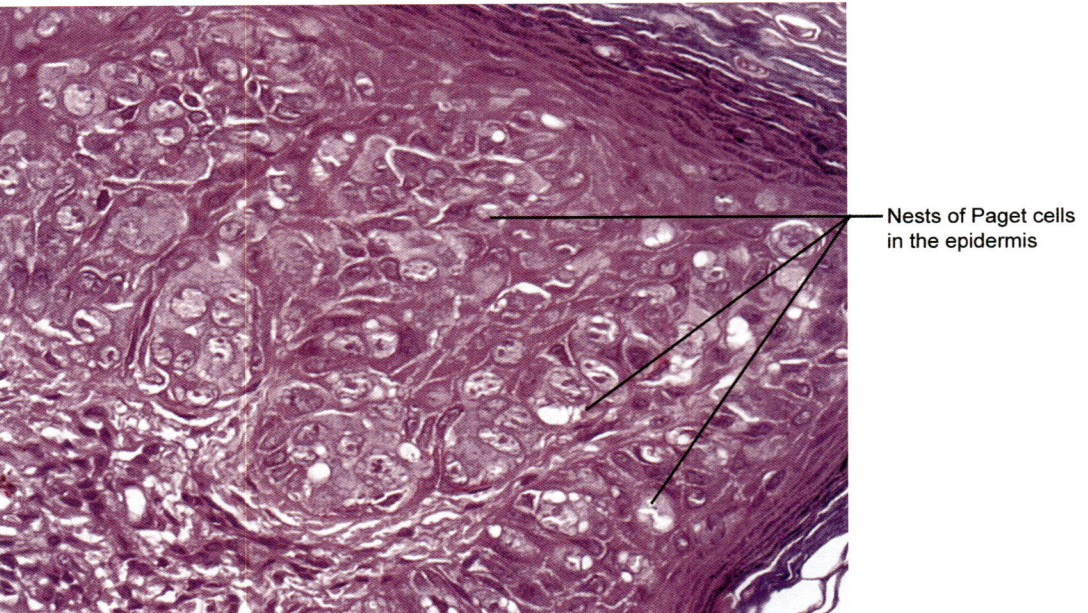

Nests of Paget cells in the epidermis

Fig. 69.4: Paget's disease (extra-mammary)

- Koilocytic atypia can be seen
- Spontaneous resolution can occur

Bowenoid Actinic Keratosis

- Can be differentiated on the basis of its smaller diameter

Erythroplasia of Queyrat

- Also called Bowen's disease (carcinoma *in situ*) of the glans penis

- Presents as a red plaque on the coronal sulcus or the inner surface of prepuce
- Has similar histopathology as of the Bowen's disease, with only the site being different

Paget's Disease (Figs 69.3 and 69.4)

- Vacuolated cells with clear cytoplasm
- Paget's cells are PAS positive and diastase resistant, show mucicarmine, Her-2-neu and CK-7 positivity

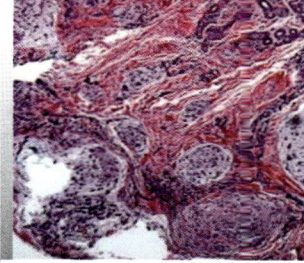

Squamous Cell Carcinoma (SCC)

INTRODUCTION

- Predisposing factors—sun-damaged skin; burns scar, stasis ulcers or osteomyelitis sinuses (Marjolin's ulcer); immune-suppression; HPV—infection of genitals
- Associated conditions—actinic keratosis, dystrophic epidermolysis bullosa, epidermolysis bullosa acquisita, lichen sclerosus, poikiloderma, balanitis xerotica obliterans, lymphogranuloma inguinale
- Presents as an ulcer with elevated border or as an fungating growth (Fig. 70.1)
- Etiology—ultraviolet B radiation, radiation therapy, arsenic, smoking

HISTOPATHOLOGY (Figs 70.2 and 70.3)

- Irregular masses comprising of malignant squamous cells arising from epidermis and invading into the dermis

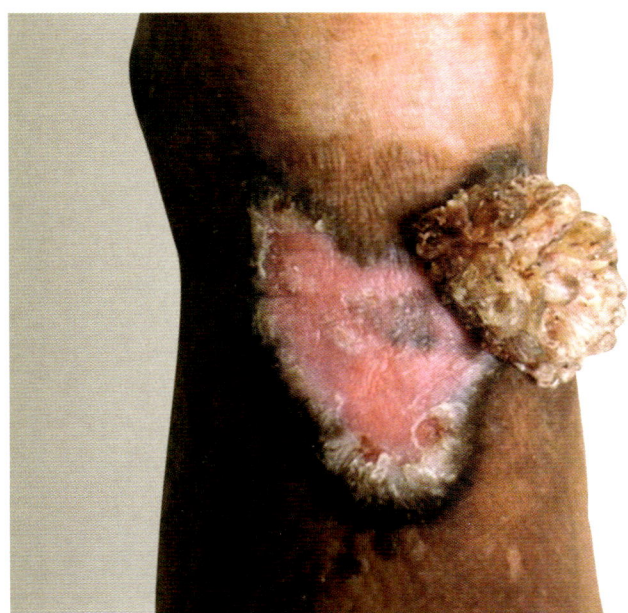

Fig. 70.1: Squamous cell carcinoma. Indurated, hyperkeratotic plaque developing on a lesion of lichen planus

- Malignant squamous cells have hyperchromatic, pleomorphic nuclei and can show abnormal mitosis
- On the basis of differentiation—they can be well, moderately or poorly differentiated
- Well-differentiated SCC—tumor cells show keratinization with formation of horn pearls
- As differentiation decreases (becomes poor)—keratinization decreases and atypical mitotically active squamous cells with bizarre nuclear features predominate

DIFFERENTIAL DIAGNOSIS

Actinic Keratosis

- Dermal invasion of atypical epidermal squamous cells is absent

Metastatic Squamous Cell Carcinoma

- Absence of carcinoma *in situ* component
- Connection of dermal tumor cell nests with the epidermis is absent
- Increased cytological atypia of tumor cells

Keratoacanthoma

- Tumor with keratinocyte proliferation with a central crater
- Peripheral extension of epidermis surrounding the tumor (cupping)
- Absence of keratinocytic atypia and mitosis

Pseudoepitheliomatous Hyperplasia

- Epithelial hyperplasia with epithelial cell nests invading into the deeper dermis
- Absence of keratinocytic atypia and mitosis

Basal Cell Carcinoma

- Basaloid cells arising from epidermis and infiltrating into the dermis as nodular masses
- Basaloid cells show peripheral palisading
- Presence of retraction clefts between the epithelium and stroma

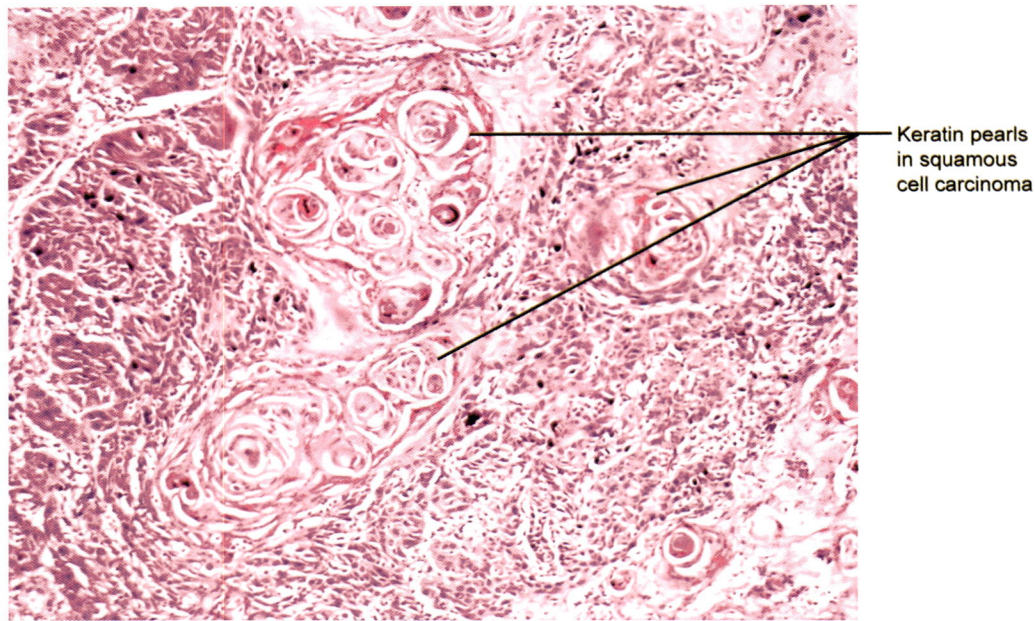

Keratin pearls
in squamous
cell carcinoma

Fig. 70.2: Well-differentiated squamous cell carcinoma

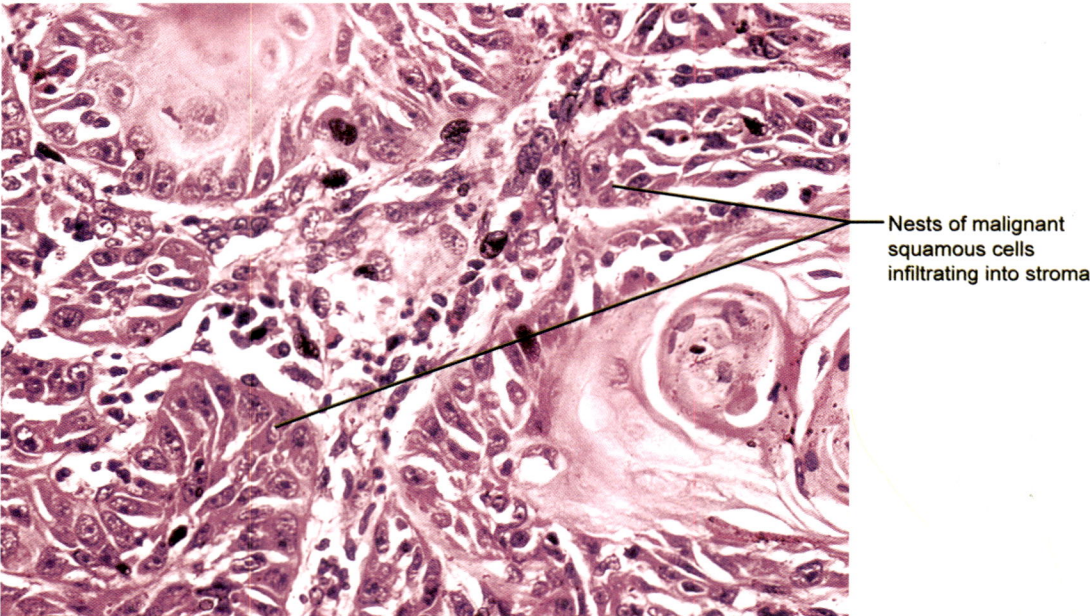

Nests of malignant
squamous cells
infiltrating into stroma

Fig. 70.3: Squamous cell carcinoma

Atypical Fibroxanthoma and Malignant Fibrous Histiocytoma

- Has to be differentiated from poorly differentiated squamous cell carcinoma
- Tumor cells show vimentin positivity in contrast to malignant squamous cells that show cytokeratin positivity

Malignant Melanoma

- Has to be differentiated from poorly differentiated squamous cell carcinoma
- Melanoma cells show S-100 positivity

Malignant Lymphoma

- Lymphoma cells show leukocyte common antigen (LCA) positivity

VARIANTS

Adenoid Squamous Cell Carcinoma

- Most common sites—head and neck
- Epithelial cells form glandular lumina and can show squamous differentiation
- Glandular lumina is filled with acantholytic cells

Spindle Cell Squamous Cell Carcinoma

- Spindle cells have large vesicular nucleus and scanty eosinophilic cytoplasm
- Squamous differentiation is also seen

Mucin Producing Squamous Cell Carcinoma

- Mucin producing tumor cells showing keratinous differentiation

Basaloid Squamous Cell Carcinoma

- Affects head and neck, ano-genital areas
- Associated with human papillomavirus-16 (HPV-16) infection
- Composed of small basaloid cells with high mortality rates

Verrucous Carcinoma

- Low grade squamous cell carcinoma
- Plantar lesions (exophytic) are the most common form
- Can involve oral cavity, genital regions (condyloma acuminatum of Buschke and Lowenstein), larynx, esophagus and skin
- Predisposing factors—tobacco chewing or betel-nut chewing, human papillomavirus 6 and 11

Histopathology (Figs 70.4 to 70.7)

- Acanthosis, hyperkeratosis and parakeratosis
- Tumor cells form broad strands and show downward proliferation as large bulbous masses
- Bulbous masses appear blunted and can compress the collagen bundles
- Nuclear atypia and keratin pearls are absent

Other Variants

- Pigmented SCC, inflammatory SCC, follicular SCC, infiltrative SCC, desmoplastic SCC, poorly differentiated SCC

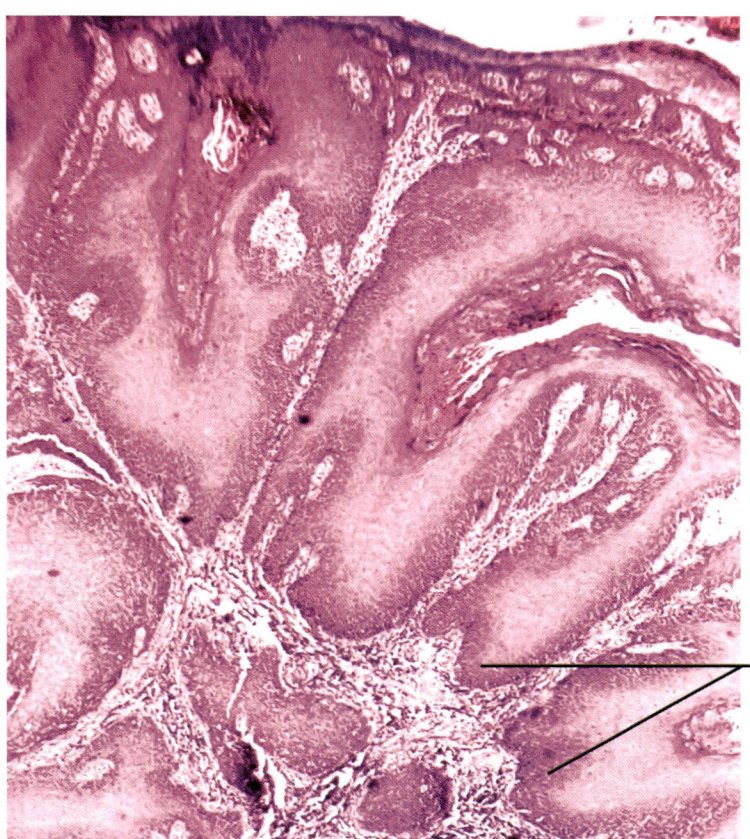

Bulbous expansion of rete ridges that push into the dermis

Fig. 70.4: Verrucous carcinoma

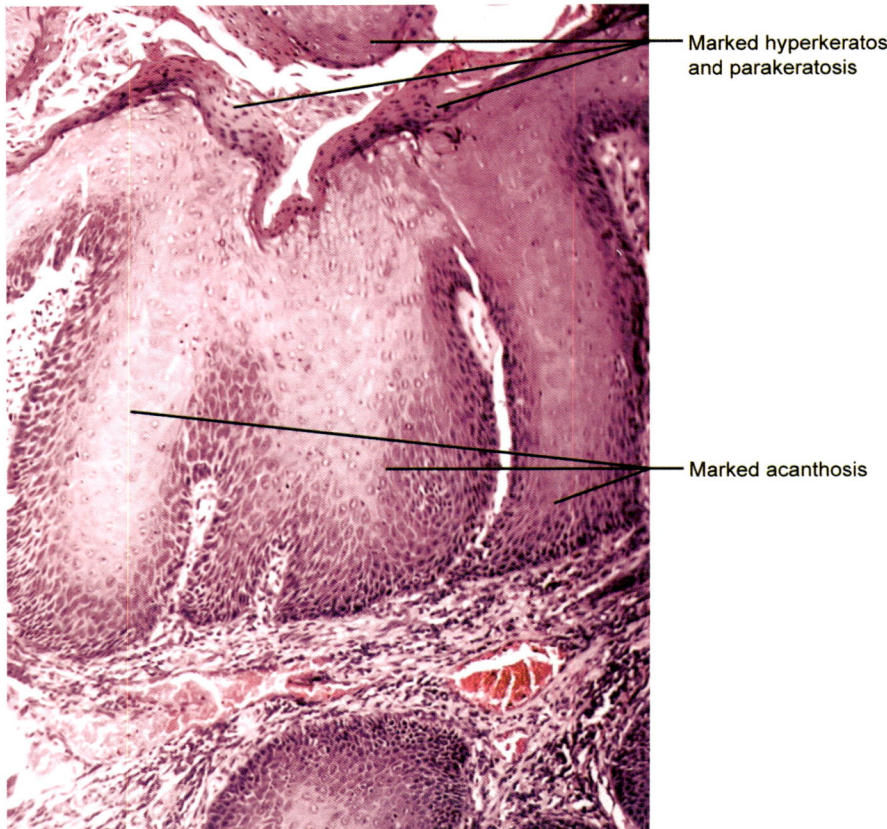

Marked hyperkeratosis and parakeratosis

Marked acanthosis

Fig. 70.5: Verrucous carcinoma

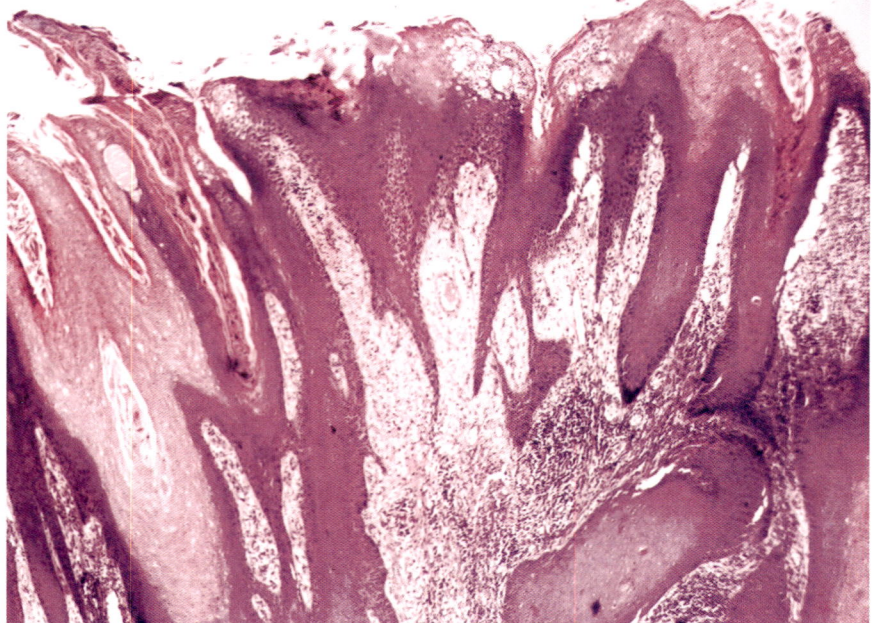

Fig. 70.6: Another case of verrucous carcinoma

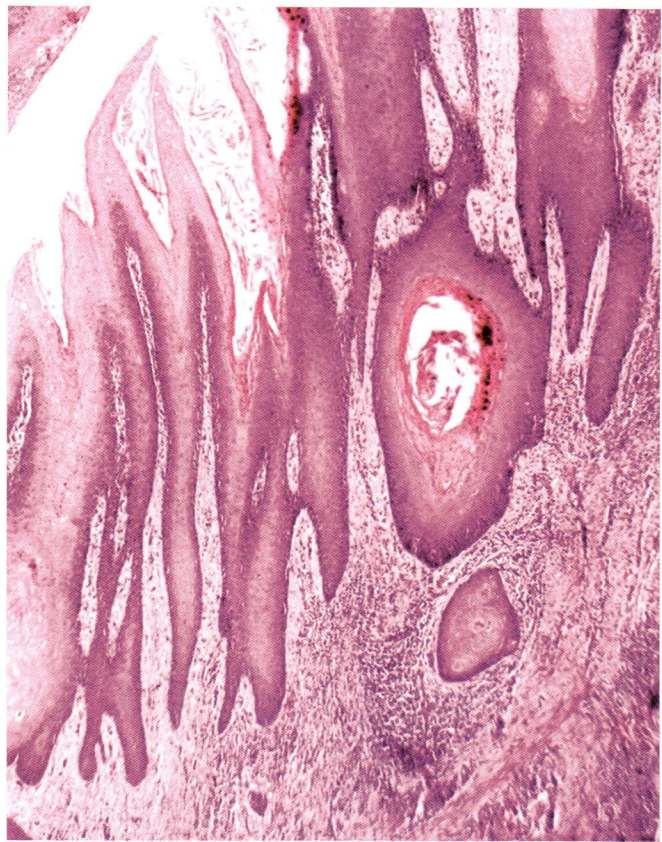

Fig. 70.7: Verrucous carcinoma

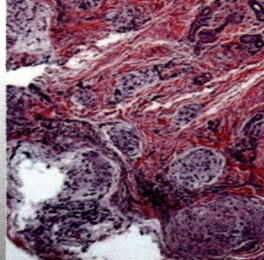

Keratoacanthoma

INTRODUCTION

- Age group—affects elderly individuals
- Solitary, flesh colored, dome-shaped nodule with a central keratin plug (Fig. 71.1)
- Size—measures 1– 2 cm in diameter
- Most common site—nose and eyelids
- Etiology—Human papillomavirus
- Predisposing factors—sunlight, immune-suppressed state, trauma, chronic renal failure
- Spontaneous resolution can occur

HISTOPATHOLOGY (Figs 71.2 to 71.5)

- Epidermis shows a central crater filled with keratin
- At the periphery of the crater, epidermis extends over tumor (lipping/buttressing/cupping)
- Keratinocytes become large and eosinophilic, as they mature towards the islands of tumor cell nests
- Epidermal proliferations extend from the base of crater into the dermis

- Epidermal proliferations at the base show abundant keratinization which appears eosinophilic and glassy with dense inflammatory cell infiltrate
- Perineural invasion can be seen

VARIANTS

Giant Keratoacanthoma

- Rapidly enlarging lesion with size of more than 5 cm
- Results in destruction of underlying tissues
- Most common sites—nose, hands

Keratoacanthoma Centrifugum Marginatum (Multinodular Keratoacanthoma)

- Size of the lesion exceeds more than 20 cm in diameter
- Site—dorsa of hands and legs
- Histopathology—central fibrosis due to healing of the lesion, with advancing edge showing buttressing by squamous epithelium

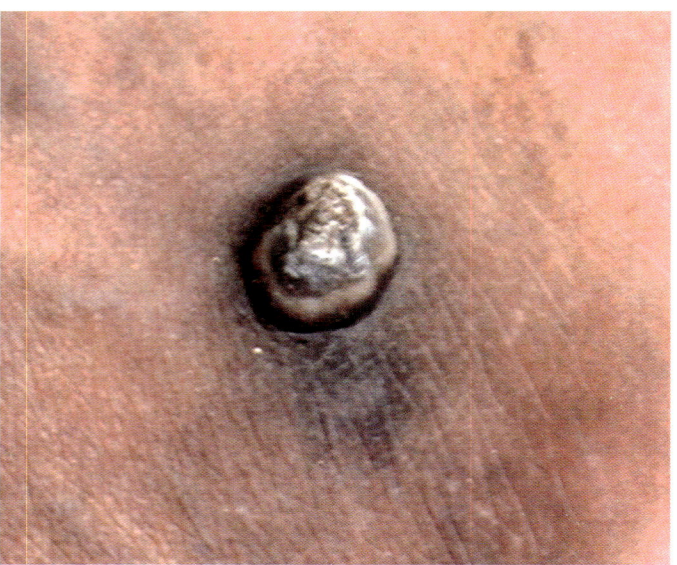

Fig. 71.1: Keratoacanthoma. Dome-shaped nodule with central keratinous plug

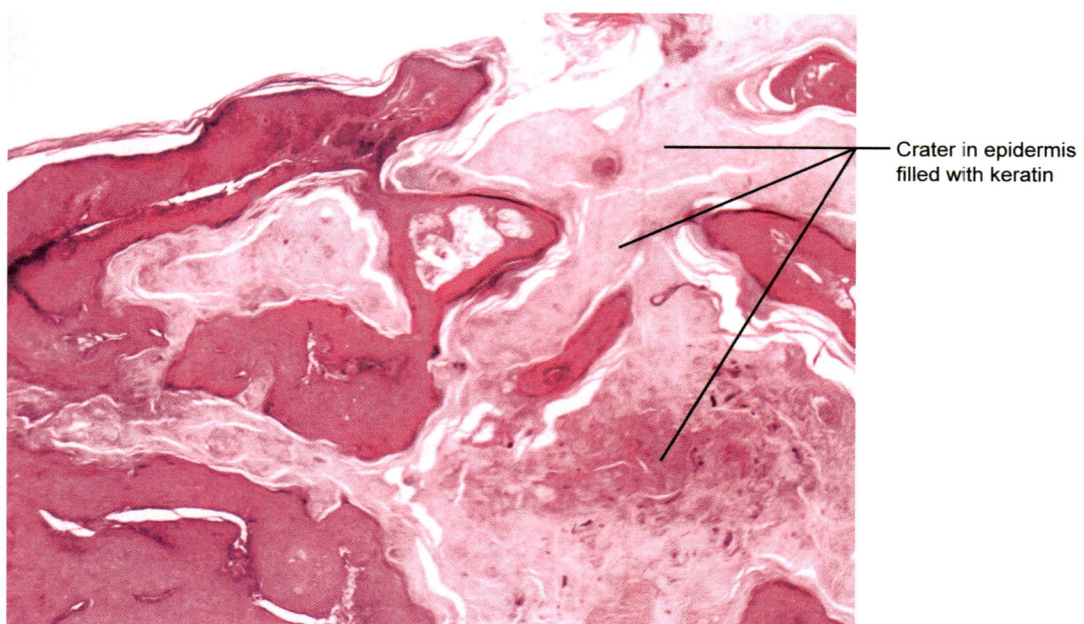

Crater in epidermis filled with keratin

Fig. 71.2: Keratoacanthoma

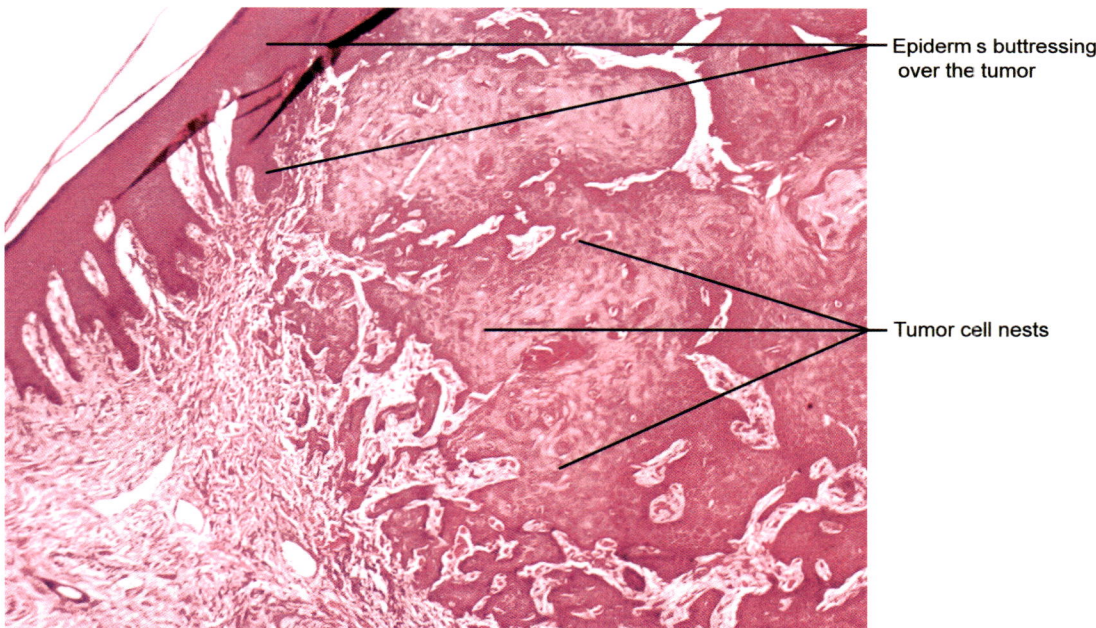

Epiderm s buttressing over the tumor

Tumor cell nests

Fig. 71.3: Keratoacanthoma

Subungual Keratoacanthoma

- Affects the distal portion of the fingernails
- Destruction of the underlying bone is seen
- Spontaneous regression can occur
- Histopathology shows dyskeratotic cells

Eruptive Keratoacanthoma

- Multiple follicular papules over skin measuring 2–3 mm in diameter

DIFFERENTIAL DIAGNOSIS

Squamous Cell Carcinoma

- Cytological atypia of squamous cells which also show individual cell keratinization
- Irregular pushing margins with features of invasion

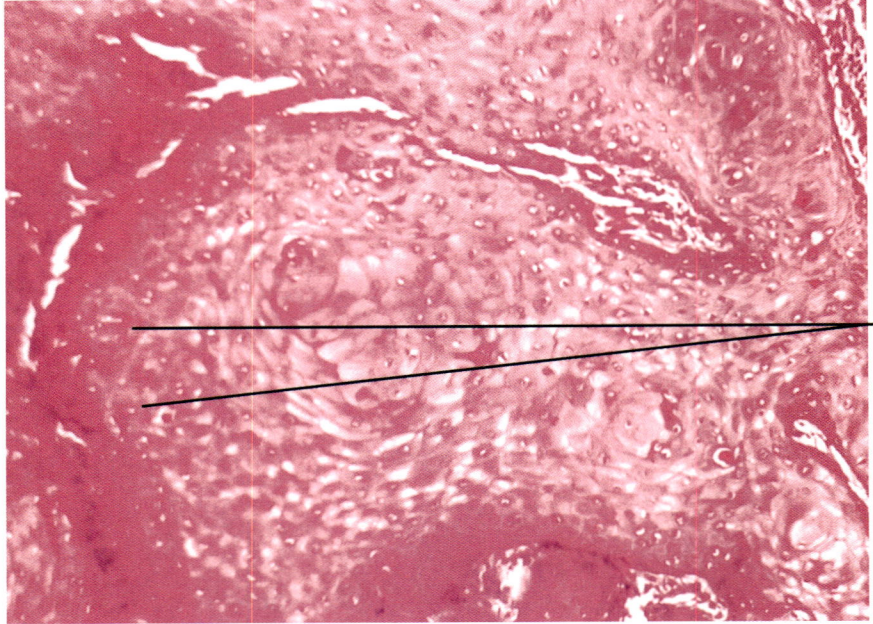

Keratinocytes become
more eosinophilic as
they mature towards
the tumor cell islands

Fig. 71.4: Keratoacanthoma

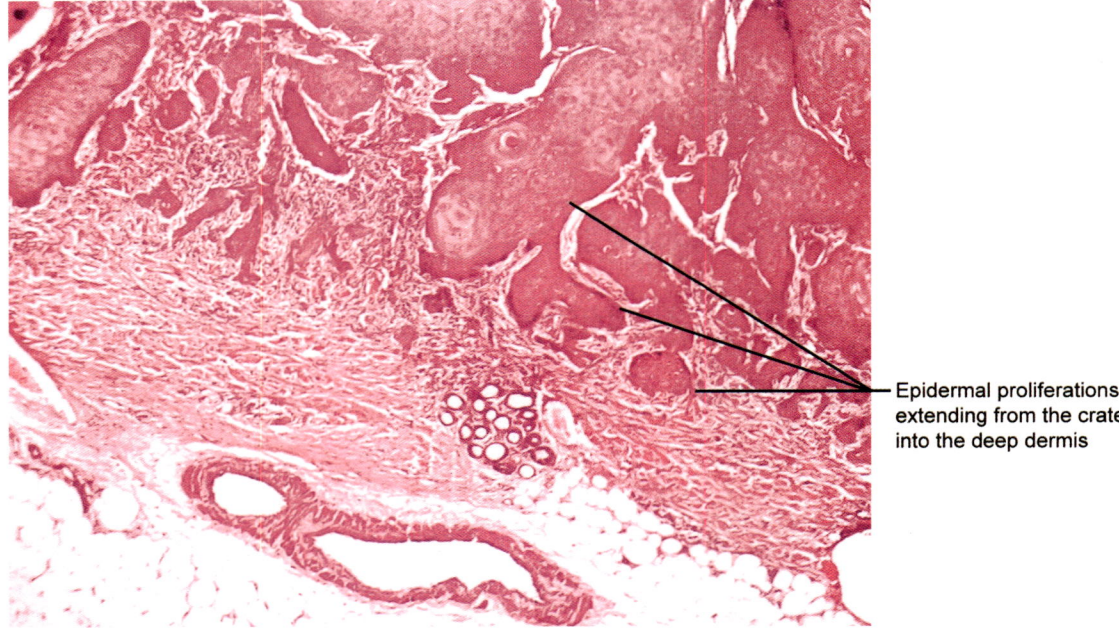

Epidermal proliferations
extending from the crater
into the deep dermis

Fig. 71.5: Keratoacanthoma

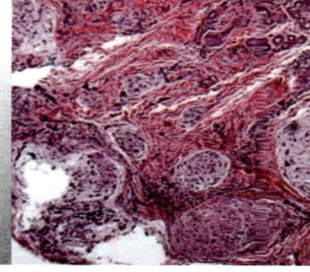

Fibroepithelial Polyp

INTRODUCTION

- Also called skin tag or acrochordon or fibroma
- Sites—axilla, neck, groin, vulva, anus, penis (Fig. 72.1)

HISTOPATHOLOGY (Figs 72.2 and 72.3)

- Polypoidal lesion
- Epidermal acanthosis and papillomatosis
- Subepithelium shows collagen bundles, adipocytes and blood vessels

DIFFERENTIAL DIAGNOSIS

Pedunculated Lipoma

- Shows mature adipocytes in the dermis

Condylomata Accuminata

- Acanthosis, parakeratosis, koilocytes

Seborrheic Keratosis

- Acanthosis, papillomatosis, horn cysts

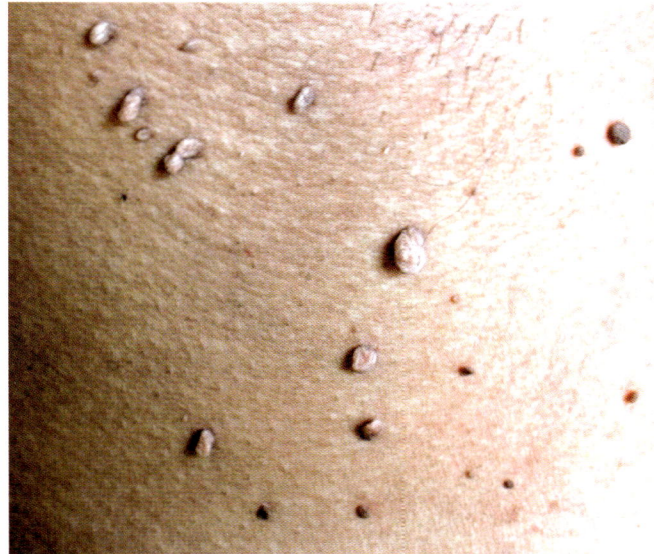

Fig. 72.1: Skin tags (acrochordon). Pedunculated skin-colored, soft papules with a narrow stalk

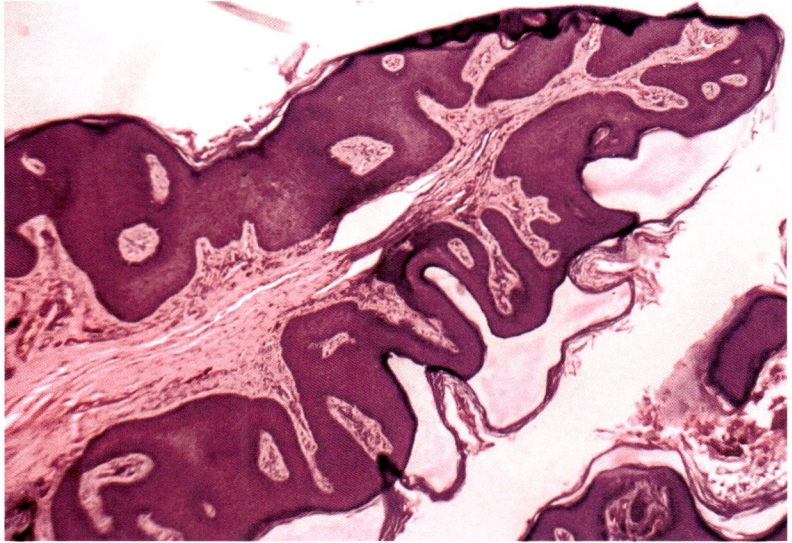

Fig. 72.2: Fibroepithelial polyp

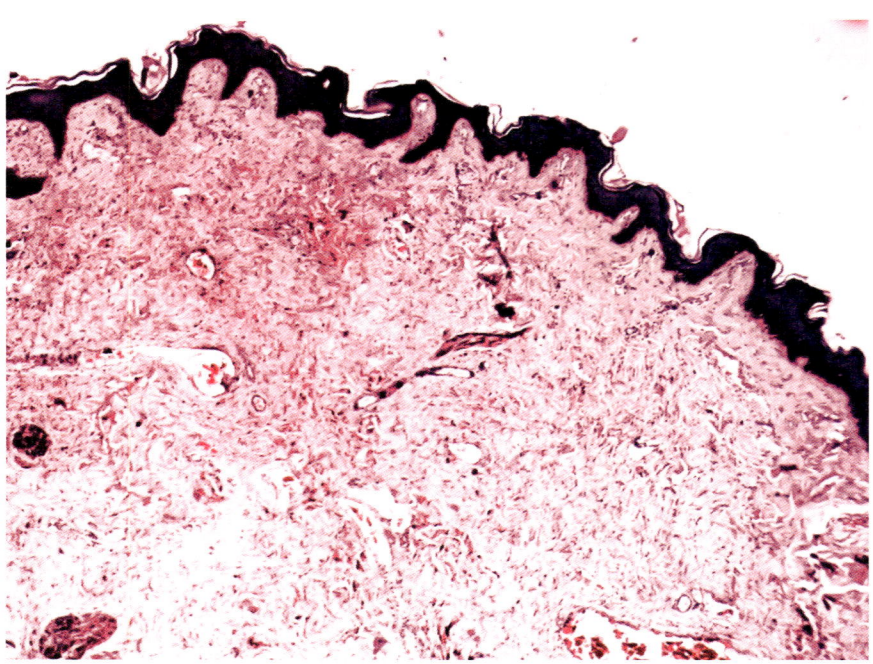

Fig. 72.3: Fibroepithelial polyp

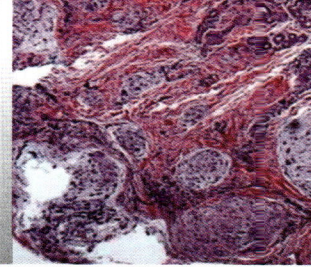

Paget's Disease

MAMMARY PAGET'S DISEASE

Introduction

- Site—most commonly affects female breast
- Unilateral lesion, seen in nipple or areola of the breast (Fig. 73.1)
- Associated with underlying carcinoma of breast

Histopathology (Figs 73.2 and 73.3)

- Paget cells are scattered singly or in groups in the epidermis
- Paget cells are large rounded cells with ample cytoplasm and large nucleus
- PAS and alcian blue stains are used to demonstrate Paget cells

- Immunohistochemistry (IHC) studies—Paget cells show cytokeratin-7, CEA, EMA and HER2-neu positivity

Differential Diagnosis

Bowen Disease

- Full thickness epithelial dysplasia
- Cells show nuclear hyperchromasia, multinucleation and atypical mitotic figures

Melanoma (Superficial Spreading Type)

- Melanoma cells can invade the dermis unlike Paget cells
- Melanocytes unlike Paget cells show S-100, HMB-45 and Melan-A positivity

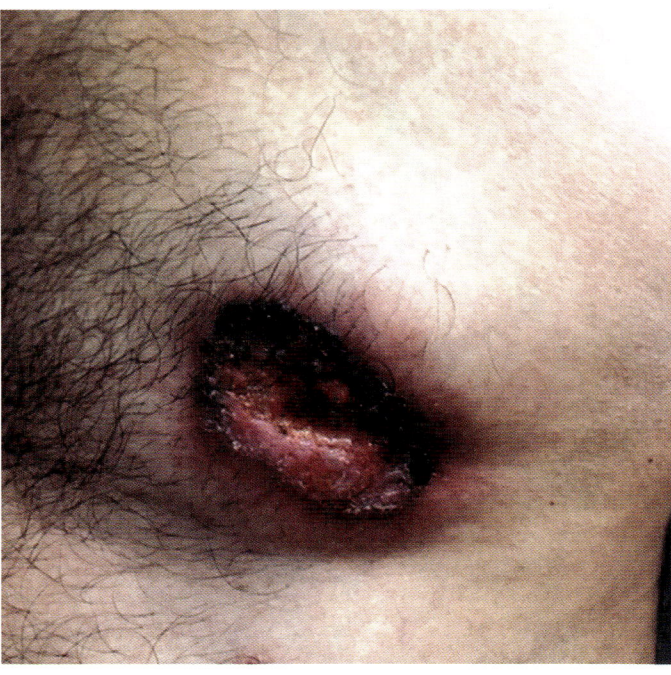

Fig. 73.1: Paget's disease of the breast. Scaly, raw, ulcerated lesion spreading to the areolar region

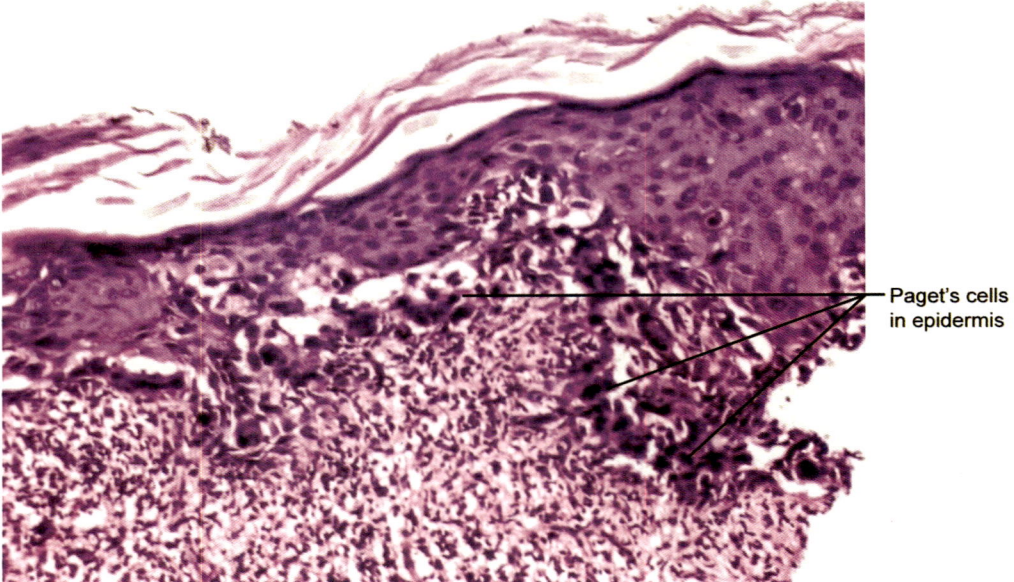

Fig. 73.2: Paget's disease

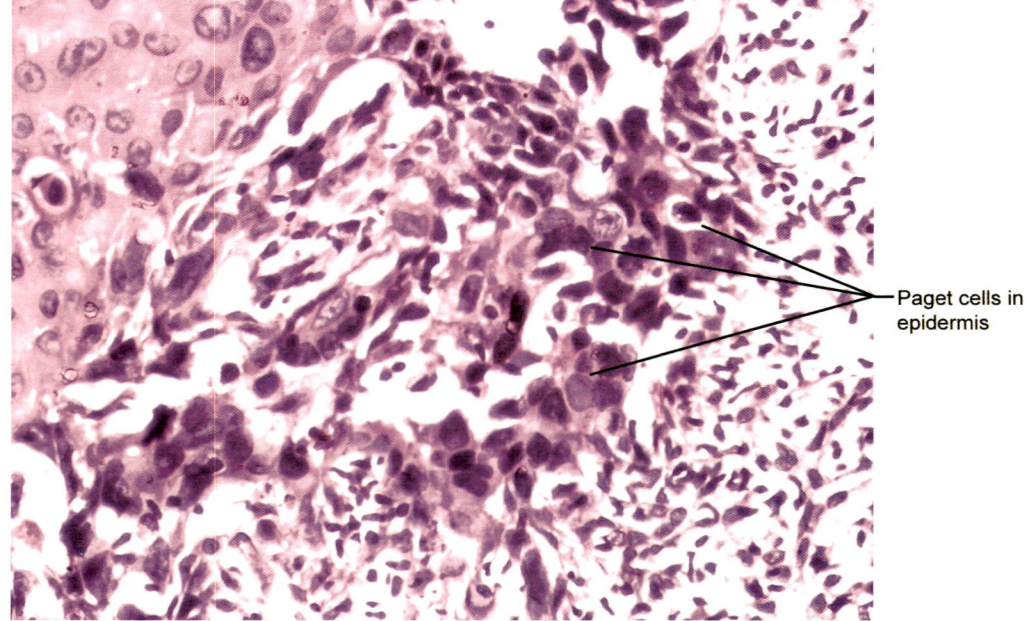

Fig. 73.3: Paget's disease

EXTRA-MAMMARY PAGET'S DISEASE

- Most commonly affects the vulva
- Other sites—male genitals, perianal area
- Paget cells invade the dermis from epidermis
- Paget cells are PAS-positive and diastase resistant
- Paget cells stain with alcian blue at pH 2.5, mucicarmine and cytokeratin-7
- Differential diagnosis—Bowen disease, melanoma (superficial spreading type)

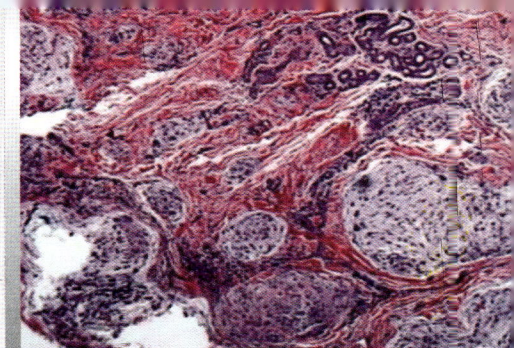

Melanocytic Lesions

Part

13

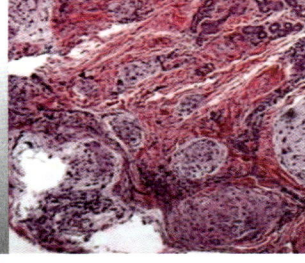

Benign Pigmented Lesions

Chapter 74

DIFFERENCES BETWEEN MELANOCYTES, NEVUS CELLS AND MELANOMA CELLS

	Melanocytes	Nevus cells	Melanoma cells
Cells	Solitary	Arranged in clusters	Arranged in clusters and sheets
Nuclei	Small, regular	Small, regular	Large, hyper-chromatic, irregular
Cytoplasm	Dendritic	Rounded or spindle	Rounded or spindle
Mitosis	Rare	Rare	Usually present

FRECKLES

- Represent hyperplastic and hyperactive response of melanocytes to UV light
- Tan or brown lesion which shows increased melanin pigment in the basal layer keratinocytes without increase in number of melanocytes

LENTIGINES

- Present as a pigmented macule, measuring few mm in diameter
- Histopathology—increase in the number of epidermal melanocytes in the basal cell layer without any nests of melanocytes. This pattern is termed 'Lentiginous pattern'

NEVI

- Increased number of epidermal melanocytes arranged in nests

MUCOSAL MELANOTIC MACULE

INTRODUCTION

- Uniformly pigmented light brown macules, less than 6 mm in diameter (Fig. 74.1)

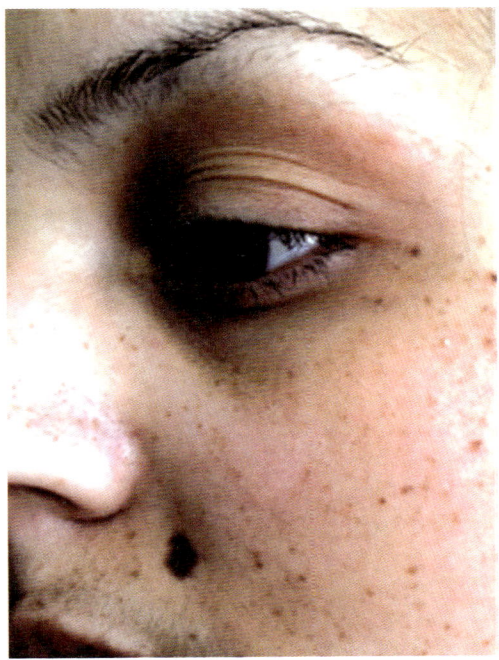

Fig. 74.1: Mucosal melanotic macule

- Sites—lower lip, oral cavity, vulva, penis
- Etiology—reactive hyperplasia

HISTOPATHOLOGY

- Mild acanthosis
- Hyper-pigmentation of basal keratinocytes
- Papillary dermis shows scattered melanophages due to pigment incontinence
  Note: Differentiation from atypical/malignant melanocytic lesions can be done easily

LENTIGO SIMPLEX

INTRODUCTION

- Most commonly affects children

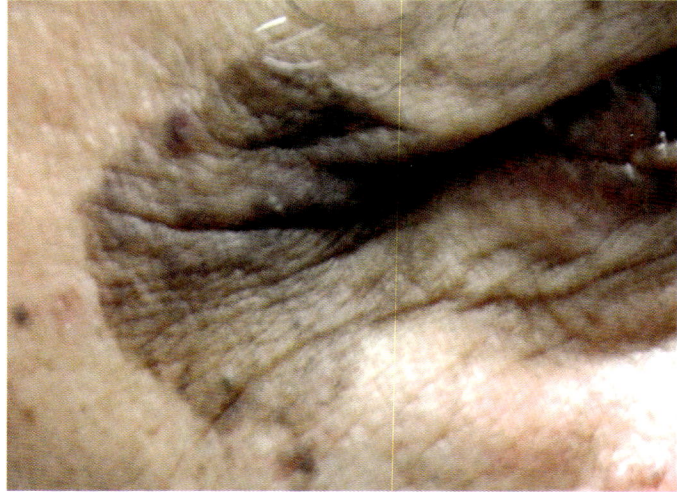

Fig. 74.2: Lentigo simplex. Sharply circumscribed, round to oval, brown macule

- Brown, well-circumscribed pigmented macules (Fig. 74.2)

HISTOPATHOLOGY (Figs 74.3 and 74.4)

- Basal layer shows hyperpigmentation
- Increased melanin in melanocytes

- Papillary dermis shows sparse mononuclear inflammatory cell infiltrate and scattered melanophages
- Absence of nevus cell nests or atypical cells
- **Lentiginous melanocytic proliferation**—melanocytes proliferation seen in basal cell layer
- **Lentiginous junctional nevus** – presence of diffusely arranged single nevus cells in the lowermost epidermis

DIFFERENTIAL DIAGNOSIS

Solar Lentigo (Senile Lentigo)

- Seen in sun-exposed areas
- Affects older individuals
- Most common site—face
- Presents as dark-brown to black macules
- Histopathology—rete ridges are elongated and bulbous and shows hyperpigmentation

MELANOCYTIC NEVI

INTRODUCTION

- Benign neoplastic proliferation of melanocytes
- Presents in adolescence and early adulthood

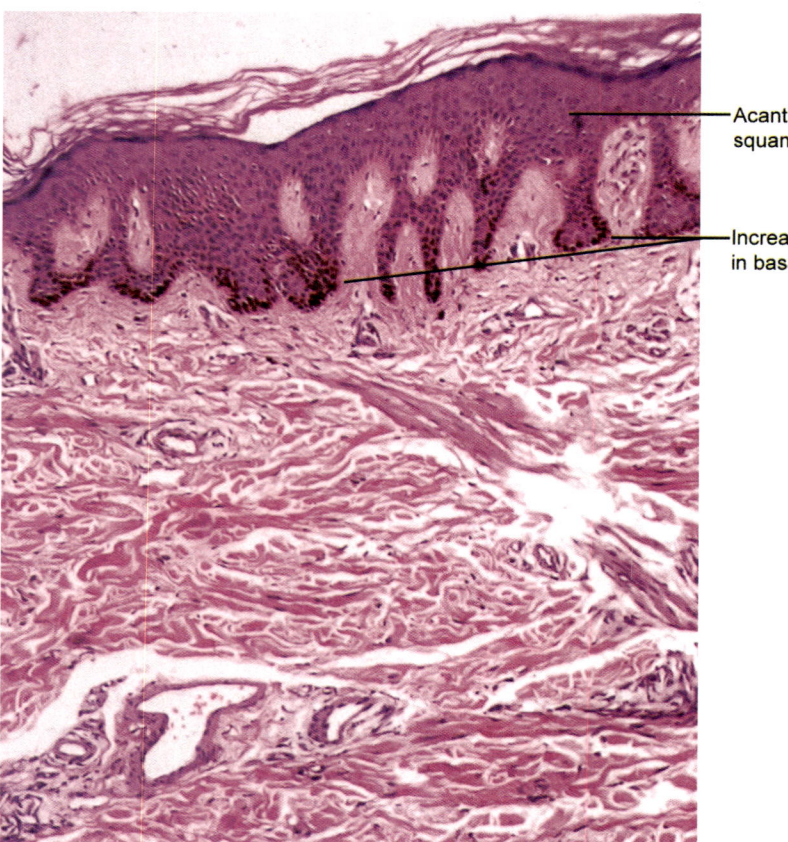

Acanthotic stratified squamous epithelium

Increased melanin in basal cell layer

Fig. 74.3: Lentigo simplex

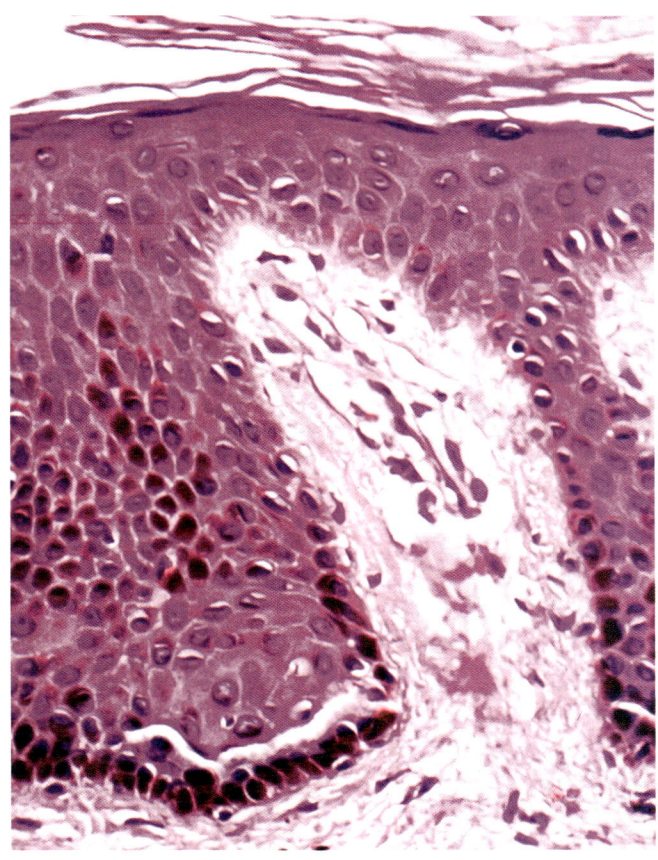

Fig. 74.4: Lentigo simplex. Increased melanin pigment in basal cell layer with intraepidermal melanophages

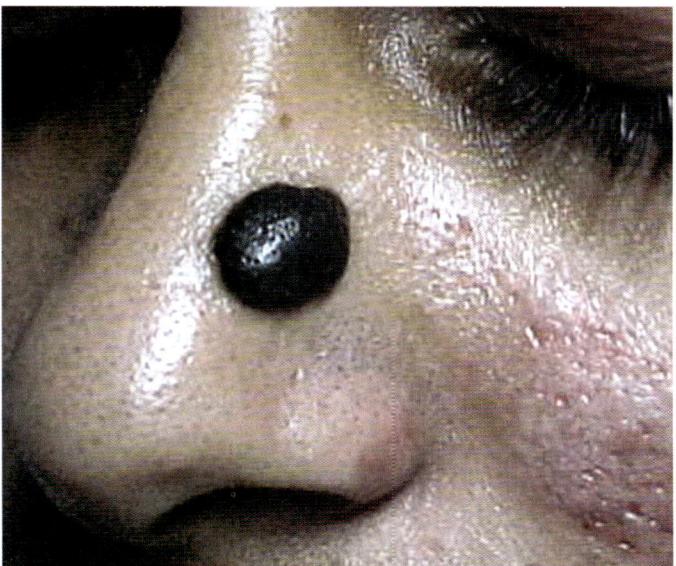

Fig. 74.5: Compound melanocytic nevus. Evenly pigmented, round to oval lesion with homogenous surface and sharply demarcated border

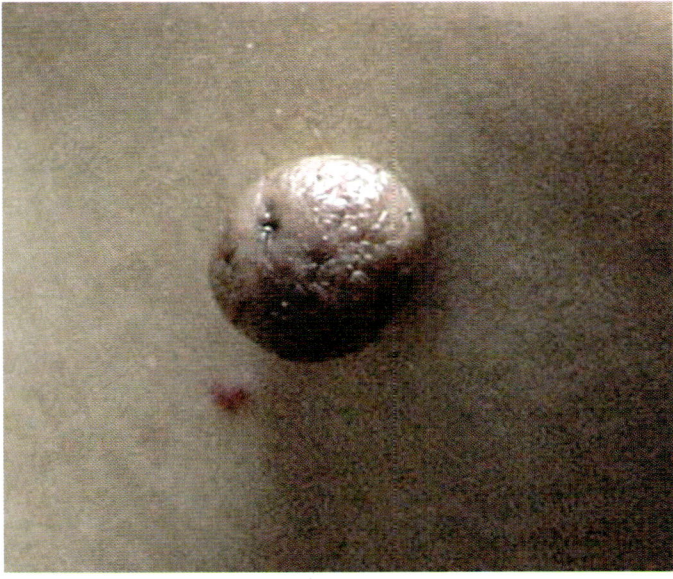

Fig. 74.6: Dermal melanocytic nevus

- Presents as tan-brown macules or papules
- On histological examination—nevi are classified into junctional nevus, compound nevus or an intra-dermal nevus
- Associated with BRAF and RAS mutations

Junctional Nevus

- Presents as a well-circumscribed brown to black macule
- Seen during childhood or early adulthood
- Melanocytes or nevus cells are arranged in well-circumscribed nests at dermo-epidermal junction
- Nevus cell contains melanin granules
- Absence of atypia and mitosis

Compound Nevus

- Presents as a pigmented papule or plaque (Fig. 74.5)
- Seen in children and adolescents
- Microscopy—nevus cell nests are present at the dermoepidermal junction and in the upper dermis (Figs 74.10 and 74.11)

MATURATION OF NEVUS CELLS

- Upper dermis shows **Type A** nevus cells with abundant cytoplasm

- Mid-dermis shows **Type B** nevus cells (which are of the size of lymphocytes) interspersed within the collagen bundles
- Deep dermis shows **Type C** nevus cells (resembling fibroblasts or Schwann cells) that appear elongated with spindle-shaped nucleus (neurotized dermal/melanocytic nevus) and can form corpuscles resembling "Wagner-Meissner body"
- Presence of maturation suggests benign nature

Intradermal Nevus (Figs 74.6 to 74.9)

- Most common type of melanocytic nevi

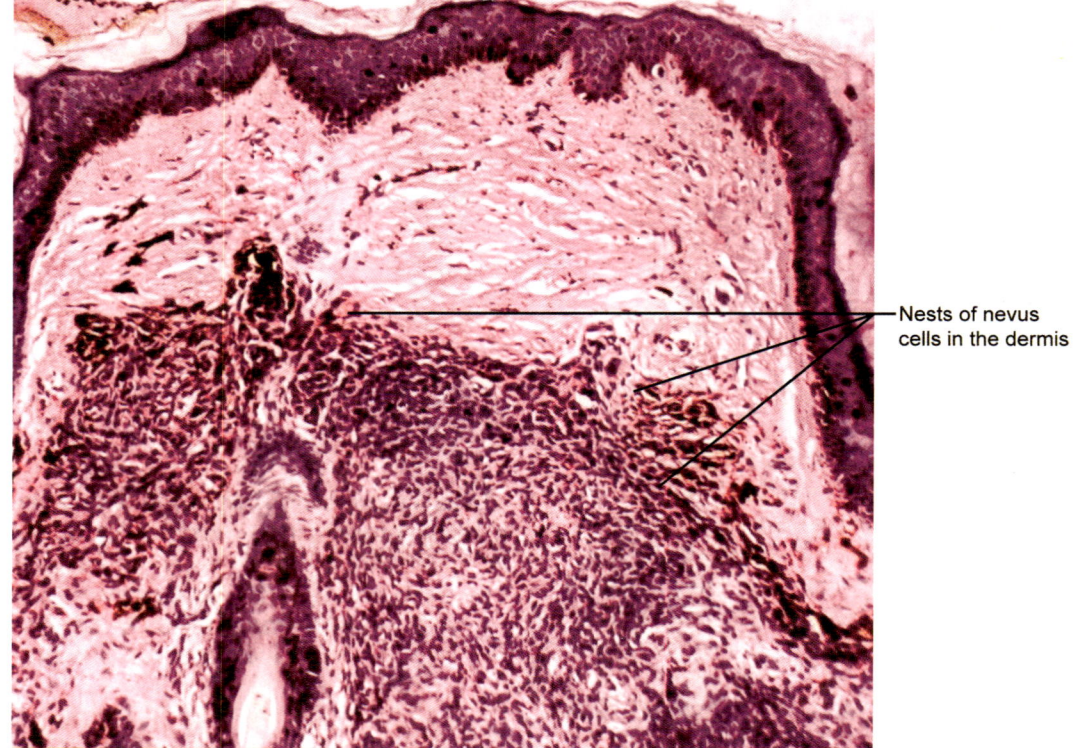

Nests of nevus cells in the dermis

Fig. 74.7: Intradermal nevus

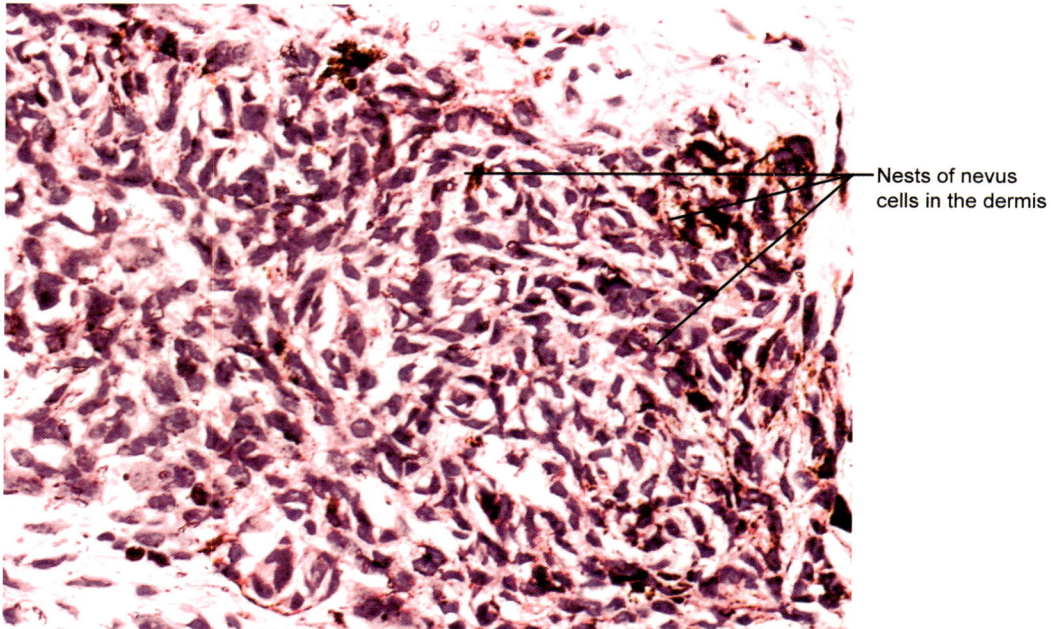

Nests of nevus cells in the dermis

Fig. 74.8: Intradermal nevus

- Presents as polypoidal or nodular lesions
- Upper dermis contains nests and cords of nevus cells with no junctional activity
- Consists of Type A, B and C nevus cells
- Absence of nuclear atypia and mitosis
- Has to be differentiated from neurofibroma, which can be done with the help of immunohistochemical markers

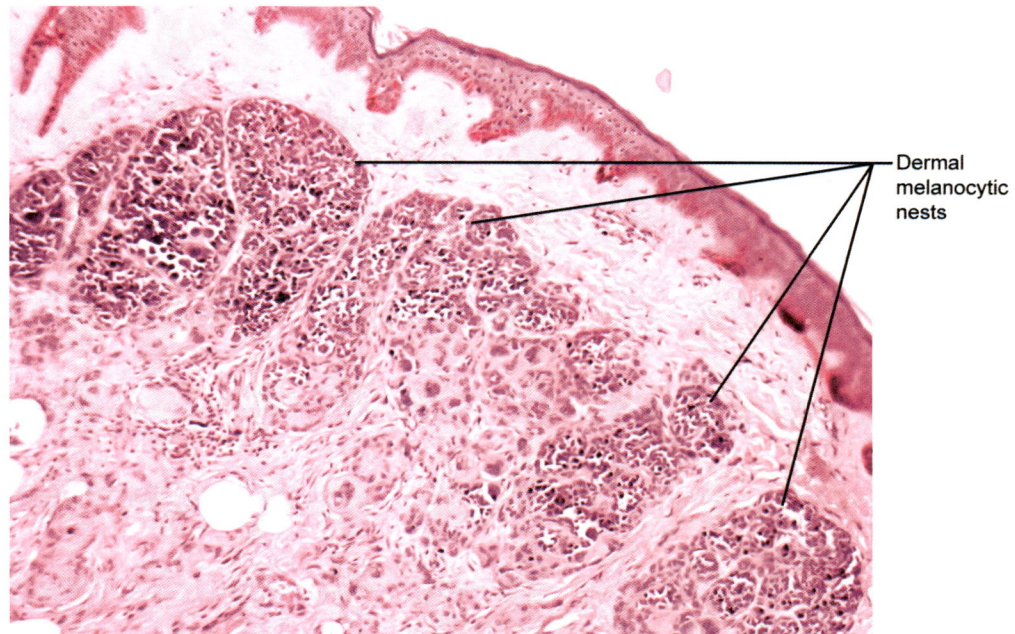

Fig. 74.9: Intradermal nevus

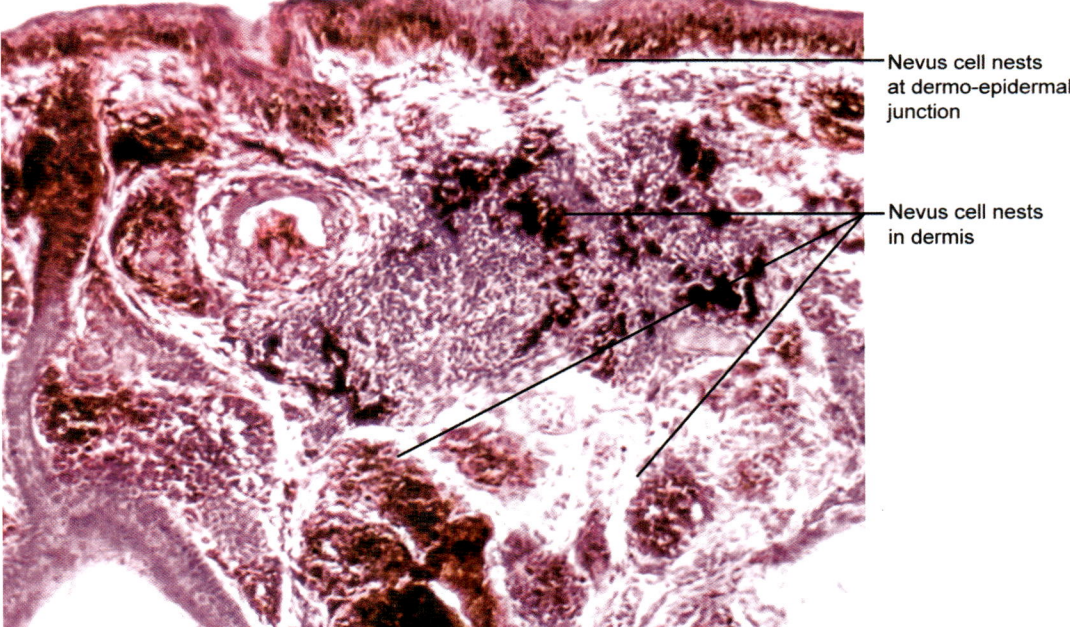

Fig. 74.10: Compound nevus

BLUE NEVUS

- Three types—common blue nevus, cellular blue nevus and combined blue nevus
- Reticular dermis shows pigmented spindle and dendritic melanocytes

COMMON BLUE NEVI

Introduction

- Presents as a small, well-circumscribed, dome-shaped nodule, blue-black in color
- Sites—extremities, hand, feet, scalp
- Size—less than 1 cm

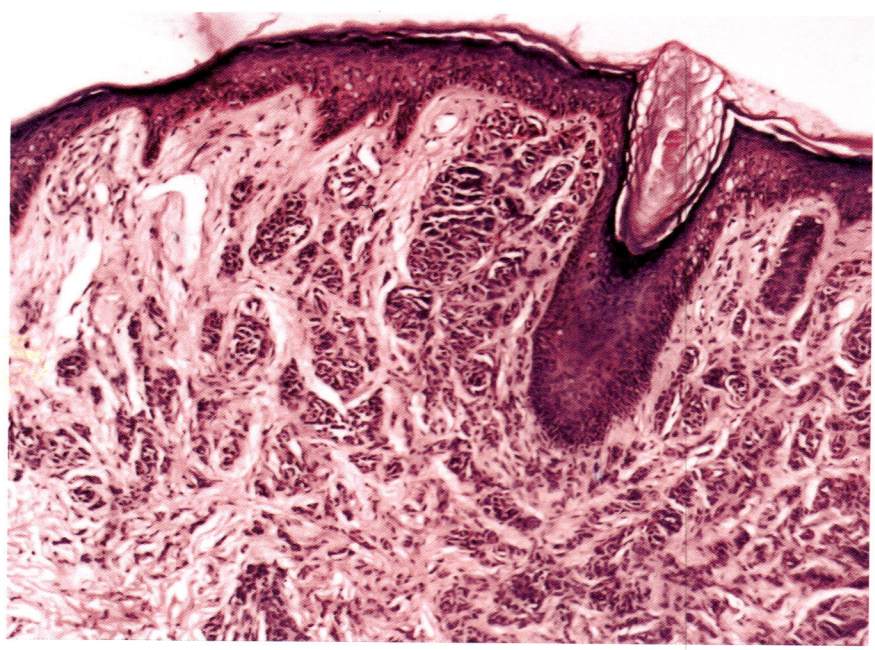

Fig. 74.11: Compound nevus. Nevus cells and nevus cell nests appear to be arising from dermoepidermal junction and are seen extending up to the deep dermis

Histopathology

- Spindle-shaped melanocytes in the reticular dermis
- Melanocytes are heavily pigmented, and are present amongst the collagen bundles, arranged parallel to the epidermis
- Melanocytes are positive for S-100, HMB-45 and Melan-A

CELLULAR BLUE NEVUS

Introduction

- Measures 1–3 cm in diameter (Fig. 74.12)
- Site—buttocks, sacrococcygeal region
- Rarely, malignant transformation can occur

Histopathology (Figs 74.13 and 74.14)

- Lesion spans reticular dermis
Following patterns can be seen
1. Lesion comprises spindle-shaped cells, which lie in contiguity with one another and can penetrate into the subcutaneous fat in a dumbbell-shaped pattern
2. Epithelioid blue nevus—lesion can present as sheets of cuboidal cells with pale cytoplasm
3. Biphasic pattern—comprising of ovoid islands of epithelioid/polygonal cells with clear cytoplasm, alternating with fascicles of spindle cells (pigmented)
Note: Features favoring malignant blue nevus include frequent mitosis, high grade cytological atypia, presence of tumor necrosis

COMBINED NEVUS

- Two or more types of melanocytic nevi in a single lesion
- Example—epithelioid blue nevus (first component) and spitz or congenital or desmoplastic (second component)

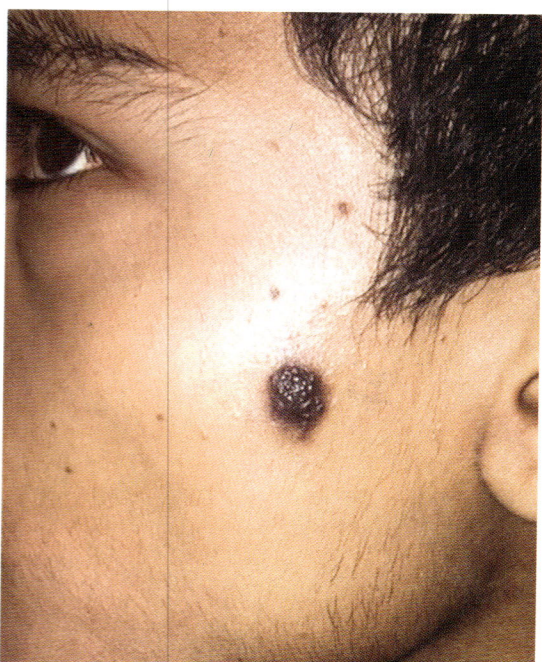

Fig. 74.12: Blue nevus. Solitary, blue-black, dome-shaped papule

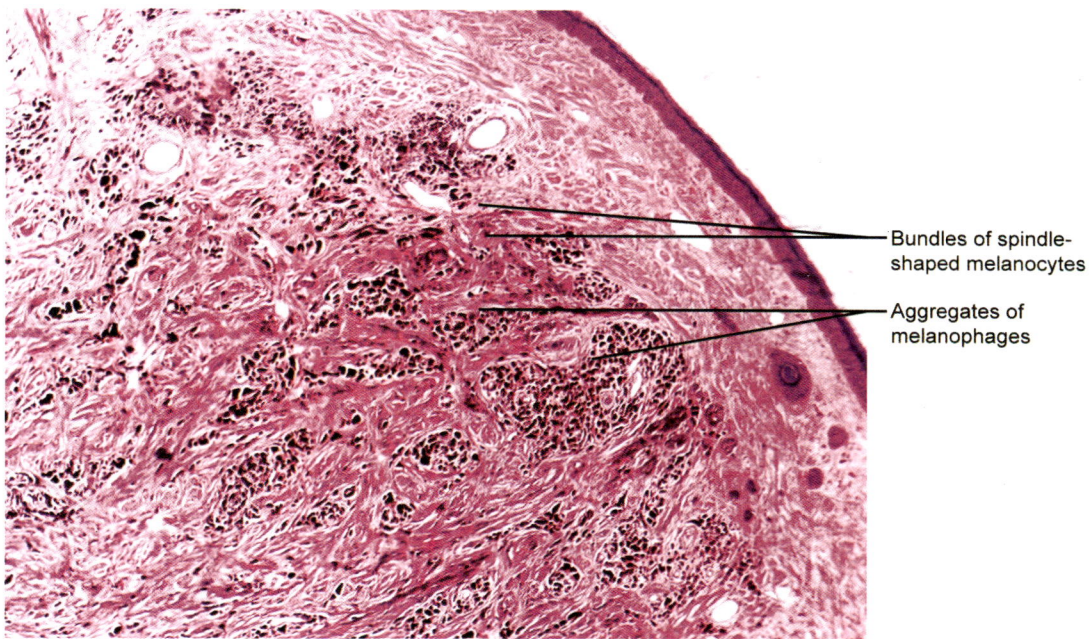

Fig. 74.13: Cellular blue nevus

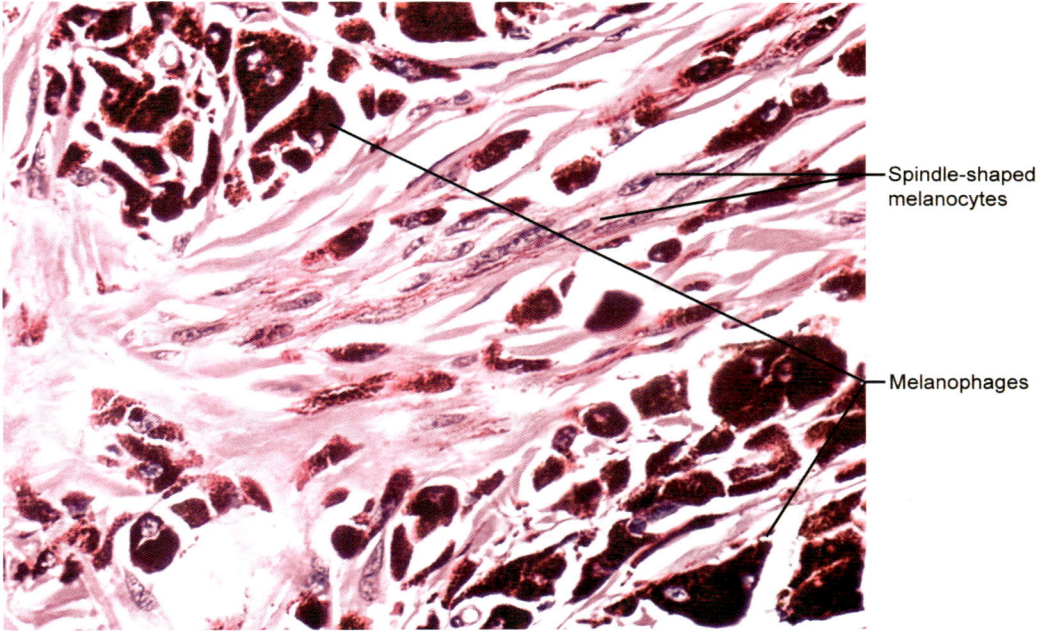

Fig. 74.14: Cellular blue nevus

SPITZ NEVUS

INTRODUCTION

- Also called **"spindle-cell nevus"** or **"epithelioid-cell nevus"**
- Site—extremities and face
- Presents as a solitary, symmetrical, well-circum-scribed, pink nodule or papule

HISTOPATHOLOGY

- Usually a compound nevi, but can be junctional or intradermal nevi
- Lesion appears symmetrical and lacks pagetoid spread of single melanocytes
- Comprises large spindle cells and/or epithelioid cells, spindle cells can be plump

- Epidermis—acanthosis (pseudoepitheliomatous hyperplasia can be seen) and can show Kamino bodies (PAS—positive homogenous globules)
- Melanocytic tumor of unknown malignant potential (MELTUMP) – > 2 mitosis/mm^2 in the dermal nevus cells or mitosis within the lower half of dermal component
- Maturation from larger cells near surface to smaller cells at the base and uniformity of the cells are features that favor Spitz nevus
- Features favoring Spitz nevus over melanoma include small size, circumscription, symmetry, lack of marked cytological and nuclear atypia, absence of mitosis

DIFFERENTIAL DIAGNOSIS

Epithelioid Histiocytoma or Juvenile Xanthogranuloma

- Histiocytic lesions show CD68 positivity, whereas Spitz nevus cells show Melan-A and HMB-45 positivity

Malignant Melanoma

- > 6 mm in diameter, asymmetrical lesion, tumor cells arranged in nests and fascicles which can show lateral extension, heavy pigmentation is common
- Presence of high mitotic count, atypical mitosis, hyperchromatic and clumped nuclei with irregular nuclear margins

VARIANTS

Desmoplastic Spitz Nevus

- Spindle-shaped nevus cells in a desmoplastic stroma
- Nevus cells show no junctional activity, nesting and pigmentation
- Nevus cells are negative for HMB-45 and Melan-A

Pigmented Spindle Cell Nevus/Reed Nevus

- Presents as a pigmented papule
- Most common site—extremities
- Elongated spindle-shaped cells containing abundant coarse melanin pigment
- Spindle cells are arranged in nests and are vertically oriented

HALO NEVUS

INTRODUCTION

- Also called Sutton's nevus or nevus depigmentosa centrifugum
- Pigmented nevus surrounded by a halo/depigmented zone (Fig. 74.15)

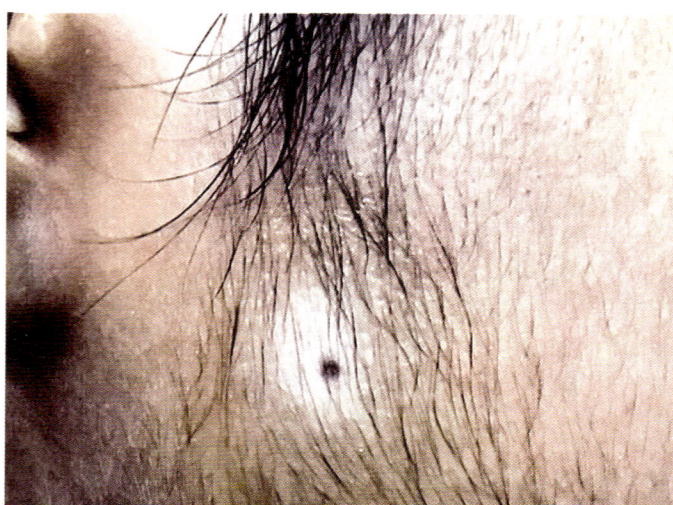

Fig. 74.15: Halo nevus. A melanocytic nevus surrounded by a round to oval, symmetric halo of depigmentation

- Most common site—back
- Seen in children or young adults

HISTOPATHOLOGY (Figs 74.16 to 74.18)

- Early stage—nests of nevus cells in a dense inflammatory cell infiltrate comprising predominantly of lymphocytes
- Nevus cells contain melanin pigment
- A few nevus cells show enlarged ovoid nucleoli (reactive atypia)
- Mitosis is absent
- Nevus cells mature and become small from superficial dermis to deep dermis
- Later stage—nevus cells and inflammatory cells disappear

DIFFERENTIAL DIAGNOSIS

Melanoma

- Presents as a large size, asymmetrical nodule
- Less pronounced inflammatory cell infiltrate
- Absence of maturation of lesional/ nevus cells
- Presence of high grade nuclear atypia and mitotic activity

DYSPLASTIC NEVUS

INTRODUCTION

- Presents as a macule of large size, with size of more than 5 mm with irregular margins (borders), and irregular pigmentation within the lesion
- Most common site—trunk

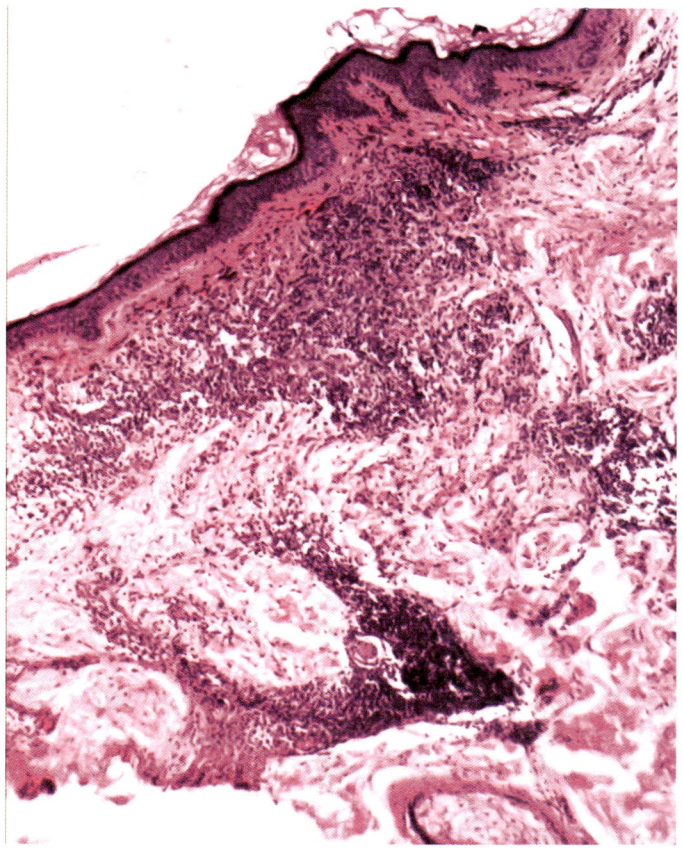

Fig. 74.16: Halo nevus (early stage) in which nevus cells with melanin pigment are interspersed throughout upper dermis with accompanying dense inflammatory cell infiltrate

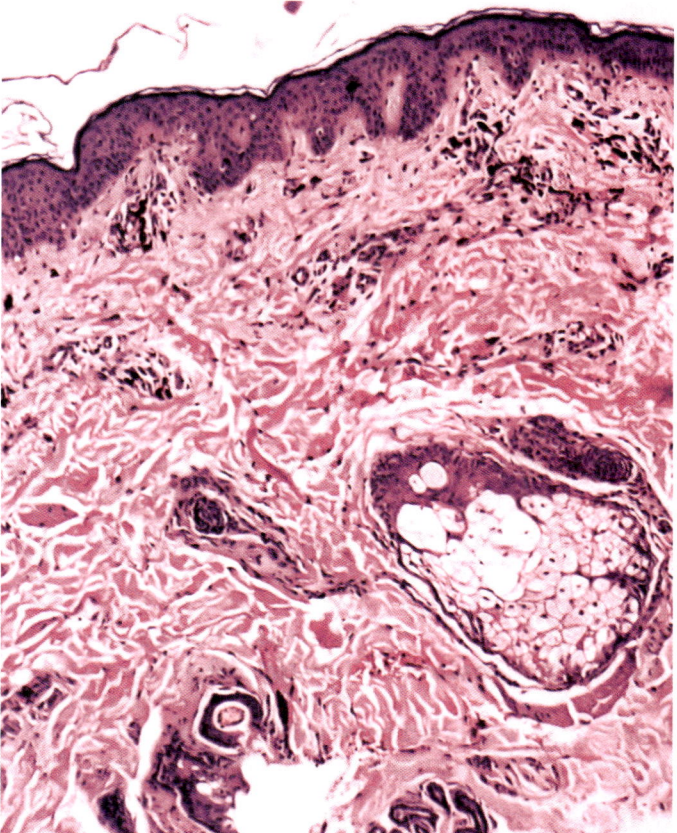

Fig. 74.17: Halo nevus with upper dermis demonstrating a few nevus cell nests containing melanin pigment and reduced inflammatory cell component

- Associated with increased risk of melanoma
- Associated with NRAS, BRAF, CDKN2A mutations and increased TERT expression
- Dysplastic nevus syndrome—autosomal dominant disorder, in which the patients are at increased risk of developing multiple dysplastic nevi and melanomas

HISTOPATHOLOGY (Figs 74.19 and 74.20)

- Can involve both epidermis and dermis
- Junctional component—single nevus cells replace normal basal cell layer along the dermoepidermal junction
- Lentiginous hyperplasia—lentiginous proliferation of nevus cells in the epidermis
- Nevus cells are arranged in nests and are present at sides of elongated rete ridges
- Bridging—confluence of nevus cell nests present at the tips of adjacent rete ridges
- Shoulder phenomenon—nevus cell nests in the junctional component extend laterally and beyond the underlying dermal component

- Nevus cells exhibit architectural and cytological atypia
- Cytological atypia—cells present with nuclear enlargement, angulated nuclear contours and hyperchromasia
- Dermis underlying atypical cells shows lamellar fibrosis
- Melanin incontinence is seen

CRITERIA FOR DIAGNOSIS
(Diagnosis requires presence of both major criteria and at least two minor criteria)

Major Criteria

- Lentiginous melanocytic hyperplasia
- Focal melanocytic atypia

Minor Criteria

- Shoulder phenomenon
- Fusion of rete ridges
- Subepidermal lamellar fibrosis
- Superficial perivascular lymphocytic infiltrate

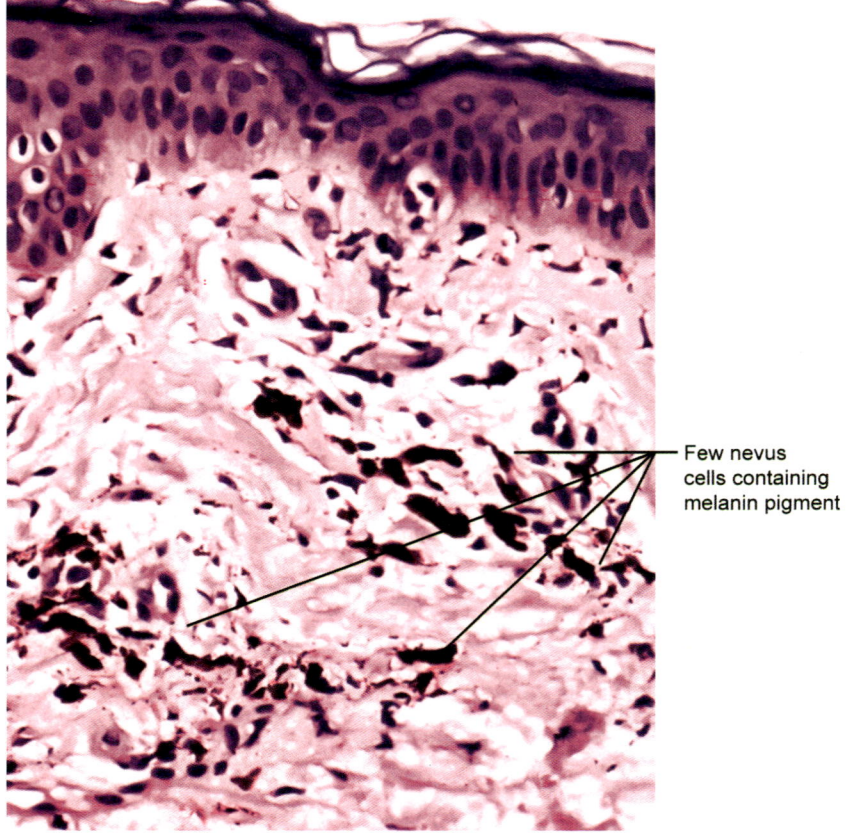

Few nevus cells containing melanin pigment

Fig. 74.18: Halo nevus (late stage)

CONGENITAL NEVUS

INTRODUCTION
- Present since birth
- Site—lower extremities, scalp
- Measures >1.5 cm in diameter

VARIANTS
1. *Giant congenital melanocytic nevus*
- Can measure more than 20 cm in diameter
- Usually, covers large areas of skin (garment nevi)
- Areas of increased pigmentation is commonly seen
- Increased risk of cutaneous melanoma
2. *Other variants*—non-giant melanocytic nevus, cerebriform congenital melanocytic nevus, congenital acral melanocytic nevus, and desmoplastic pigmented nevus

HISTOPATHOLOGY
- Greater size and depth of the lesion
- Nevus cells nests in the reticular dermis, can reach up to the subcutis

- Involvement of skin appendages, hair follicles and sebaceous glands by nevus cells can be seen
- Melanomas most commonly arising in congenital nevus are of superficial spreading type

BECKER'S NEVUS

INTRODUCTION
- Most commonly affects adults but can be seen since birth (Note—we have seen twin sisters affected by the same)
- Site—most commonly affects trunk and extremities
- Associations—scleroderma, neurofibromatosis, lichen planus, skeletal deformities, basal cell carcinoma, melanocytic nevus

HISTOPATHOLOGY (Figs 74.21 and 74.22)
- Acanthosis, mild papillomatosis, flattened elongated rete ridges
- Hyperpigmentation of the basal cell layer of the epidermis with melanophages in dermis

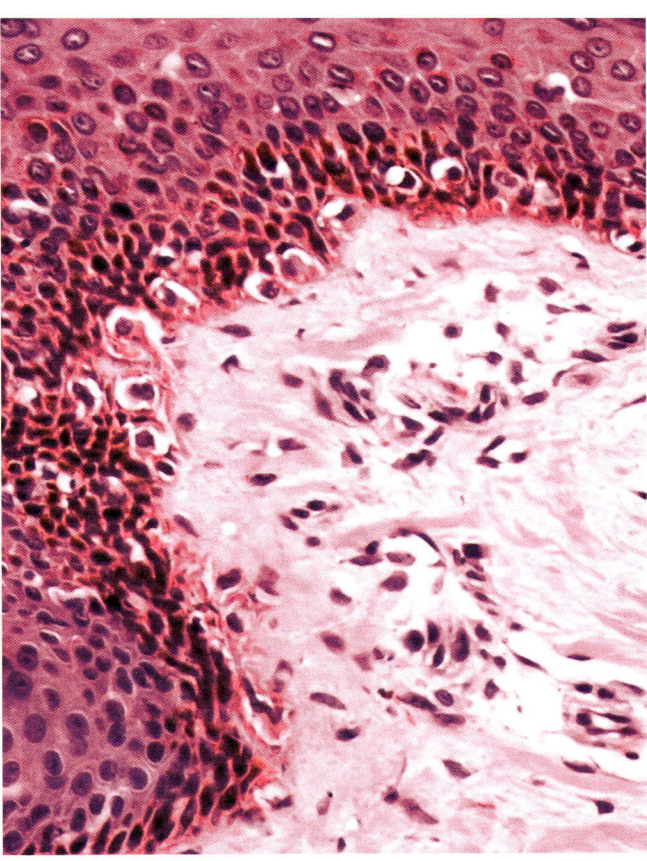

Fig. 74.19: Dysplastic nevi (lentiginous hyperplasia with atypical melanocytes, superficial perivascular lymphocytic infiltrate)

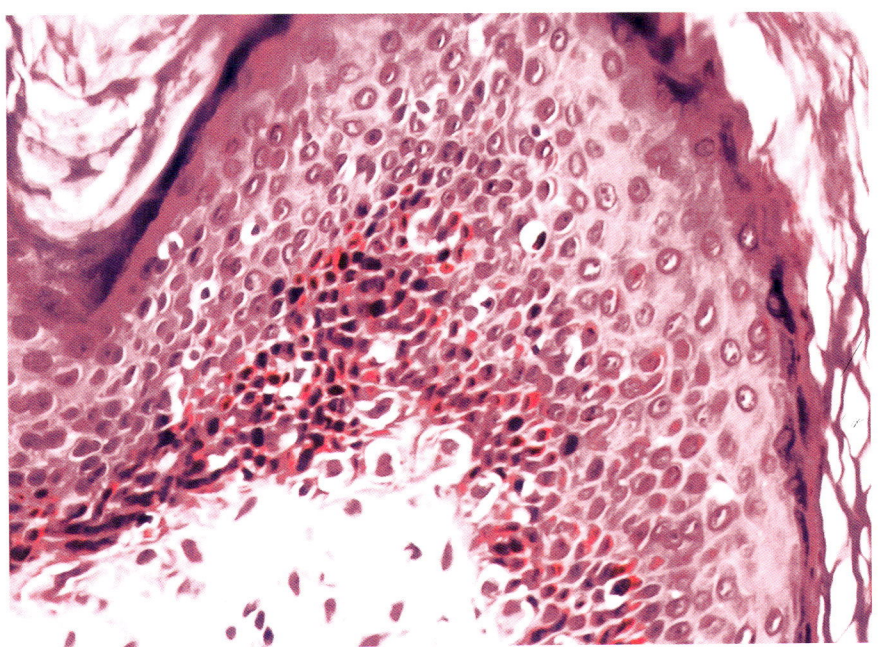

Fig. 74.20: Dysplastic nevi (lentiginous hyperplasia with atypical melanocytes)

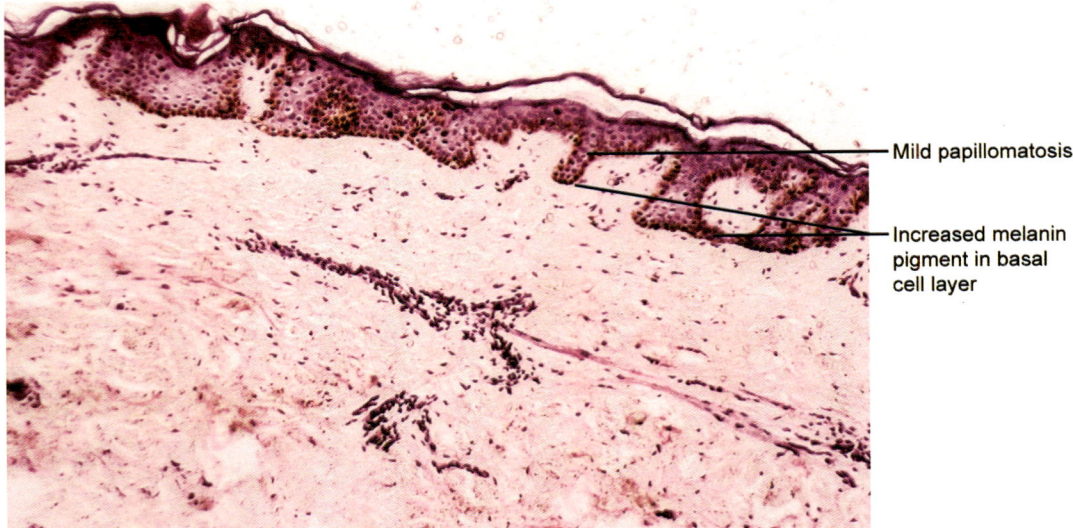

Fig. 74.21: Becker's nevus

Mild papillomatosis

Increased melanin pigment in basal cell layer

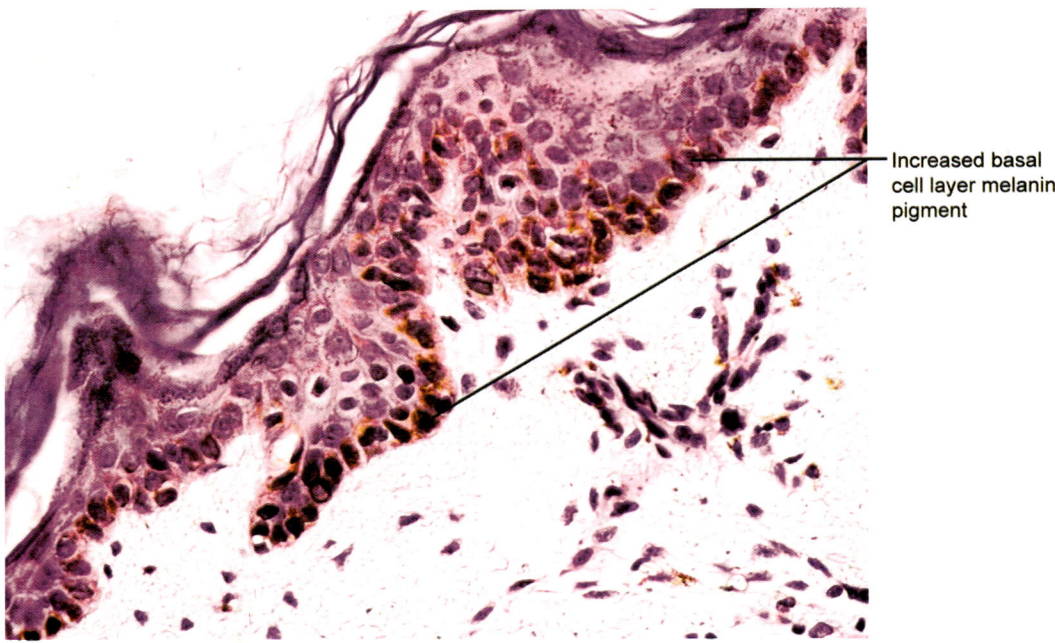

Fig. 74.22: Becker's nevus

Increased basal cell layer melanin pigment

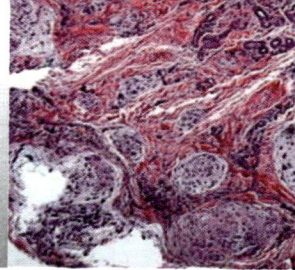

Malignant Pigmented Lesions (Melanoma)

INTRODUCTION

- Sites—skin (most common), oral mucosa, nasal cavity and sinuses, gastrointestinal tract, genitourinary tract
- Predisposing factor—exposure to UV radiation, presence of nevi and freckles, immune-suppression
- Pathogenesis—CDKN2A gene mutations (loss of p16/INK4a), BRAF and RAS mutations, PTEN mutations, reactivation of telomerase enzyme can be seen
- Warning signs—ABCDE of melanoma (**A**symmetry, irregular **b**orders, variegated **c**olor, increasing **d**iameter (>6 mm), **e**volution of change over time)

MORPHOLOGY

Two Phases

1. **Radial growth phase**—intra-epidermal proliferation of atypical melanocytes. Includes superficial spreading melanoma, lentigo melanoma, acral lentiginous melanoma
2. **Vertical growth phase**—characterized by invasion of papillary and/or reticular dermis by nests of atypical melanocytes. Includes nodular melanoma and desmoplastic melanoma
   Note: In vertical growth phase, dermal nests are larger than epidermal melanoma cells with presence of mitosis

NONTUMOROGENIC MELANOMAS

- Patterns of presentation of tumor cells—pagetoid or lentiginous

SUPERFICIAL SPREADING MELANOMA

Introduction

- Also called pagetoid melanoma
- Most frequent form of melanoma
- Presents as elevated lesion with irregular outline
- Sites—upper back in men and lower legs in women
- Arise from the junctional nevus cells

Histopathology

- Alternate thickening and thinning of epidermis
- Large, round melanocytes scattered throughout the epidermis in pagetoid pattern
- Tumor cells showing nuclear atypia and mitoses are present in nests in the lower epidermis and singly in upper epidermis
- *In situ* lesion—basement membrane is intact
- Invasive radial growth phase or micro-invasive melanoma (non-tumorogenic)—cells similar to melanoma cells in epidermis are present in dermis, but these melanoma cell nests in dermis are not larger than melanoma cell nests in epidermis

Differential Diagnosis

Junctional Nevus

- Absence of mitosis, nuclear atypia, pagetoid spread and significant inflammatory cell infiltrate

Junctional Melanocytic Dysplasia

- Small size (< 6 mm), symmetrical, normal stratum corneum, absence of pagetoid spread of lesional cells, no mitosis

Lentiginous Melanoma

- Atrophic epidermis, absence of pagetoid spread of melanoma cells, replacement of the basal cell layer by atypical melanocytes

Paget's Disease

- Presence of basal cells beneath the tumor cells (differentiate it from melanoma)
- Tumor cells demonstrate cytokeratin, carcinoembryonic antigen (CEA) positivity and are negative for Melan-A and HMB-45

Bowen's Disease

- Well-preserved basal cell layer
- Tumor cells show positivity for anti-keratin antibodies
- Tumor cells do not stain for S-100, Melan-A, HMB-45

LENTIGO MALIGNA MELANOMA

- Seen in elderly people
- Site—most commonly affects face
- Lesion starts as a macule and can attain diameter of several centimetres
- Borders are impalpable and indistinct (unlike superficial spreading melanoma)
- Arise from spindle-shaped junctional melanocytes

Histopathology

- Also called melanoma *in situ*
- Atrophic epidermis
- Contiguous replacement of basal cell layer by atypical melanocytes
- Atypical melanocytes in nests are spindle-shaped and often hang down like rain droplets
- Upper dermis shows degeneration, contains numerous melanophages and band-like inflammatory cell infiltrate

ACRAL LENTIGINOUS MELANOMA

Introduction

- Site—palms and soles
- Presents as plaques or nodules
- Occurs due to cyclin D-1 gene amplification

Histopathology

- Irregular acanthosis
- Lentiginous pattern—lesional cells are located near the dermo-epidermal junction
- Lesional (tumor) cells can be spindle-shaped or round pagetoid type
- Dense inflammatory cell infiltrate at dermo-epidermal junction
- Upper dermis shows melanophages

TUMORIGENIC MELANOMA

NODULAR MELANOMA

Introduction

- Most common in older men
- Presents as small, symmetrical, well-circumscribed, dark-brown or blue-black papules or nodules (Fig. 75.1)

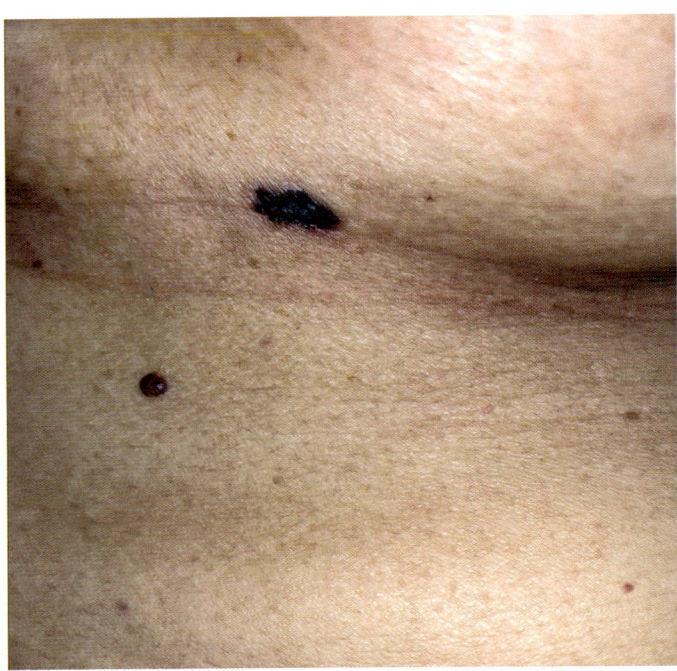

Fig. 75.1: Melanoma. Variably pigmented, irregular macule with shades of gray and black

Histopathology (Figs 75.2 to 75.4)

- Proliferation of tumor cells in the dermis
- Tumor cells grow in nests or sheets in the papillary dermis or can invade the coarse collagen fibers of reticular dermis
- Tumor cells in dermis can be epithelioid cell type or spindle cell type
- Epithelioid cells are also seen in nodular melanomas and superficial spreading melanomas
- Spindle cells are also seen in lentigo maligna melanoma and acral lentiginous melanoma
- Tumor cells show irregular nuclear membranes, hyperchromasia, prominent nucleoli (irregular in shape, size and number) and presence of mitotic figures
- Immunohistochemistry—melanoma cells are positive for S-100, HMB-45, Melan-A

Differential Diagnosis

Spitz Nevus

- Lesions are of small size, circumscribed, symmetrical and lack marked cytological atypia
- Epidermis—pseudoepitheliomatous hyperplasia with presence of Kamino bodies
- Comprising of spindle cells or epithelioid cells with large nuclei, pale delicate nuclear chromatin and smooth nuclear membranes with eosinophilic nucleoli

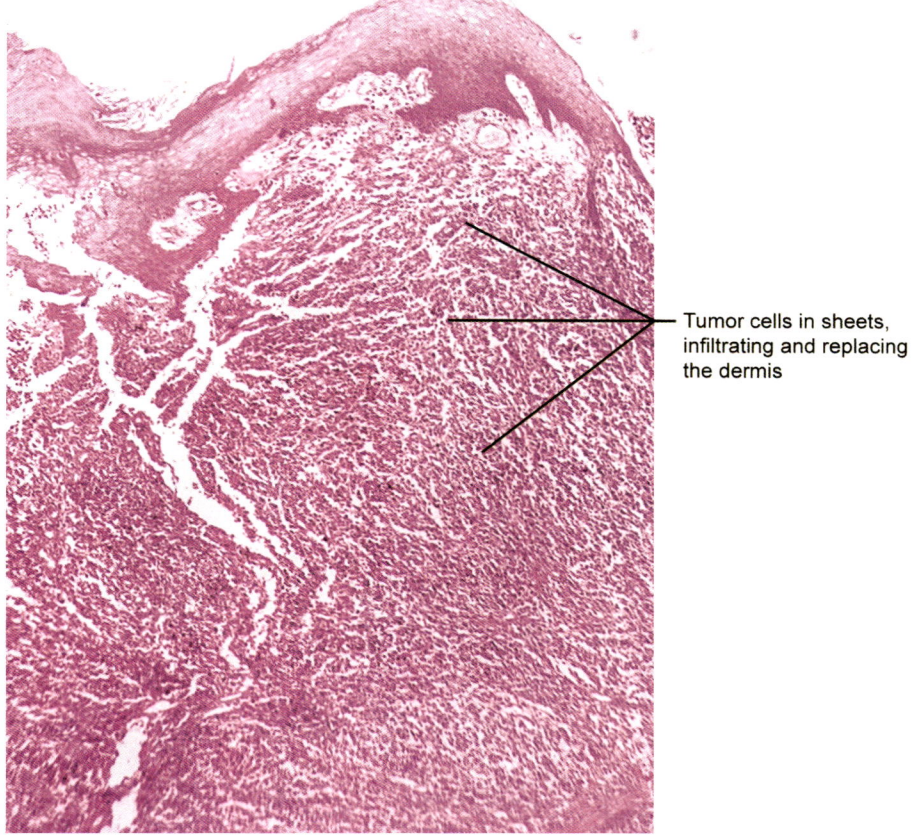

Tumor cells in sheets, infiltrating and replacing the dermis

Fig. 75.2: Nodular melanoma

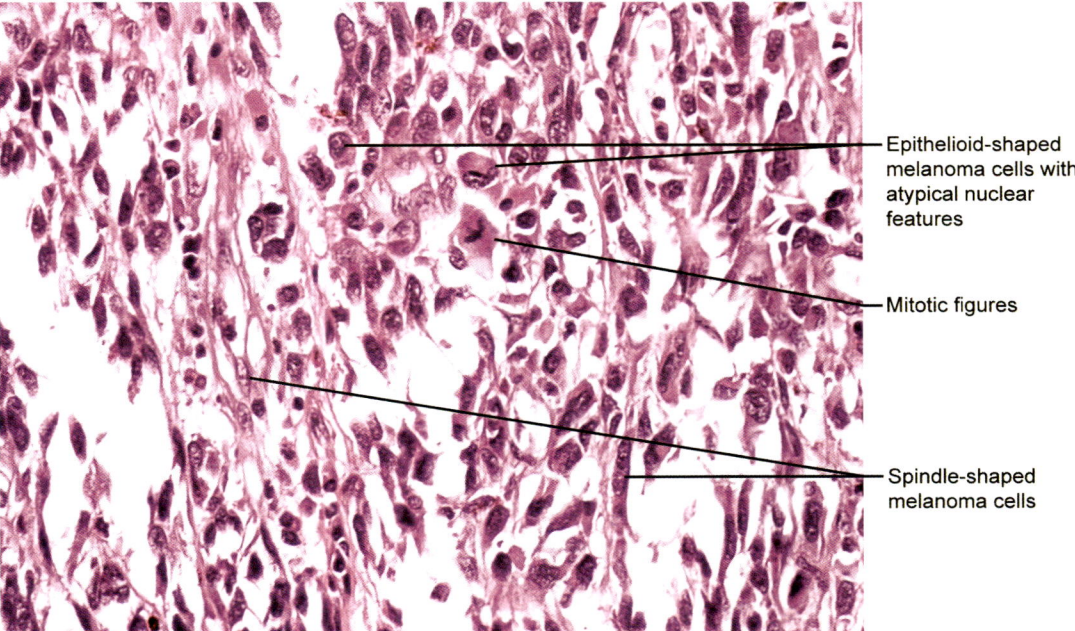

Epithelioid-shaped melanoma cells with atypical nuclear features

Mitotic figures

Spindle-shaped melanoma cells

Fig. 75.3: Nodular melanoma (melanoma cells with atypical nuclear features)

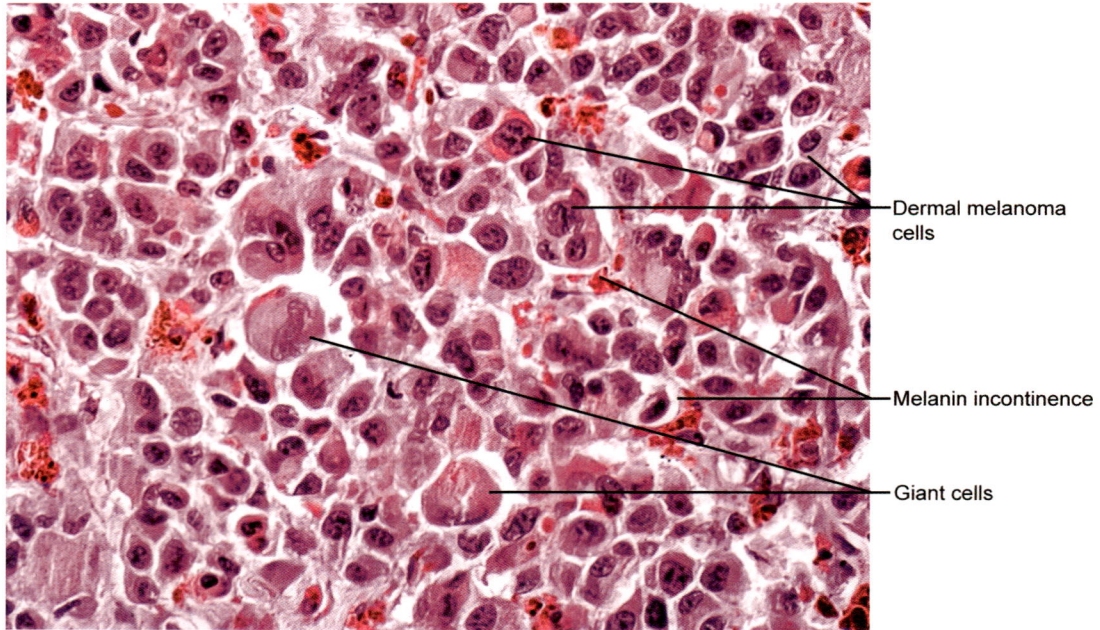

Fig. 75.4: Malignant melanoma

Labels on figure:
- Dermal melanoma cells
- Melanin incontinence
- Giant cells

- Diffuse HMB-45 positivity is seen in nevus cells in comparison to melanoma cell clusters, which show patchy positivity

Non-Hodgkin Lymphoma (Anaplastic Large Cell Lymphoma)

- Can involve skin
- Shows CD-30 and LCA positivity

Juvenile Xanthogranuloma

- Presence of Touton's giant cells/foam cells

DESMOPLASTIC MELANOMA

Introduction

- Affects elderly individuals
- Sites—head and neck, lower lip

Histopathology (Figs 75.5 and 75.6)

- Dermis shows atypical spindle cells arranged in loose fascicles, that can extend into the deep dermis and subcutis
- Lymphocytic aggregates are seen within the tumor
- Neurotropism (neurotropic melanoma)—spindle-shaped melanoma cells arranged in a concentric fashion around small nerves in deep dermis
- Spindle-shaped tumor cells show S-100 positivity and Melan-A, HMB-45 negativity

Differential Diagnosis

Neurofibromatosis

- Absence of nuclear atypia, mitotic activity and lymphocytic infiltrate in the dermal component

Desmoplastic Nevi

- Affects head and neck
- Absence of mitotic figures
- Decreased HMB-45 expression

Cellular Dermatofibroma

- Cells are negative for S-100

Dermatofibroma Sarcoma Protuberans

- Cells show CD34 positivity

PROGNOSIS OF MELANOMA

1. TNM staging
2. Levels of Invasion (Clarke)

   Level I—melanoma cells confined to the epidermis (*in situ* melanoma)

   Level II—invasion of the papillary dermis (micro-invasive)

   Level III—invasion to the papillary/reticular dermal interface

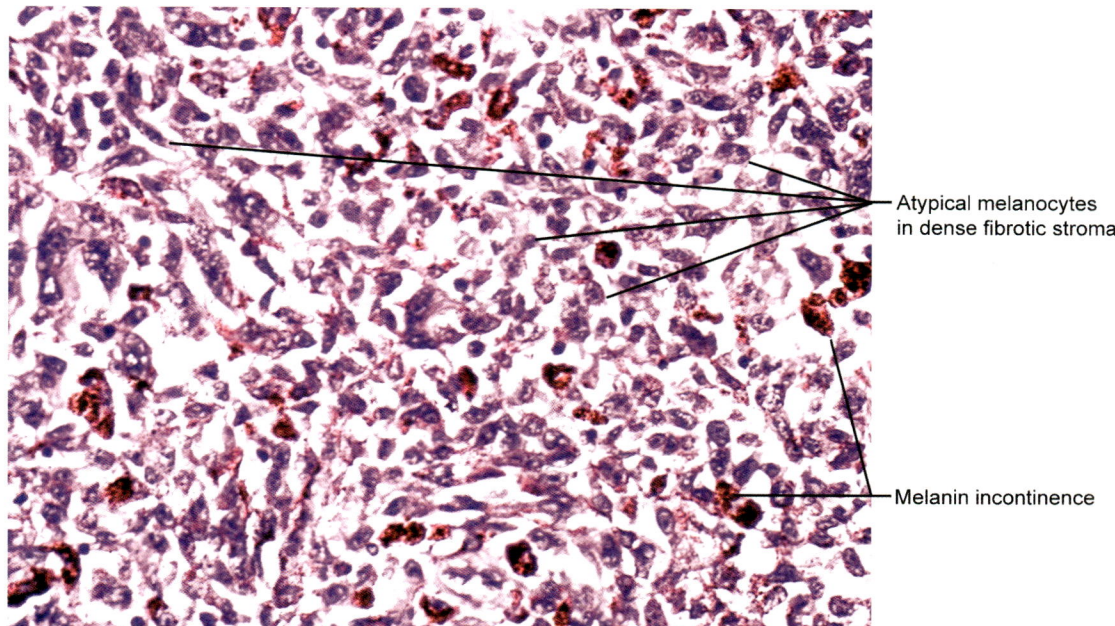

Fig. 75.5: Desmoplastic melanoma

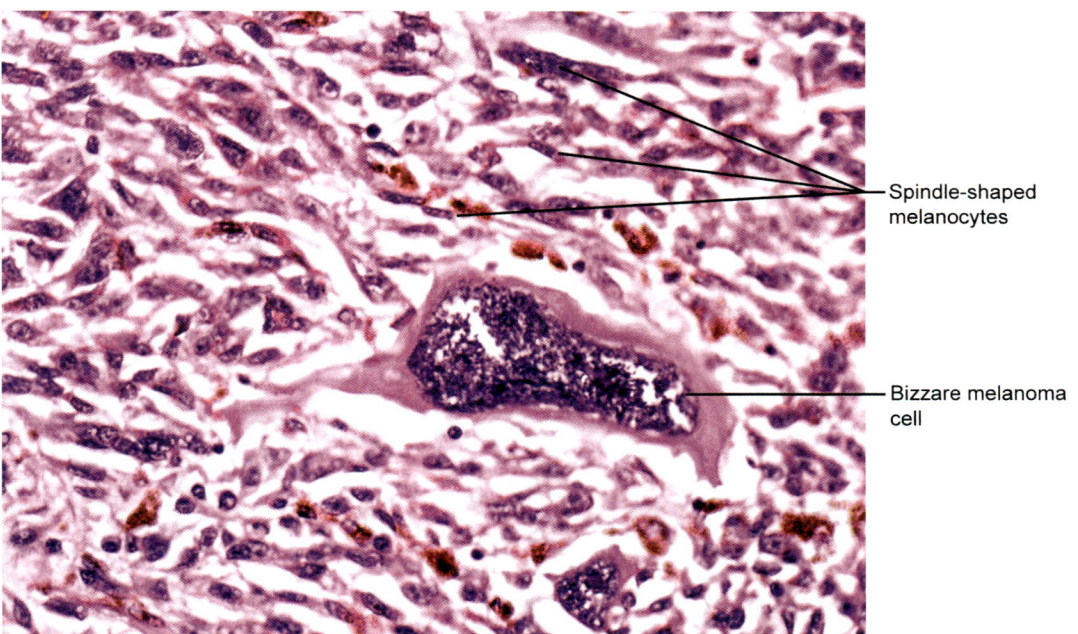

Fig. 75.6: Desmoplastic melanoma

Level IV—invasion into the reticular dermis
Level V—invasion into the subcutaneous fat

3. Thickness of tumor

- Breslow's thickness—distance from the superficial epidermal granular cell layer to the deepest intradermal tumor cells
- Melanomas less than 1 mm have excellent prognosis

4. Regression

- Defined as presence of degenerated tumor cells with lymphocytic infiltrate
- Melanoma may be present in epidermis and/or papillary dermis, but not within the area of regression
- Most commonly seen in non-tumorogenic compartment called radial growth phase regression
- Absence of regression—good prognosis

5. **Tumor infiltrating lymphocytes**
   - Lymphocytes forming a continuous band beneath the tumor
   - Tumors with brisk tumor infiltrating lymphocytes have good prognosis

6. **Mitotic figures**
   - Presence of > 6 mitosis/mm^2 is associated with worse prognosis

7. **Ulceration of overlying skin**
   - Absence of ulceration confers good prognosis

8. **Micrometastasis**
   - Microscopic involvement of a sentinel lymph node even with a small number of melanoma cells confer worse prognosis

9. **Gender**
   - Females have better prognosis than males

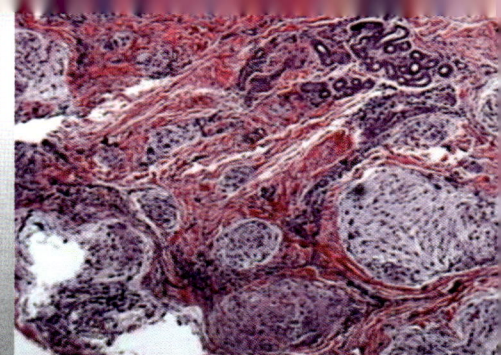

Adnexal Tumors

Part 14

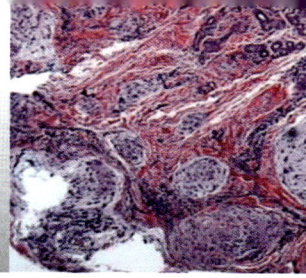

Sebaceous Hyperplasia

INTRODUCTION

- Sites of involvement—nose, forehead and cheeks. Vulva, vagina and areola being the rare sites
- Age group—affects elderly individuals
- Presents as yellow colored papules measuring 2–3 mm in diameter (Fig. 76.1)
- Cause—decrease in circulating androgen levels

HISTOPATHOLOGY (Figs 76.2 and 76.3)

- Four or more sebaceous lobules attached to the infundibulum of each pilosebaceous unit
- Sebaceous lobules show normal peripheral rim of basaloid cells

VARIANT

Montgomery's Tubercle

- Ectopic mature sebaceous glands located on the areola of breasts

- Histopathology—mature sebaceous lobule in continuity with the epidermis of the nipple

Differential Diagnosis

Sebaceous Adenoma (Fig. 76.4)

- Enlarged sebaceous lobules of varying shapes and sizes
- Sebaceous lobules comprising of mature sebaceous cells with basaloid cells at the periphery
- Absence of cytological atypia or mitosis

Sebaceoma (Sebaceous Epithelioma) (Figs 76.5 and 76.6)

- Large size and is located more deeply (in comparison to sebaceous adenoma)
- Can present as well-circumscribed or an ill-circumscribed nodule
- Composed of basaloid cells (undifferentiated) and mature sebaceous cells

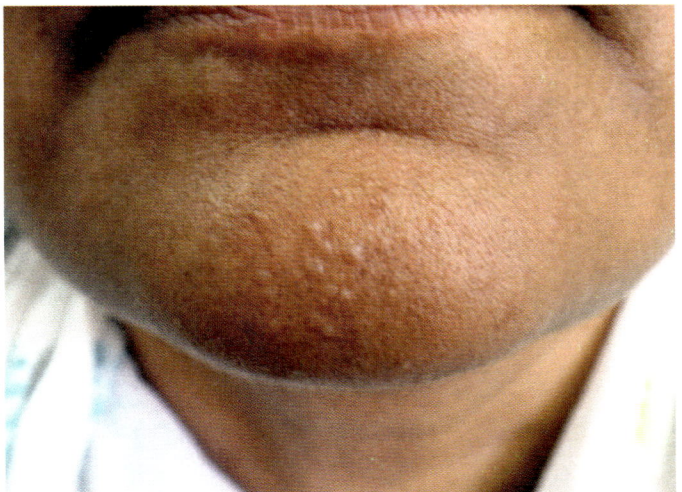

Fig. 76.1: Sebaceous hyperplasia. Umblicated, skin-colored to yellowish papules

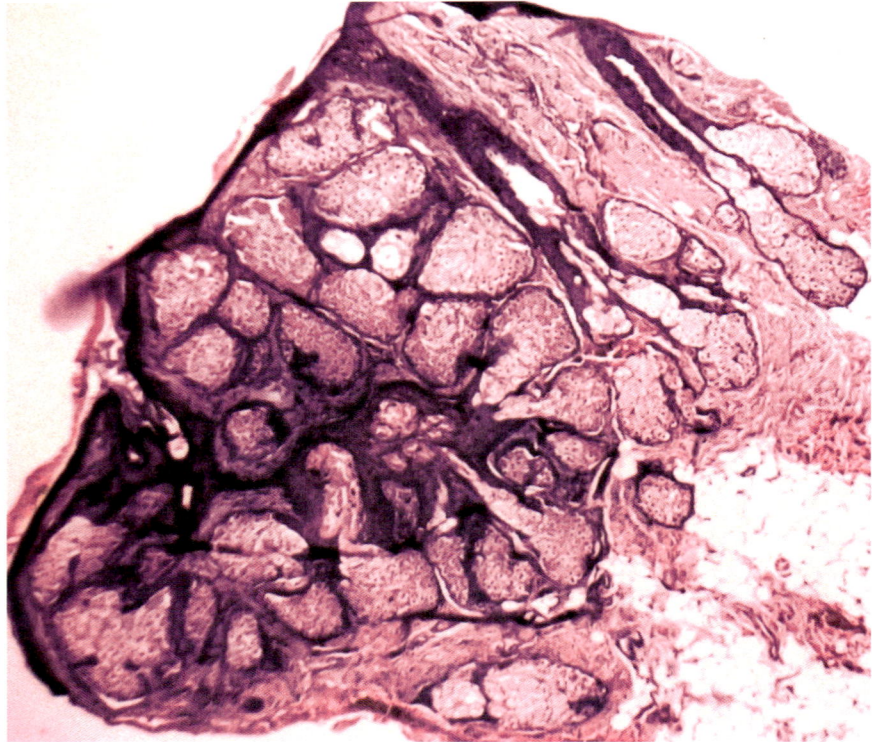

Fig. 76.2: Sebaceous hyperplasia

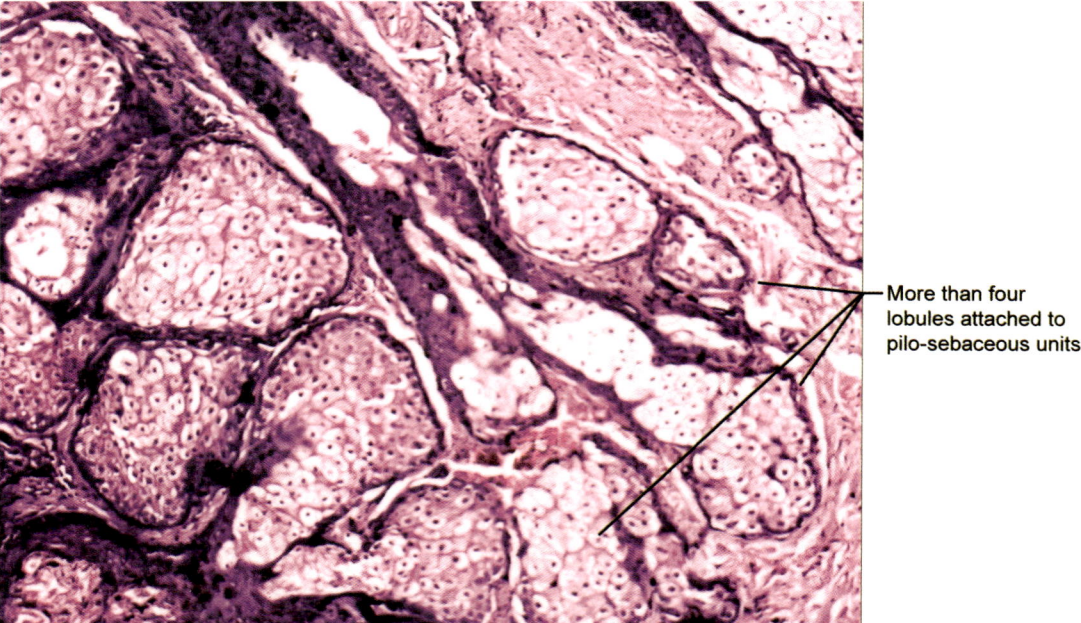

More than four lobules attached to pilo-sebaceous units

Fig. 76.3: Sebaceous hyperplasia

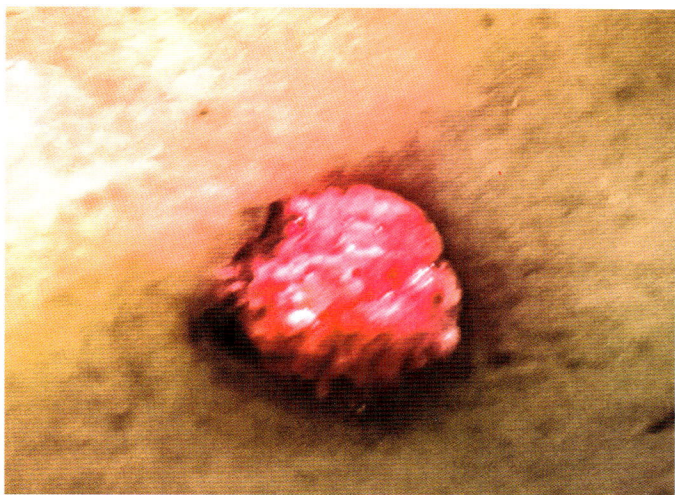

Fig. 76.4: Sebaceous adenoma

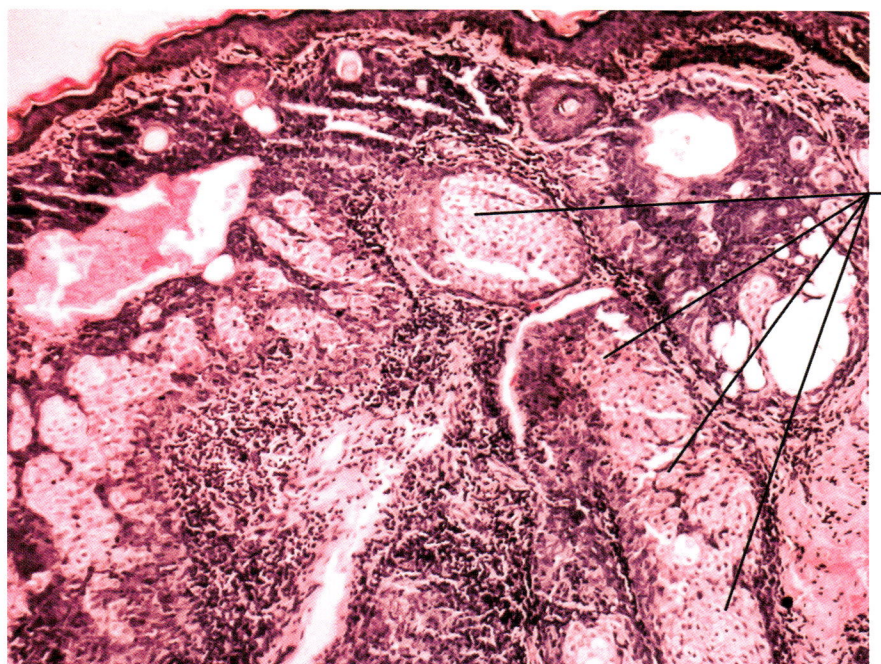

Dermis showing mature sebaceous cells and basaloid cells at periphery

Fig. 76.5: Sebaceoma

- Absence of nuclear atypia
- Presence of numerous mitotic figures

SEBACEOUS CARCINOMA

INTRODUCTION

- Most common site—ocular adnexa (upper eyelids)
- Age group—affects elderly individuals
- More common in females

HISTOPATHOLOGY (Fig. 76.7)

- Lobules or sheets of malignant cells separated by fibrovascular stroma
- Tumor cells have vacuolated or foamy cytoplasm
- Vacuolated cells contain lipid and are stained with Oil-red-O or Sudan black
- Infiltrative growth pattern, vascular and lymphatic invasion can occur
- Malignant sebaceous cells show EMA and Ber-EP4-positivity
- Mitotic count is high

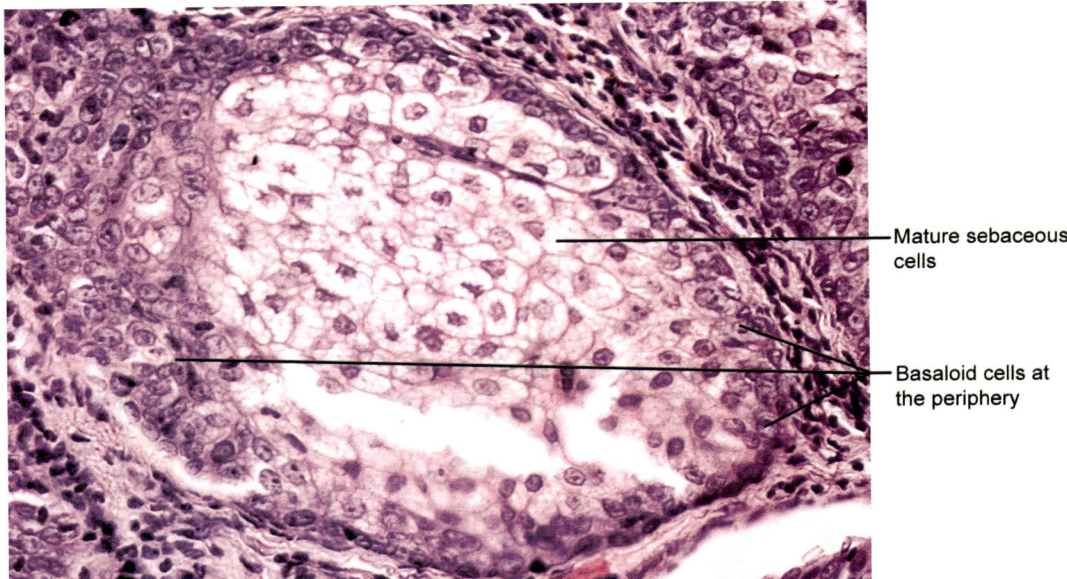

Fig. 76.6: Sebaceoma

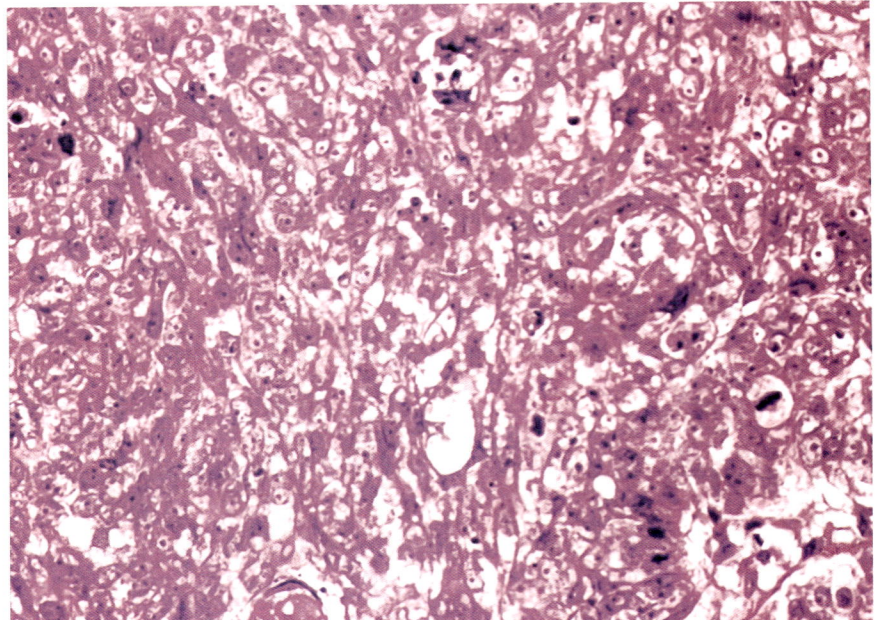

Fig. 76.7: Sebaceous carcinoma: Malignant sebaceous cells with increased mitotic count

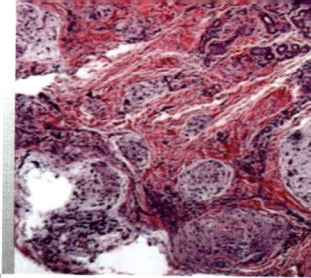

Pilomatricoma

- Also called calcifying epithelioma of Malherbe
- Adnexal tumor with follicular differentiation
- Sites—affects head and neck, upper extremities
- Age group—children and adolescents
- Clinical presentation—presents as solitary, firm, dermal nodule
- Genetic mutation—associated with beta catenin gene mutation

HISTOPATHOLOGY (Figs 77.1 to 77.4)

- Well circumscribed, encapsulated lesion
- Composed of basaloid cells and shadow cells
- Basaloid cells transforming into shadow cells are seen at the center of the lesion
- Basaloid cells resemble hair matrix cells and shadow cells represent a central unstained shadow at the site of the lost nucleus

- Keratinization seen at the centre of the lesion is abrupt and complete
- Calcium deposits can be seen in the stroma of tumor, which can be demonstrated by von Kossa stain
- Also seen within the stroma are numerous foreign body giant cells surrounding keratin

DIFFERENTIAL DIAGNOSIS

Basal Cell Carcinoma

- Presence of clefting and peripheral palisading of tumor cells

Trichilemmal Cysts

- Peripheral layer of basophilic cells can show peripheral palisading
- Absence of shadow cells

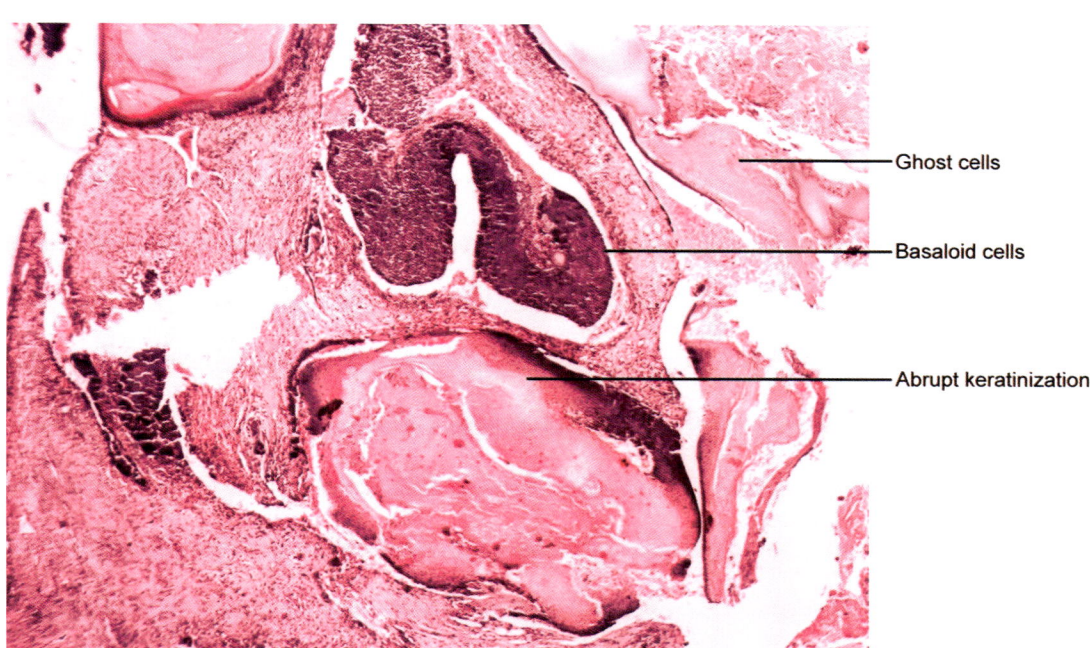

Ghost cells

Basaloid cells

Abrupt keratinization

Fig. 77.1: Pilomatricoma

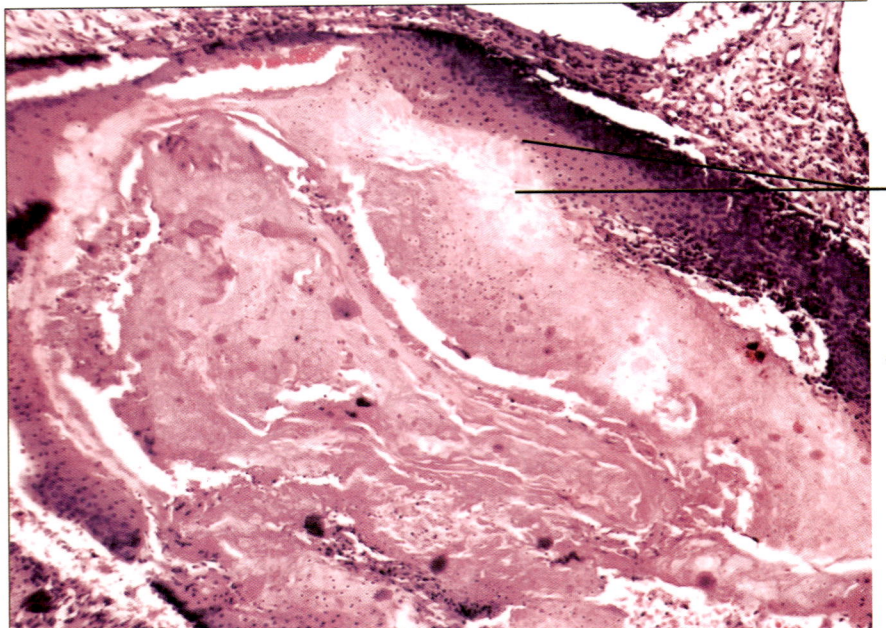

Trichilemmal keratinization at the center of the lesion

Fig. 77.2: Pilomatricoma

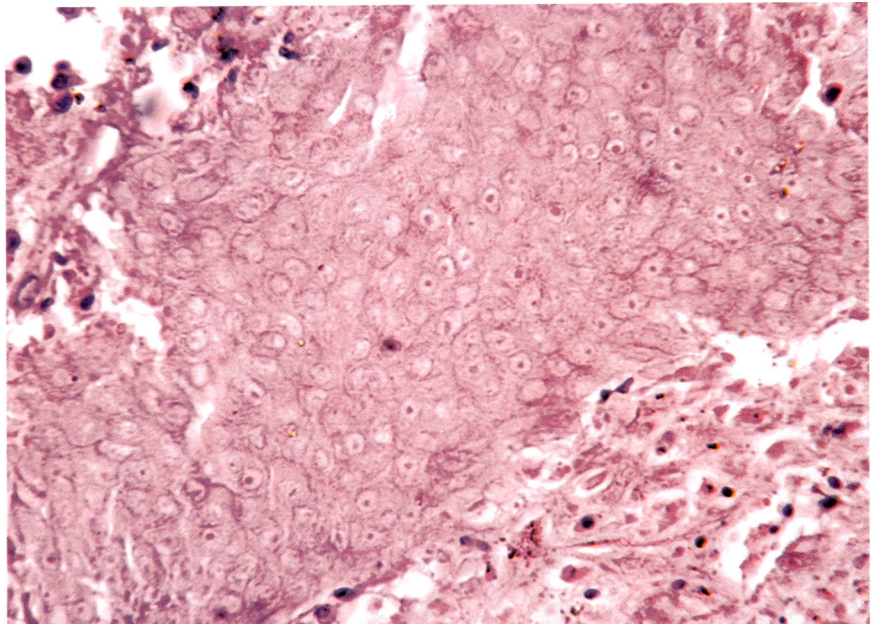

Fig. 77.3: Ghost cells with adjacent inflammatory cell infiltrate in pilomatricoma

PILOMATRIX CARCINOMA

- Malignant counterpart of pilomatricoma
- Poorly circumscribed
- Infiltrative growth pattern
- Proliferation of pleomorphic hyperchromatic basophilic cells
- Frequent mitotic figures

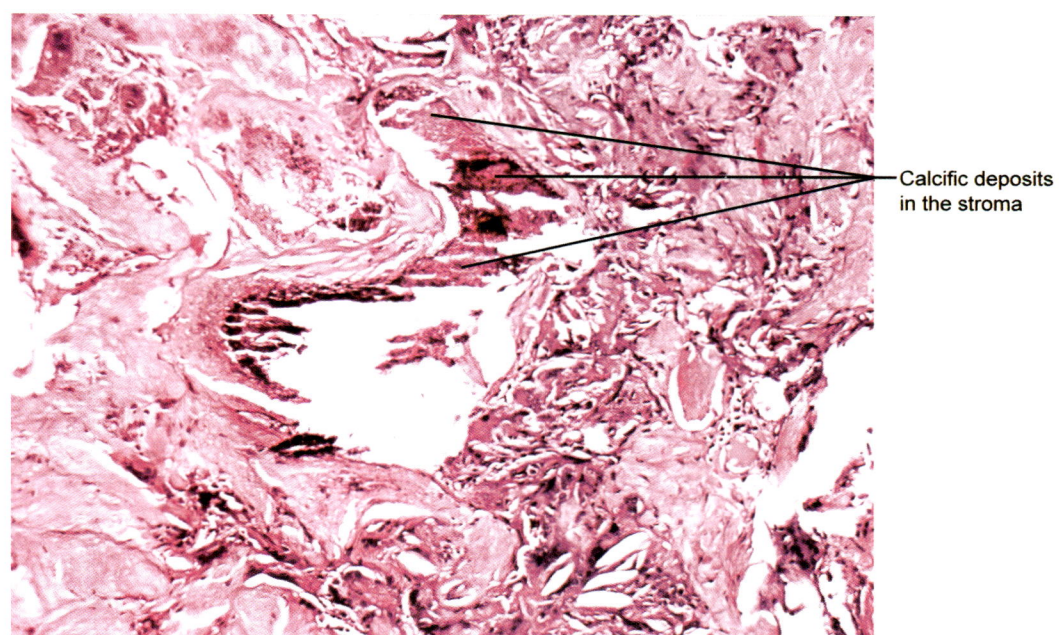

Calcific deposits
in the stroma

Fig. 77.4: Pilomatricoma

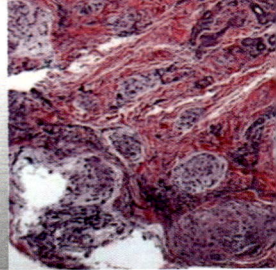

Syringoma

INTRODUCTION

- Also called eccrine duct adenoma
- More common in women
- Seen around puberty
- Sites—lower eyelids, cheeks, thigh, axilla, abdomen, vulva
- Lesions are skin colored and can be solitary or multiple

HISTOPATHOLOGY (Figs 78.1 to 78.3)

- Upper dermis and mid-dermis show numerous small ducts, lined by two layers of cuboidal epithelial cells in fibrous stroma
- Duct lining epithelial cells can show clear cell change, due to glycogen deposition (glycogen shows PAS positivity)

- Ducts have a characteristic coma like tail of epithelial cells (giving it a tadpole-like appearance)
- Duct lumina contains amorphous debris
- Cells show CEA positivity and involucrin negativity

DIFFERENTIAL DIAGNOSIS

Desmoplastic Trichoepithelioma

- Cords and nests of basaloid cells embedded in a dense stroma
- Multiple horn cysts lined by stratified squamous epithelium can be seen

Microcystic Adnexal Carcinoma

- Large sized poorly circumscribed tumors
- Located in deep dermis

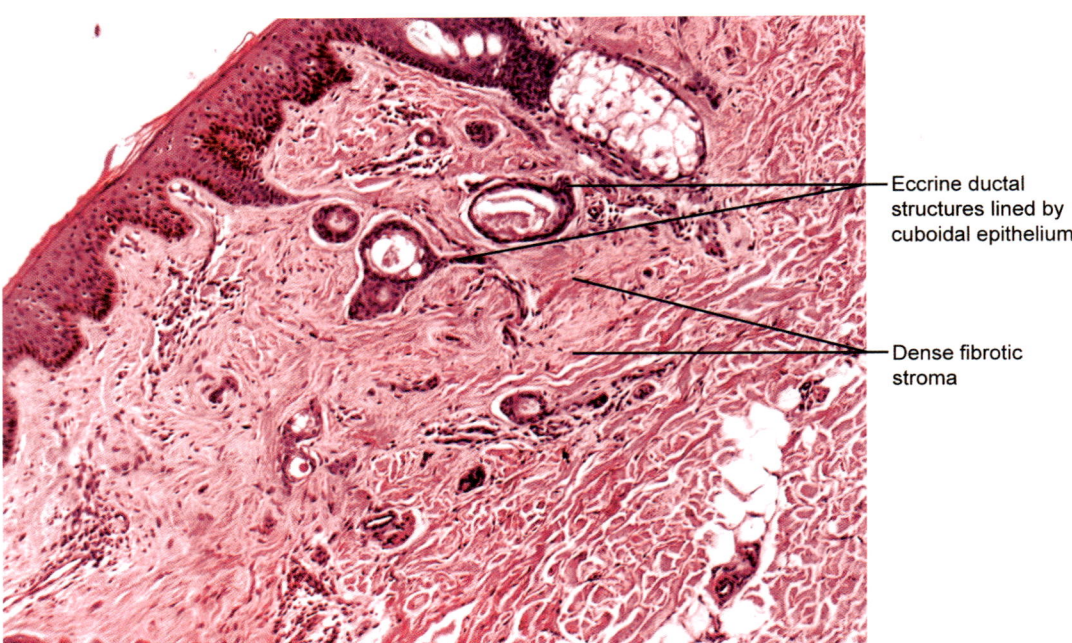

Eccrine ductal structures lined by cuboidal epithelium

Dense fibrotic stroma

Fig. 78.1: Syringoma

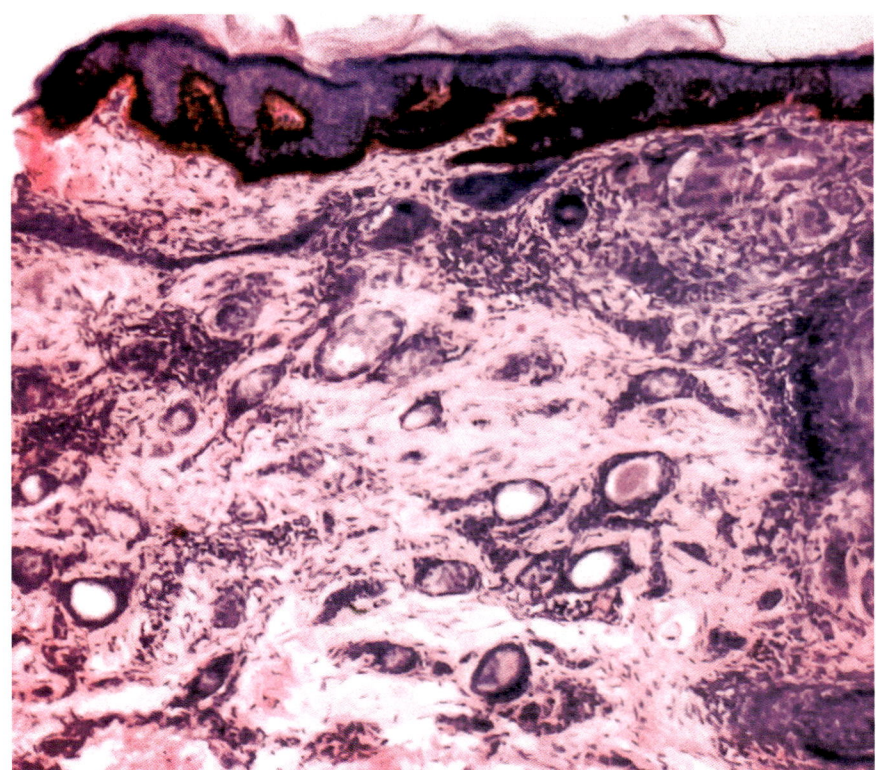

Fig. 78.2: Syringoma. Numerous eccrine ductal structures, lined by cuboidal epithelium in a dense fibrotic stroma

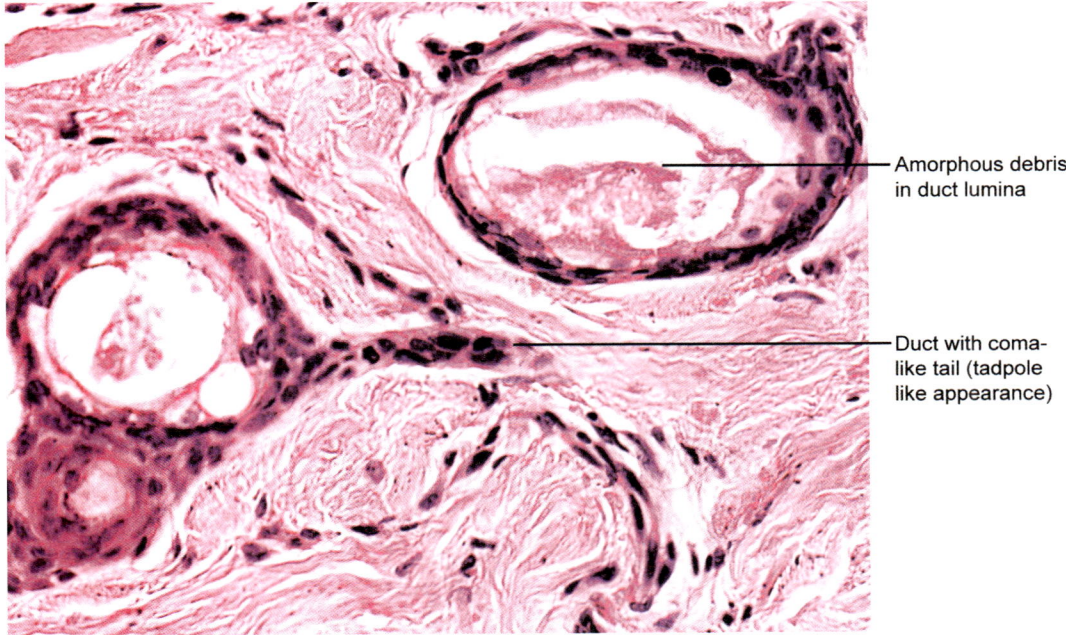

— Amorphous debris in duct lumina

— Duct with coma-like tail (tadpole like appearance)

Fig. 78.3: Syringoma

- Tumor is composed of proliferating tubular structures that extend into the subcutis
- Perineural invasion is commonly seen
- Horn cysts can be seen

Sclerosing Basal Cell Carcinoma

- Infiltrative basaloid cells
- Prominent sclerotic stroma
- Cells show CEA negativity and involucrin positivity

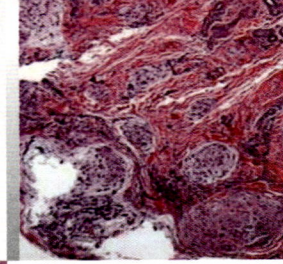

Syringocystadenoma Papilliferum

INTRODUCTION

- Sites—scalp or face
- Presents as papules or plaques measuring 1–3 cm in diameter
- Predisposing factor—nevus sebaceous
- p16 tumor suppressor gene mutation is a common finding
- Malignant variant—syringocystadenocarcinoma papilliferum

HISTOPATHOLOGY (Figs 79.1 to 79.3)

- Tumor with multiple epithelial invaginations extending down from the epidermis and contains numerous papillae

- These papillary structures are composed of squamous epithelium lining in upper portions
- In lower portion, these papillae are lined by luminal columnar cell layer with decapitation secretions and outer cuboidal cell layer
- Fibrous cores contain dense plasmacytic inflammatory cell infiltrate
- Rarely can transform into syringocystadenocarcinoma papilliferum

DIFFERENTIAL DIAGNOSIS

Hidradenoma Papilliferum

- Affects predominantly females
- Sites—vulva and perianal regions

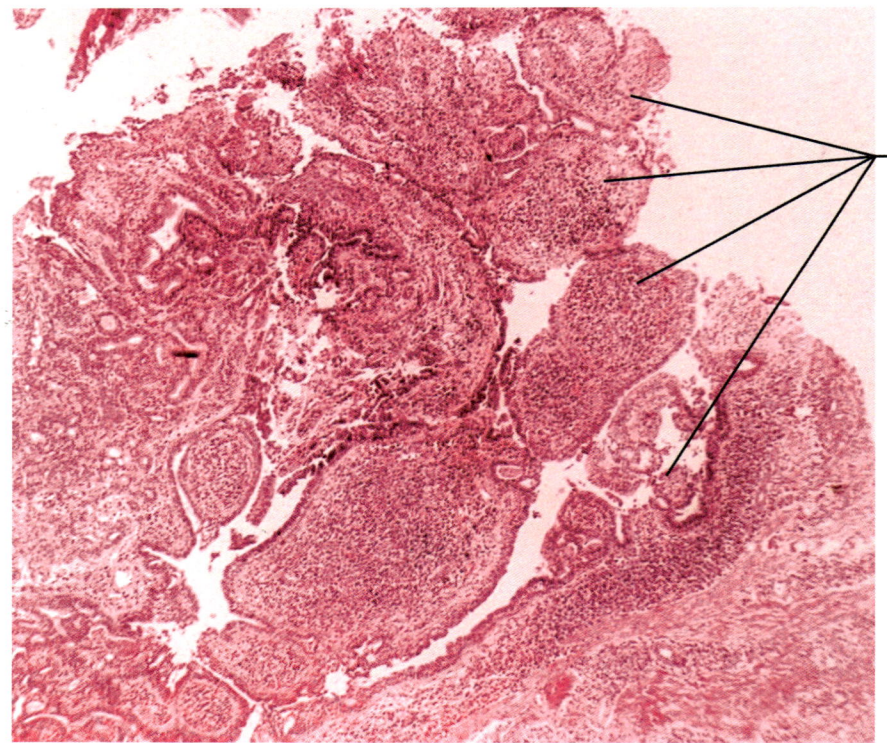

Epithelial invaginations extending down from epidermis containing numerous papillae

Fig. 79.1: Syringocystadenoma papilliferum

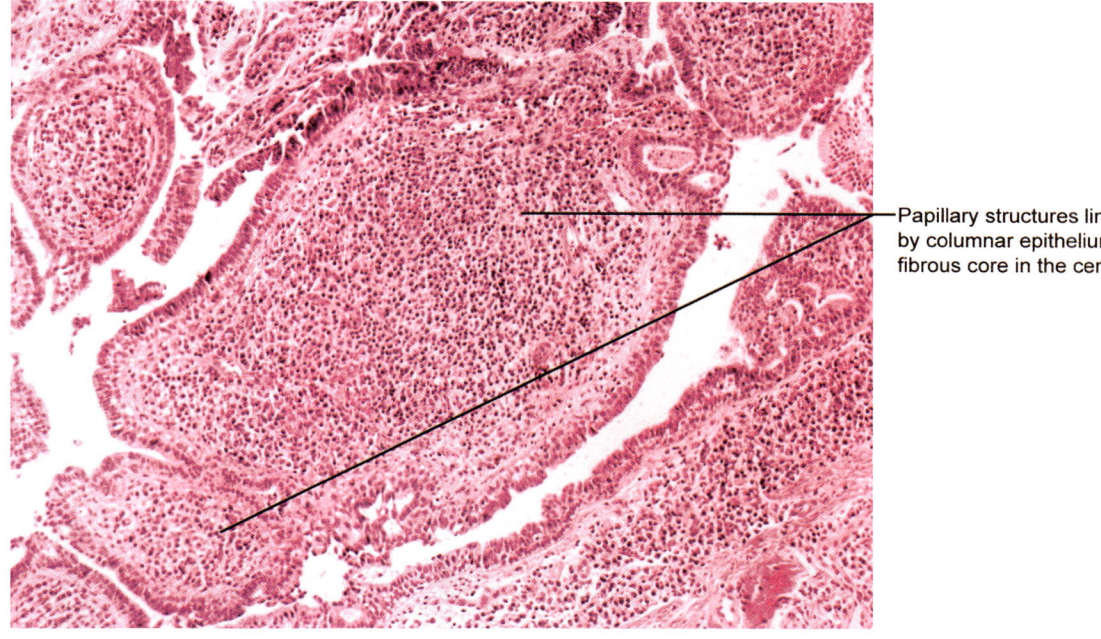

Papillary structures lined
by columnar epithelium with
fibrous core in the center

Fig. 79.2: Syringocystadenoma papilliferum

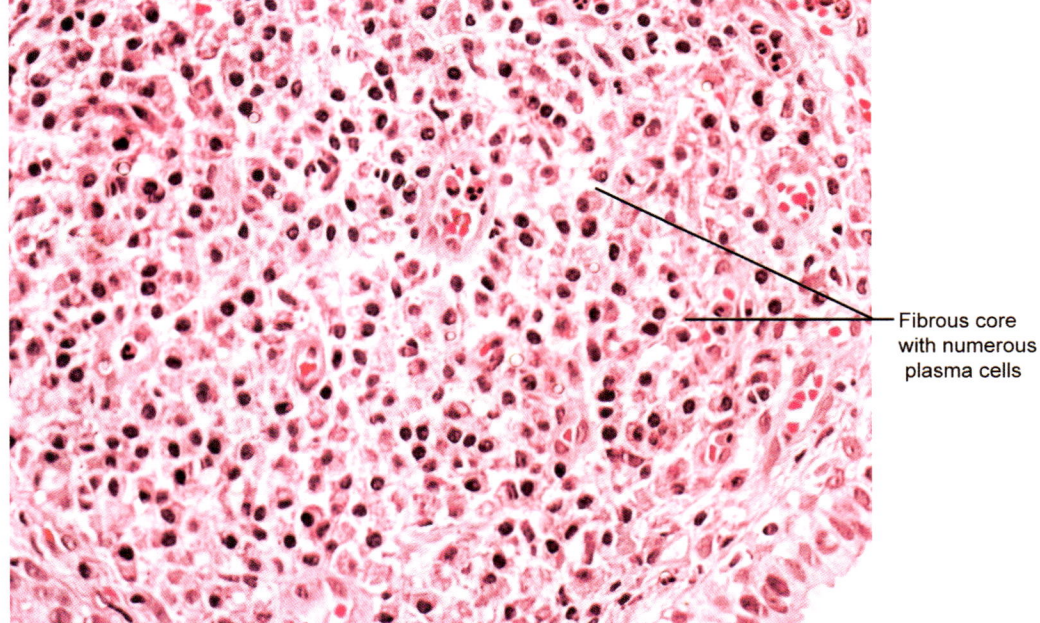

Fibrous core
with numerous
plasma cells

Fig. 79.3: Syringocystadenoma papilliferum

• Microscopy—elongated fronds forming an arborising pattern and are lined by inner cuboidal or low columnar epithelial cells with apical secretions and an outer myoepithelial cell layer.

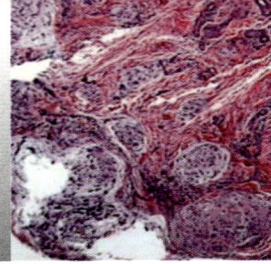

Eccrine Poroma

Chapter 80

INTRODUCTION

- Solitary pink or red exophytic tumor nodule
- Soles, being the most favored site, others being hands and fingers
- Neck, chest, nose and eyelids being less frequently involved
- Tumor is firm in consistency and pedunculated
- Size—less than 2 cm in diameter

HISTOPATHOLOGY (Figs 80.1 to 80.3)

Three Subtypes

1. Poroma—confined to both epidermis and dermis
2. Hidroacanthoma simplex (intra-epidermal eccrine poroma)—poroma confined within the epidermis, and comprises well-circumscribed nests of basaloid cells
3. Dermal duct tumor (dermal eccrine poroma)—poroma limited to the dermis with prominent duct-like structures

Characteristic Features of Tumor Cells

- Cords of basaloid cells extend from undersurface of epidermis into the dermis
- Cytoplasm of tumor cells can be eosinophilic to clear
- Tumor cells are PAS-positive and diastase sensitive
- Ducts within the tumor cell columns can be seen

DIFFERENTIAL DIAGNOSIS

Basal Cell Carcinoma

- Palisading of tumor cells
- Clefts around the tumor cell islands
- Absence of intercellular bridges and ductal lumina

Seborrheic Keratosis

- Hyperkeratotic stratified squamous epithelium
- Presence of horn cysts

Porocarcinoma (Malignant Eccrine Poroma)
(Figs 80.4 to 80.6)

- Asymmetrical, solid, nodular growth pattern of tumor cells
- Tumor cells have infiltrative or pushing margins

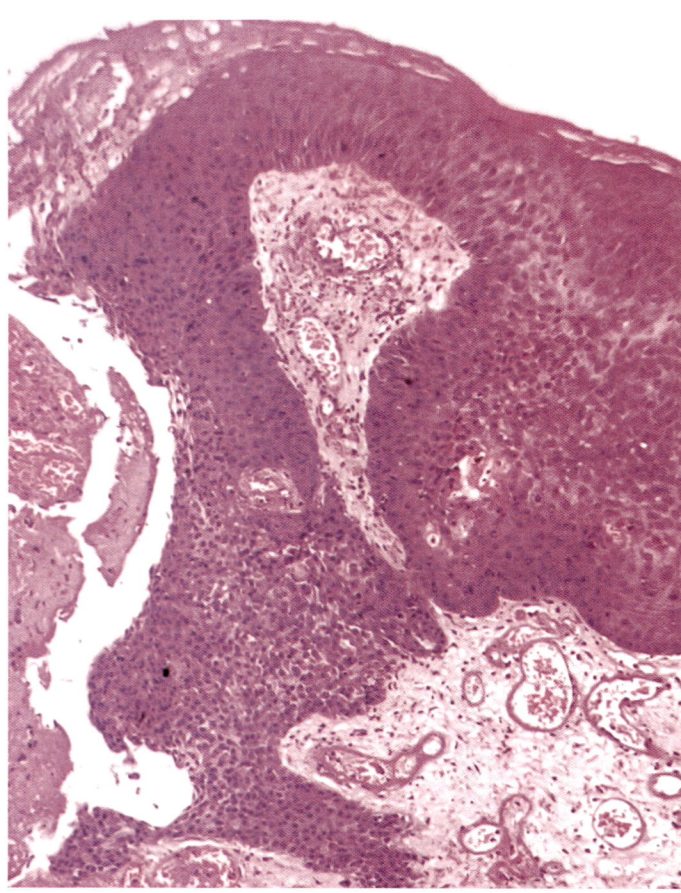

Fig. 80.1: Eccrine poroma. Cords of basaloid cells extending from epidermis into the dermis with stroma showing telangiectatic blood vessels

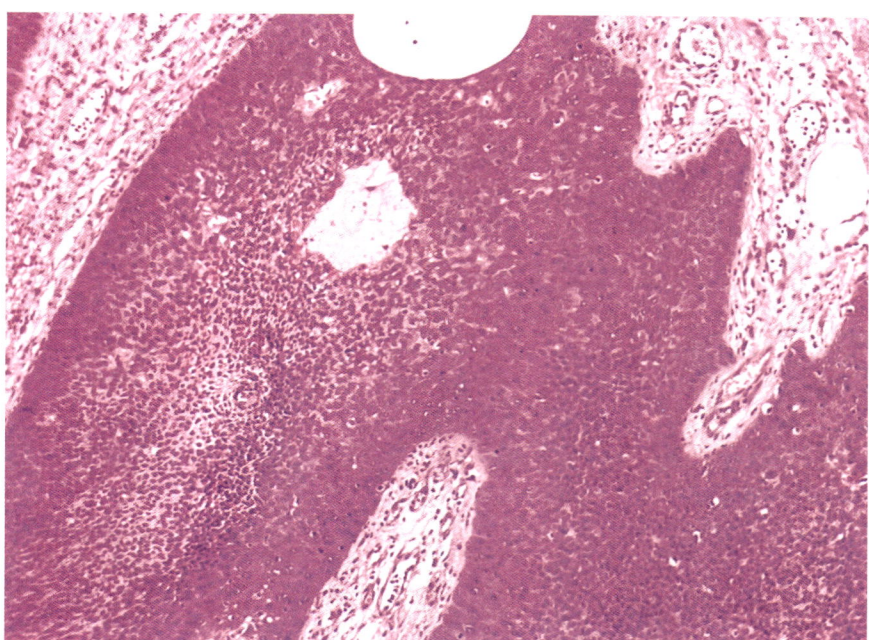

Fig. 80.2: Eccrine poroma. Nests of basaloid cells in the superficial dermis

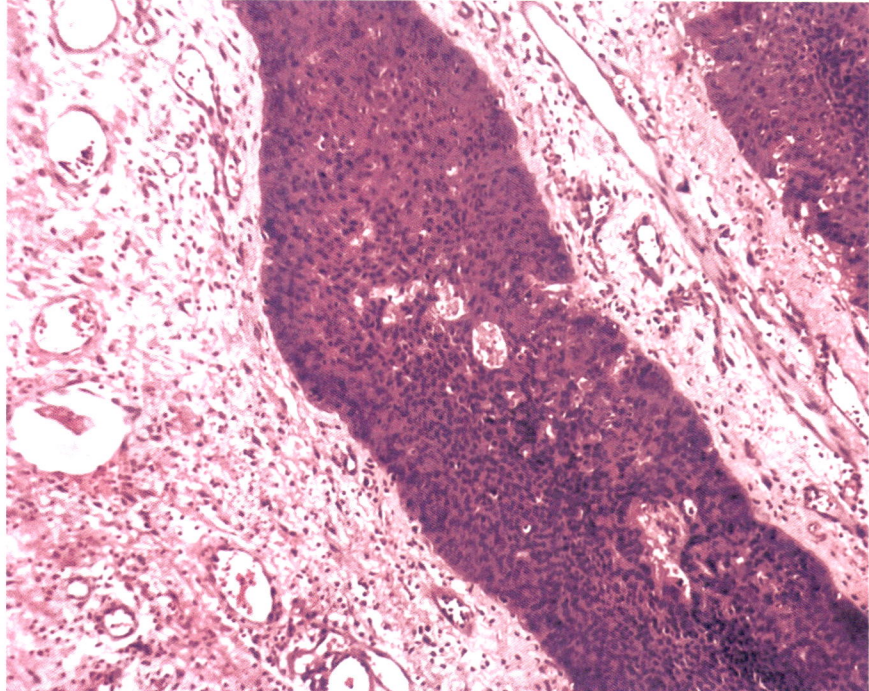

Fig. 80.3: Eccrine poroma. Basaloid cell nests with duct-like structures and stroma showing numerous vascular channels

- Basaloid cells with cytological and nuclear atypia
- Necrosis is also evident
- Clear cell change and duct formation can be seen
- Can show distant metastasis

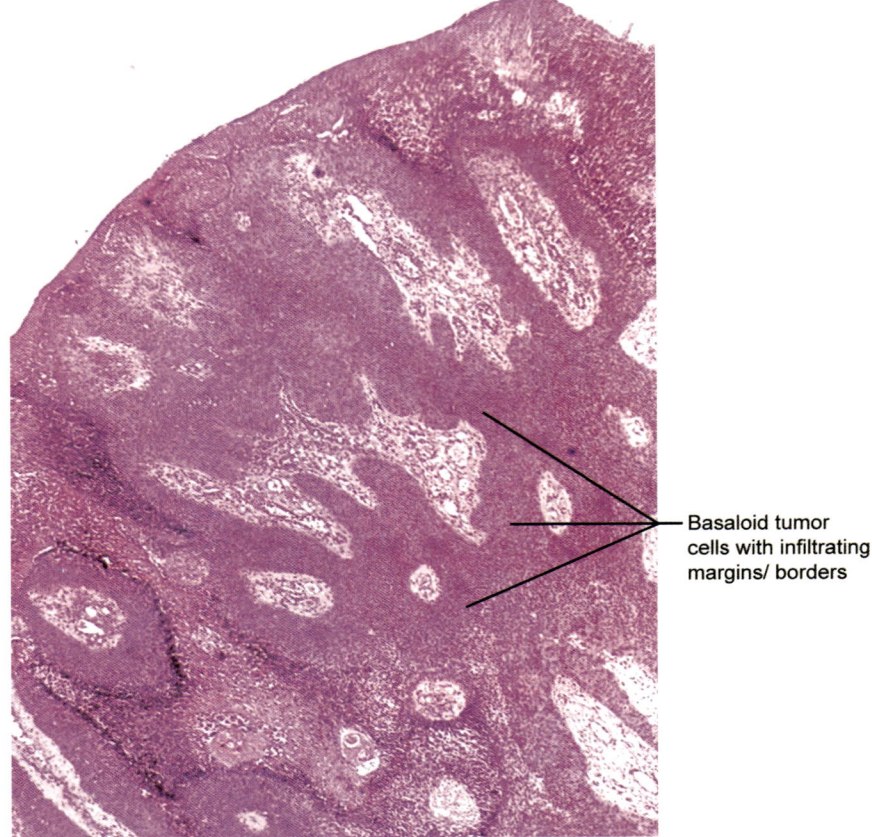

Basaloid tumor cells with infiltrating margins/ borders

Fig. 80.4: Eccrine porocarcinoma

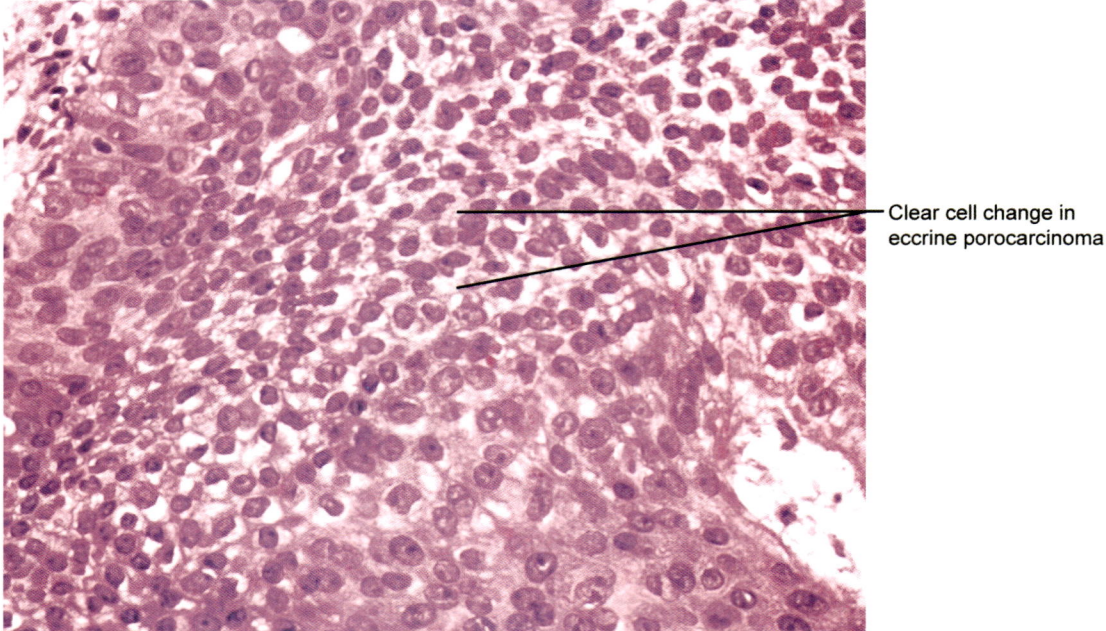

Clear cell change in eccrine porocarcinoma

Fig. 80.5: Eccrine porocarcinoma

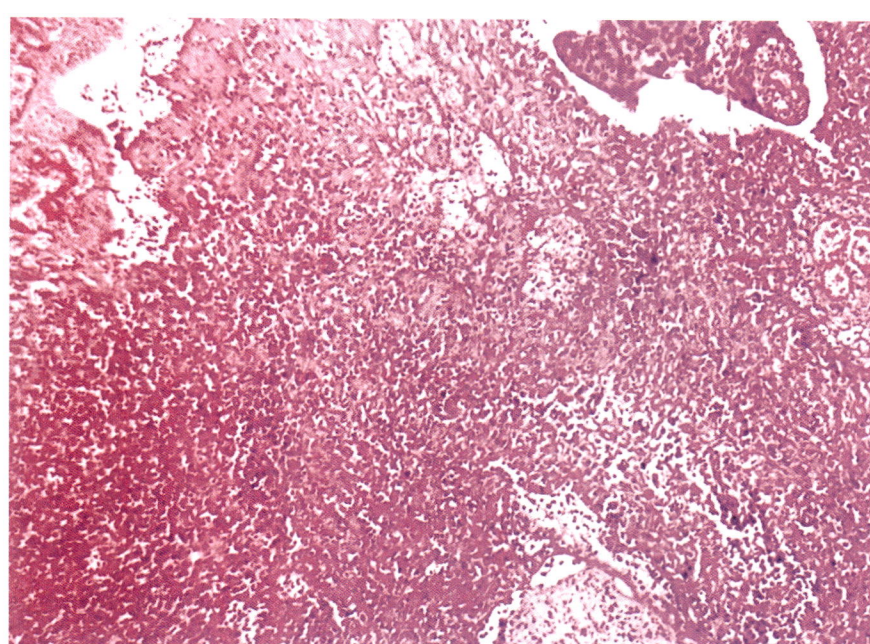

Fig. 80.6: Eccrine porocarcinoma with areas of cellular necrosis

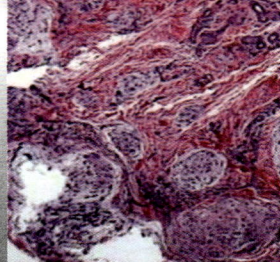

Nodular Hidradenoma

INTRODUCTION

- Synonyms—clear cell/apocrine hidradenoma, clear cell myoepithelioma, eccrine acrospiroma, solid-cystic hidradenoma
- Clinical features—presents as solitary, skin covered nodule measuring 2–3 cm in diameter
- Sites—head and neck, extremities

HISTOPATHOLOGY (Figs 81.1 to 81.3)

- Well-circumscribed, non-encapsulated, multi-lobular dermal tumor
- Dermis shows nests and nodules of neoplastic epithelial cells
- Nodules shows two-cell population—polygonal cells with eosinophilic cytoplasm and round cells with clear cytoplasm
- Nodules comprise tubular lumina, which are lined by cuboidal cells or columnar secretory cells
- Clear cells contain glycogen, which is PAS-positive and diastase resistant
- Large cystic areas can be seen in tumor nodules
- Eosinophilic hyalinized stroma is seen within tumor nodules

DIFFERENTIAL DIAGNOSIS

Poroma

- Basaloid cells with eosinophilic cytoplasm arranged in solid sheets and nodules
- Tumor cells are connected by intercellular bridges
- Tumor cells can show narrow duct lumina

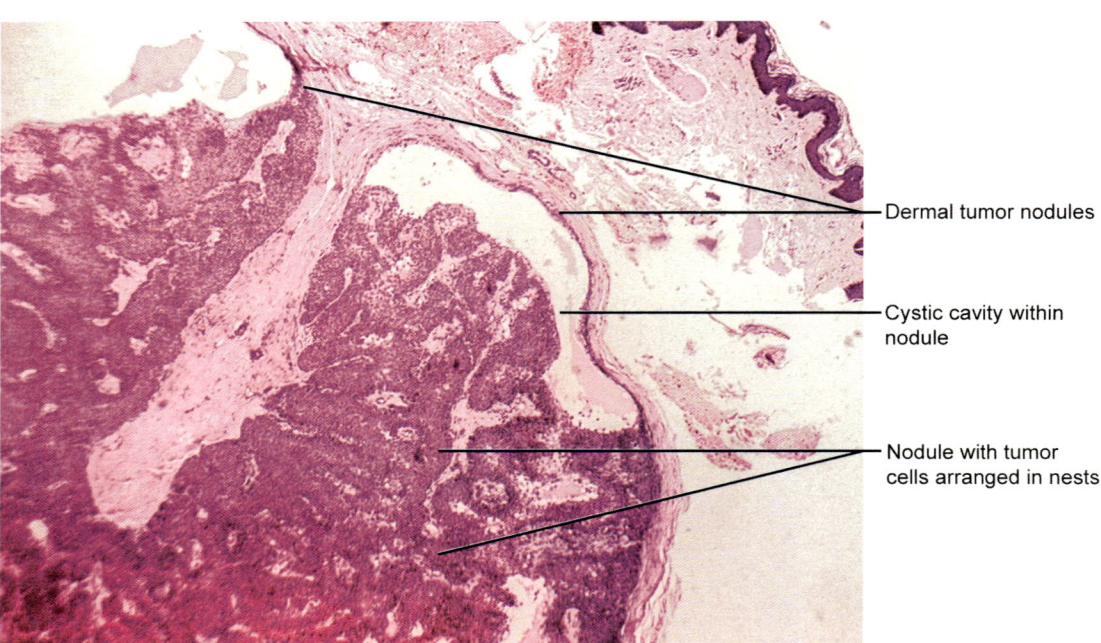

Dermal tumor nodules

Cystic cavity within nodule

Nodule with tumor cells arranged in nests

Fig. 81.1: Nodular hidradenoma

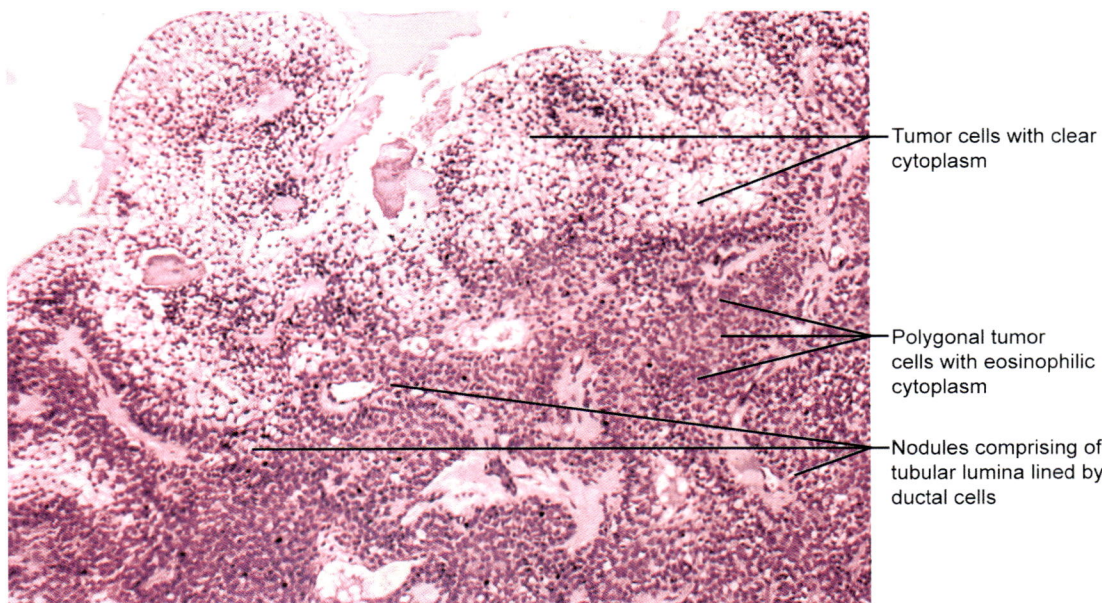

Tumor cells with clear cytoplasm

Polygonal tumor cells with eosinophilic cytoplasm

Nodules comprising of tubular lumina lined by ductal cells

Fig. 81.2: Nodular hidradenoma

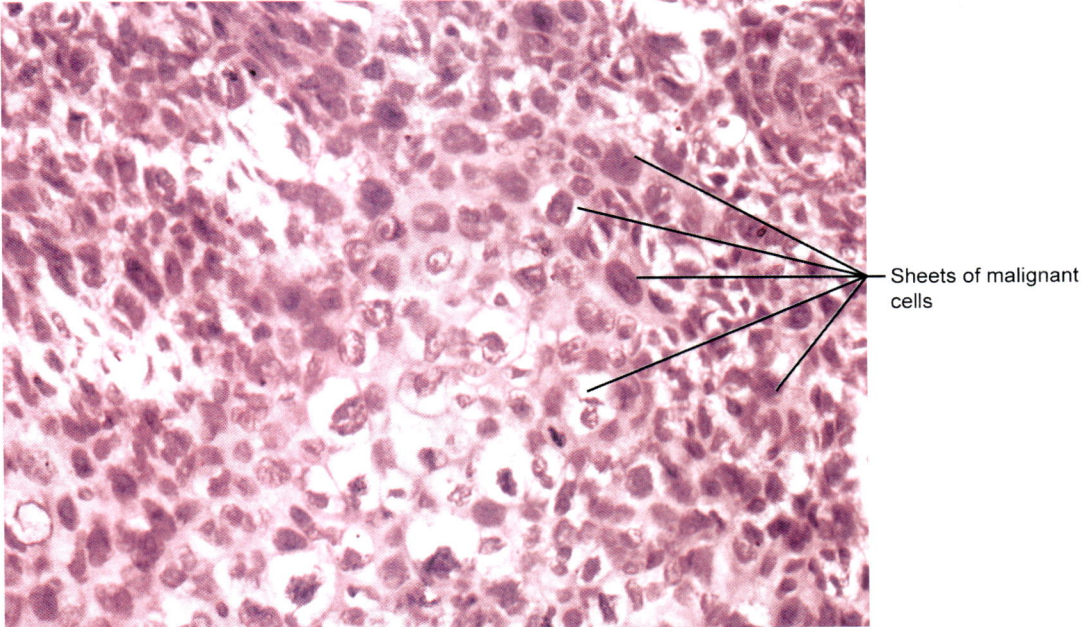

Sheets of malignant cells

Fig. 81.3: Malignant nodular hidradenoma

Trichilemmoma

- Hyperkeratosis with papillomatosis
- Down growth of epithelial cells from the epidermis into the dermis
- These cells show clear cell change
- Peripheral palisading of tumor cells

Basal Cell Carcinoma

- Peripheral palisading of tumor cells
- Clefts around the tumor cell islands
- Absence of intercellular bridges and ductal lumina

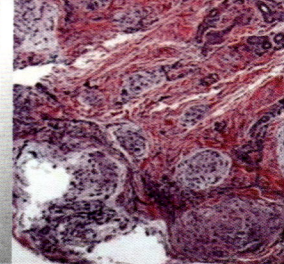

Eccrine Spiradenoma

INTRODUCTION

- Presents as a painful, solitary skin colored intra-dermal nodule
- Size varies from 0.5 to 1 cm
- Sites—head and neck, trunk, extremities
- Age group—20–40 years

HISTOPATHOLOGY (Figs 82.1 and 82.2)

- Multiple, well-circumscribed, basophilic dermal lobules surrounded by a fibrous capsule
- Intact overlying epidermis, absence of overlying epidermal connections
- Dermal lobules comprises two types of epithelial cells—(a) small basaloid cells with scant cytoplasm at the periphery (b) large cells with eosinophilic cytoplasm in the center
- Large cells, can be seen arranged around the tubular lumina
- Lumina contains eosinophilic PAS-positive and diastase resistant material
- Stroma contains hyaline material, dilated blood vessels and lymphocytic infiltrate
- Tumor cells are positive for cytokeratin (CK) and S-100
- Tumor cells are negative for CEA (carcinoembry-onic antigen) and SMA (smooth muscle antigen)

DIFFERENTIAL DIAGNOSIS

Cylindroma

- Circumscribed nests of basaloid cells surrounded by PAS-positive membrane, arranged in a jigsaw puzzle pattern

Basal Cell Carcinoma

- Basaloid tumor cells show peripheral palisading
- Retraction clefts around the tumor cell nests

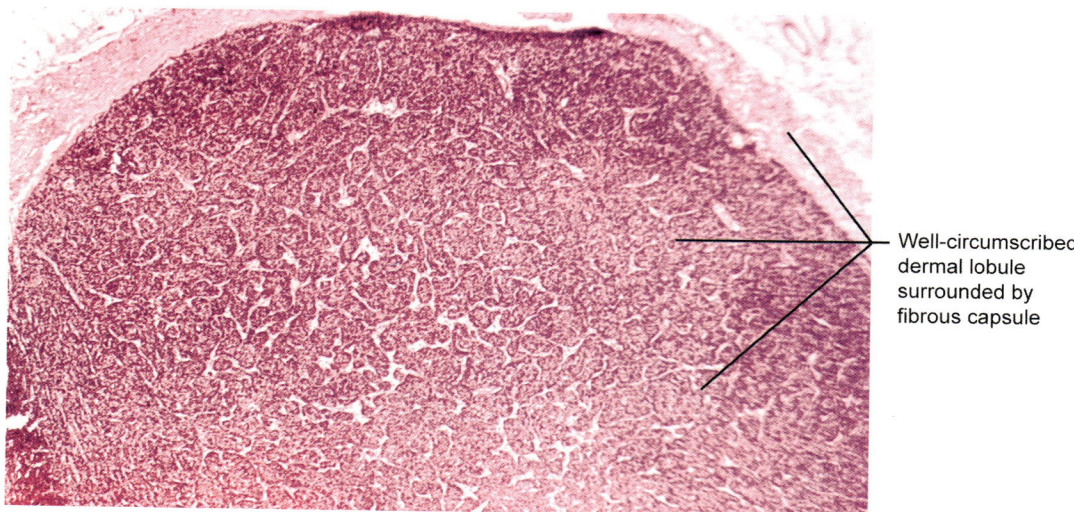

Well-circumscribed dermal lobule surrounded by fibrous capsule

Fig. 82.1: Eccrine spiradenoma

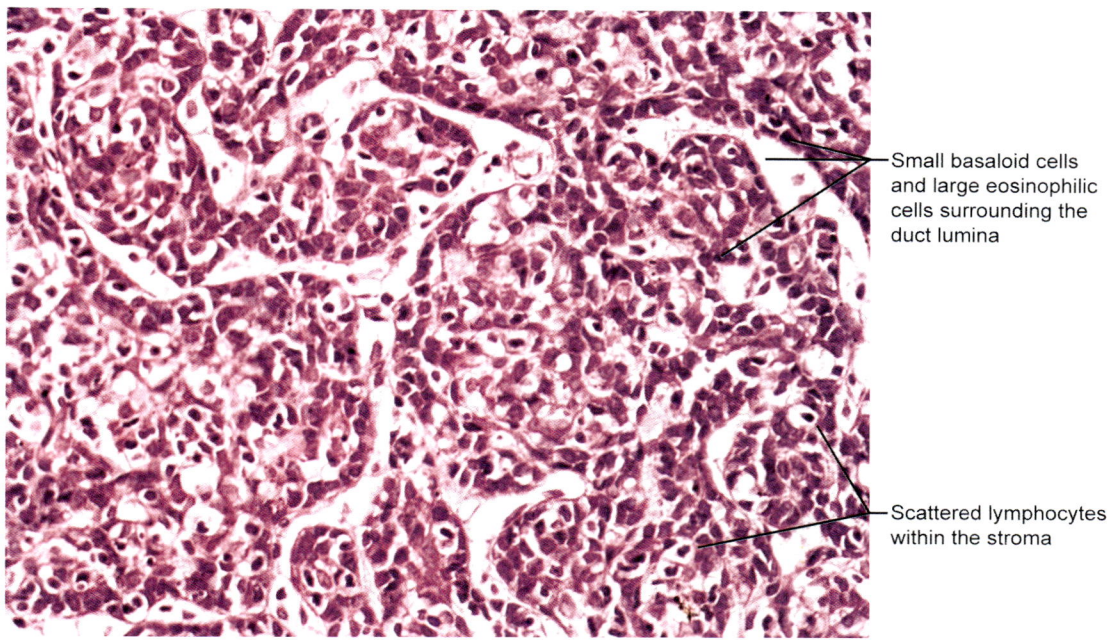

Small basaloid cells and large eosinophilic cells surrounding the duct lumina

Scattered lymphocytes within the stroma

Fig. 82.2: Eccrine spiradenoma

MALIGNANT ECCRINE SPIRADENOMA

- Loss of two-cell populations

- Tumor cells have increased nuclear to cytoplasmic ratio and are hyperchromatic with high mitotic activity

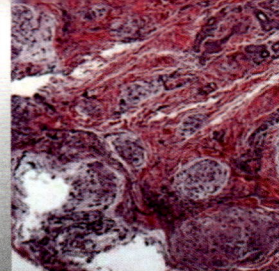

Cylindroma

INTRODUCTION

- Lesion presents as dome-shaped nodule
- Size—varies from few mm to cm
- Most favored site—scalp
- **Turban tumor**—multiple scalp cylindromas, that cover the entire scalp like a turban
- **Brooke-Spiegler syndrome**—autosomal dominant disorder associated with multiple skin adnexal tumors, i.e. trichoepithelioma, cylindromas and spiradenomas

HISTOPATHOLOGY

- Tumor is composed of epithelial cells, arranged in nests ("jigsaw puzzle like pattern") or cords and are surrounded by hyaline material (PAS-positive, diastase resistant)

- Epithelial cells of two types are seen—peripheral basaloid cells (small dark nuclei) showing palisading and central cuboidal cells with large pale nuclei
- Tubular lumina lined by ductal epithelial cells are often present, and contains PAS-positive amorphous material

DIFFERENTIAL DIAGNOSIS

Eccrine Spiradenoma

- Absence of jigsaw puzzle like arrangement of tumor cell islands

Basal Cell Carcinoma

- Basaloid tumor cells showing peripheral palisading
- Presence of retraction clefts

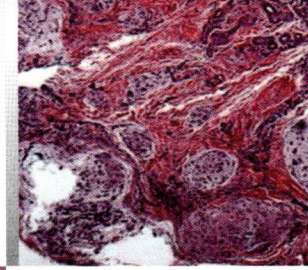

Trichoblastoma

INTRODUCTION

- Benign skin adnexal tumor showing hair follicular differentiation
- Clinical feature—presents as a solitary, skin colored nodule measuring 1 cm in diameter
- Site—most commonly affects scalp

HISTOPATHOLOGY (Fig. 84.1)

- Dermis shows islands of basaloid epithelial cells showing peripheral palisading in a fibrous stroma (resembling hair follicular structure)
- Subcutaneous extension of the basaloid cells can be seen
- Malignant counterpart of trichoblastoma is called trichoblastic carcinoma (irregular epithelial islands, tumor cells with cytological atypia and increased mitotic activity)

DIFFERENTIAL DIAGNOSIS

Basal Cell Carcinoma

- Asymmetrical lesion
- Absence of follicular differentiation of basaloid tumor cells
- Presence of clefting between tumor cells and stroma
- Prominent peripheral palisading

Pilomatricoma

- Basophilic epithelial tumor cells and shadow cells
- Presence of calcification and giant cell reaction

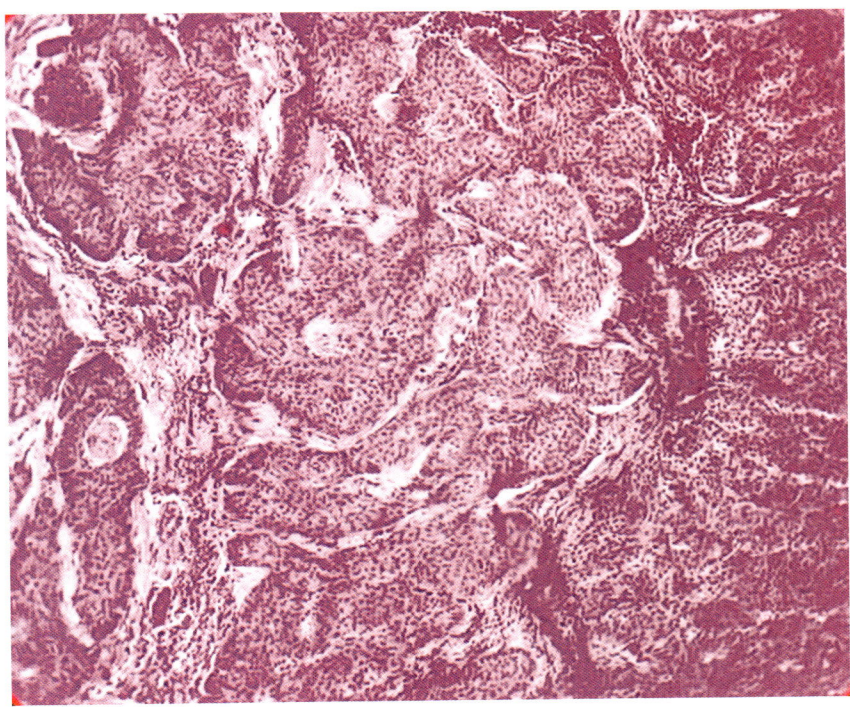

Fig. 84.1: Trichoblastoma. Basaloid cell nests in mid-dermis with intervening fibrous stroma

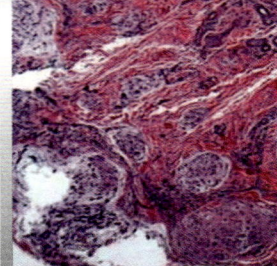

Trichoepithelioma

INTRODUCTION

- Three types—solitary, multiple and desmoplastic
- Origin—hair follicle
- Solitary lesion (more common)—firm, elevated, flesh colored nodule, measuring less than 2 cm in diameter or,
- Multiple skin colored papules measuring 2–8 mm in diameter (Fig. 85.1)
- Sites—face, nasolabial folds, nose, forehead, upper lip, scalp, neck and upper trunk

HISTOPATHOLOGY (Figs 85.2 to 85.4)

- Horn cysts of varying sizes, filled with keratinous material, showing abrupt keratinization (trichilemmal type) and are surrounded by basaloid cells

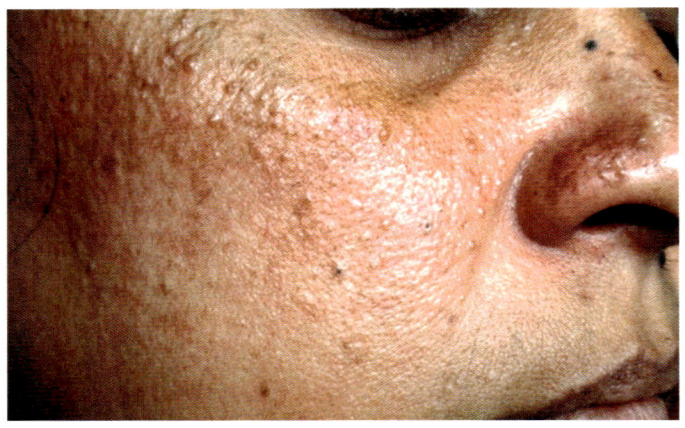

Fig. 85.1: Trichoepithelioma. Smooth, non-ulcerated, skin-colored papules

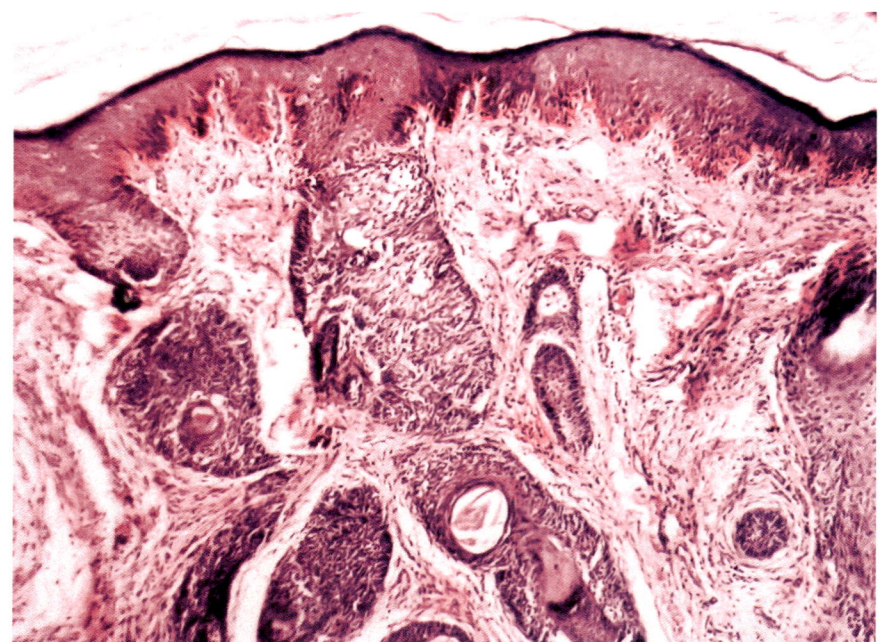

Fig. 85.2: Trichoepithelioma. Tumor comprises basaloid cell nests and keratinous cysts

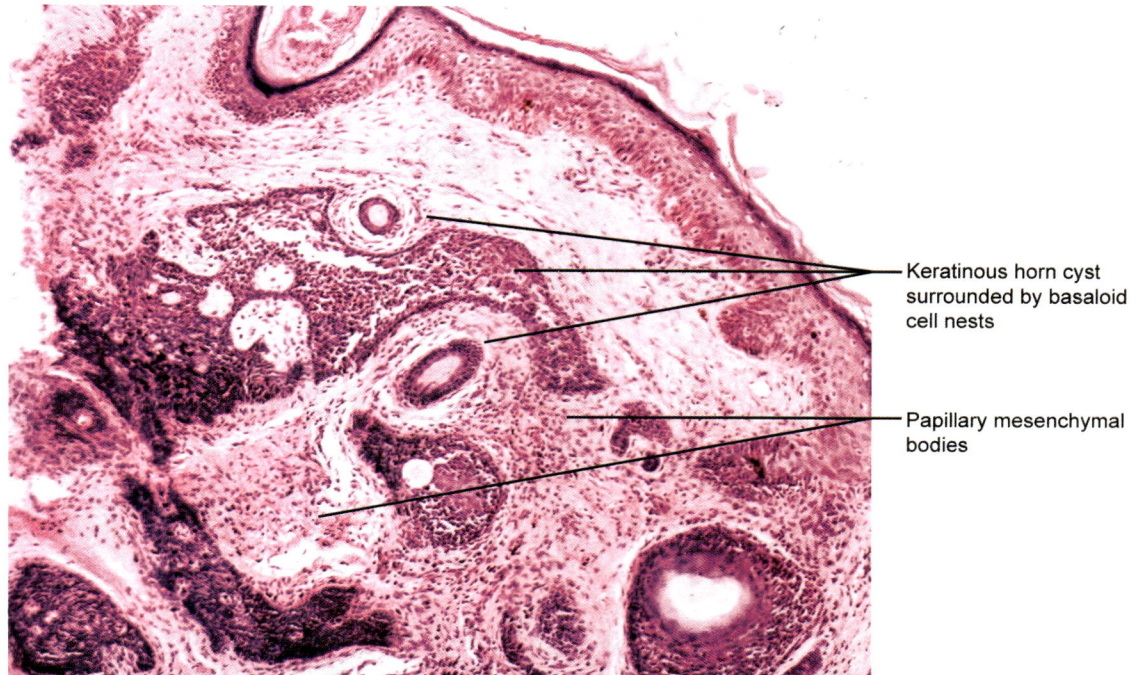

Keratinous horn cyst surrounded by basaloid cell nests

Papillary mesenchymal bodies

Fig. 85.3: Trichoepithelioma

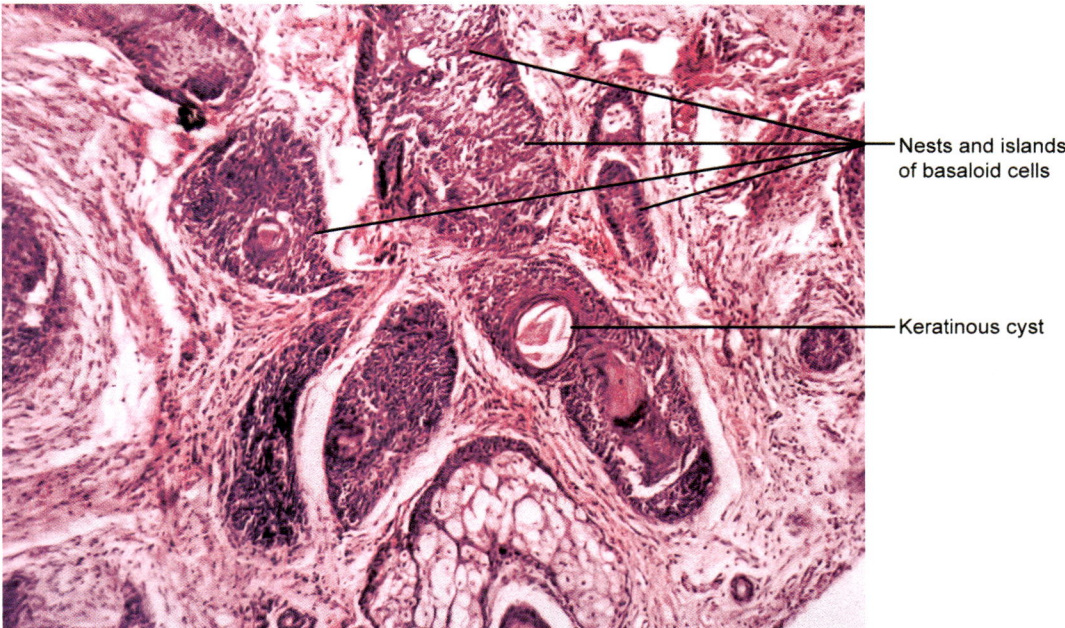

Nests and islands of basaloid cells

Keratinous cyst

Fig. 85.4: Trichoepithelioma

- Ruptured horn cysts with foreign body type giant cell reaction can be seen
- Basaloid cells are arranged in nests, islands, showing peripheral palisading without retraction clefts
- Basaloid cell islands are surrounded by distinct fibroblastic aggregations (papillary mesenchymal bodies)
- Peri-tumoral stroma and papillary mesenchymal bodies show CD-10 positivity

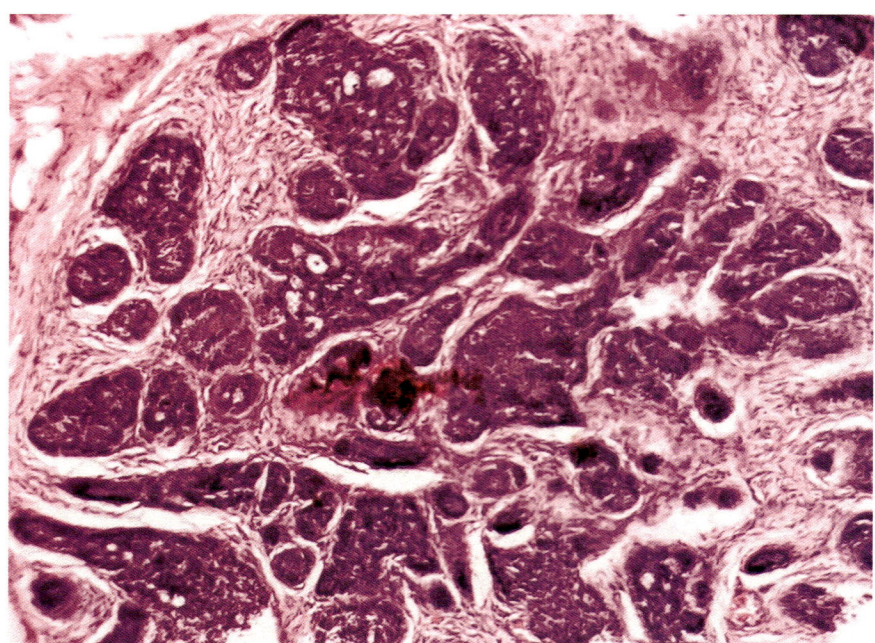

Fig. 85.5: Desmoplastic trichoepithelioma mimicking basal cell carcinoma

DIFFERENTIAL DIAGNOSIS

Basal Cell Carcinoma

- Basaloid cells showing retraction clefts
- Absence of keratinous cysts
- Stroma is negative for CD10, however, basaloid cells stain strongly for CD10

Trichofolliculoma

- Nodular lesion with a central pore containing immature hair follicle

DESMOPLASTIC TRICHOEPITHELIOMA

INTRODUCTION

- Solitary lesion, measuring 3–8 mm in diameter
- Site—face

HISTOPATHOLOGY (Fig. 85.5)

- Triad of basaloid tumor cells arranged in strands/islands/nests, horn cysts and desmoplastic stroma

- Foreign body granulomas in response to cyst rupture and calcification can be seen
- Basaloid tumor cells are one to three epithelial cell layer thick

DIFFERENTIAL DIAGNOSIS

Microcystic Adnexal Carcinoma

- Presence of horn cysts, strands of basaloid cells and dense desmoplastic stroma
- Presence of ductal structures, infiltrative growth pattern and perineural invasion

Basal Cell Carcinoma (Fibrosing/Morphea Like)

- Absence of horn cysts
- Presence of mitosis, necrosis, retraction clefts, fibroblasts showing stromelysin-3 positivity
- Stromal cells of basal cell carcinoma does not stain for CD34, however, stromal cells of desmoplastic trichoepithelioma show strong CD34 positivity

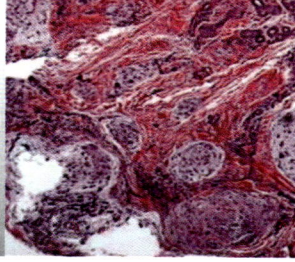

Basal Cell Carcinoma

INTRODUCTION

- Cell of origin—lower epidermal layer cells or follicular epithelial cells
- Site of origin—surface epidermis
- Associated with PTCH gene mutations (component of nevoid basal cell carcinoma syndrome), BAX gene and p53 gene mutations
- Most common site— face (head and neck)
- More common in males
- Etiological factor—ultraviolet light (UV-B) exposure
- Lesion presents as a pearly papule with prominent dilated subepidermal blood vessels
- Rodent ulcers—locally aggressive cancer, which can spread and result in destruction of the bone and facial sinuses (Fig. 86.1)

HISTOPATHOLOGY (Figs 86.2 and 86.3)

- Basaloid cells originate from epidermis forming islands or nests, infiltrating the dermis

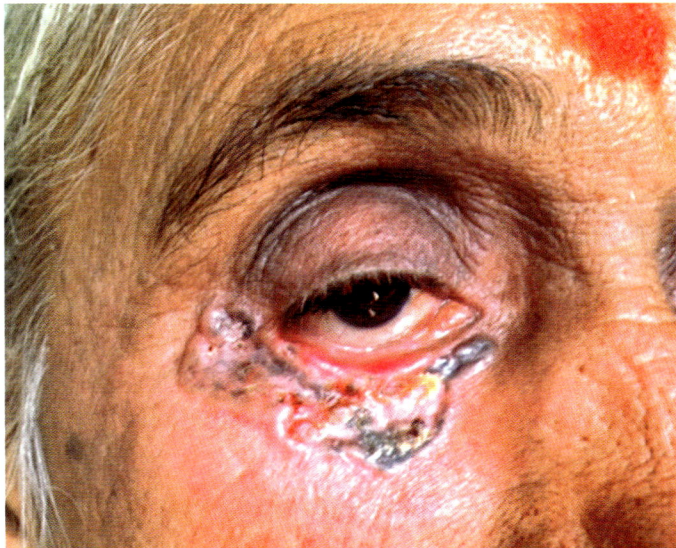

Fig. 86.1: Basal cell carcinoma. Ulcer with rolled out borders and patchy hyperpigmentation

- These haphazardly arranged basaloid tumor cells show peripheral palisading
- These cells have large, oval to elongated hyperchromatic nuclei with scant cytoplasm
- Tumor cells can show numerous mitotic figures
- Retraction cleft between epithelium and stroma is seen
- Stromal fibroblasts demonstrate stromelysin-3 positivity
- Basaloid tumor cells demonstrate diffuse Bcl-2 positivity and CD-10 expression
- Tumor cells stain diffusely for Ber-EP4, unlike squamous cell carcinomas

VARIANTS

- Solid/nodular basal cell carcinoma (circumscribed and infiltrative)
- Keratotic basal cell carcinoma
- Basal cell carcinoma with sebaceous differentiation
- Nodular basal cell carcinoma
- Micro-nodular basal cell carcinoma
- Pigmented basal cell carcinoma
- Adenoid basal cell carcinoma
- Fibroepithelioma of Pinkus (fibroepithelial basal cell carcinoma)
- Basal cell carcinoma with follicular differentiation
- Morphea like or fibrosing variant
- Superficial basal cell carcinoma

DIFFERENTIAL DIAGNOSIS

Squamous Cell Carcinoma (SCC)

- Squamous cells in SCC appear eosinophilic due to keratinization
- Cells with high mitotic count and pleomorphism indicate poorly differentiated squamous cell carcinoma
- Absence of retraction clefts
- Tumor cells show p63 positivity

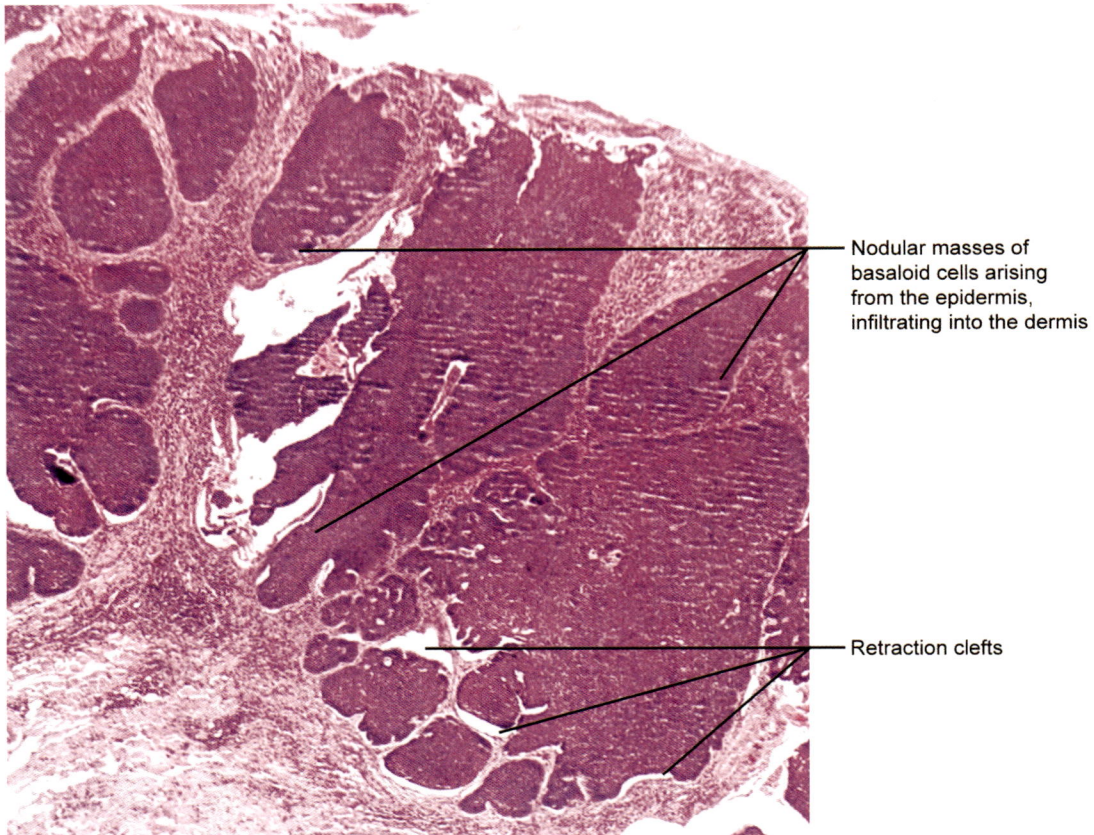

Nodular masses of
basaloid cells arising
from the epidermis,
infiltrating into the dermis

Retraction clefts

Fig. 86.2: Basal cell carcinoma

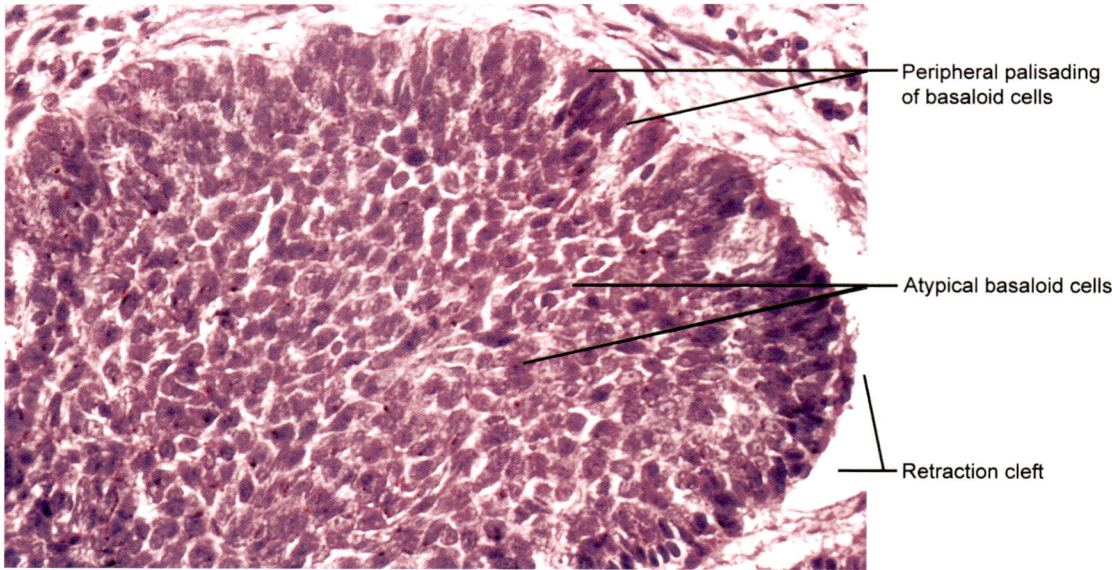

Peripheral palisading
of basaloid cells

Atypical basaloid cells

Retraction cleft

Fig. 86.3: Basal cell carcinoma

- Ber-EP4 antigen is negative (basal cells in BCC show Ber-EP4 positivity)

Trichoepithelioma

- Horn cysts filled with keratinous material, showing abrupt keratinization
- Basaloid cells arranged in islands, show peripheral palisading without retraction clefts
- Presence of papillary mesenchymal bodies
- CD-10 expression is seen in stroma and not in basaloid cell nests
- Bcl-2 positivity is seen in basaloid keratinocytes

Trichoblastoma

- Symmetrical tumor
- Follicular differentiation of basaloid cells can be seen
- Absence of retraction clefts

- Absence of epidermal connections

Microcystic Adnexal Carcinoma

- Presence of horn cysts and strands of basaloid cells with dense desmoplastic stroma
- Presence of ductular structures, infiltrative growth pattern and perineural invasion

FIBROEPITHELIOMA OF PINKUS

- Also called fibroepithelial basal cell carcinoma
- Presents as soft nodular lesion on the lower back

Histopathology

- Superficial tumor showing long, thin, branching anastomosing strands of basaloid cells arising from the epidermis
- Epidermal nests infiltrate into the dense fibrous and vascular stroma

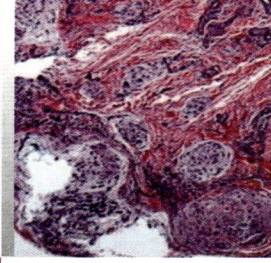

Chondroid Syringoma

INTRODUCTION

- Also called cutaneous mixed tumor, due to the presence of epithelial and mesenchymal elements
- Clinical features—lesion presents as a firm, intradermal or subcutaneous nodule and measures 0.5–3 cm in diameter
- Sites—head and neck

HISTOPATHOLOGY (Figs 87.1 and 87.2)

Epithelial Element

- Arranged in a tubular pattern with lumina, lined by luminal layer of cuboidal cells and a peripheral layer of flattened cells

- Tubular lumina contains eosinophilic amorphous material, that is, PAS-positive and diastase resistant
- Islands of squamous epithelium can be present
- Other metaplastic changes like mucinous, columnar, oxyphilic, hobnail and clear cell can be seen
- Luminal epithelial cells stain with cytokeratin, CEA, EMA
- Peripheral layer cells are stained with vimentin, S-100

Stromal Component

- Stroma has mucoid, basophilic appearance, that stains with alcian blue or mucicarmine
- Epithelial cells in the stroma are scattered and are surrounded by a halo (resembling cells of cartilage)

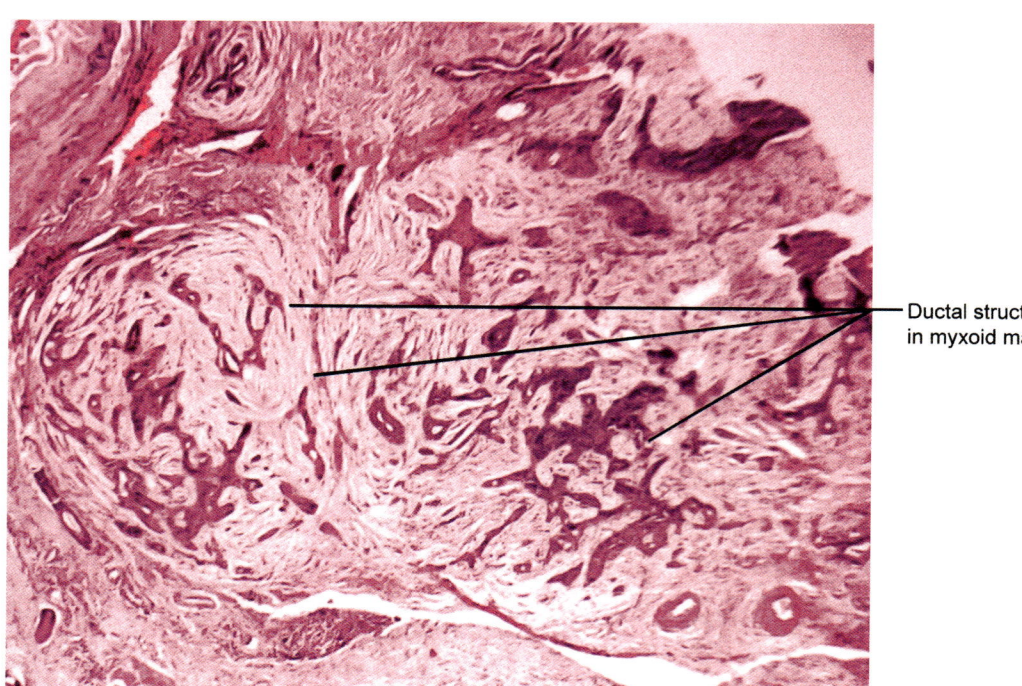

Ductal structures in myxoid matrix

Fig. 87.1: Chondroid syringoma

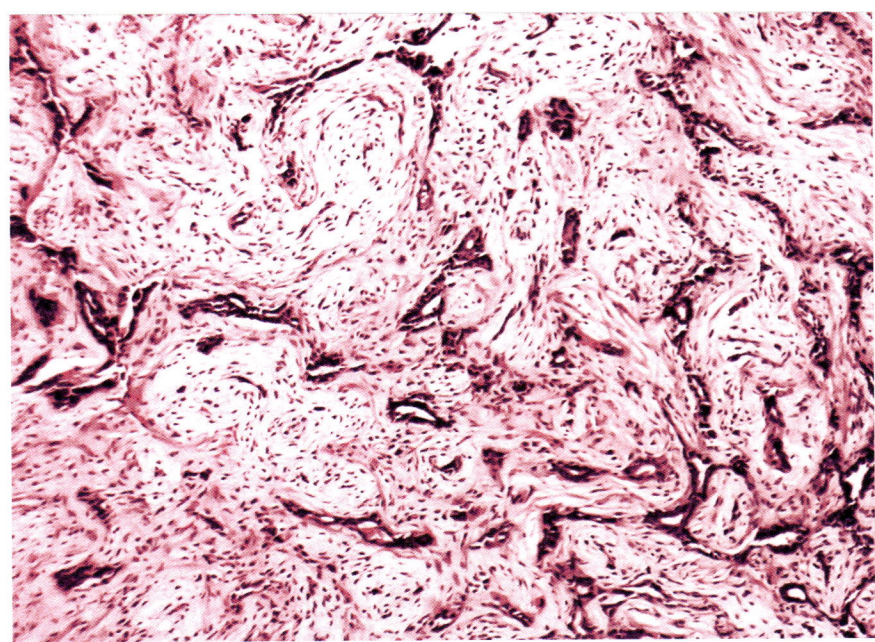

Fig. 87.2: Chondroid syringoma. Ductal structures in a myxoid background

- Presence of small ducts scattered throughout the hyaline stroma gives it an appearance of syringoma

MALIGNANT CHONDROID SYRINGOMA (MALIGNANT MIXED TUMOR)

- Sites—trunk and extremities

- Comprises malignant cells with or without glandular differentiation
- Sheets of atypical cells with anaplastic features can be seen
- Mucinous stroma with spindle-shaped cells are seen

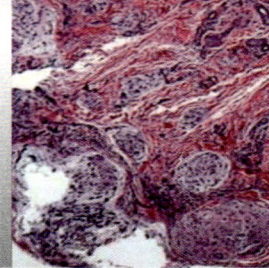

Trichofolliculoma

INTRODUCTION

- Most commonly affects adults
- Most common sites—face, scalp and neck
- Presents as a small, skin covered, dome-shaped nodule

HISTOPATHOLOGY (Figs 88.1 and 88.2)

- Dermis shows keratin-filled cyst, lined by stratified squamous epithelium

- Radiating from these cystic structures, numerous small hair follicles are seen
- Stroma is rich in fibroblasts

VARIANT

Sebaceous Trichofolliculoma (Figs 88.3 and 88.4)

- Most common site—nose
- Central cystic cavity lined by stratified squamous epithelium, with radially arranged pilosebaceous follicles (sebaceous lobules and hair follicles) arising from it

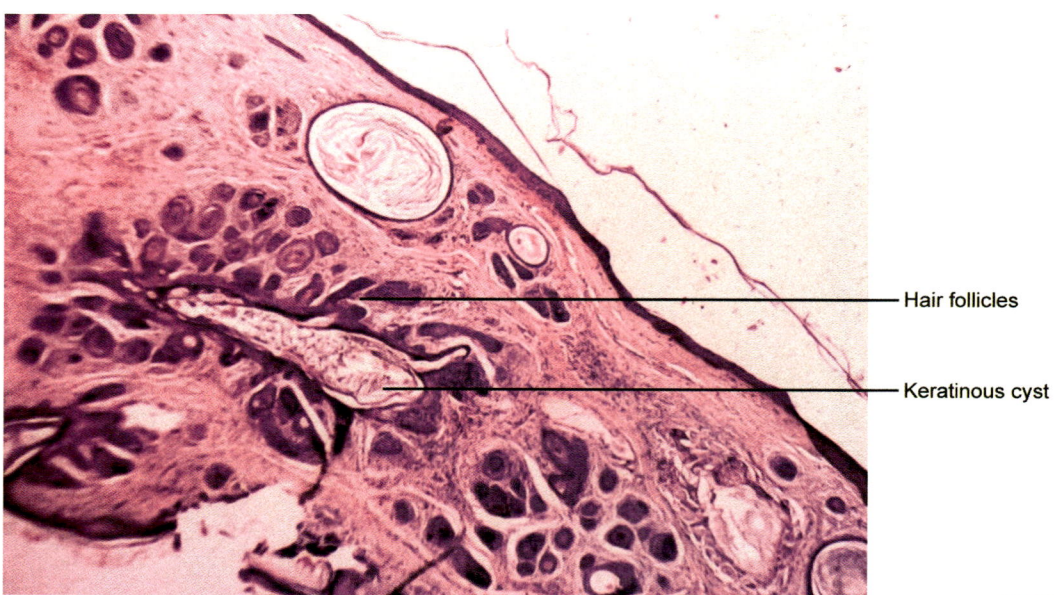

Hair follicles

Keratinous cyst

Fig. 88.1: Trichofolliculoma. Keratin-filled cysts surrounded by numerous small hair follicles

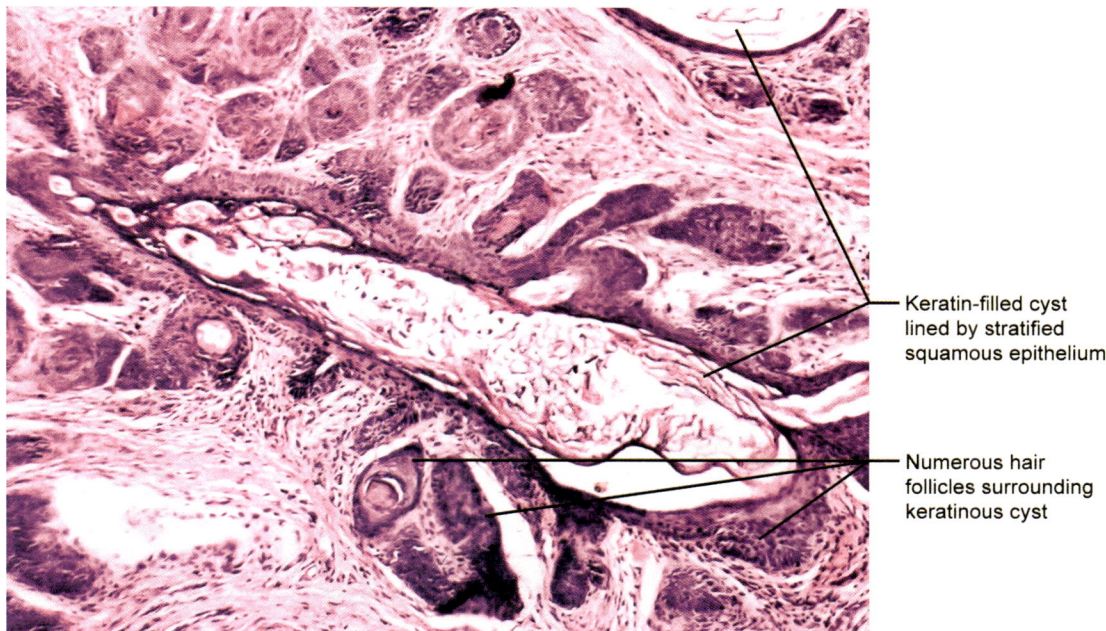

Keratin-filled cyst lined by stratified squamous epithelium

Numerous hair follicles surrounding keratinous cyst

Fig. 88.2: Trichofolliculoma

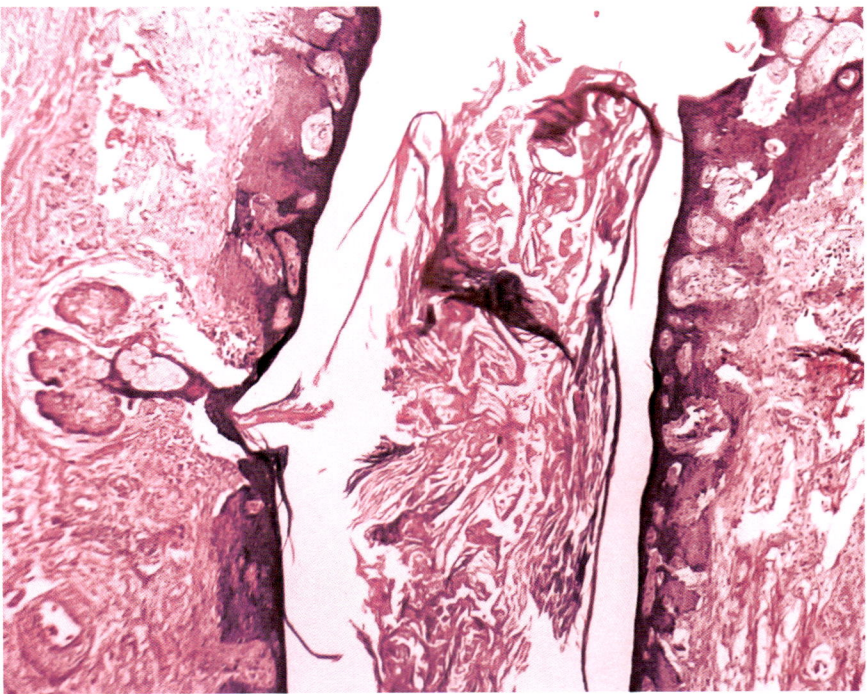

Fig. 88.3: Sebaceous trichofolliculoma. Central cystic cavity, lined by stratified squamous epithelium containing keratin in its lumen, surrounded by pilo-sebaceous units

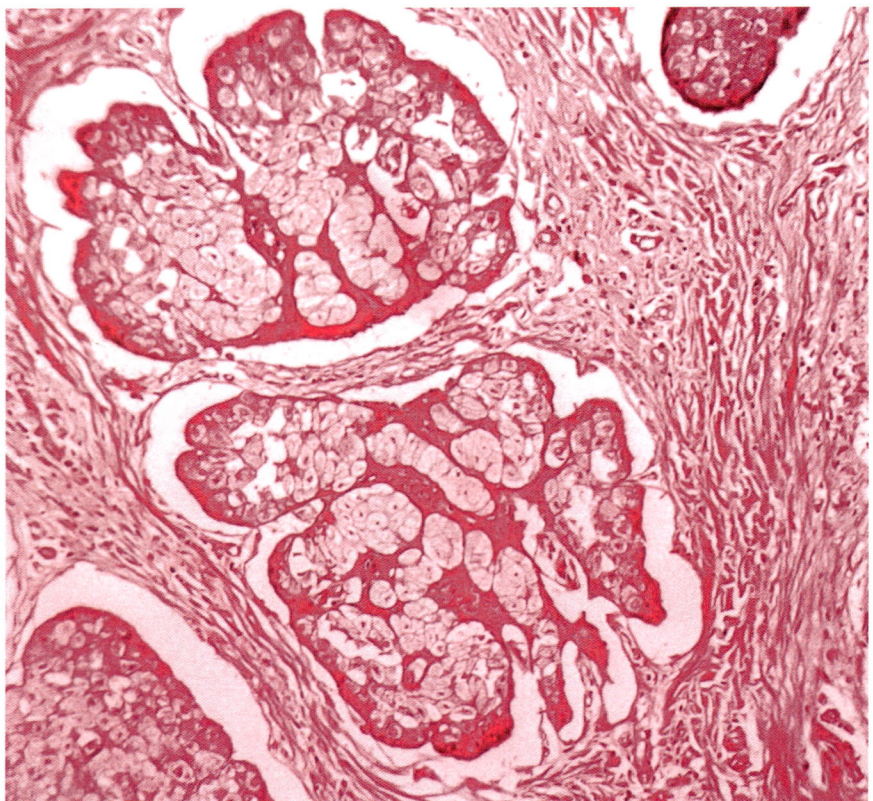

Fig. 88.4: Proliferation of sebaceous lobules adjacent to the keratinous cyst in sebaceous trichofolliculoma

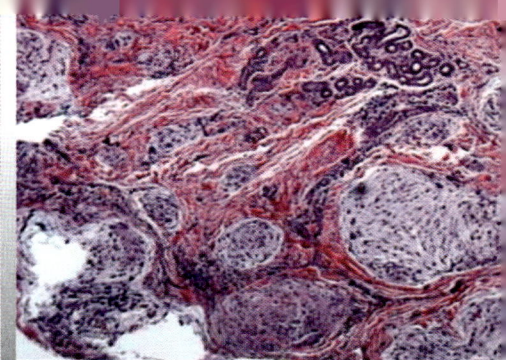

Soft Tissue Proliferation and Neoplasms

Part 15

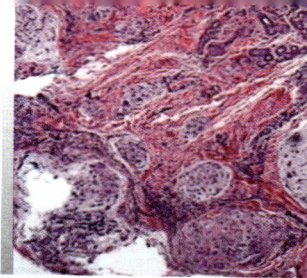

Scar

- Repair mechanism by which the damaged tissue is replaced by fibrosis
- Lesion can be elevated, depressed or flat (Fig. 89.1)

HISTOPATHOLOGY

- Epidermis—acanthotic, but can show atrophy in late stages
- Collagen fibers in dermis are oriented parallel to the skin surface
- Increased number of fibroblasts, myofibroblasts and capillaries
- Inflammatory cell infiltrate

KELOID SCAR

INTRODUCTION

- Raised lesion, that extends beyond the limits of original wound
- Age group—affect individuals younger than 30 years
- More common in dark skinned individuals
- Sites—ear lobes, cheek, upper arms, back and sternal regions (Fig. 89.2)
- Presents as well-circumscribed, erythematous papules or plaques

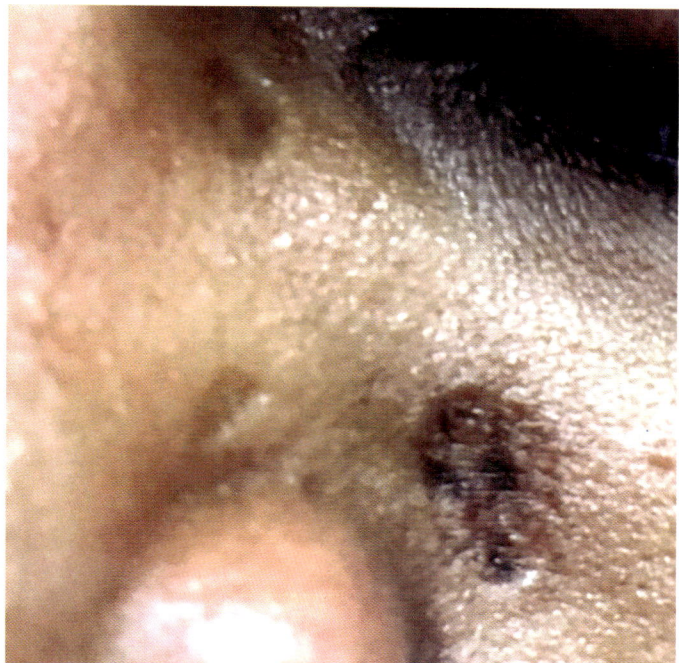

Fig. 89.1: Scar. Atrophic plaque showing color change

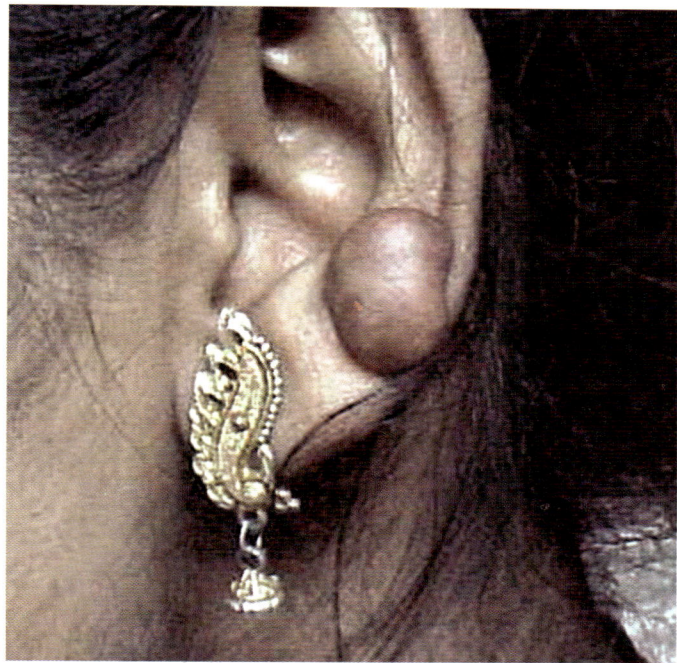

Fig. 89.2: Keloid. Firm, fleshy, plaque extending beyond the margin of the original wound

- Lesions appear during puberty and tend to enlarge during pregnancy
- High recurrence rates after surgical removal

ETIOLOGY

Fibroblastic proliferation is brought about by
- Increased transforming growth factor—beta and platelet-derived growth factor levels
- Reduction in interferon-alpha levels
- Inhibition of collagenase activity

HISTOPATHOLOGY (Figs 89.3 and 89.4)

- Normal to thinned out epidermis
- Early keloid—abundant collagen
- Late keloid—deeper dermis shows dense collagen bundles (keloidal collagen), arranged haphazardly, with irregular borders
- Along the collagen bundles, increased fibroblasts are also seen
- Periphery of lesion may show telangiectatic vessels, which are surrounded by chronic inflammatory cell infiltrate

HYPERTROPHIC SCAR

INTRODUCTION

- Raised scar, that does not extend beyond the limits of original wound

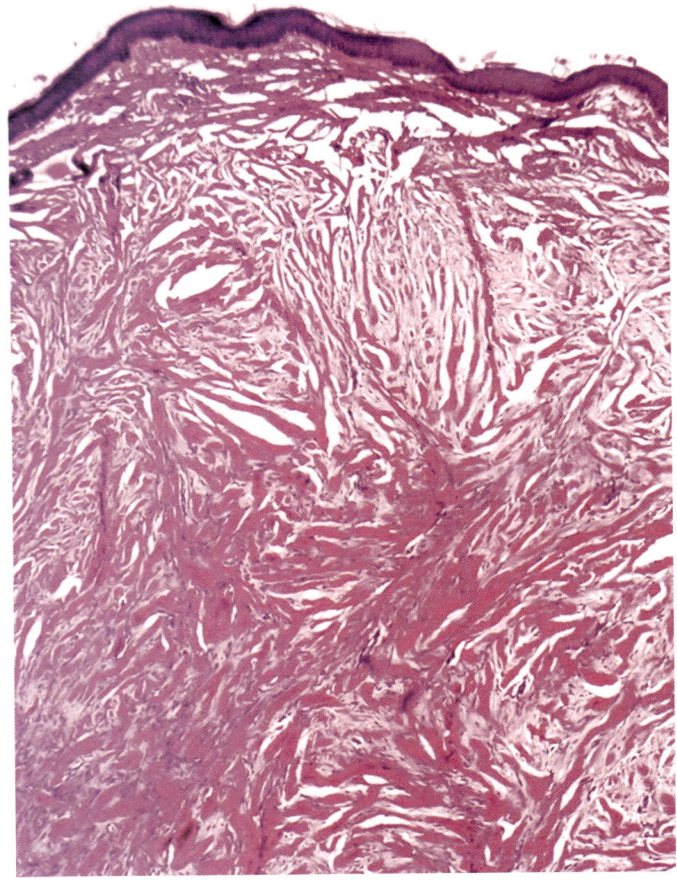

Fig. 89.3: Keloid. Dermis shows dense collagen bundles

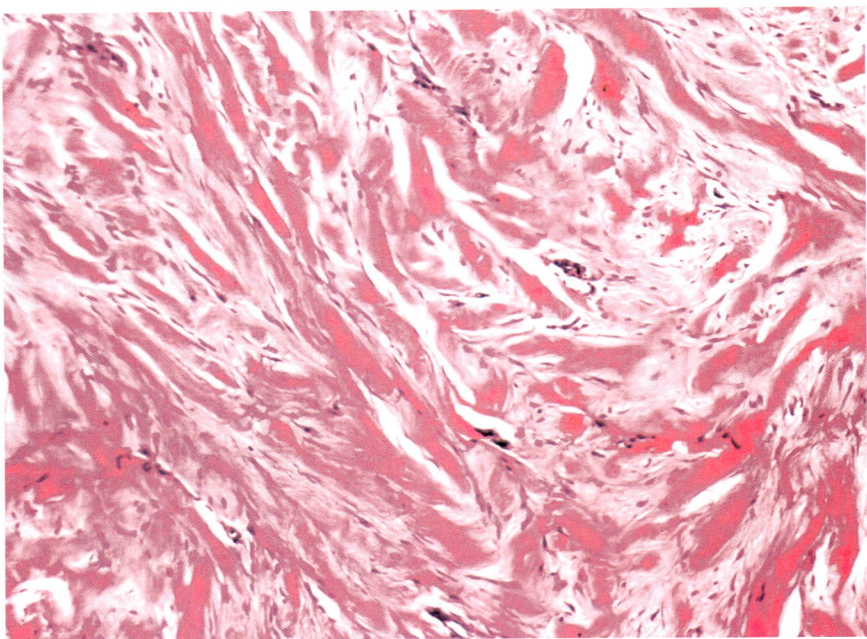

Fig. 89.4: Keloidal collagen in keloid

- Predisposing factors—occur following surgery and burns
- Sites—flexure aspects of joints and abdomen (Fig. 89.5)
- Spontaneous regression can occur
- Lower recurrence rates in comparison to keloids, following their removal

HISTOPATHOLOGY (Figs 89.6 and 89.7)

- Dermis shows thick collagen bundles arranged parallel to the skin surface
- Blood vessels amongst the collagen fibers are perpendicularly arranged to the epidermis
- Increased number of fibroblasts in the collagen bundles
- Mast cells and dystrophic calcification can be seen

DIFFERENTIAL DIAGNOSIS OF HYPERTROPHIC SCAR AND KELOID

Dermatofibroma

- Acanthotic epidermis

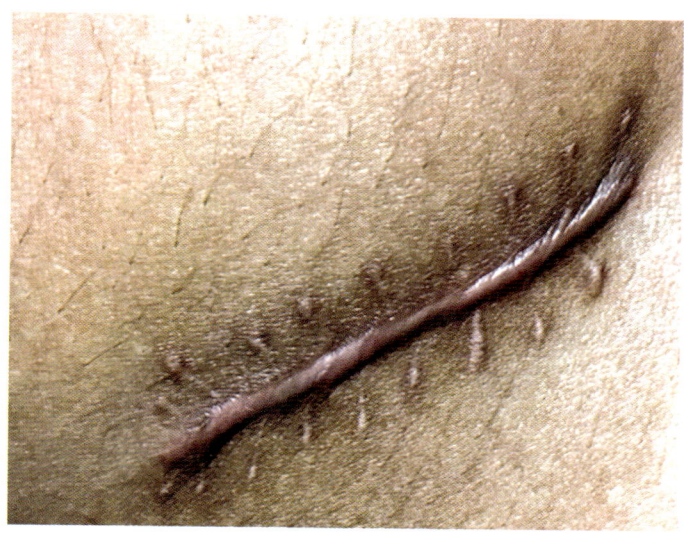

Fig. 89.5: Hypertrophic scar. Firm, skin-colored plaque with margins not exceeding beyond the original wound

- Dermal proliferation of myofibroblasts and fibroblasts, entrapping the collagen bundles at the periphery

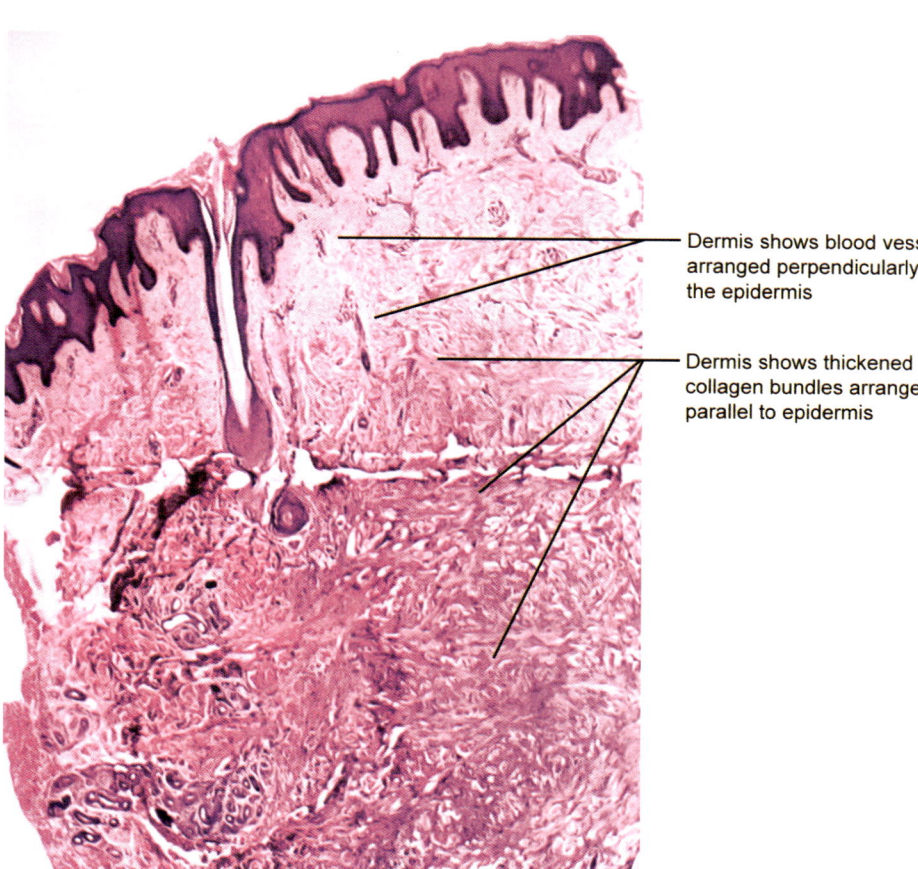

Dermis shows blood vessels arranged perpendicularly to the epidermis

Dermis shows thickened collagen bundles arranged parallel to epidermis

Fig. 89.6: Hypertrophic scar (10X)

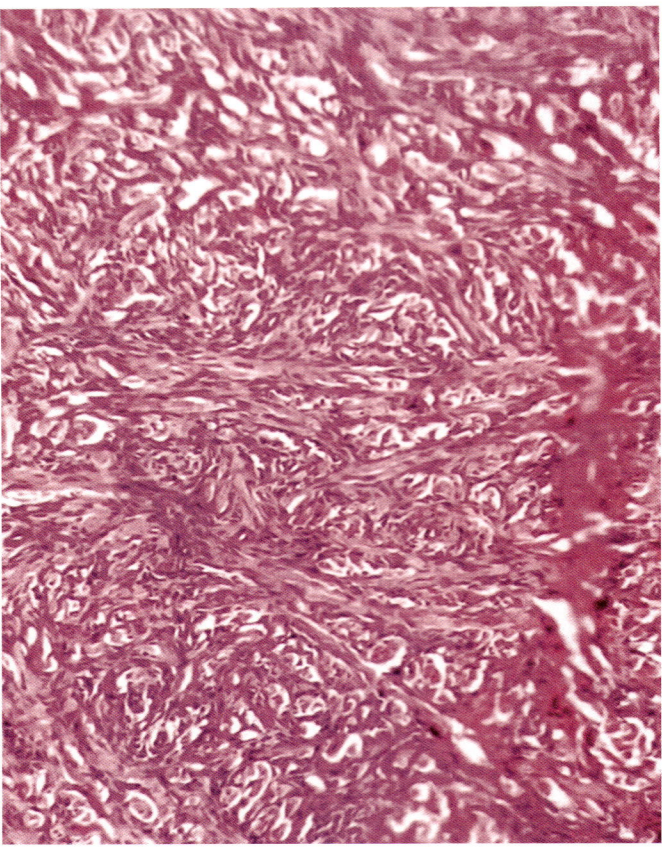

Fig. 89.7: Hypertrophic scar (40X)

Dermatofibrosarcoma Protuberans

- Spindle-shaped tumor cells arranged in storiform pattern, which are reaching up to the subcutis
- Tumor cells demonstrate CD34 positivity

Dermatomyofibroma

- Dermis shows spindle-shaped tumor cells (myofibroblasts), arranged in fascicles, with parallel orientation to the epidermis

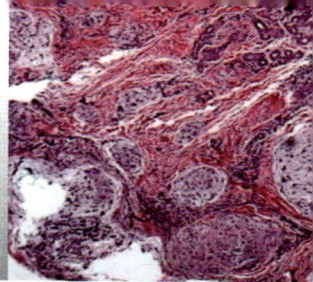

Dermatofibroma

INTRODUCTION

- Also called benign fibrous histiocytoma (BFH)
- Age group—3rd to 4th decade
- Sites—trunk and extremities (lower)
- Presents as well-circumscribed, skin covered, round or ovoid, firm nodules (Fig. 90.1)
- Lesions are usually small, but larger lesions can also be encountered
- Cell of origin—histiocytes or endothelial cells, or dermal dendrocytes

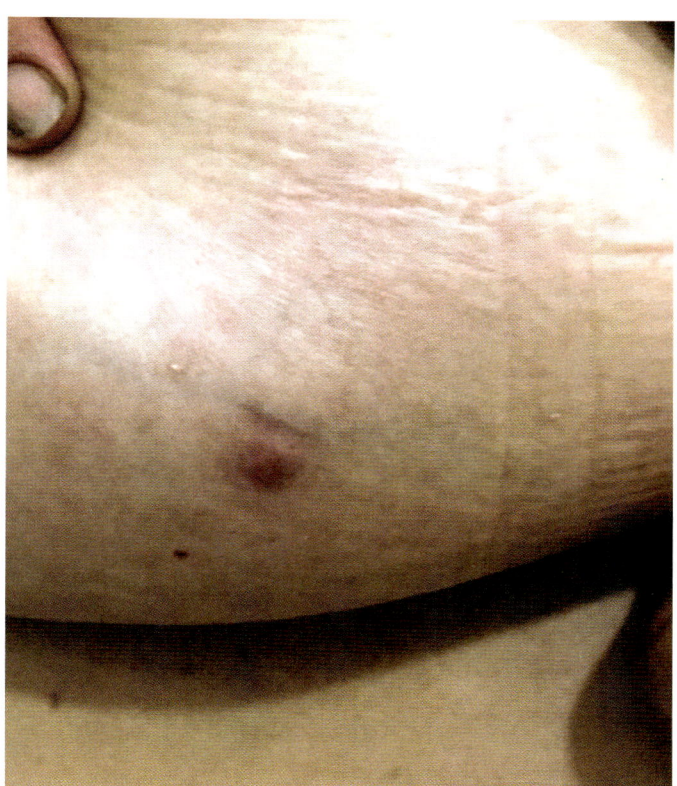

Fig. 90.1: Dermatofibroma. Firm, round to oval lesion

HISTOPATHOLOGY (Figs 90.2 to 90.5)

- Hyperplastic epidermis, with basal layer showing hyperpigmentation
- Tumor is located in the dermis and is separated from the epidermis by a grenz zone
- Tumor is composed of fibroblasts, histiocytes, foam cells, Touton's giant cells and capillaries
- Storiform pattern of spindle shaped/fibroblastic tumor cells can be seen
- Tumor margins are ill-defined and show entrapped collagen bundles at the periphery
- Variants include—cellular fibrous dermatofibroma, aneurysmal dermatofibroma, angiomatous derma- tofibroma, sclerotic dermatofibroma, hemosiderotic dermatofibroma, histiocytic dermatofibroma, granular cell dermatofibroma, atypical fibrous histiocytoma
- Tumor cells demonstrate stromelysin-3 positivity
- Fibroblasts express factor XIIIa and vimentin positivity

DIFFERENTIAL DIAGNOSIS

Dermatofibrosarcoma Protuberans (DFSP)

- Larger lesion, with multiple nodules
- Spindle-shaped cells with wavy nuclei, and expre- sses CD34 positivity
- Distinction from cellular dermatofibroma is extre- mely difficult

Leiomyosarcoma

- Plump spindle shaped cells with cigar-shaped nuclei
- Tumor cells demonstrate cytological atypia, nuclear pleomorphism, hyperchromasia and increased mitotic figures
- Tumor cells demonstrate SMA (smooth muscle actin) and desmin positivity
- Cellular dermatofibroma closely mimics this lesion

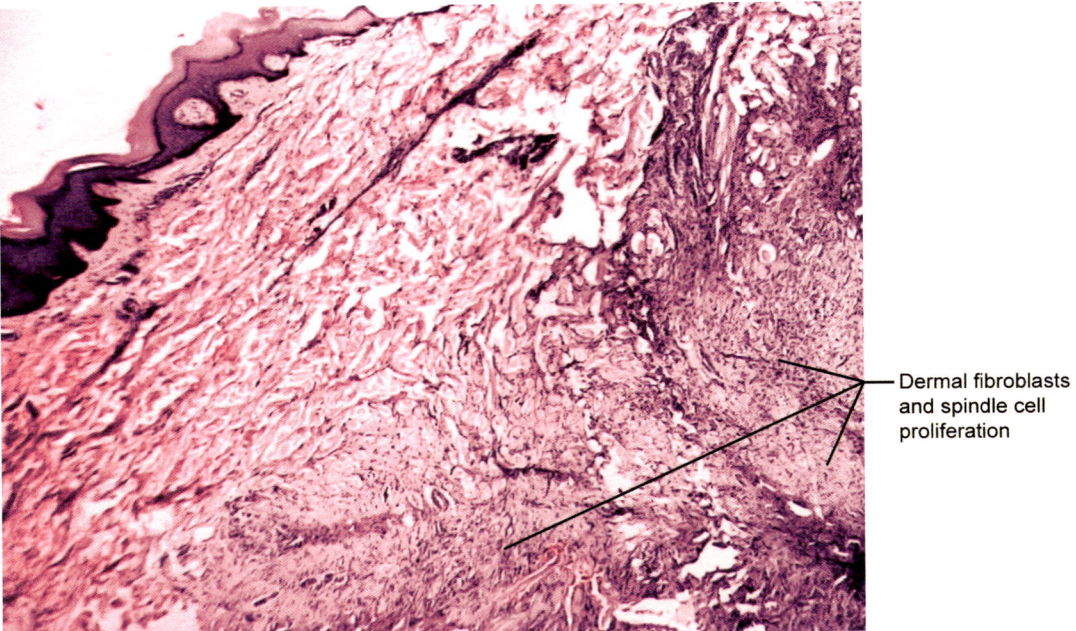

Fig. 90.2: Benign fibrous histiocytoma (BFH)

Dermal fibroblasts and spindle cell proliferation

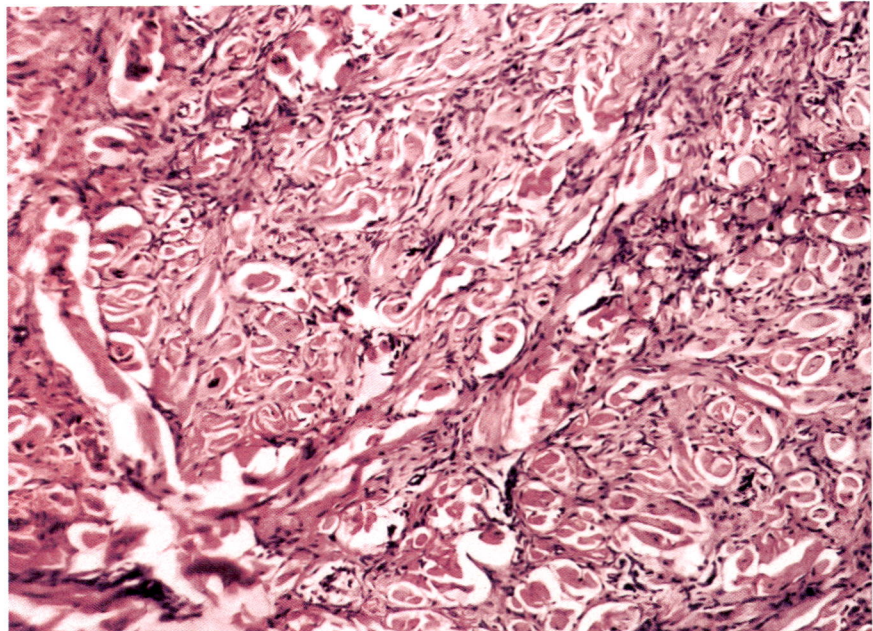

Fig. 90.3: Benign fibrous histiocytoma. Lesion entrapping collagen bundles at periphery

Kaposi Sarcoma

- Distinction from aneurysmal dermatofibroma is difficult
- Demonstrate closely packed spindle-shaped cells and cleft-like spaces filled with RBCs
- Endothelial cells express CD34, CD31 and factor VIII positivity

Xanthogranuloma

- Thinned out epidermis
- Proliferation of epithelioid macrophages, foam cells, Touton's giant cells
- Presence of neutrophils, eosinophils

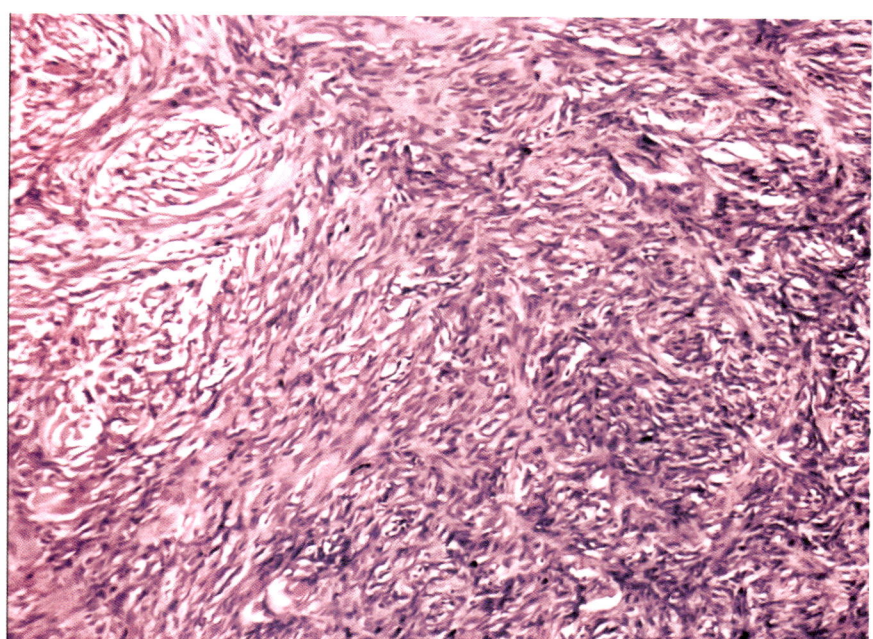

Fig. 90.4: Benign fibrous histiocytoma. Storiform and whorling pattern of spindle cell proliferation

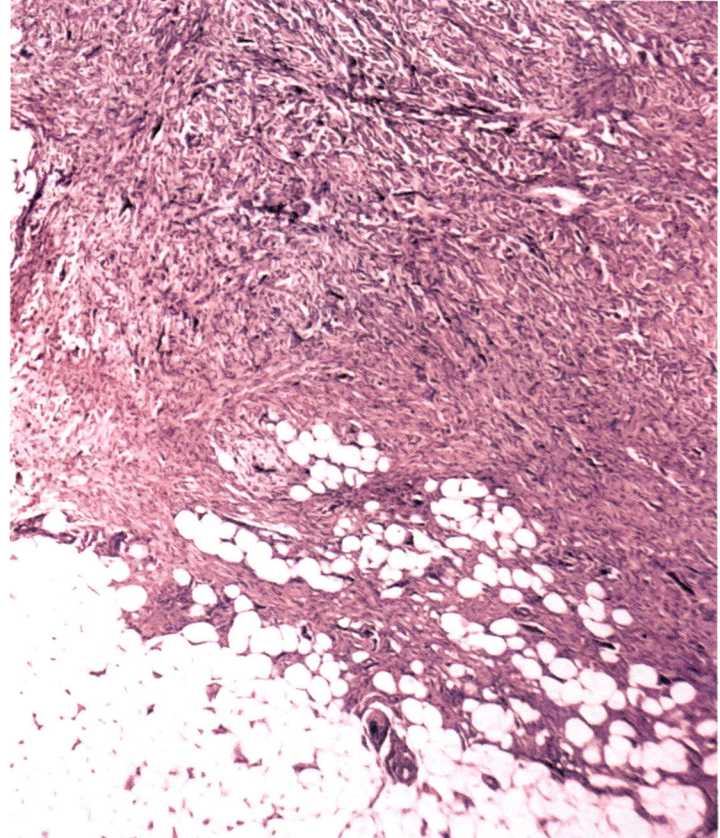

Fig. 90.5: Benign fibrous histiocytoma. Fibrous histiocytes reaching up to the subcutis, but characteristic honeycomb pattern of dermatofibrosarcoma protuberans is not seen

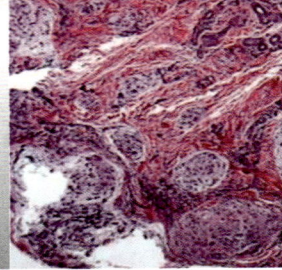

Epithelioid Cell Histiocytoma

INTRODUCTION

- Variant of dermatofibroma (fibrous histiocytoma)
- Presents as an elevated nodule
- Sites—extremities
- Age group—seen in adults
- Cell of origin—endothelial cells

HISTOPATHOLOGY (Figs 91.1 to 91.3)

- Presence of an epidermal collarette
- Perivascular epithelioid and spindle-shaped cells are seen
- Xanthoma cells, giant cells and mononuclear inflammatory cell infiltrate can be seen

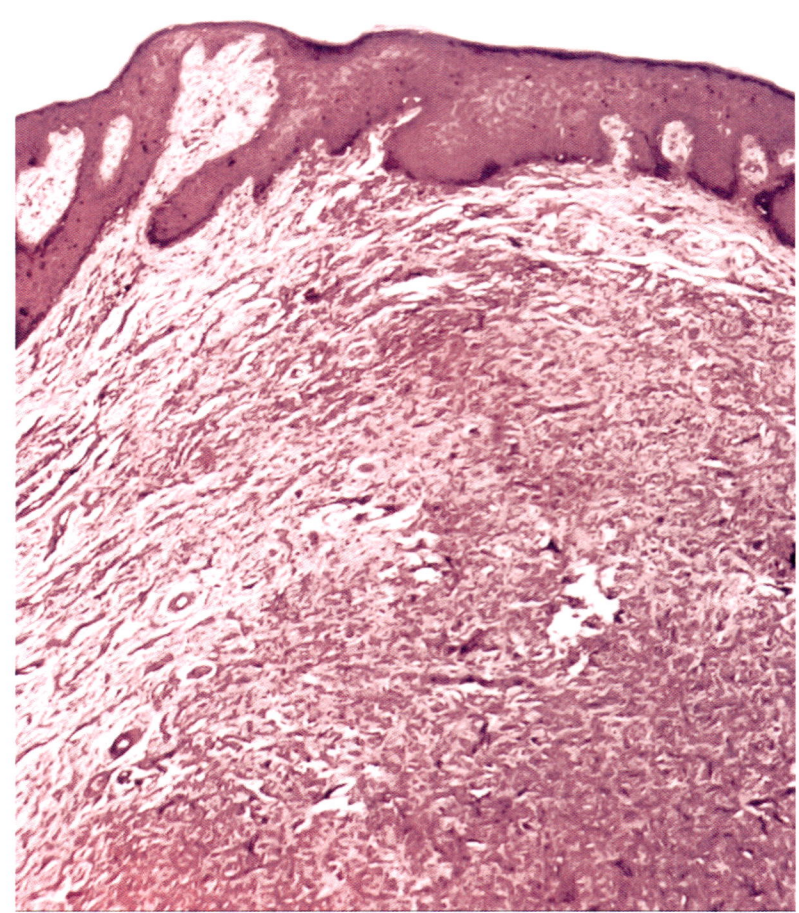

Fig. 91.1: Epithelioid cell histiocytoma

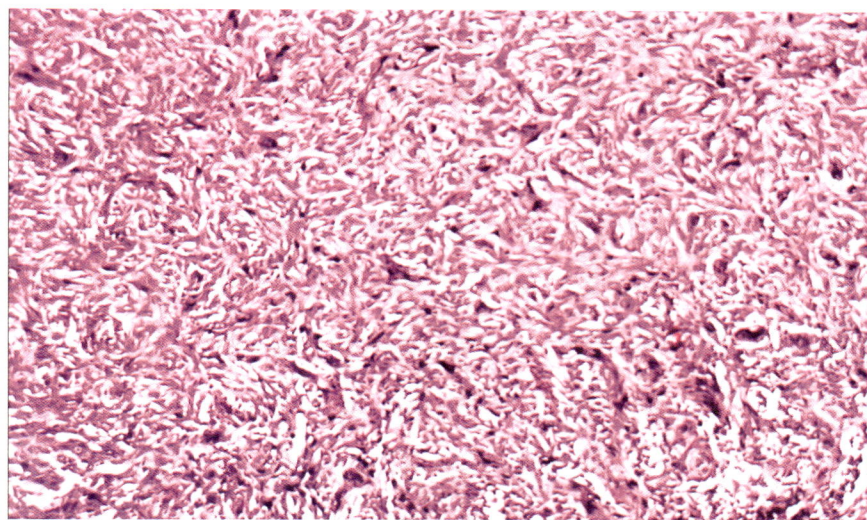

Fig. 91.2: Epithelioid cell histiocytoma. Dermal epithelioid histiocytes, xanthocytes and inflammatory cells

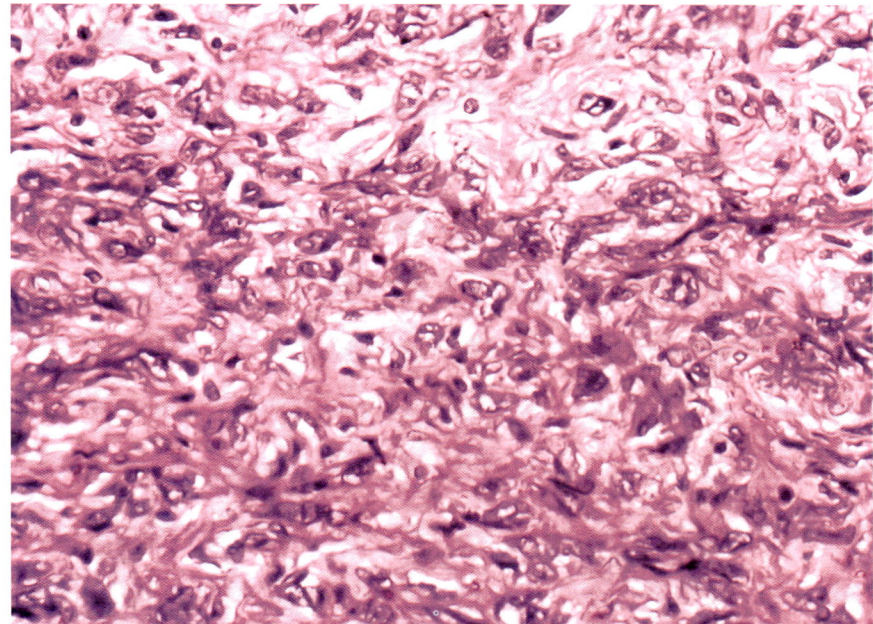

Fig. 91.3: Epithelioid cell histiocytoma. Epithelioid cells, xanthocytes and inflammatory cells in dermis

IMMUNOHISTOCHEMISTRY

- Cells express factor XIIIa positivity
- Vascular channels express CD31 or CD34 positivity

DIFFERENTIAL DIAGNOSIS

Pyogenic Granuloma

- Capillary channel proliferation, forming lobules

- Stroma is composed of mixed inflammatory cell infiltrate composed of neutrophils, lymphocytes and eosinophils

Spitz Nevus

- Epidermis shows pseudoepitheliomatous hyperplasia
- Dermis shows large spindle-shaped cells or epithelioid cells

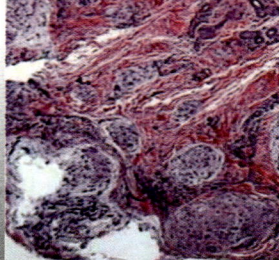

Atypical Fibroxanthoma

INTRODUCTION

- Presents as an exophytic, solitary, dome-shaped nodule
- Size—measures less than 2 cm in diameter
- Sites—head and neck, dorsum of hand
- Affects most commonly elderly individuals
- Associated with ultraviolet radiation, trauma, and in transplant recipient patients
- Cell of origin—undifferentiated mesenchymal cell

HISTOPATHOLOGY (Figs 92.1 to 92.4)

- Cellular neoplasm of the dermis
- Tumor is surrounded by an epidermal collarette
- Tumor cells do not reach up to the squamous epithelium
- Tumor is composed of plump spindle-shaped cells, epithelioid cells and bizarre cells arranged in fascicular and storiform pattern
- Other cell types—clear cells, giant cells (multinucleated/osteoclastic, mononucleated)
- Xanthoma cells (foam cells) can be seen
- Adnexal structure involvement can occur
- Extension into the subcutis is an indicator of recurrence
- Variants—clear cell, granular cell, osteoid, chondroid

IMMUNOHISTOCHEMISTRY

- Tumor cells demonstrate CD10 (strong), vimentin, actin and CD68 positivity
- Tumor cells are negative for cytokeratin, CEA, S-100, Melan-A and desmin

DIFFERENTIAL DIAGNOSIS

Malignant Fibrous Histiocytoma (MFH)

- Tumor cells invade into the muscle, fascia and subcutis
- Tumor necrosis is present
- Vascular and perineural invasion is seen

Leiomyosarcoma

- Tumor cells are arranged in fascicles, with blunt end nuclei

Dermatofibrosarcoma Protuberans (DFSP)

- Uniform population of fibroblasts arranged in a storiform-pattern
- Tumor cells demonstrate CD34 positivity

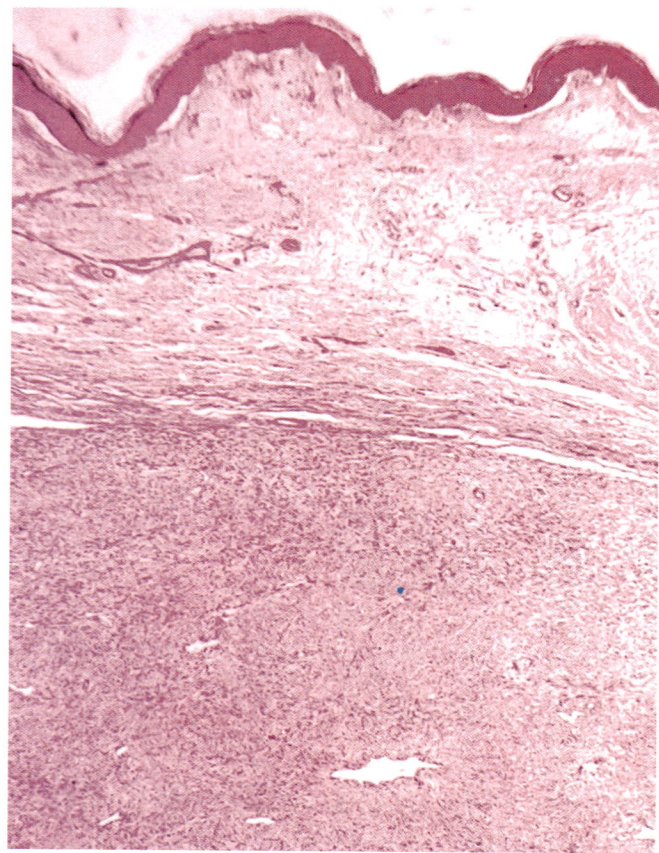

Fig. 92.1: Atypical fibroxanthoma. Well-circumscribed dermal lesion with clear cut separation from the epidermis

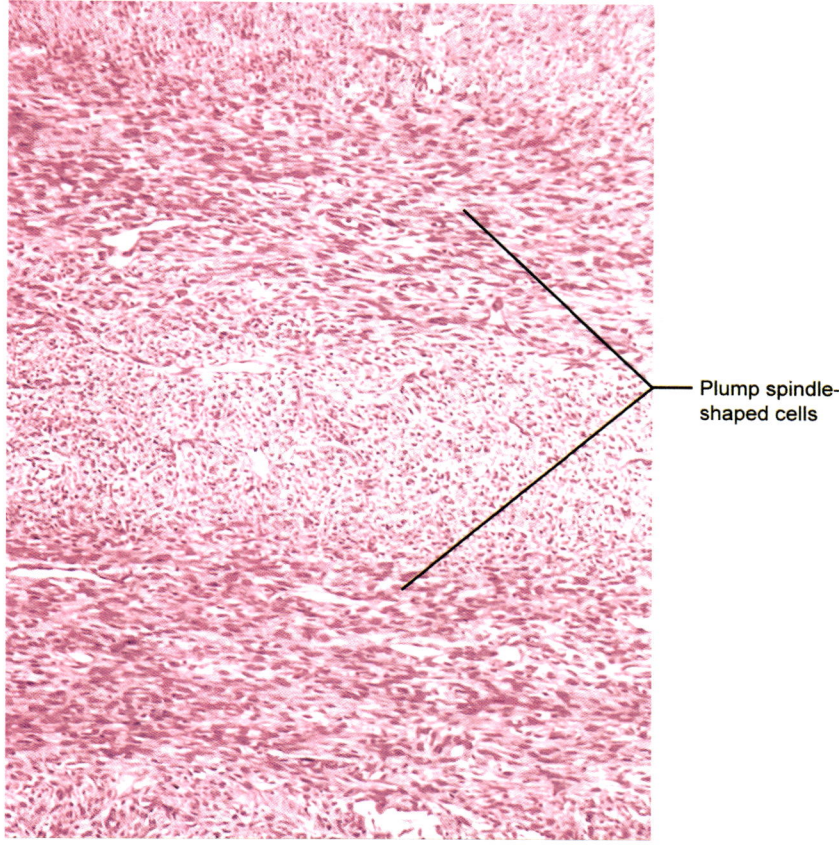

Plump spindle-shaped cells

Fig. 92.2: Atypical fibroxanthoma

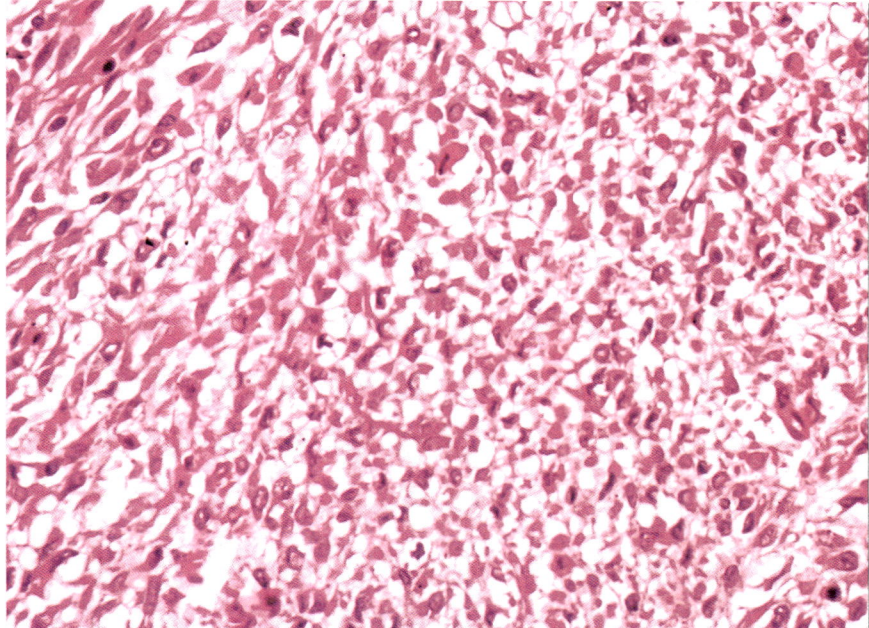

Fig. 92.3: Atypical fibroxanthoma. Foci of epithelioid and polygonal tumor cells

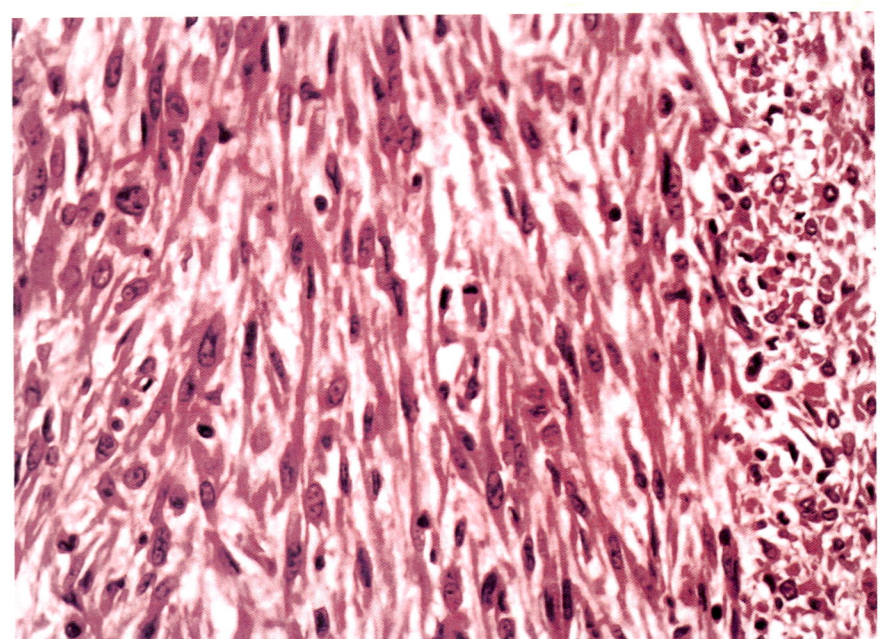

Fig. 92.4: Atypical fibroxanthoma. Atypia and mitosis are seen in spindle cell population of tumor

Squamous Cell Carcinoma

- Tumor cells demonstrate cytokeratin positivity

Nodular Melanoma

- Tumor cells demonstrate S-100 and Melan-A positivity

Table 92.1 Differential diagnosis of important soft-tissue neoplasms on immunohistochemical basis

Antibody	Atypical fibroxanthoma	Malignant fibrous histiocytoma	Leiomyo-sarcoma	Squamous cell carcinoma	Malignant melanoma	DFSP
Cytokeratin, EMA	–	–	–	Positive	–	–
S–100, HMB–45, MART–1, Melan A	–	–	–	–	+	–
SMA, Desmin, Calponin	+/–	+/–	+	–	–	–
CD68	+	+	–	–	–	–
Vimentin	+	+	+	–	+	+
CD10	++	+	+	–	–	+

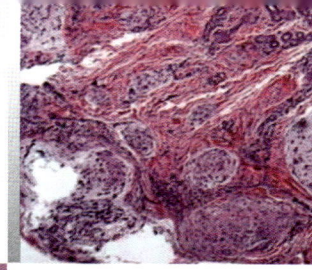

Dermatofibrosarcoma Protuberans (DFSP)

INTRODUCTION

- Age group—young adults, although can affect children
- Sites—trunk, proximal extremities and rarely head and neck
- Presents as red to tan-brown or flesh colored, firm plaque or nodule (Fig. 93.1)
- Lesion can show rapid growth during pregnancy
- Increased risk of local recurrence
- Associated with reciprocal translocation, t (17; 22)

HISTOPATHOLOGY (Figs 93.2 to 93.5)

- Epidermis does not show hyperplastic change
- Presence of superficial grenz zone
- Deep dermis shows spindle-shaped tumor cells arranged in storiform or in cartwheel pattern
- Tumor cells diffusely infiltrate the subcutis, and produce a characteristic honeycomb pattern
- Bednar tumor (pigmented dermatofibrosarcoma protuberans)—scattered melanocytes within the tumor and these pigment-laden cells show S-100 positivity
- Tumor cells demonstrate CD34 positivity
- Variants—myxoid, atrophic, sclerosing, granular cell, palisaded, fibrosarcomatous, fibrosarcomatous with myxoid change

DIFFERENTIAL DIAGNOSIS

Dermatofibroma

- Hyperplastic epidermis
- Presence of grenz zone
- Ill-defined tumor margins with entrapment of collagen bundles

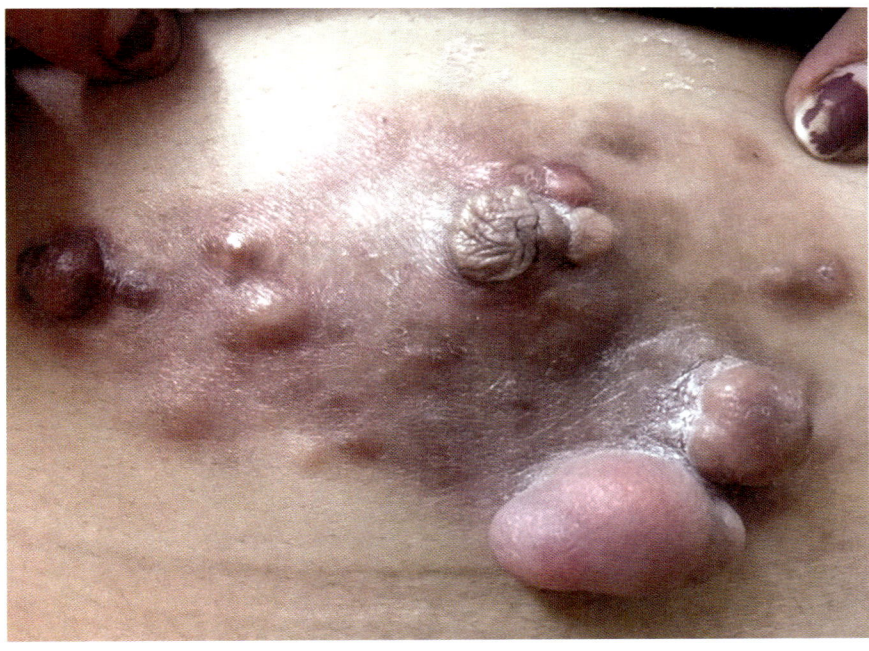

Fig. 93.1: Dermatofibrosarcoma protuberans. Indurated plaque covered by skin-colored, red-tinged, sclerodermiform or telangiectatic atrophic skin

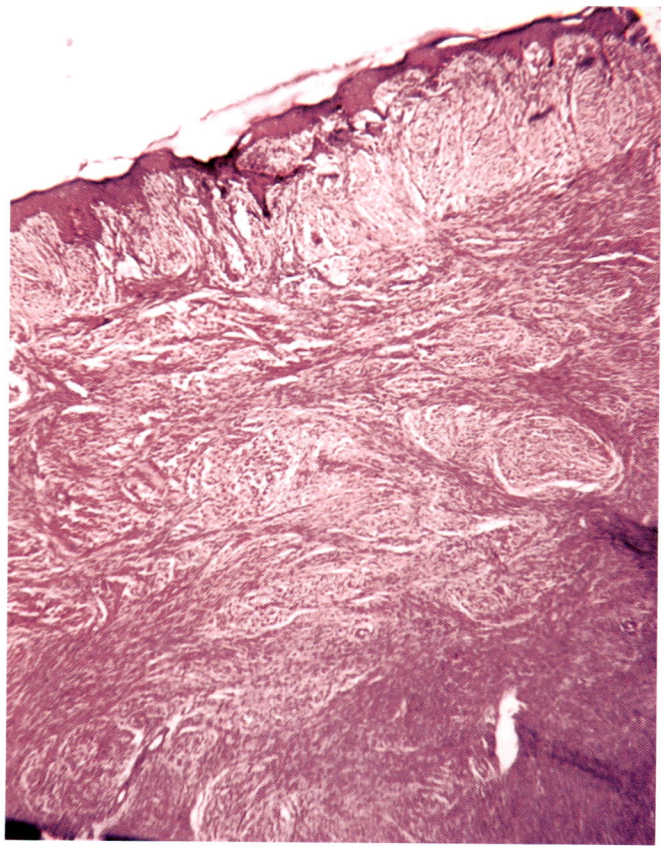

Fig. 93.2: Dermatofibrosarcoma protuberans. Dermis shows spindle-shaped tumor cells arranged in whorled and storiform pattern

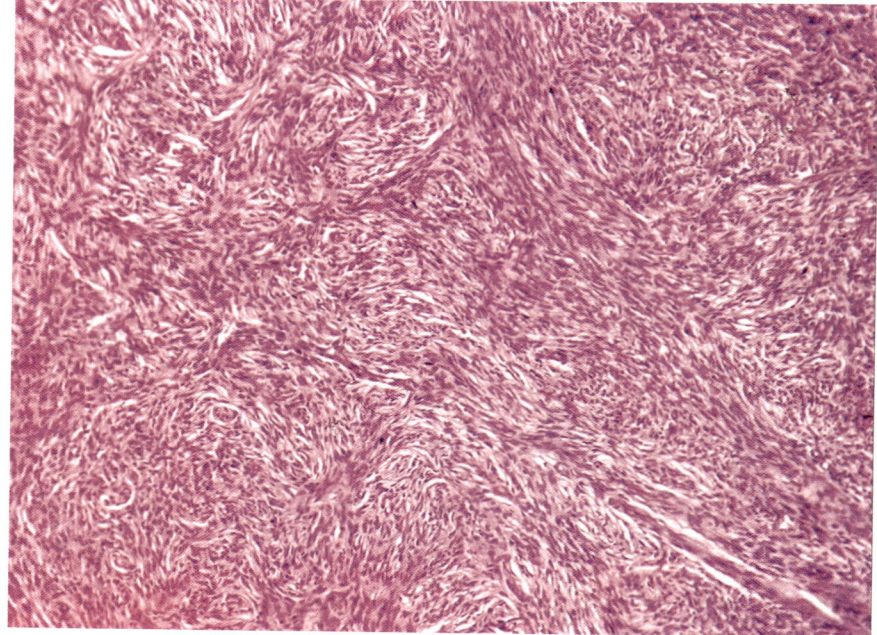

Fig. 93.3: Dermatofibrosarcoma protuberans. Dermis shows spindle cells arranged in storiform and whorled pattern

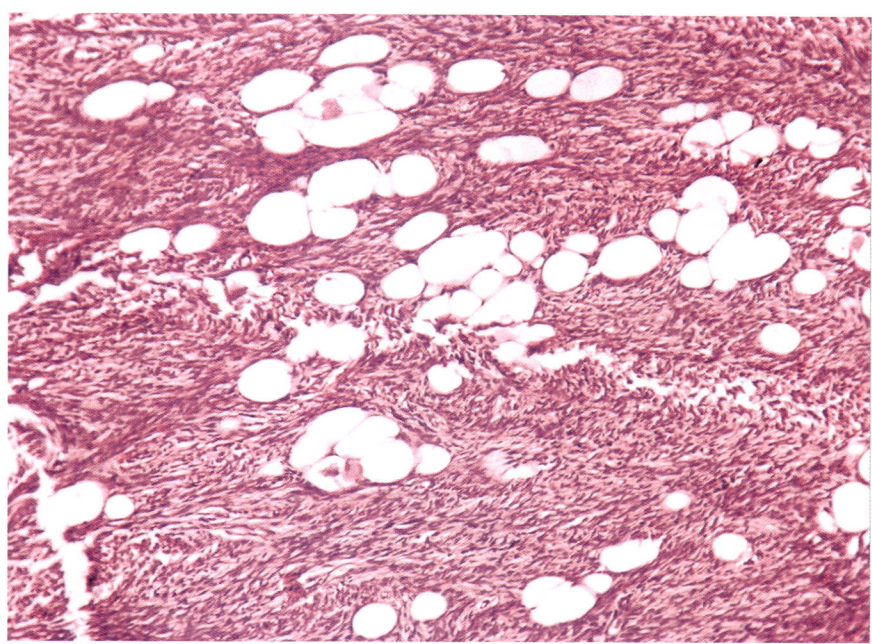

Fig. 93.4: Dermatofibrosarcoma protuberans with subcutis showing a characteristic honeycomb pattern of arrangement of tumor cells

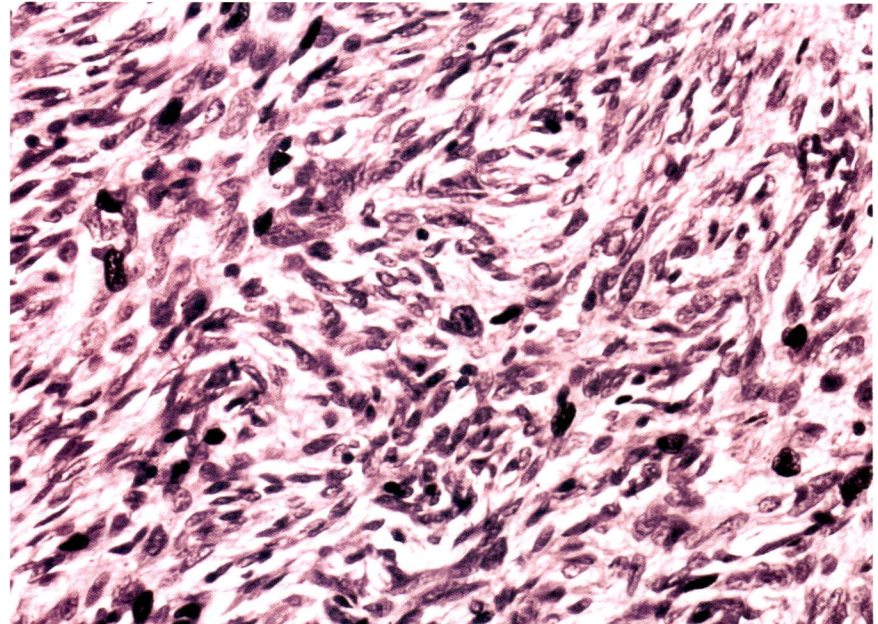

Fig. 93.5: Dermatofibrosarcoma protuberans. Tumor is composed of plump spindle-shaped tumor cells showing mild-nuclear pleomorphism

Leiomyosarcoma

- Plump spindle-shaped tumor cells demonstrating SMA and desmin positivity

Neurofibroma

- Neural cells showing S-100 positivity

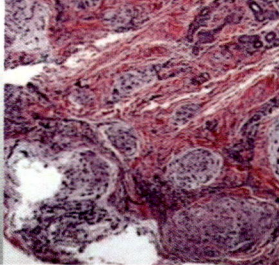

Leiomyoma

Chapter **94**

INTRODUCTION

- Benign mesenchymal tumor showing smooth muscle differentiation
- Shows autosomal dominant pattern of inheritance

TYPES

Multiple Pilar Leiomyomas

- Site of origin—arrector pili muscle
- Most common type of leiomyoma
- Clinical features—presents as small, firm, brown or red intradermal nodules (Fig. 94.1)
- Painful lesions
- Sites—trunk and extremities

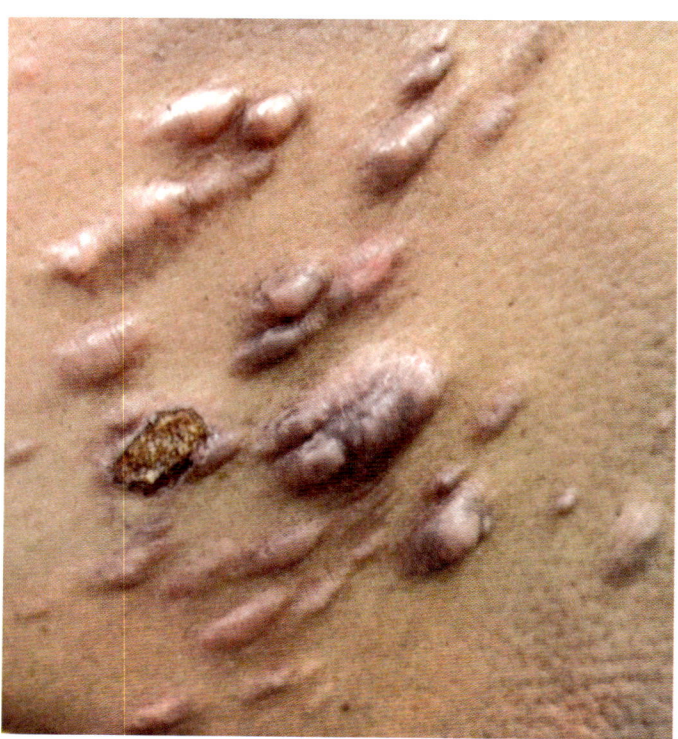

Fig. 94.1: Leiomyoma. Firm, flesh-colored skin nodules

Solitary Pilar Leiomyoma

- More common in females
- Presents as painful solitary lesions
- Measuring up to 2 cm in diameter

Solitary Genital Leiomyoma

- Located on the scrotum, labia majora and nipples arising from dartoic, vulvar or mammary smooth muscles, respectively
- Presents as firm, solitary, asymptomatic nodules

Solitary Angioleiomyoma

- Painful subcutaneous lesions
- Size—less than 4 cm in diameter
- Most common site—lower extremities, most commonly on lower legs

Cutaneous Angiolipoleiomyoma/Angiomyolipoma

- More common in females
- Sites—foot and toes

HISTOPATHOLOGY

Pilar Leiomyoma (Figs 94.2 to 94.4)

- Subepidermal 'grenz-zone' is seen
- Dermis—circumscribed, non-encapsulated tumor
- Tumor is composed of bundles of smooth muscle cells arranged in interlacing pattern
- Smooth muscle cells have abundant eosinophilic cytoplasm, elongated nuclei with blunt ends
- Nuclear pleomorphism is absent

Angioleiomyoma

- Encapsulated tumor
- Tumor is composed of interlacing bundles of smooth muscles between numerous vascular channels

Angiolipoleiomyoma/Angiomyolipoma

- Subcutaneous, well-circumscribed tumor composed of benign smooth muscle fibers, vascular spaces and mature fat

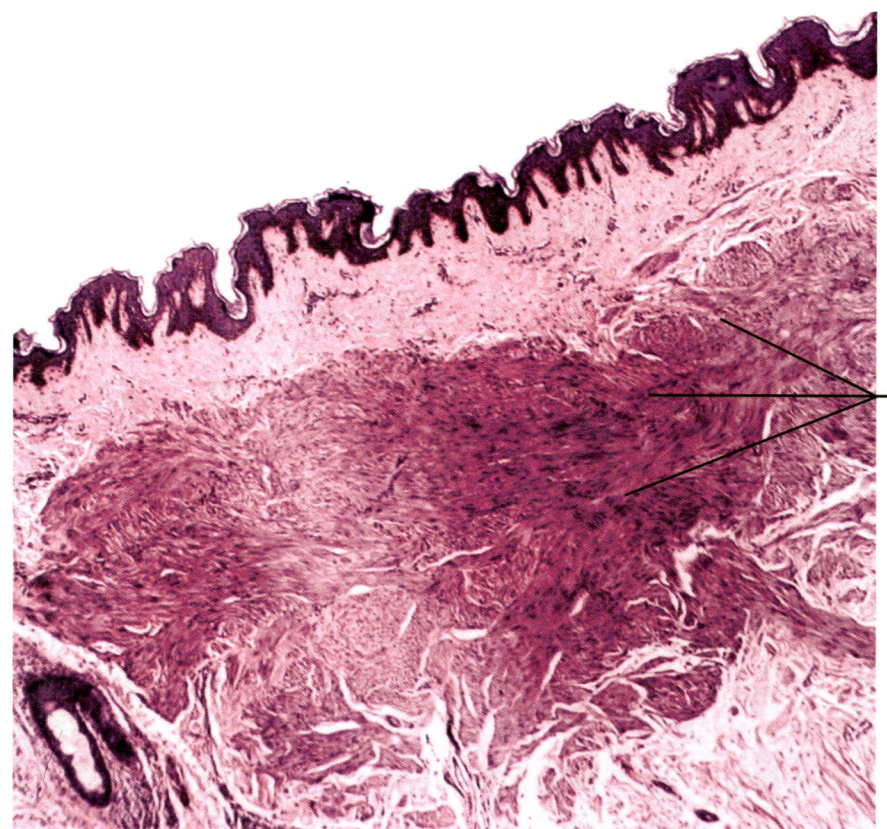

Unencapsulated
dermal tumor comprising
of interlacing bundles of
smooth muscle cells

Fig. 94.2: Pilar leiomyoma

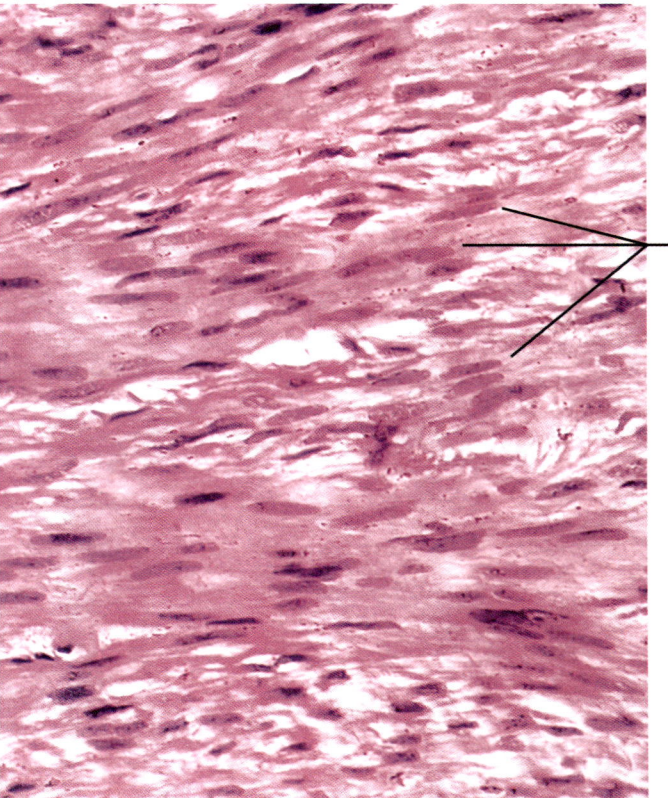

Smooth muscle
cells with cigar-
shaped nuclei in
pilar leiomyoma

Fig. 94.3: Leiomyoma

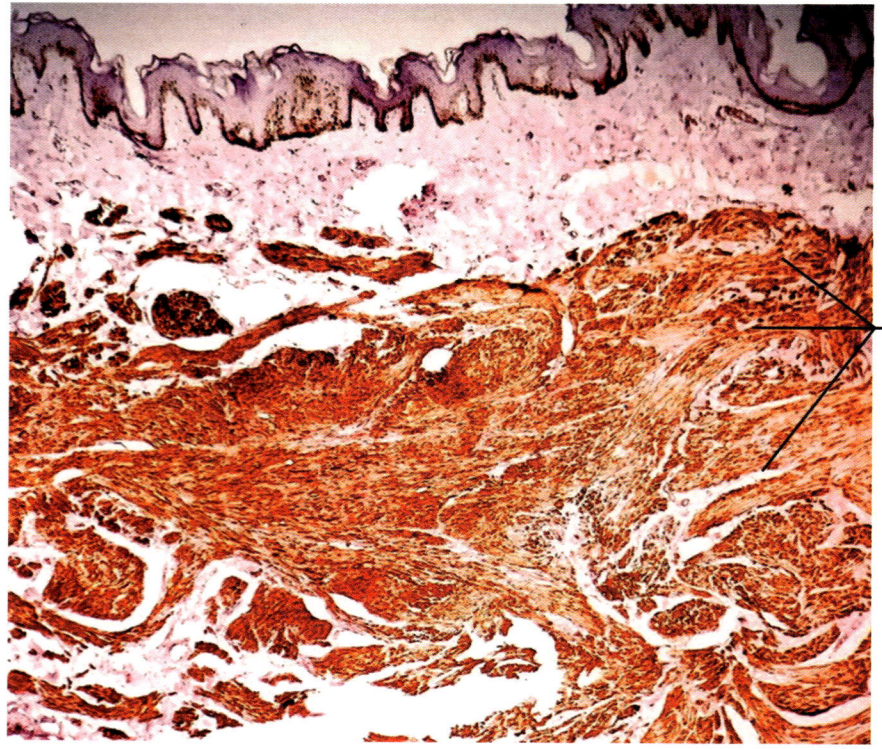

Smooth muscle cells demonstrating SMA positivity in pilar leiomyoma

Fig. 94.4: Leiomyoma

IMMUNOHISTOCHEMISTRY

- Tumor cells express vimentin, smooth muscle actin (SMA) and desmin
- Genital leiomyomas exhibit estrogen and progesterone receptor positivity

DIFFERENTIAL DIAGNOSIS

Leiomyosarcoma

- Interlacing fascicles of elongated plump spindle shaped cells.
  These cells show varying degrees of nuclear atypia, pleomorphism, hyperchromasia and increased mitotic figures

Dermatofibroma

- Fibroblastic tumor cells entrapping the collagen bundles at the periphery

Dermatofibrosarcoma Protuberans (DFSP)

- Spindle cells with wavy nuclei, extending into the subcutaneous tissue
- Tumor cells demonstrate CD34 positivity

Neurofibroma

- Tumor cells have wavy nuclei and show S-100 positivity

Smooth Muscle Hamartoma

- Bundles of smooth muscle fibers in dermis
- Smooth muscle fibers are separated by dermal collagen
- Smooth muscle fibers and collagen are demonstrated by Masson's trichrome stain

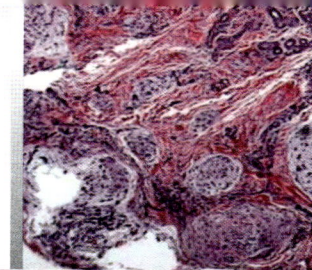

Lipoma

INTRODUCTION

- Most common mesenchymal neoplasm
- Presents as single or multiple, encapsulated tumors, that are soft, rounded and mobile against the overlying skin (Fig. 95.1)
- Sites—upper trunk, extremities, thighs
- According to the location, lipomas can be classified into—perineural lipoma, lumbosacral lipoma, tendon sheath lipoma, muscular lipoma, myolipoma and angiomyolipoma
- Cowden syndrome patients can show multiple lipomas and hemangiomas

HISTOPATHOLOGY (Fig. 95.2)

- Composed of sheets of mature adipocytes surrounded by fibrous capsule

- These adipocytes are dissected by fibrous septa containing blood vessels

VARIANTS

Intramuscular Lipoma

- Mature fat cells, infiltrate and splay around the muscle fibers

Fibrolipoma (Fig. 95.3)

- Strands of fibro-collagenous tissue, surrounding mature adipocytes

Sclerotic (Fibroma-like) Lipoma

- Sclerotic stroma (spindle or stellate-shaped cells) in a storiform pattern

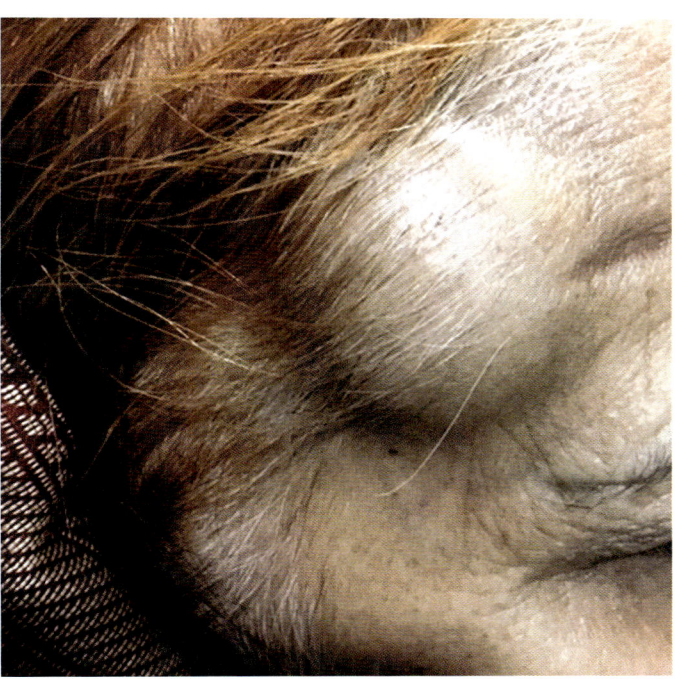

Fig. 95.1: Lipoma. Single soft painless subcutaneous nodule

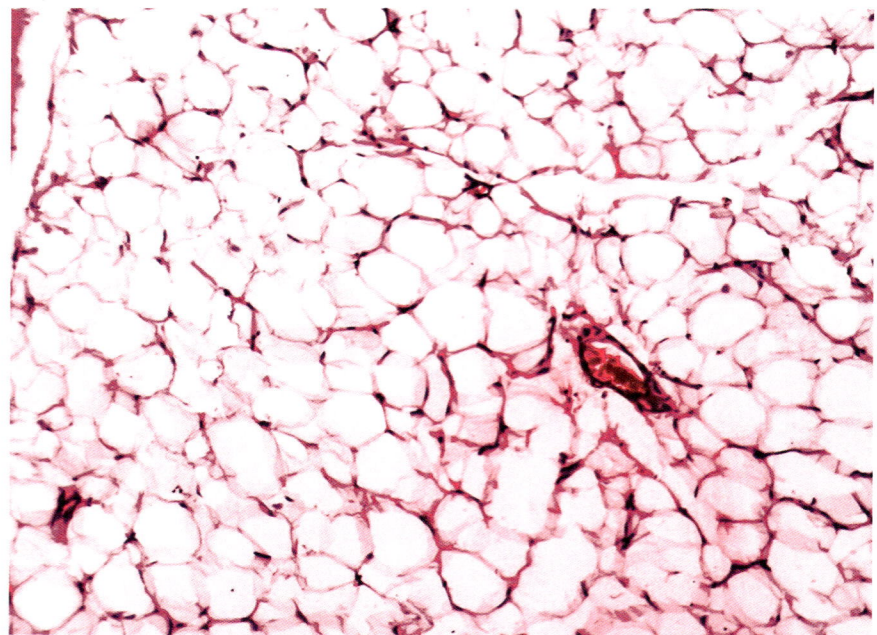

Fig. 95.2: Mature adipocytes in lipoma

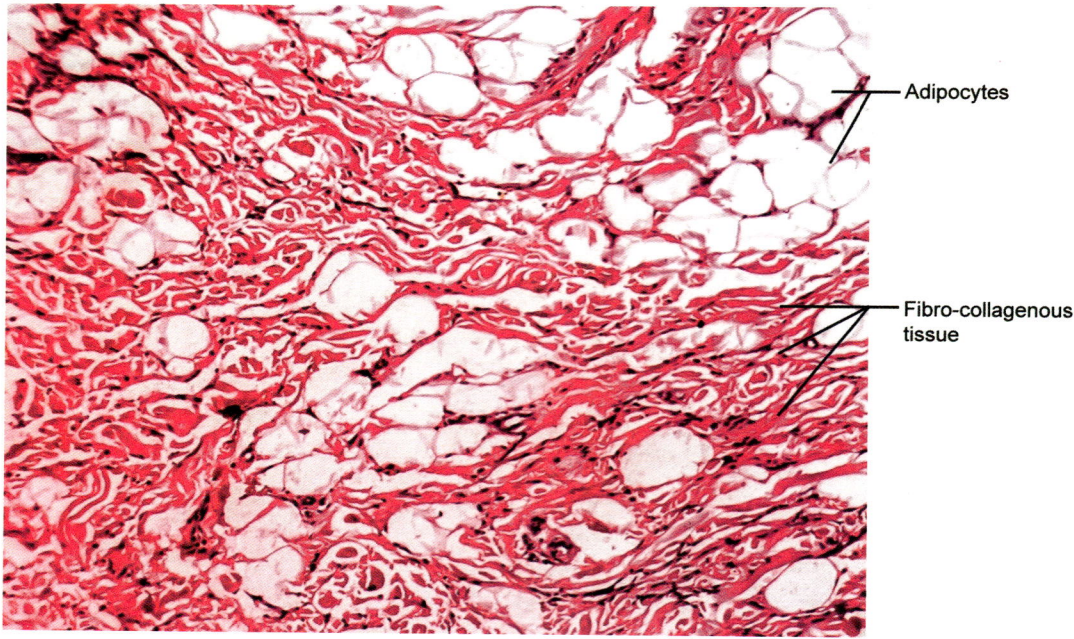

Fig. 95.3: Fibrolipoma (fibro-collagenous tissue surrounds mature adipocytes)

Myxolipoma

- Basophilic myxoid substance, between mature adipocytes

Osteolipoma

- Focal chondroid or osteoid production in a fibro-fatty background

Myolipoma

- Benign smooth muscle cells and mature adipose tissue

Angiomyolipoma

- Mature adipose tissue, smooth muscle fascicles and medium-sized blood vessels

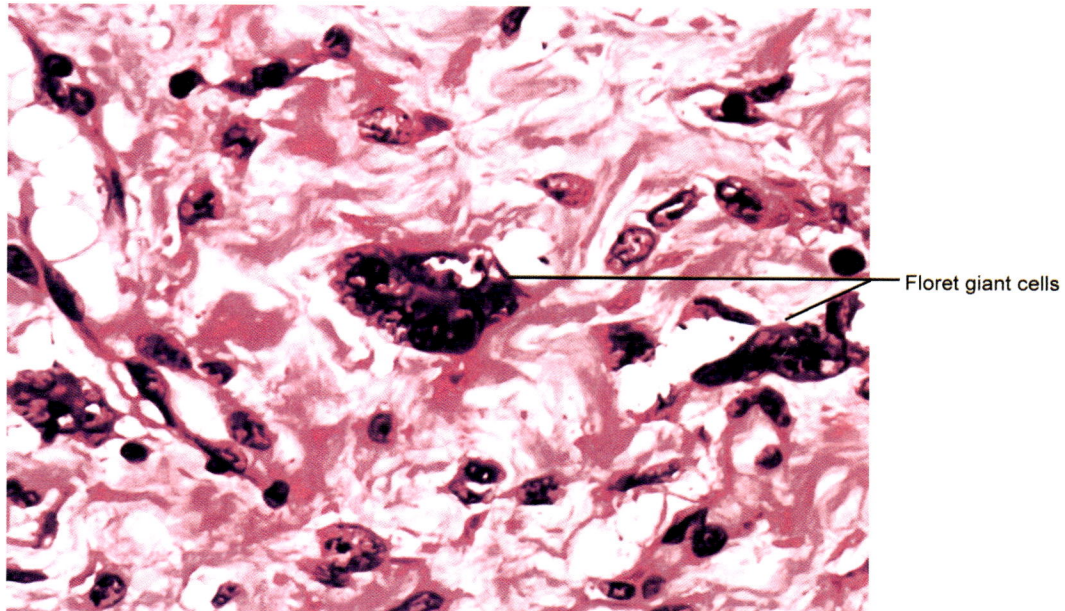

Fig. 95.4: Pleomorphic lipoma

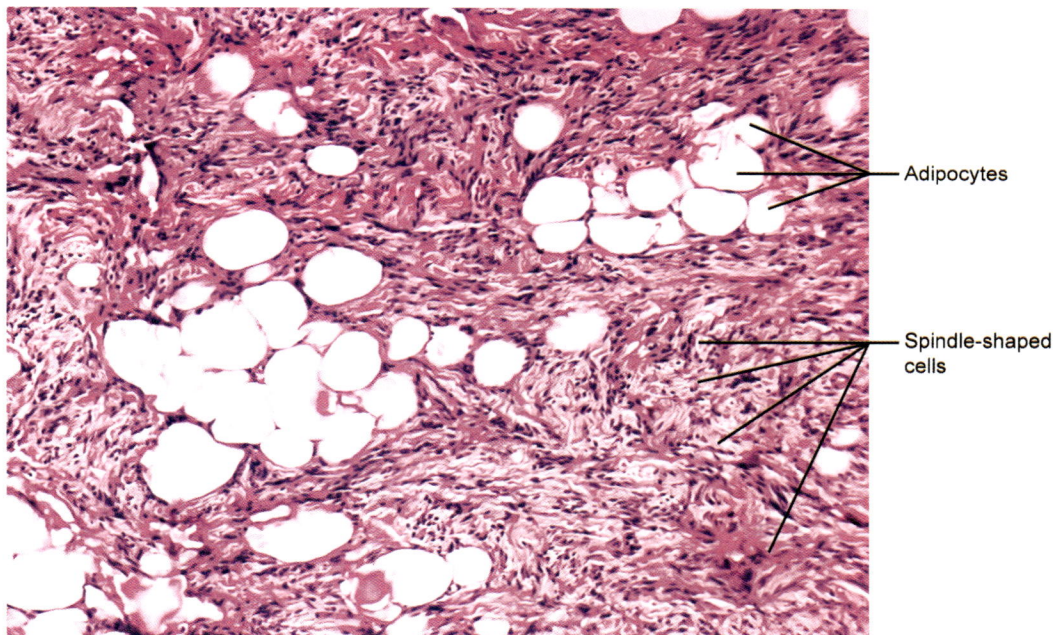

Fig. 95.5: Spindle cell lipoma (mature adipocytes with intervening spindle cells)

Adenolipoma

- Lobules of mature adipose tissue admixed with normal eccrine glands

Pleomorphic Lipoma (Fig. 95.4)

- Presents as a soft, subcutaneous mass
- Sites—shoulder, neck and back
- Adipocytes with hyperchromatic nuclei, giant cells, and floret giant cells
- Giant cells show smudgy nuclei
- Absence of mitotic figures

Spindle Cell Lipoma (Fig. 95.5)

- Affects shoulders, back, neck, extremities

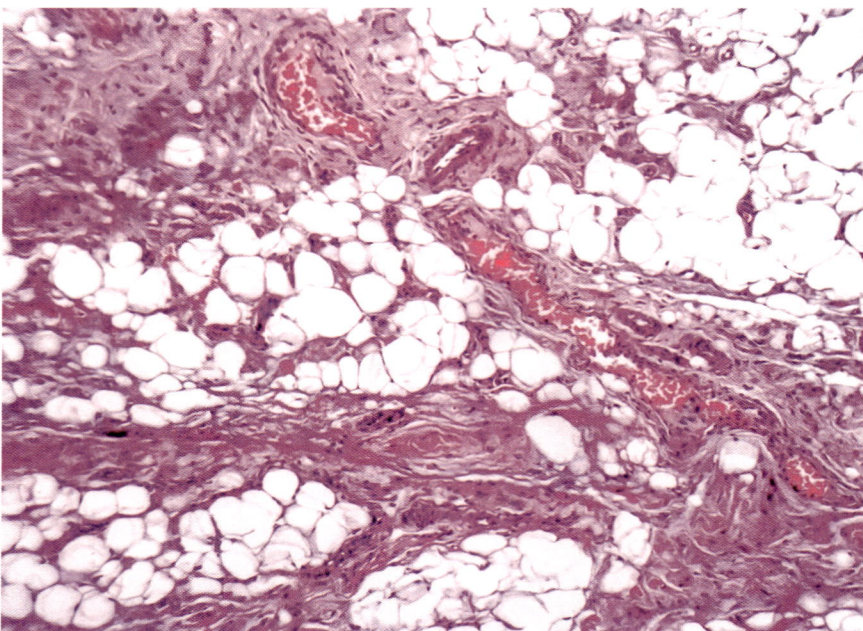

Fig. 95.6: Angiolipoma. Mature adipocytes with thin-walled blood vessels

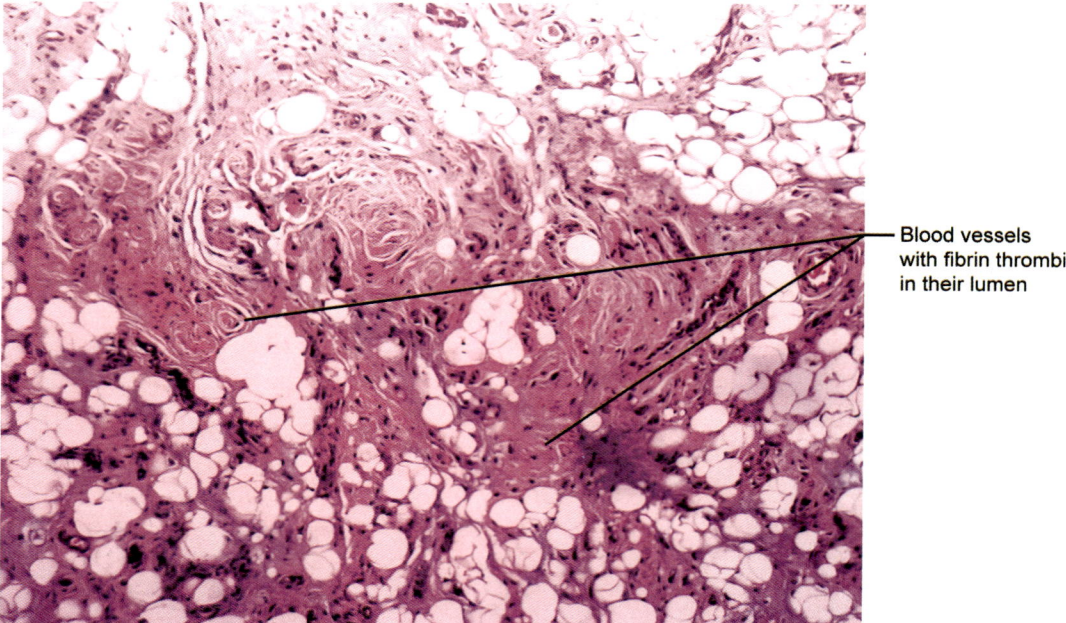

Blood vessels with fibrin thrombi in their lumen

Fig. 95.7: Angiolipoma

- Circumscribed, un-encapsulated tumors of the subcutis
- Tumor is composed of mature adipocytes and spindle cells, the latter are separated by variable amounts of collagen bundles
- Spindle cells show CD34 positivity

Angiolipoma (Figs 95.6 to 95.8)

- Sites—affects extremities and trunk
- Circumscribed tumors with a yellow–red cut surface
- Increased number of small capillaries (comprising 5–50% or more of tumor) within fat lobules
- Capillary lumen shows RBCs and may also show scattered fibrin thrombi

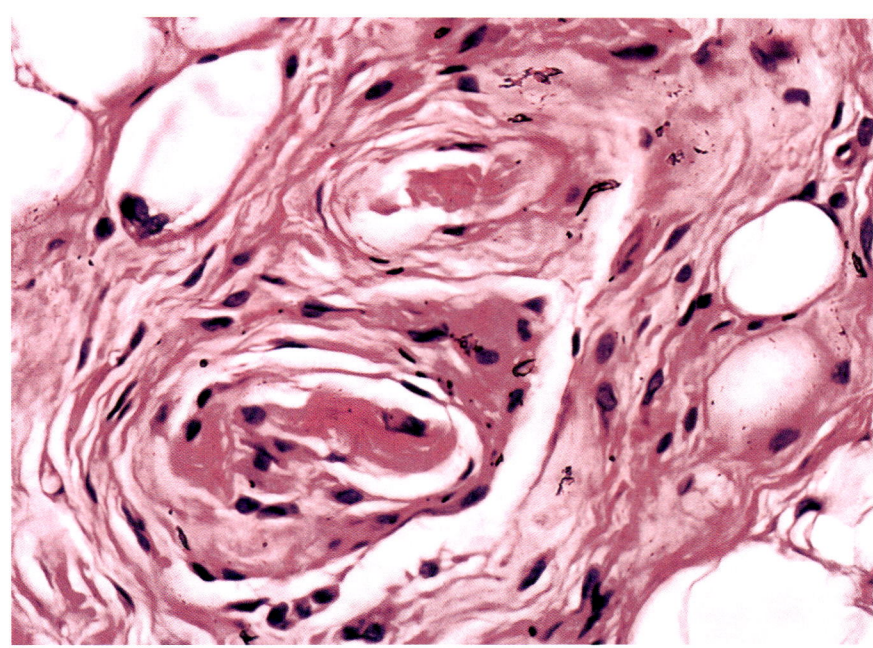

Fig. 95.8: Angiolipoma. Blood vessels with fibrin thrombi in their lumens

Angiomyxolipoma

- Mature adipocytes and small capillary channel proliferation in a myxoid stroma

Neural Fibrolipoma

- Fibro-fatty tissue surrounds and infiltrates the nerve or its branches

DIFFERENTIAL DIAGNOSIS

Liposarcoma

- Infiltrative growth pattern
- Increased cellularity, nuclear atypia, pleomorphism, mitosis, necrosis
- Presence of multi-vacuolated lipoblasts

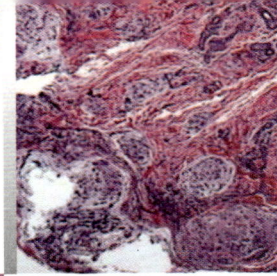

Neurofibroma

INTRODUCTION

- Presents as soft, polypoidal, skin-colored nodule (Fig. 96.1)
- Site—most commonly affects upper trunk
- Multiple cutaneous neurofibromas are seen in neurofibromatosis type 1 (NF-1)
- NF-1 is characterized by 17q11.2 mutation and the protein mutated is neurofibromin
- Plexiform neurofibroma—diffuse enlargement of peripheral nerves, seen in NF-1 patients

HISTOPATHOLOGY (Figs 96.2 to 96.5)

- Circumscribed, non-encapsulated dermal tumor

- Grenz zone separates the lesion from the under-surface of the epidermis
- Composed of axons, schwann cells and fibroblasts
- Schwann cells—spindle-shaped cells, with elongated wavy nuclei, and pointed ends
- Stroma shows collagen fibers, mucin, and mast cells
- Tumor cells demonstrate S-100 positivity

DIFFERENTIAL DIAGNOSIS

Schwannoma

- Encapsulated tumor with Antoni A and Antoni B areas
- Presence of Verocay bodies

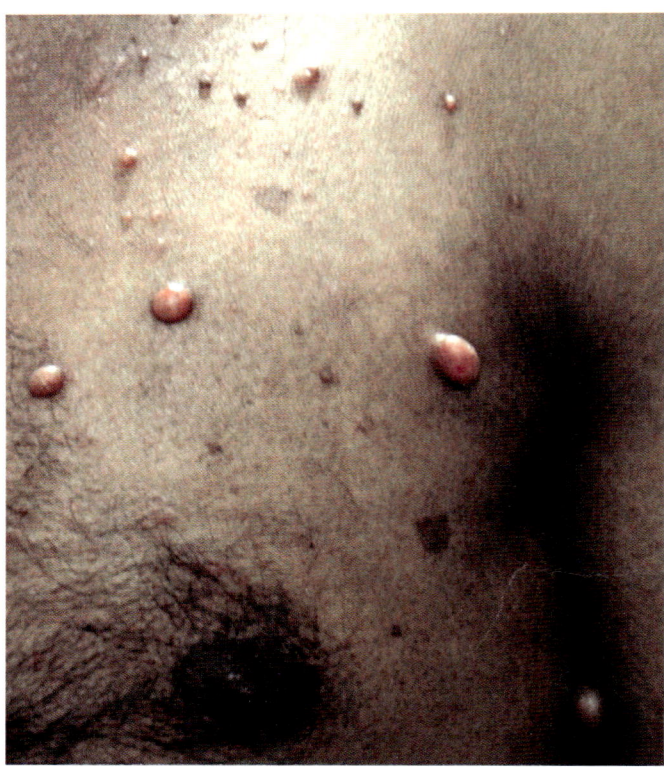

Fig. 96.1: Neurofibroma. Soft, flesh-colored and hyperpigmented nodules

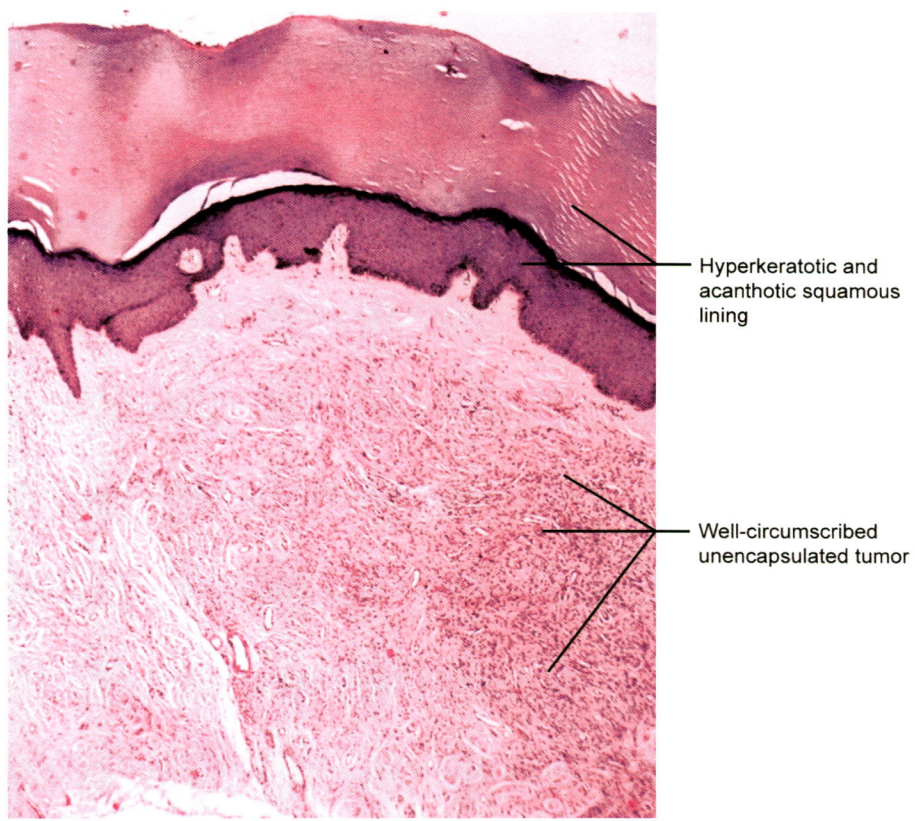

Hyperkeratotic and acanthotic squamous lining

Well-circumscribed unencapsulated tumor

Fig. 96.2: Neurofibroma

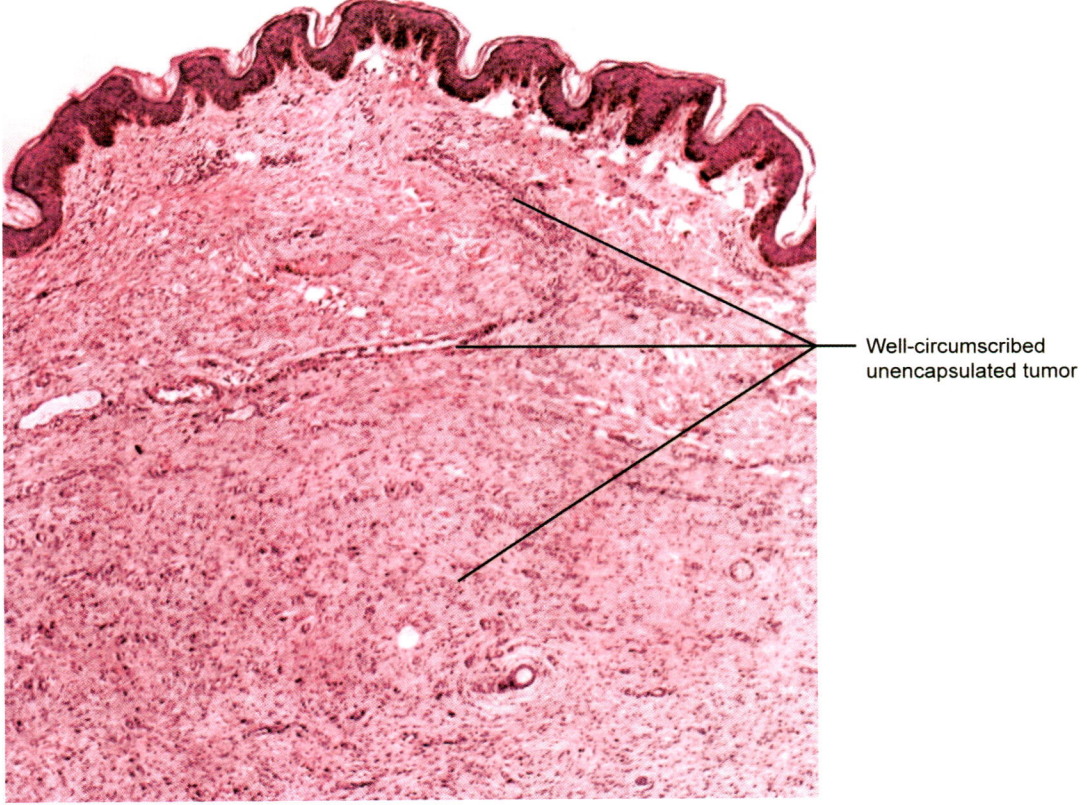

Well-circumscribed unencapsulated tumor

Fig. 96.3: Neurofibroma

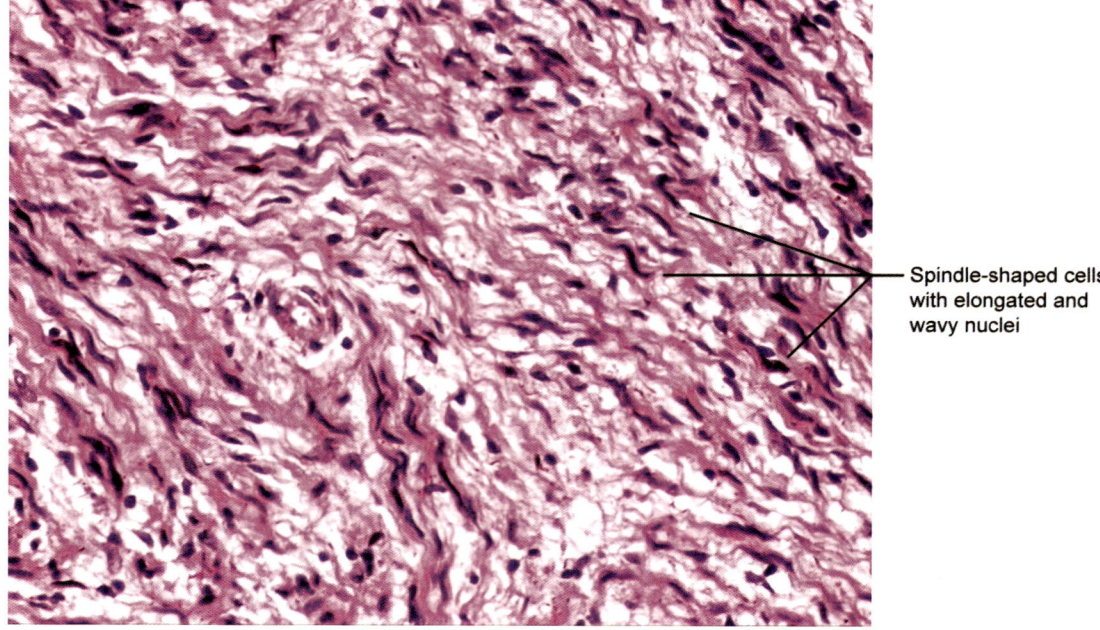

Spindle-shaped cells with elongated and wavy nuclei

Fig. 96.4: Neurofibroma

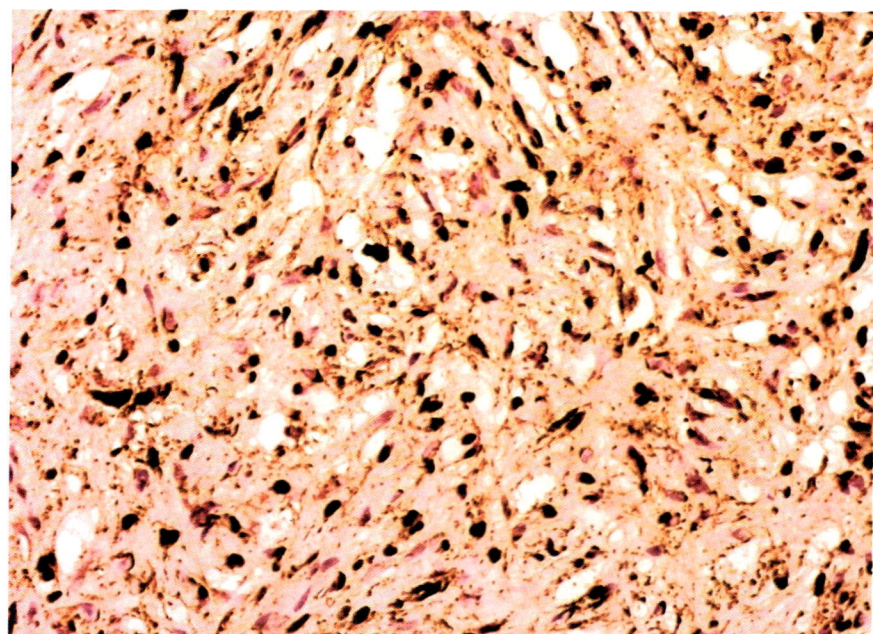

Fig. 96.5: Neurofibroma demonstrating S-100 positivity

Dermatofibrosarcoma Protuberans
- Spindle-shaped tumor cells
- Tumor cells show CD34 positivity

Malignant Peripheral Nerve Sheath Tumor
- Tumor cells show marked nuclear pleomorphism and atypical mitosis

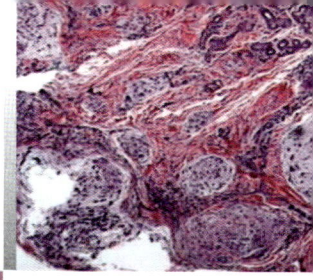

Nevus Lipomatosus Superficialis

INTRODUCTION

- Benign hamartomatous skin lesion
- Presents as skin colored polypoidal nodule or plaque (Fig. 97.1)
- Age group—present at birth or in adolescents
- Sites—trunk (most common), buttocks, thigh, flank

HISTOPATHOLOGY

- Epidermis shows acanthosis, papillomatosis and basal cell layer hyperpigmentation
- Dermis shows adipocytes in between the collagen fibers, which are irregularly distributed
- Dermis is replaced by islands of mature adipocytes
- Adipocytes can reach as high as up to undersurface of epidermis
- Increased vascular channels in the papillary dermis

DIFFERENTIAL DIAGNOSIS

Focal Dermal Hypoplasia

- Dermis is replaced by fat cells
- Collagen bundles are reduced in number

Fibrolipoma

- Variant of lipoma
- Seen in adults
- Comprises adipose tissue with interspersed fibro-collagenous tissue

Atypical Lipomatous Tumor

- Presence of lipoblasts

Fibroepithelial Polyp

- Absence of adipocytes

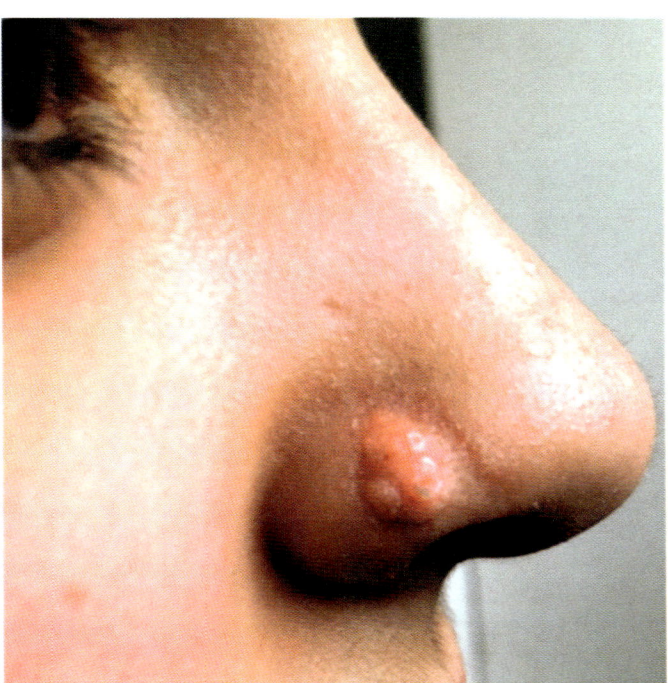

Fig. 97.1: Nevus lipomatosus superficialis. Firm, skin-colored to yellowish plaque

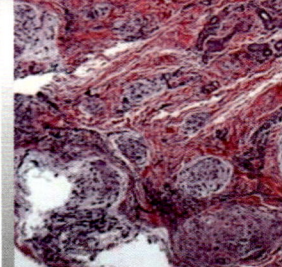

Schwannoma

- Also called neurilemmoma
- Well-encapsulated, solitary tumor and can show cystic areas on cut surface
- Sites—head and neck, flexor aspect of extremities
- Presents as painful skin colored nodules
- Associated with neurofibromatosis-2 (NF-2)
- NF-2 gene is located on chromosome 22q12, and encodes merlin protein

HISTOPATHOLOGY (Figs 98.1 to 98.3)

- Circumscribed encapsulated tumor, confined to the subcutis
- **Two patterns**
  1. **Antoni A areas**—cellular areas, with spindle-shaped schwann cells forming palisades and the areas in between the palisades are termed Verocay bodies
  2. **Antoni B areas**—Schwann cells are loosely spaced in a clear or myxoid matrix

VARIANTS

- **Ancient schwannoma**—tumor cells with bizarre hyperchromatic nuclei
- **Ceilular schwannoma**—spindle cell proliferation with absence of Verocay bodies and Antoni B areas
- **Plexiform schwannoma**—dermal nodule comprising of multiple interlacing and interconnecting fascicles of Schwann cells
- **Epithelioid schwannoma**—predominant epithelioid cell population is seen
- **Psammomatous melanotic schwannoma**—melanin and scattered psammoma bodies

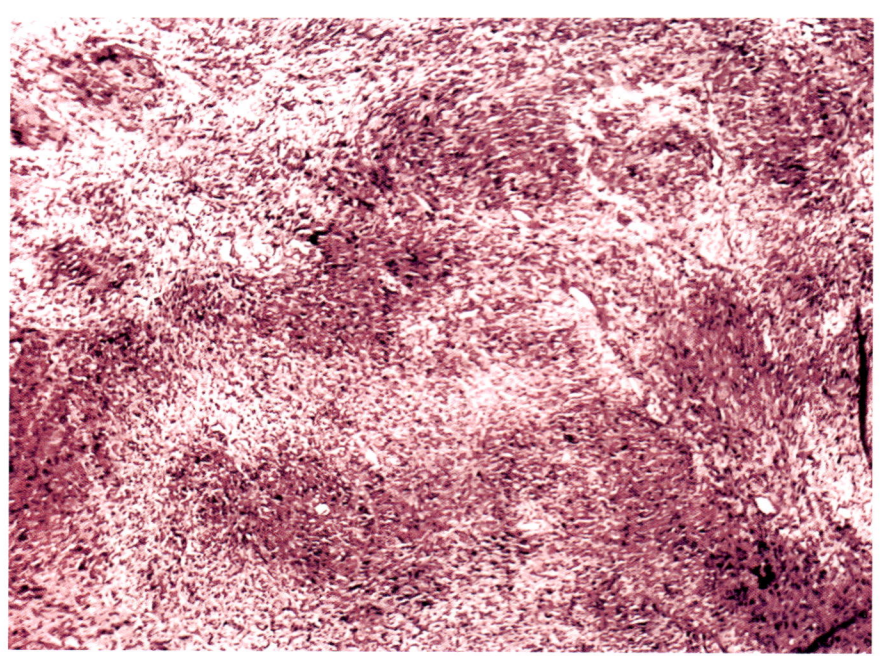

Fig. 98.1: Schwannoma, comprising of cellular and hypocellular areas

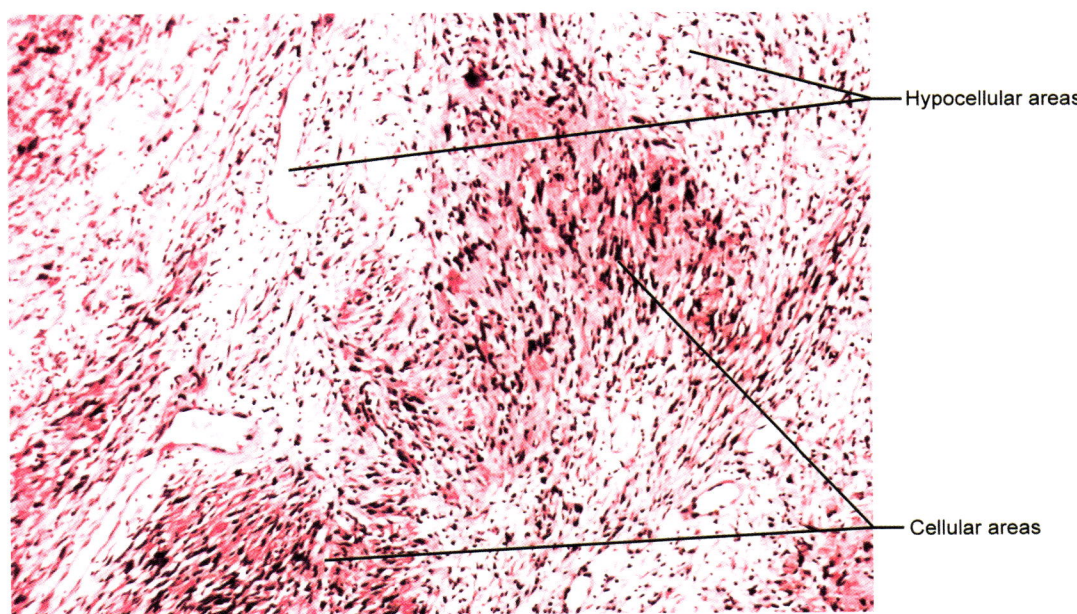

Fig. 98.2: Schwannoma

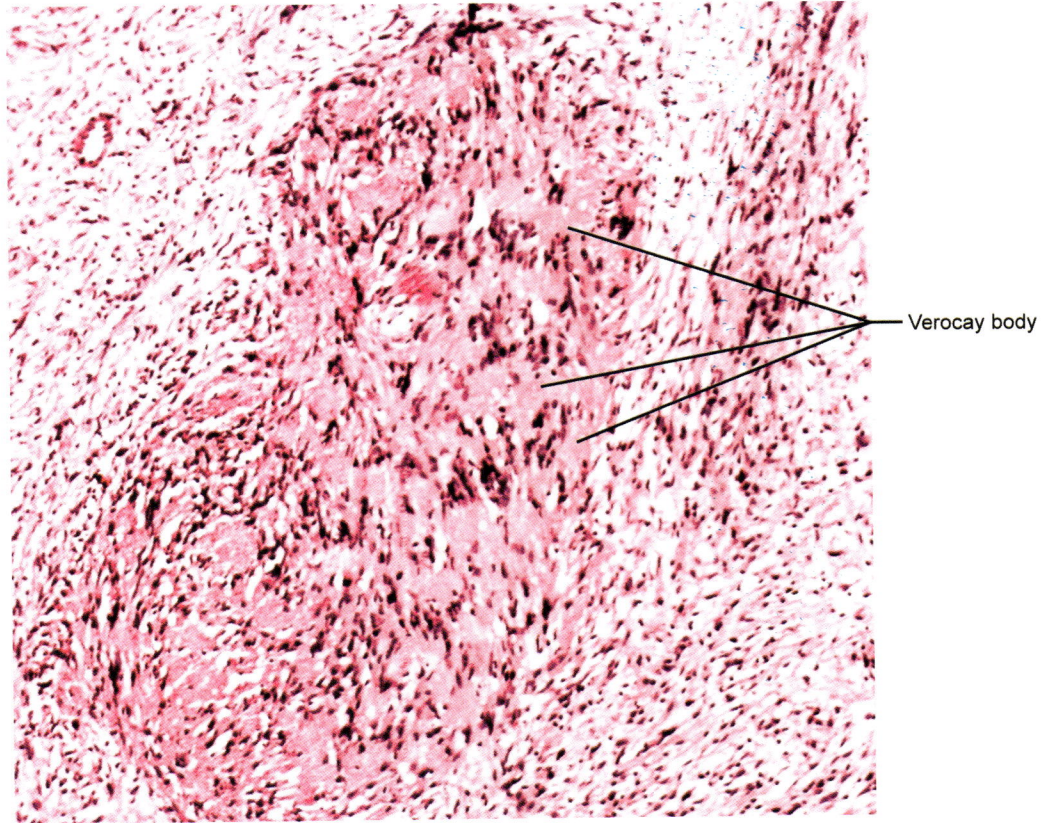

Fig. 98.3: Schwannoma

IMMUNOHISTOCHEMISTRY

- Tumor cells demonstrate S-100, calretinin, calcineurin, laminin, collagen IV positivity

DIFFERENTIAL DIAGNOSIS

Neurofibroma

- Absence of Antoni A and B areas

Perineuroma

- Unencapsulated tumor comprising of spindle-shaped tumor cells
- Tumor cells demonstrate EMA positivity

Nerve Sheath Myxoma (Figs 98.4 to 98.6)

- Circumscribed tumor with myxoid nodules
- Myxoid nodules comprise spindle-shaped tumor cells in a myxoid background
- Spindle cells demonstrate S-100 positivity

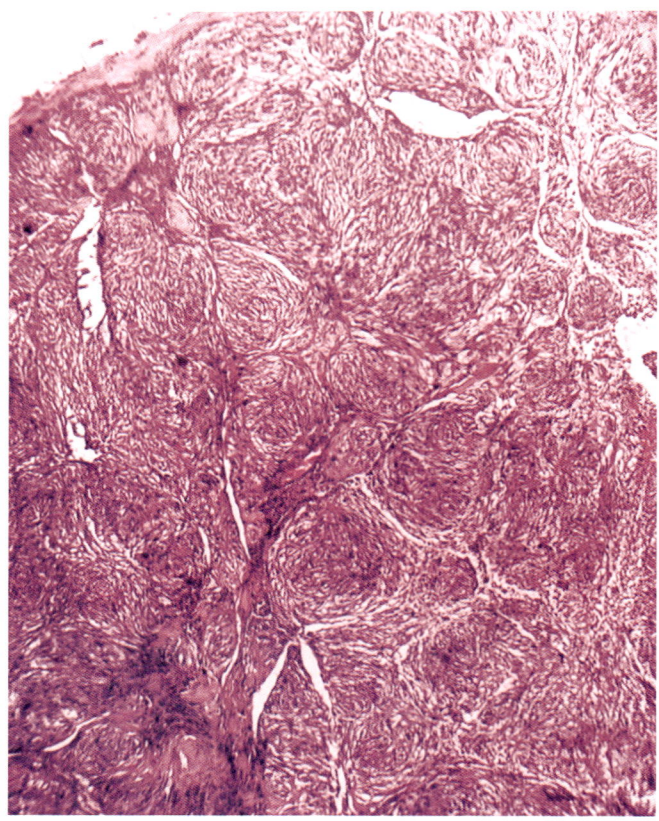

Fig. 98.4: Nerve sheath myxoma (hematoxylin and eosin)

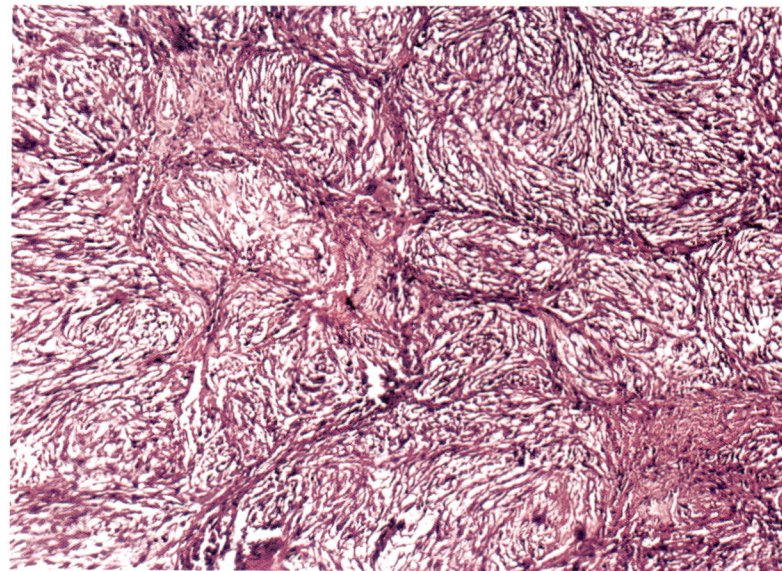

Fig. 98.5: Nerve sheath myxoma (hematoxylin and eosin)

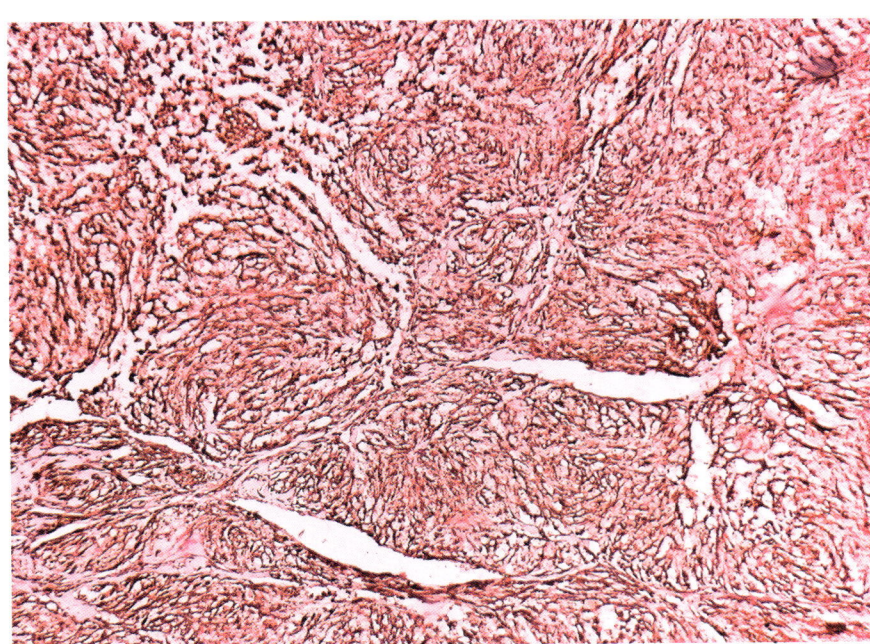

Fig. 98.6: Nerve sheath myxoma with spindle-shaped tumor cells demonstrating S-100 positivity

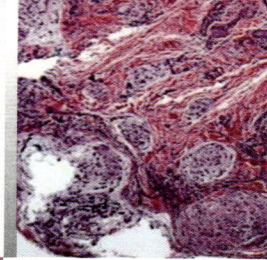

Merkel Cell Carcinoma

INTRODUCTION

- Malignant neuroendocrine cancer affecting the skin
- Cell of origin—Merkel cell
- Merkel cells—localized in basal cell layer of epidermis
- Clinical feature—presents as rapidly growing nodule or indurated plaque
- Sites—head and neck, extremities
- Age group—affects older adults
- Associated with Merkel cell polyoma virus infection
- Aggressive cancer, and can show regional lymph node and distant metastasis

HISTOPATHOLOGY (Figs 99.1 to 99.3)

- Small, round blue tumor cells within the dermis
- Tumor cells are arranged in sheets, nests or trabecular pattern and have round to oval vesicular nucleus with scant cytoplasm

- Intra-epidermal pagetoid spread can be seen
- Azzopardi phenomenon is not commonly seen

POOR PROGNOSTIC MARKERS

- Invasion of tumor cells into subcutaneous fat
- Presence of 10 or more mitosis per high power field
- Lymph node metastasis can occur
- Lymphovascular invasion can be seen

IMMUNOHISTOCHEMISTRY

- Tumor cells demonstrate perinuclear dot-like positivity for cytokeratin-20 (CK-20)
- Tumor cells demonstrate synaptophysin, chromogranin, neuron specific enolase, bombesin and PAX-5 positivity
- Tumor cells are negative for TTF-1 (TTF-1 positivity of tumor cells are seen in small cell carcinoma of lung)

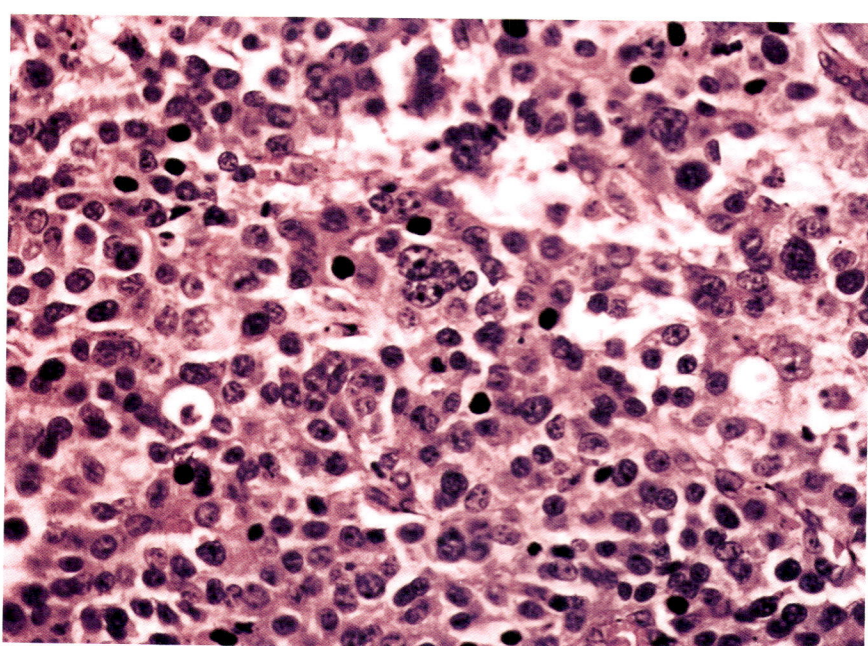

Fig. 99.1: Merkel cell carcinoma

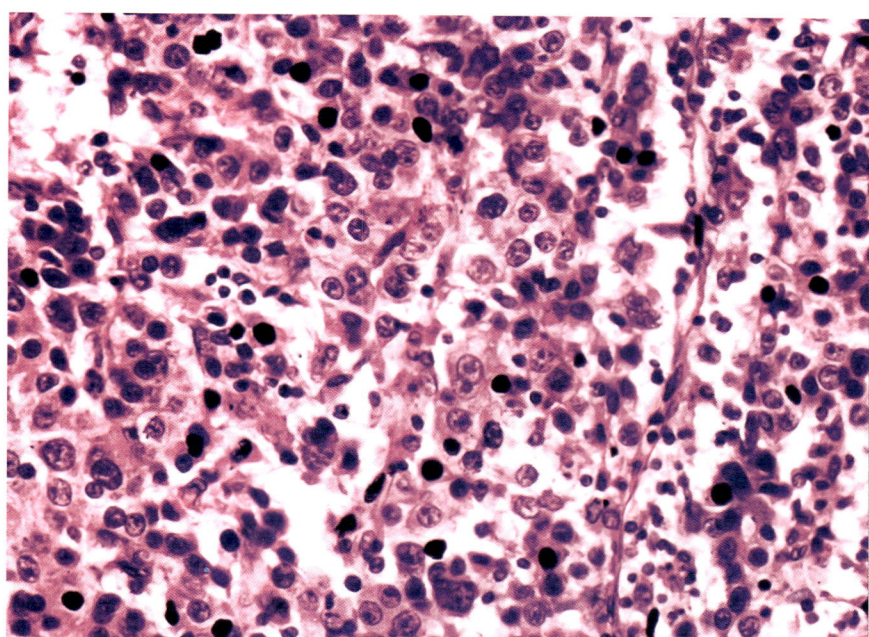

Fig. 99.2: Merkel cell carcinoma

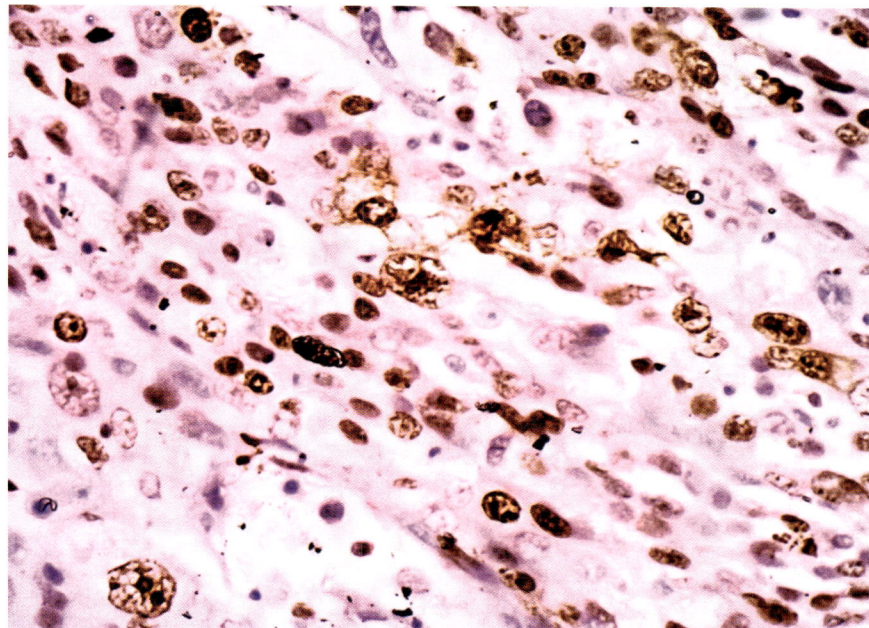

Fig. 99.3: High Ki-67 index in Merkel cell carcinoma

DIFFERENTIAL DIAGNOSIS

1. **Malignant Cutaneous B-cell Lymphoma**
   - Express B-cell markers
   - Absence of neuroendocrine cell marker positivity

2. **Metastasis** from small cell carcinoma of lung, neuroendocrine carcinoma and neuroblastoma
   - History, clinical findings and tumor specific immunohistochemical markers are helpful for differentiating these neoplasms from Merkel cell carcinoma

3. **Melanoma**
   - Tumor cells express S-100, HMB-45 and Melan-A positivity

4. **Basal cell carcinoma**
   - Basaloid cells show peripheral pallisading with adjacent retraction clefts

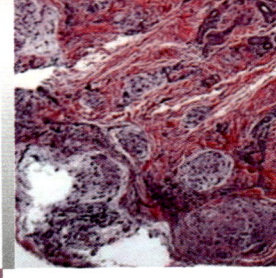

Fibrokeratoma

INTRODUCTION

- Clinical features—presents as solitary, dome-shaped lesions
- Site—fingers, toes, palms, soles
- Size—1–3 mm in diameter
- Associated with tuberous sclerosis and familial retinoblastoma

HISTOPATHOLOGY (Fig. 100.1)

- Epidermis—shows hyper-parakeratosis and acanthosis

- Papillary dermis shows thin-walled capillary channels
- Dermis shows thick collagen bundles oriented in vertical axis

DIFFERENTIAL DIAGNOSIS

Rudimentary Digit/Polydactyly

- Occurs at the base of fifth finger
- Base of the lesion shows numerous nerve bundles

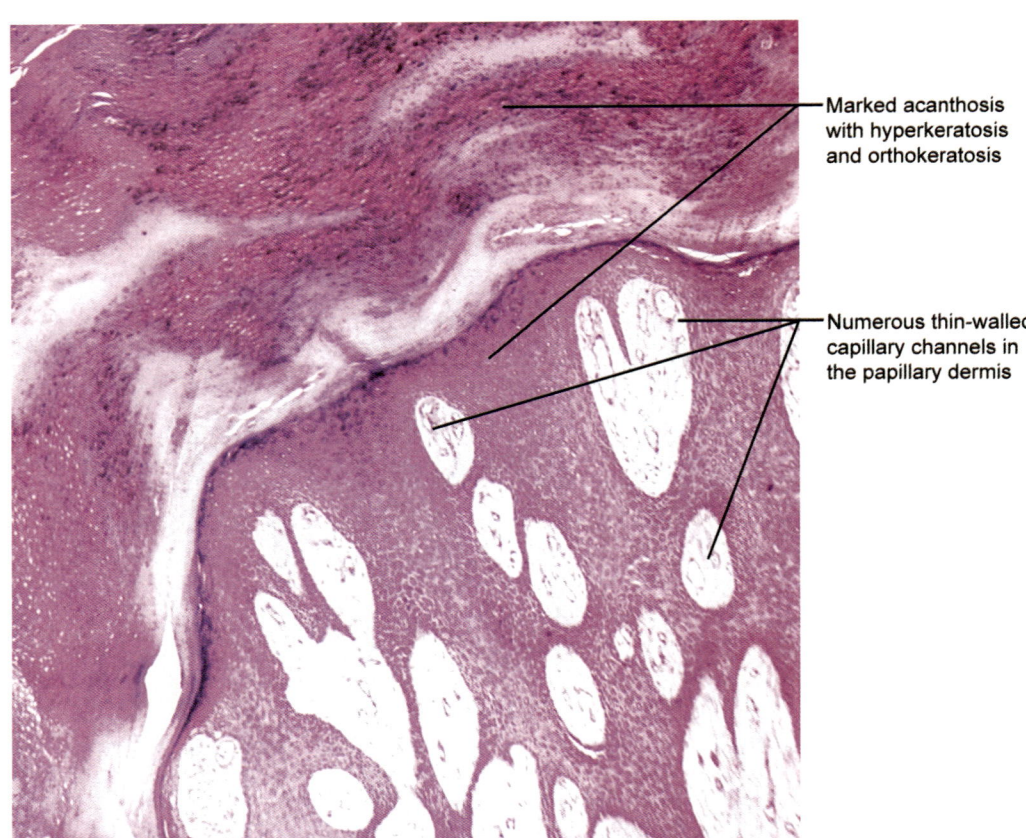

Marked acanthosis with hyperkeratosis and orthokeratosis

Numerous thin-walled capillary channels in the papillary dermis

Fig. 100.1: Fibrokeratoma

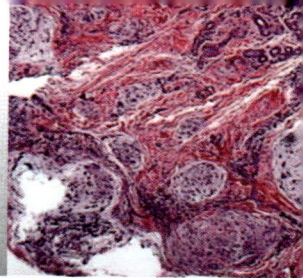

Keratoderma

INTRODUCTION

- Sites—affects palms and soles
- Most commonly affects newborn and children
- Types—diffuse, circumscribed (focal) or punctate

HISTOPATHOLOGY (Figs 101.1 and 101.2)

- Marked hyperkeratosis
- Marked orthokeratosis
- Marked acanthosis
- Thickened granular layer can be seen
- Focal parakeratosis can be seen
- Superficial dermis can show perivascular lympho-cytic infiltrate

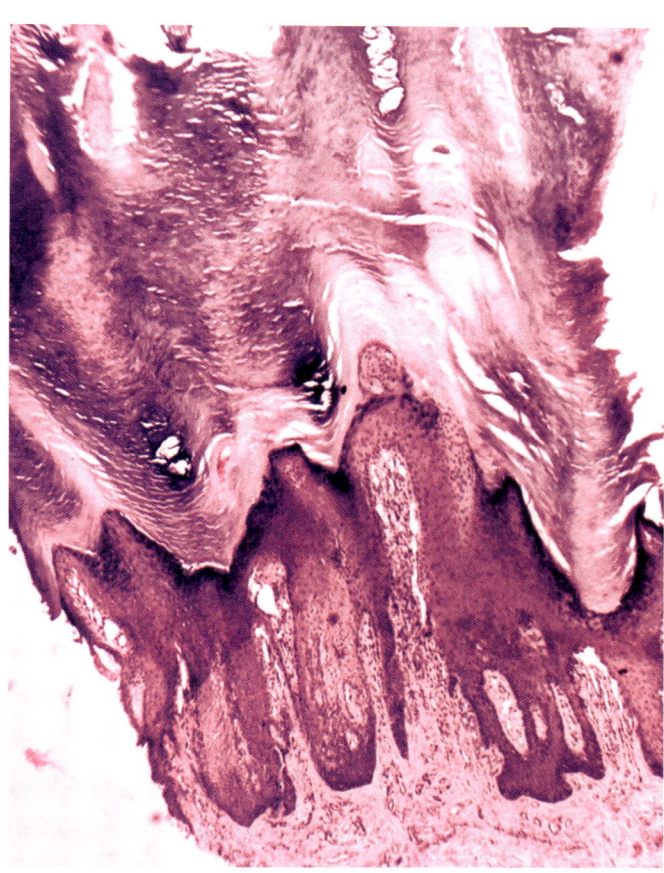

Fig. 101.1: Keratoderma

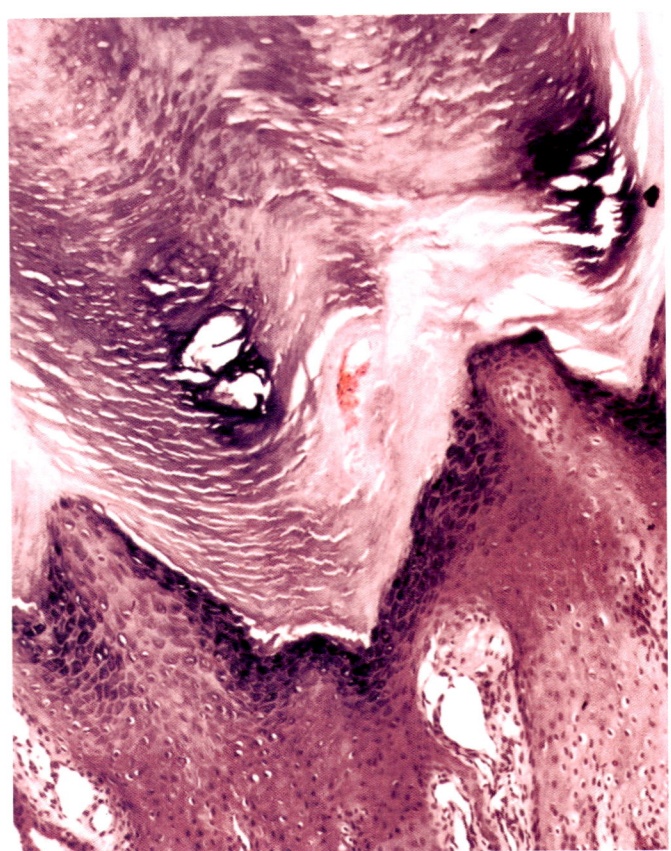

Fig. 101.2: Keratoderma

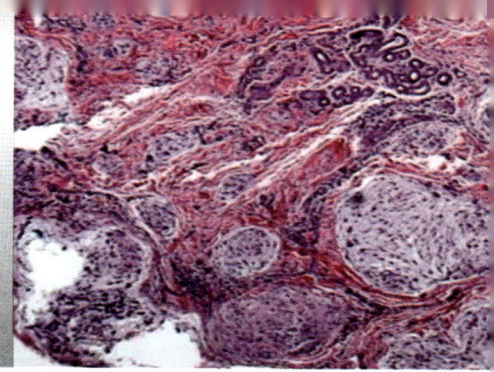

Vascular Tumors

Part 16

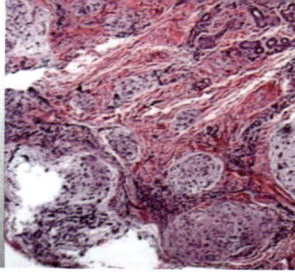

Hemangioma

INTRODUCTION

- A tumor comprising of proliferation of blood vessels
- Presents as red-blue nodules, ranging in size from mm to cm (Fig. 102.1)
- Most common tumors of infancy, with females more commonly affected than males
- Sites—skin of head and neck, trunk and extremities
- Lesions are present at birth and grows over the period of 1–2 years followed by spontaneous regression

HISTOPATHOLOGY (Figs 102.2 to 102.4)

- Upper dermis and deep dermis show numerous dilated capillary channels
- These capillaries are lined by plump endothelial cells and show increased mitosis and are surrounded by peripheral layer of pericytes

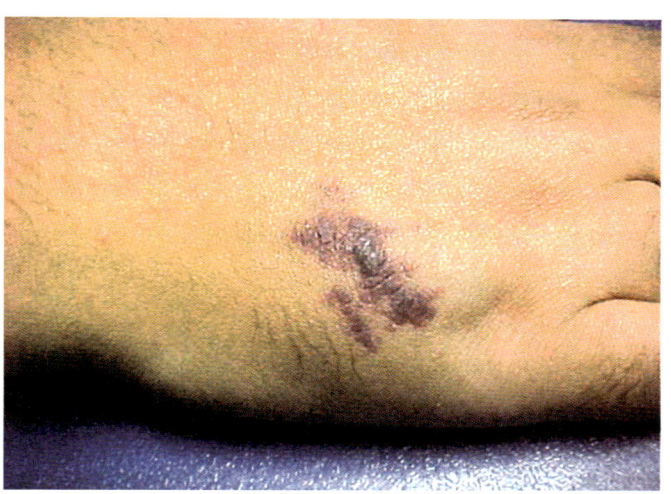

Fig. 102.1: Hemangioma. Bright red, violaceous plaque

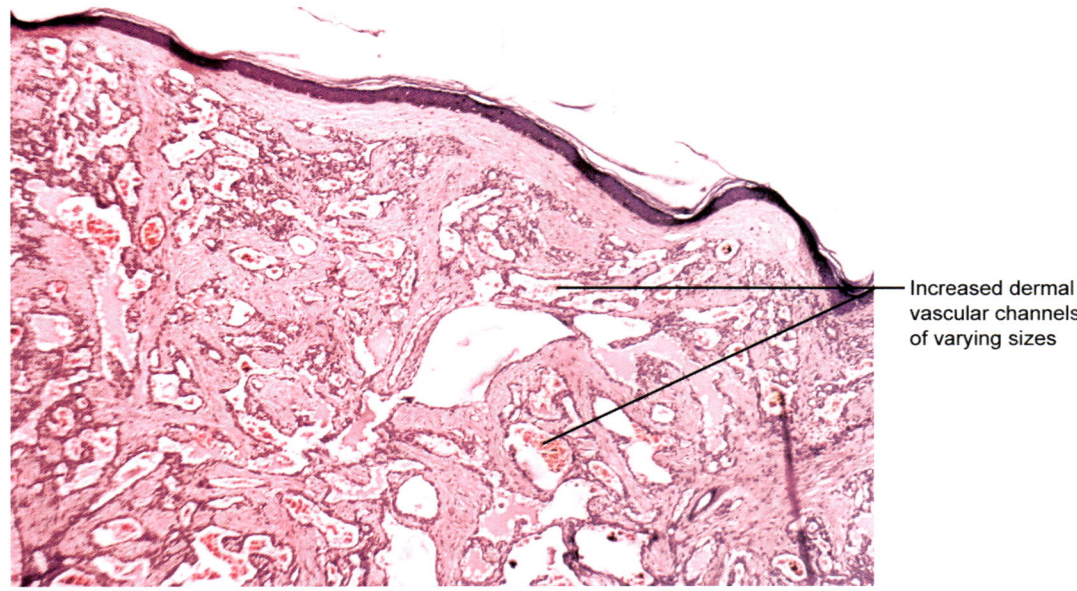

Increased dermal vascular channels of varying sizes

Fig. 102.2: Dermal hemangioma

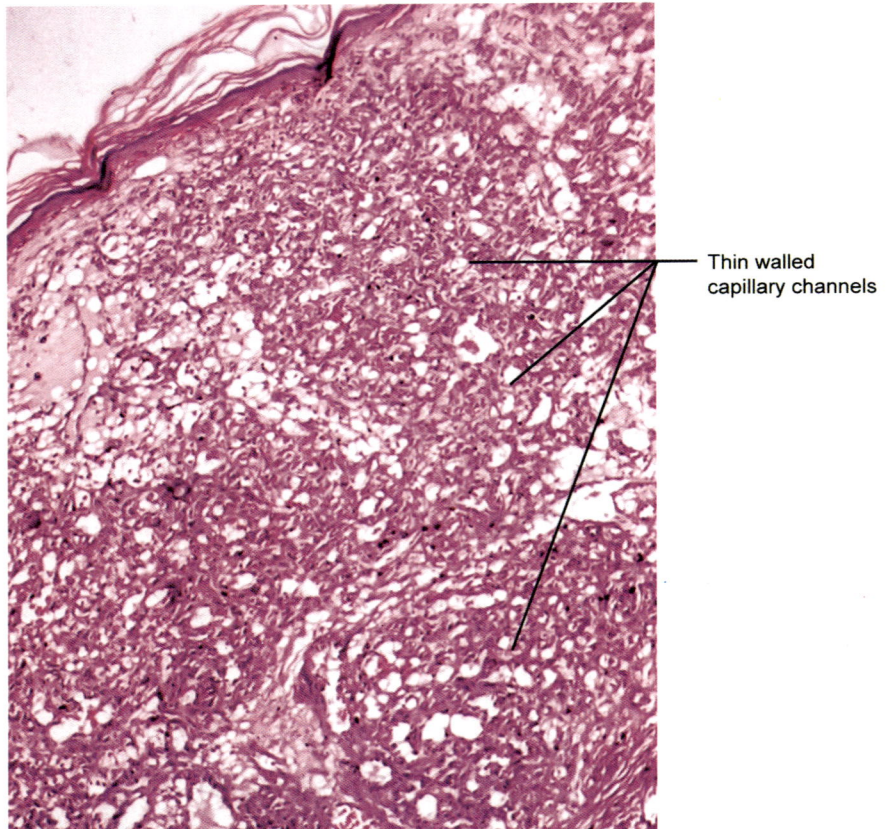

Fig. 102.3: Lobular capillary hemangioma

Thin walled
capillary channels

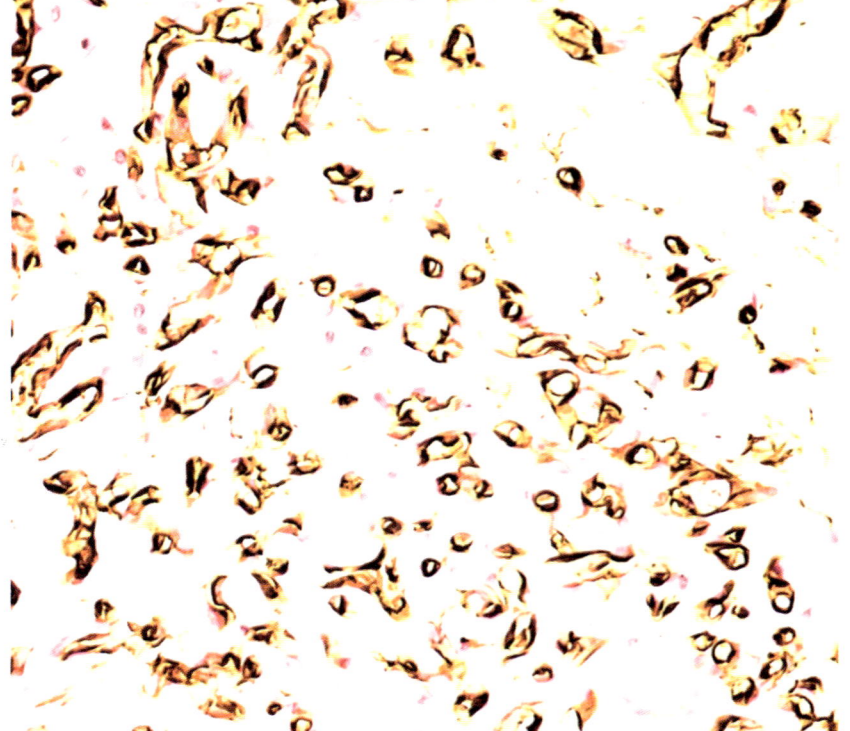

Fig. 102.4: Hemangioma. Dermal vascular channels demonstrating CD34 positivity

IMMUNOHISTOCHEMISTRY

- Endothelial cells demonstrate CD31 or CD34 positivity
- Pericytes show smooth muscle actin positivity

DIFFERENTIAL DIAGNOSIS

Pyogenic Granuloma

- Capillary hemangioma with inflammatory cell infiltrate

Kaposi Sarcoma

- Bizarre vascular spaces which transform into spindle-shaped tumor cells
- Associated with human herpes virus (HHV)-8 infection

Angiosarcoma

- Vascular spaces being lined by atypical endothelial cells, showing nuclear pleomorphism and mitosis

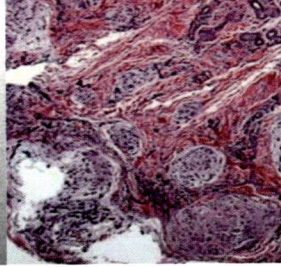

Pyogenic Granuloma

INTRODUCTION

- Also called lobular capillary hemangioma
- Age group—seen in children and young adults (multiple lesions can be seen)
- Affects males more commonly than females
- Sites—affects gingivae, lips, mucosa of the nose, fingers and face

CLINICAL FEATURES

- Presents as a papule or polyp, that bleeds easily (Fig. 103.1)
- Develops at the site of pre-existing injury or infection
- Lesions shrunk and regress by itself

HISTOPATHOLOGY (Figs 103.2 to 103.4)

- Epidermis is attenuated and forms a collarette at the periphery of the lesion
- Lesion resembles granulation tissue

- Capillary proliferation in lobular pattern, which is lined by plump endothelial cells
- Stroma is composed of mixed inflammatory cell infiltrate comprising of lymphocytes, histiocytes, plasma cells and neutrophils
- Lesion in later stages shows only fibrous tissue

IMMUNOHISTOCHEMISTRY

- Endothelial lining of the vessel walls demonstrates CD31 positivity

DIFFERENTIAL DIAGNOSIS

1. Capillary hemangioma
   - Inflammation is absent
2. Bacillary angiomatosis
   - Capillary proliferation with neutrophilic infiltrate
   - Causative organism, i.e. *Bartonella henselae* can be identified with Warthin-Starry stain

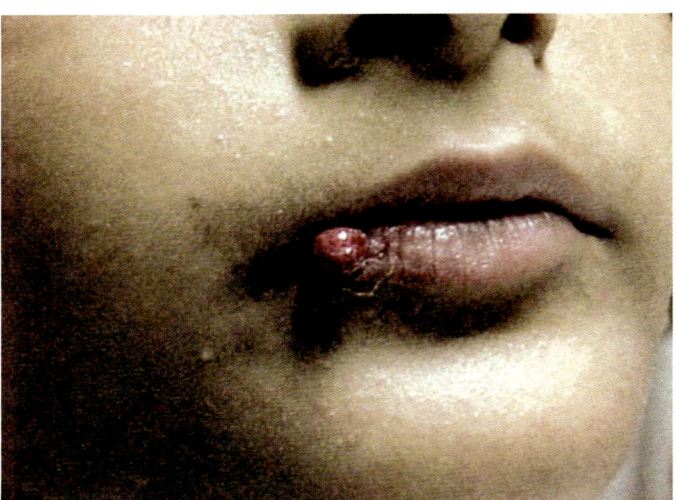

Fig. 103.1: Pyogenic granuloma. Pedunculated reddish papule

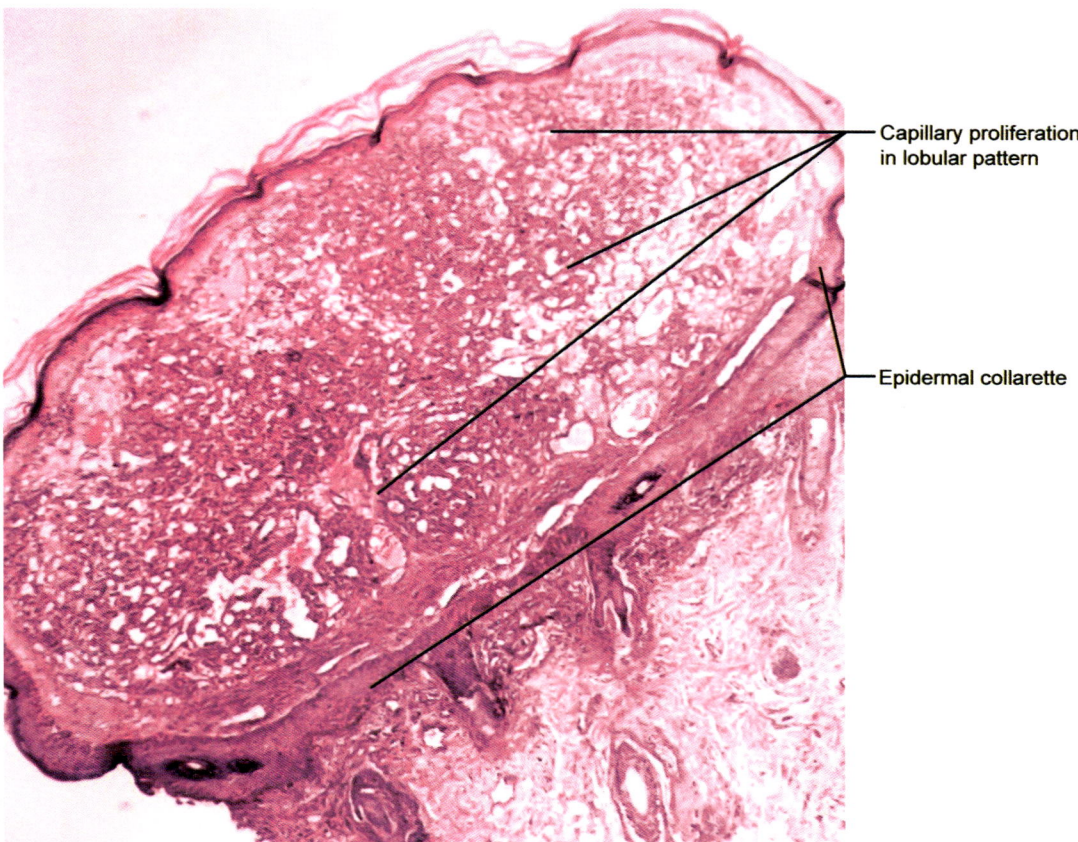

Capillary proliferation
in lobular pattern

Epidermal collarette

Fig. 103.2: Pyogenic granuloma

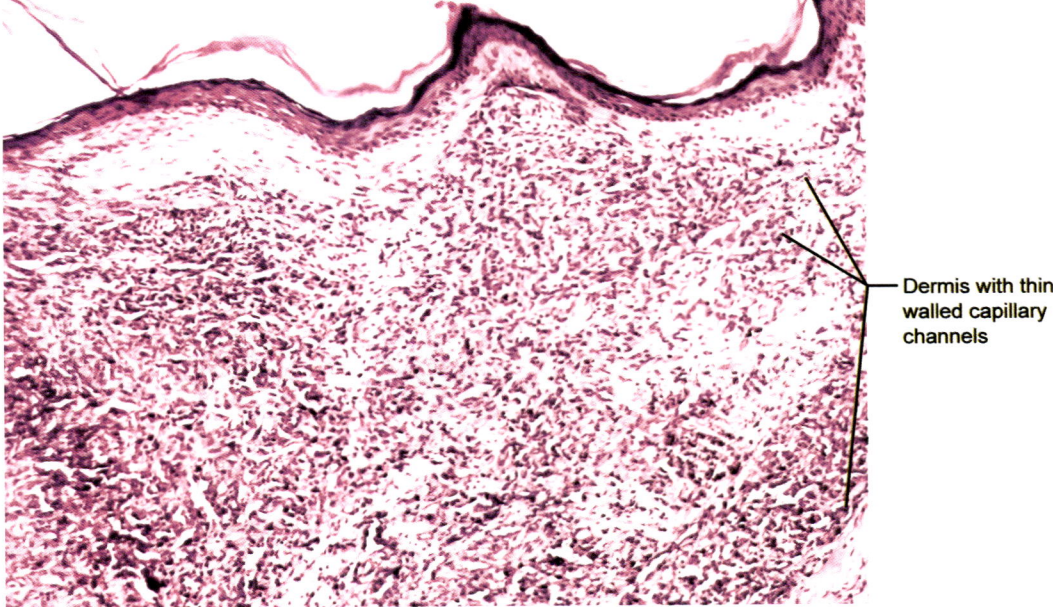

Dermis with thin
walled capillary
channels

Fig. 103.3: Pyogenic granuloma

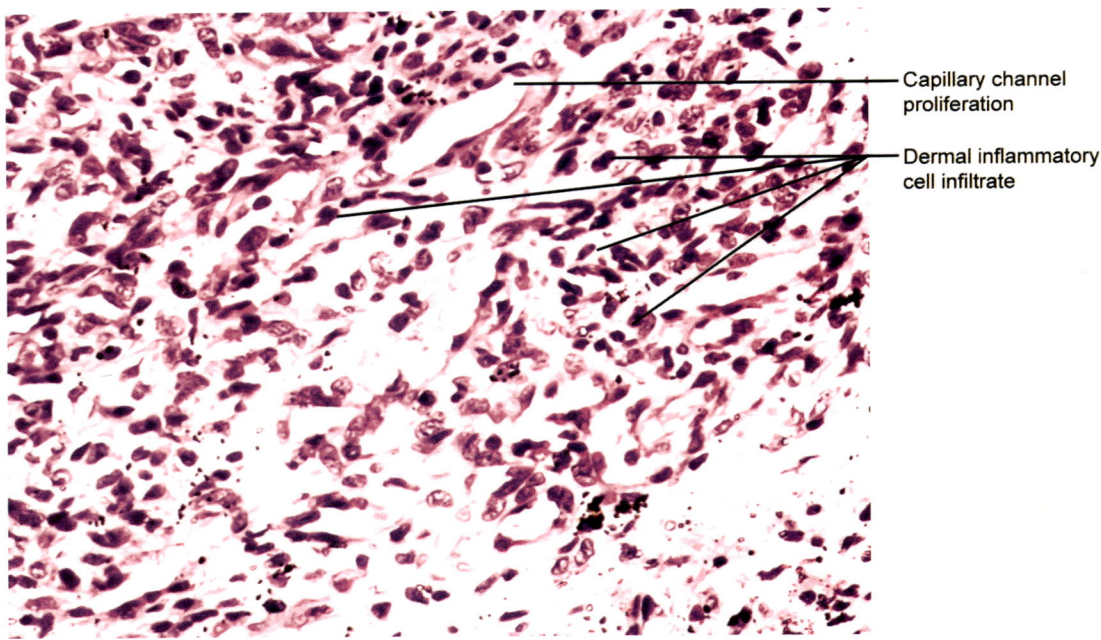

Capillary channel
proliferation

Dermal inflammatory
cell infiltrate

Fig. 103.4: Pyogenic granuloma

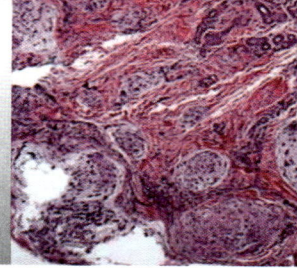

Angiokeratoma

INTRODUCTION

- Lesions occur due to injury, trauma or chronic irritation to the vessel wall of the papillary dermis
- Age group—most commonly affects young adults
- Clinical features—presents as small, warty, well-circumscribed papules
- **Four important clinical variants:** Solitary, angiokeratoma corporis diffusum, Mibelli and Fordyce
- Fabry disease is most commonly associated with angiokeratoma corporis diffusum

SITES

- Solitary angiokeratoma—most commonly affects lower limbs
- Angiokeratoma corporis diffusum—multiple papules on the trunk
- Angiokeratomas of Fordyce—most commonly affects scrotum and vulva (Fig. 104.1)
- Angiokeratomas of Mibelli—affects digits and toes

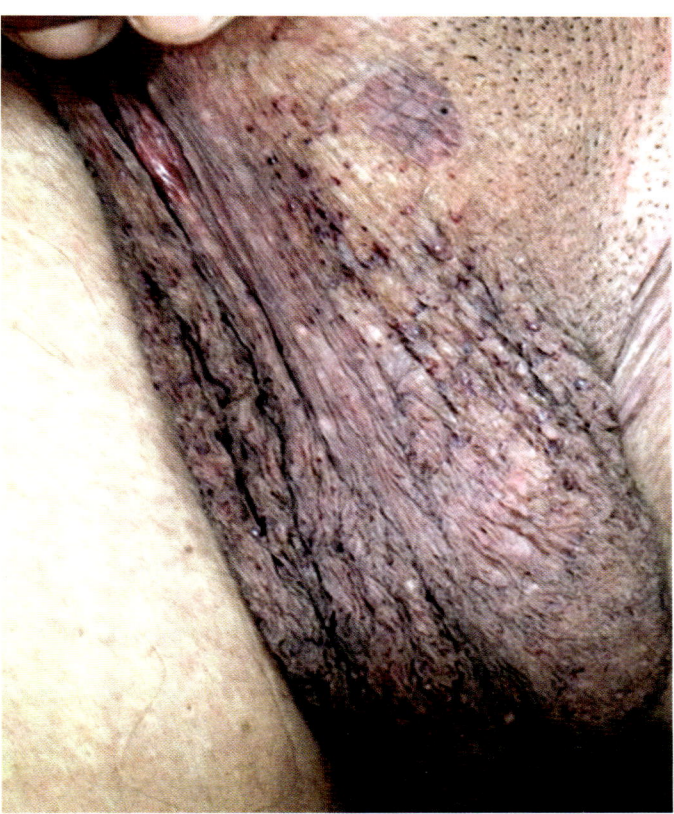

Fig. 104.1: Angiokeratoma (Fordyce type)

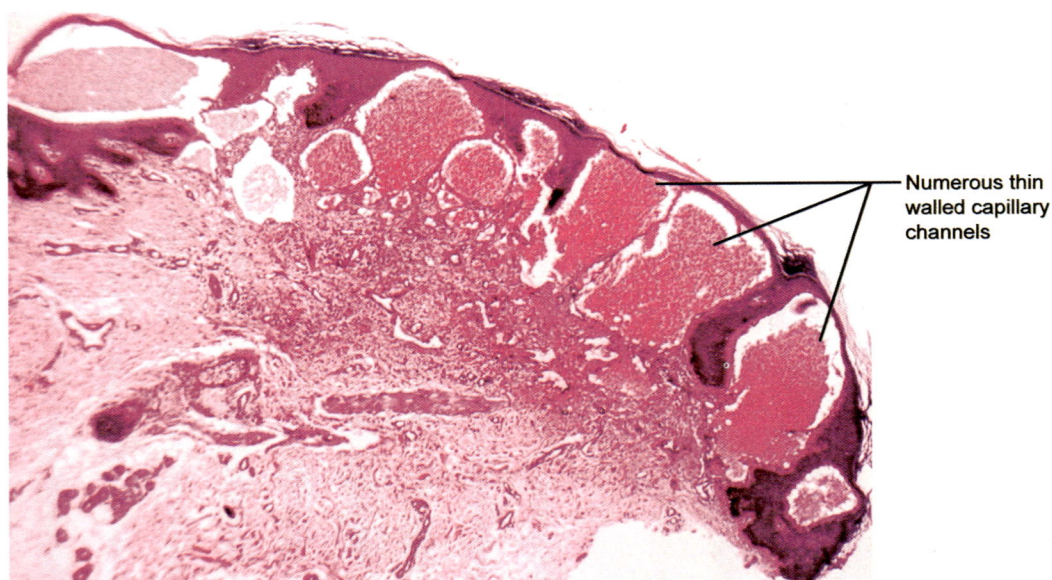

Fig. 104.2: Angiokeratoma

Numerous thin walled capillary channels

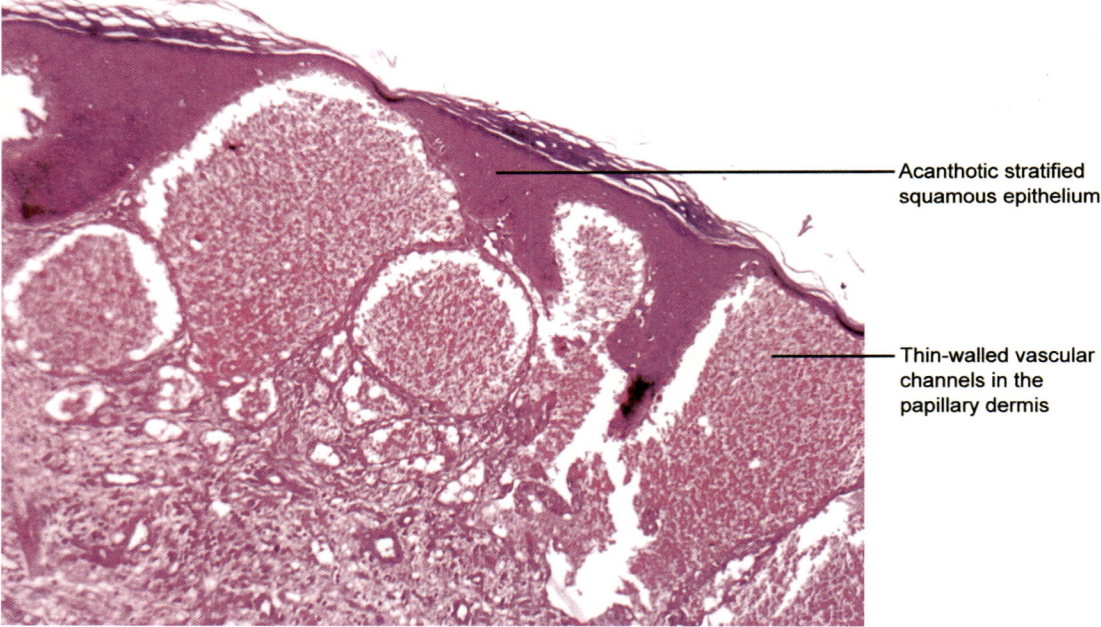

Acanthotic stratified squamous epithelium

Thin-walled vascular channels in the papillary dermis

Fig. 104.3: Angiokeratoma

HISTOPATHOLOGY (Figs 104.2 and 104.3)

- Dilated thin-walled blood vessels, lined by a layer of endothelial cells in the papillary dermis
- Overlying epidermis shows acanthosis, hyperkeratosis with elongation of rete ridges

DIFFERENTIAL DIAGNOSIS

Verrucous Hemangioma (Figs 104.4 and 104.5)

- Acanthosis, hyperkeratosis, papillomatosis, thin walled blood vessels lined by endothelial cells and filled with RBCs can be seen reaching up to the deep dermis

Telangiectasis

- Thin-walled capillaries in upper dermis with normal epidermis

Lymphangiomas

- Thin-walled vessels in the upper and mid-dermis

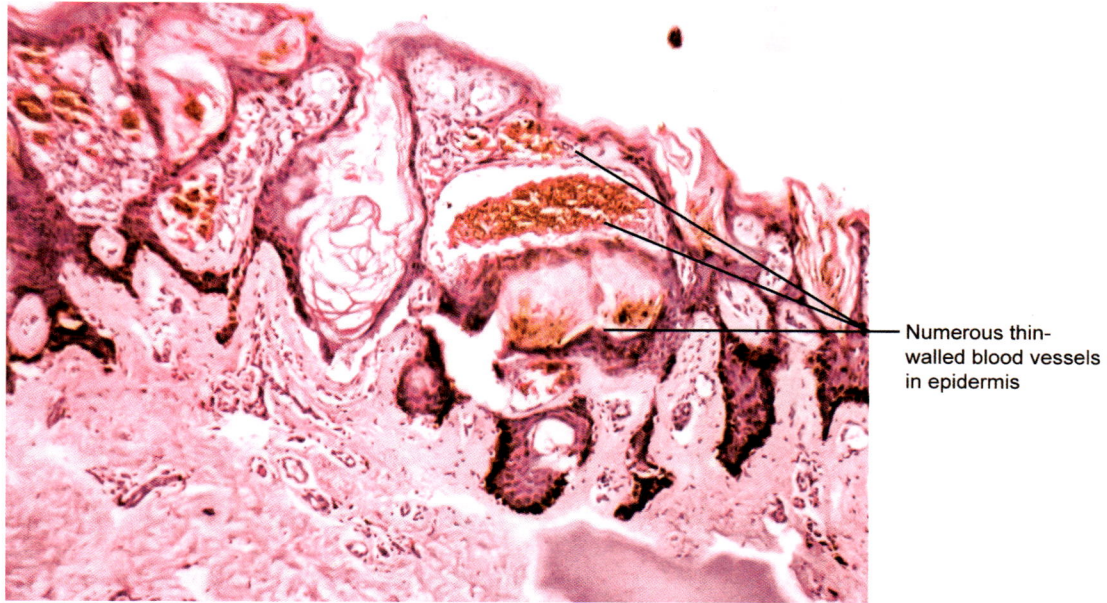

Fig. 104.4: Verrucous hemangioma

Numerous thin-walled blood vessels in epidermis

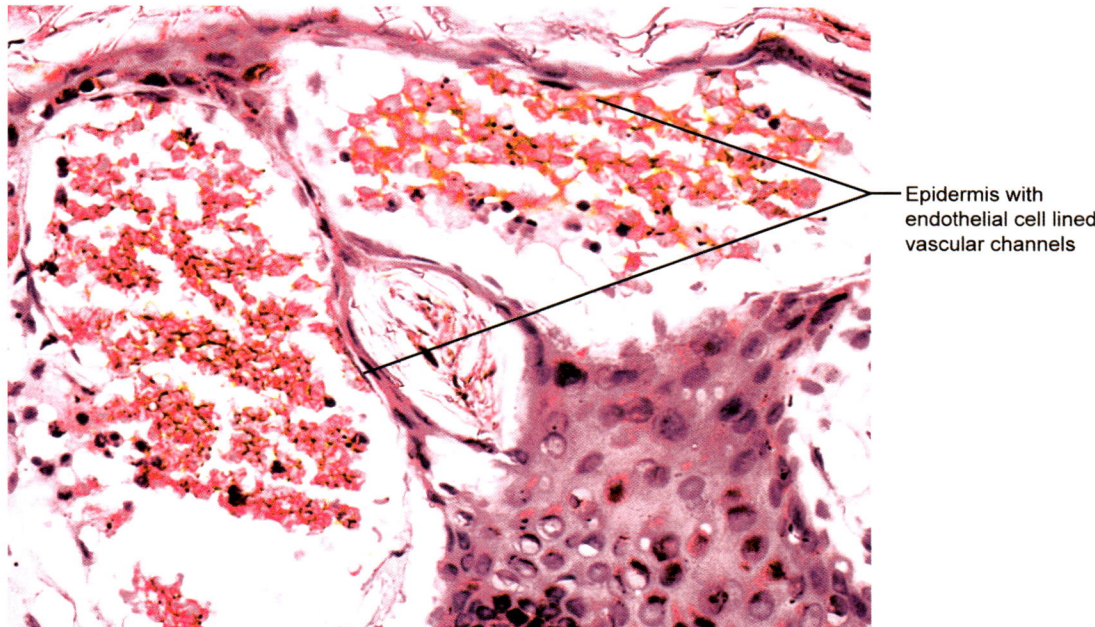

Fig. 104.5: Verrucous hemangioma

Epidermis with endothelial cell lined vascular channels

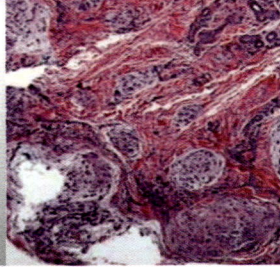

Kaposi Sarcoma

INTRODUCTION

- Slowly growing tumor
- Predisposing conditions—HIV, immunodeficiency, organ transplantation
- Associated with human herpes virus-8 (HHV-8) infection

Demonstration of HHV-8 is done by

- Detecting monoclonal antibody against viral latent nuclear antigen-1 (LNA-1)
- *In situ hybridization* technique

TYPES

Classical Type

- Affects men in fifth decade
- Sites—affects skin of extremities

African (Endemic) Type

- Can present as nodular disease or infiltrative skin lesions or can show lymph node involvement
- Associated with HHV-8 and EBV infections

Kaposi Sarcoma Associated with Immunosuppressive Therapy

- Rare complication following organ transplantation, chemotherapy or corticosteroid use

Epidemic (HIV) Associated Type

- Associated with HIV infection
- Sites—trunk, arms, head and neck

HISTOPATHOLOGY

- Stages—patch stage, plaque stage and nodular stage

Patch Stage

- Vascular channels within the dermis
- Characteristic feature—dermis shows numerous irregular vascular channels separating the collagen bundles

- Promontory sign—irregular vascular channels surround the pre-existing vessel
- Surrounding these irregular vascular channels, lymphoplasmacytic infiltrate can be seen

Plaque Stage

- Diffuse infiltrate of small blood vessels, present throughout the dermis
- Spindle cells, arranged in short fascicles are seen and produce a cleft-like space containing red blood cells
- PAS-positive and diastase resistant intracytoplasmic hyaline globules are present

Nodular Stage

- Well-formed nodules replacing the dermis
- Nodules comprise back to back arrangement of blood vessels with fascicles of spindle-shaped cells in between the vascular spaces
- Spindle cells appear elongated with well-defined cytoplasm and ovoid nuclei
- Nuclear atypia and mitotic activity are absent

IMMUNOHISTOCHEMISTRY

- Tumor cells demonstrate CD31, CD34 and podo-planin positivity
- Stromal spindle cells show HHV-8 antibody positivity

DIFFERENTIAL DIAGNOSIS

Angiosarcoma (Figs 105.1 to 105.4)

- Vascular channels are lined by atypical endothelial cells
- Endothelial cells show hyperchromasia and atypical mitosis
- These vascular channels dissect the surrounding collagen bundles

Kaposiform Hemangioendothelioma

- Seen in children

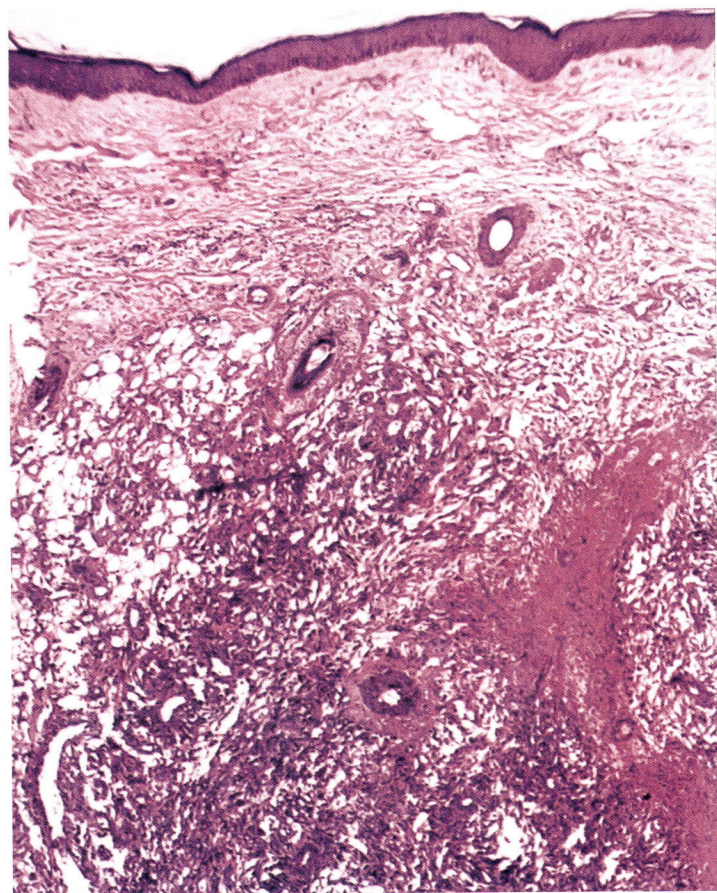

Fig. 105.1: Angiosarcoma. Vascular channels are lined by atypical endothelial cells

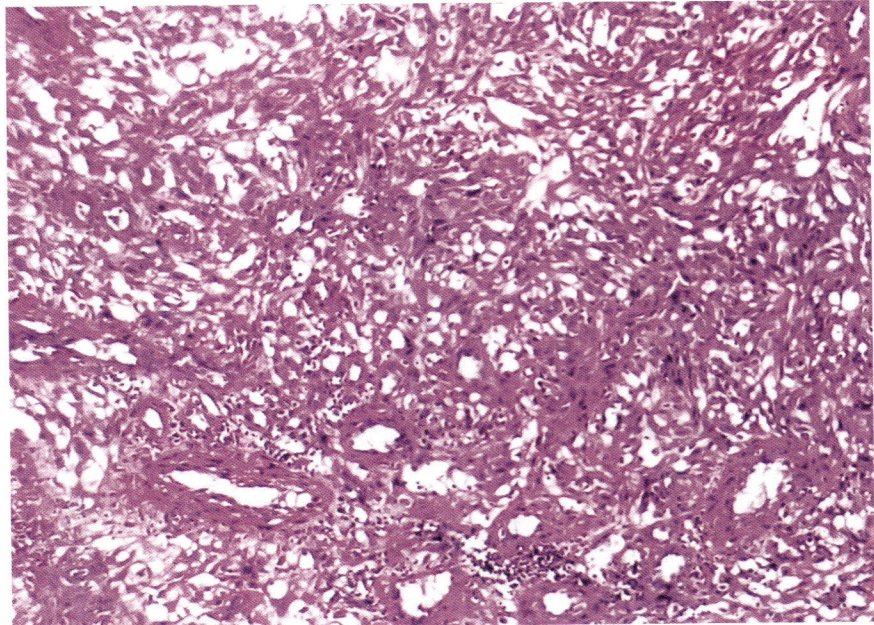

Fig. 105.2: Angiosarcoma. Irregular vascular channels are seen dissecting the surrounding collagen bundles

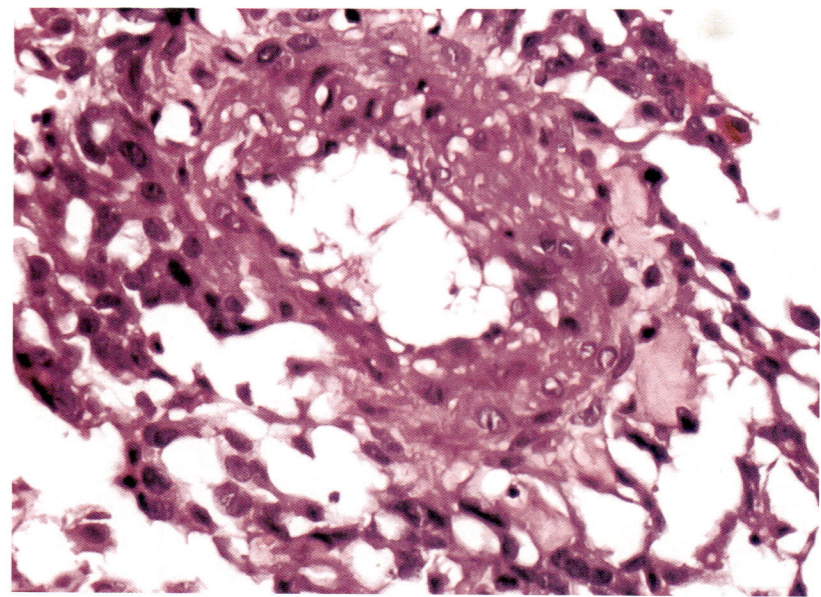

Fig. 105.3: Vascular channel in angiosarcoma with atypical lining endothelial cells

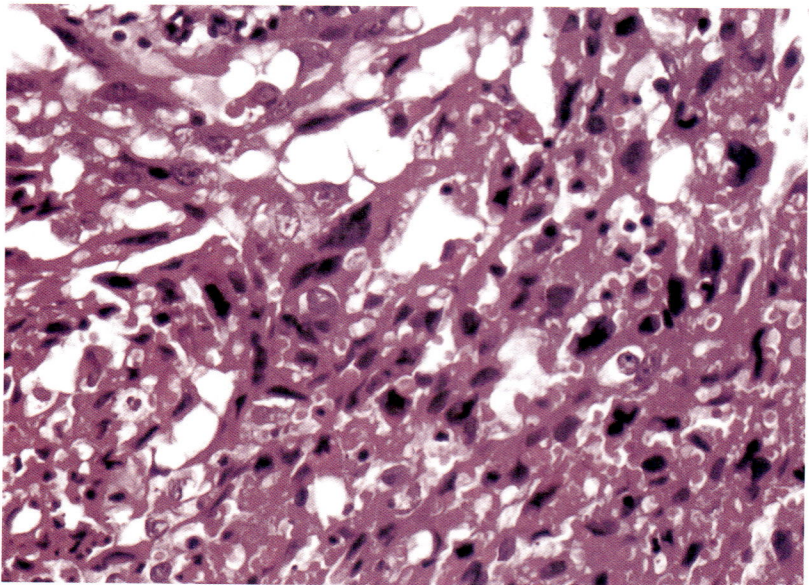

Fig. 105.4: Marked cytological atypia of endothelial cells in angiosarcoma

- Tumor shows lobular growth pattern, and characteristic epithelioid endothelial cells

Lymphangioma
- Difficult to distinguish from Kaposi sarcoma
- Comprises dilated channels lined by flattened endothelial cells

Spindle Cell Hemangioendothelioma
- Vessels appear cavernous
- Endothelial cells appear epithelioid and vacuolated

Pyogenic Granuloma
- HHV-8 antibody demonstration is not seen

Dermatofibroma, Spindle Cell Hemangioendothelioma
- Smooth muscle/spindle cells demonstrate SMA positivity

Aneurysmal Fibrous Histiocytoma
- Presence of foamy macrophages and multinucleated giant cells

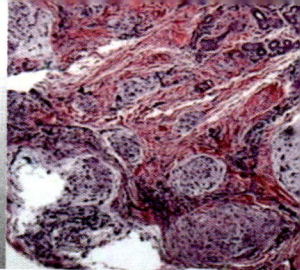

Glomus Tumor

INTRODUCTION

- Presents as a painful, solitary, small, purple dermal nodule
- Most common sites—subungual region, extremities (fingers and toes), forearms and knee

HISTOPATHOLOGY (Figs 106.1 to 106.4)

- Well-circumscribed dermal tumor
- Characterized by solid aggregates of glomus cells surrounding the blood vessels
- Glomus cells have eosinophilic cytoplasm and round to oval nuclei
- Each cell is surrounded by basal lamina
- Characteristically, the tumor cells lack pleomorphism
- Symplastic glomus tumor—tumor cells showing striking nuclear atypia (degenerative change)
- Stroma is characteristically fibrous and contains mast cells
- Immunohistochemistry—tumor cells demonstrate cytoplasmic vimentin and smooth muscle actin positivity

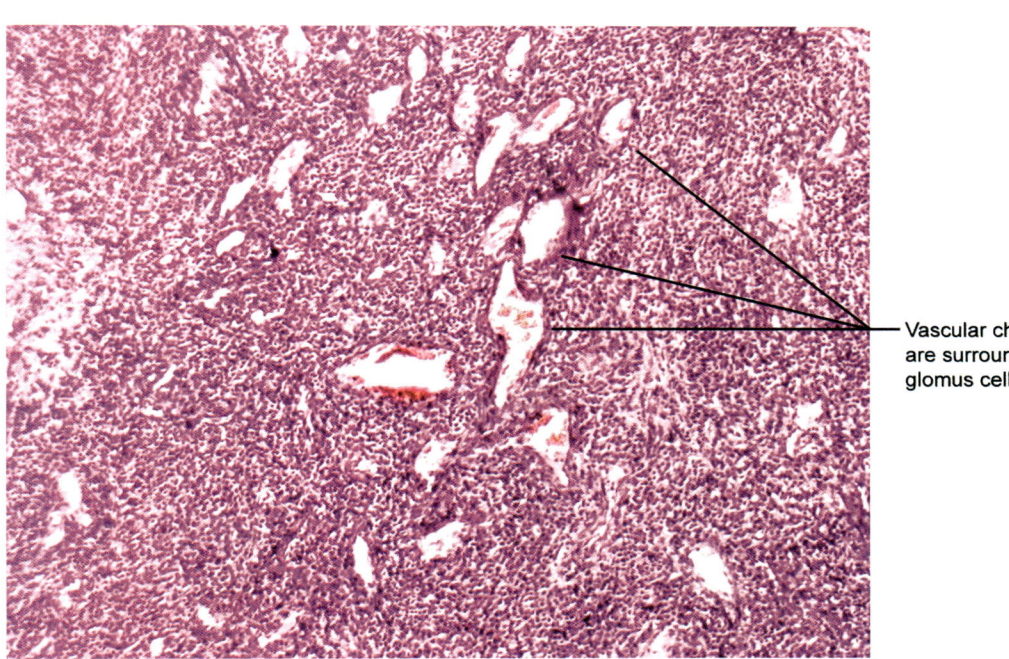

Vascular channels are surrounded by glomus cells

Fig. 106.1: Glomus tumor

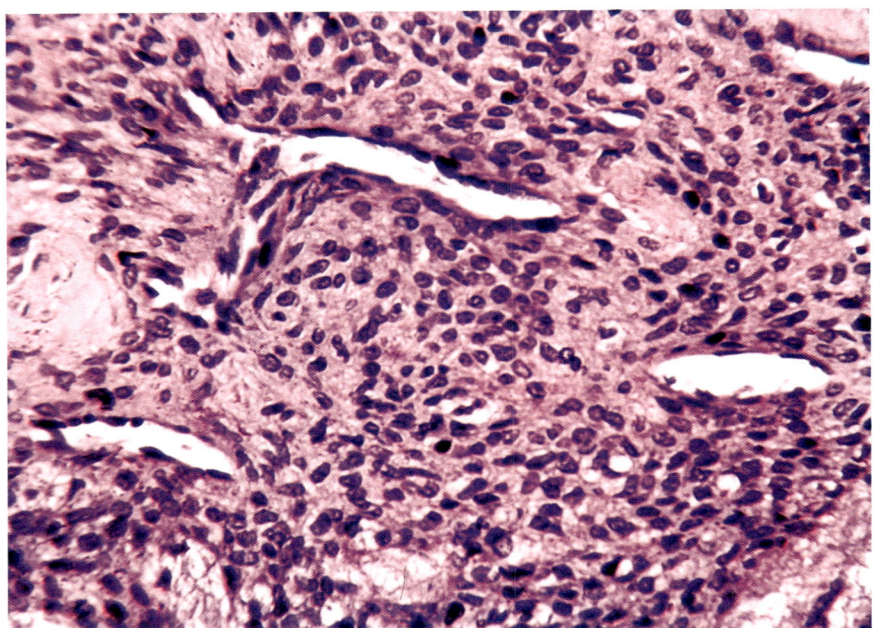

Fig. 106.2: Glomus tumor with glomus cells being small, round and regular with central blue nucleus

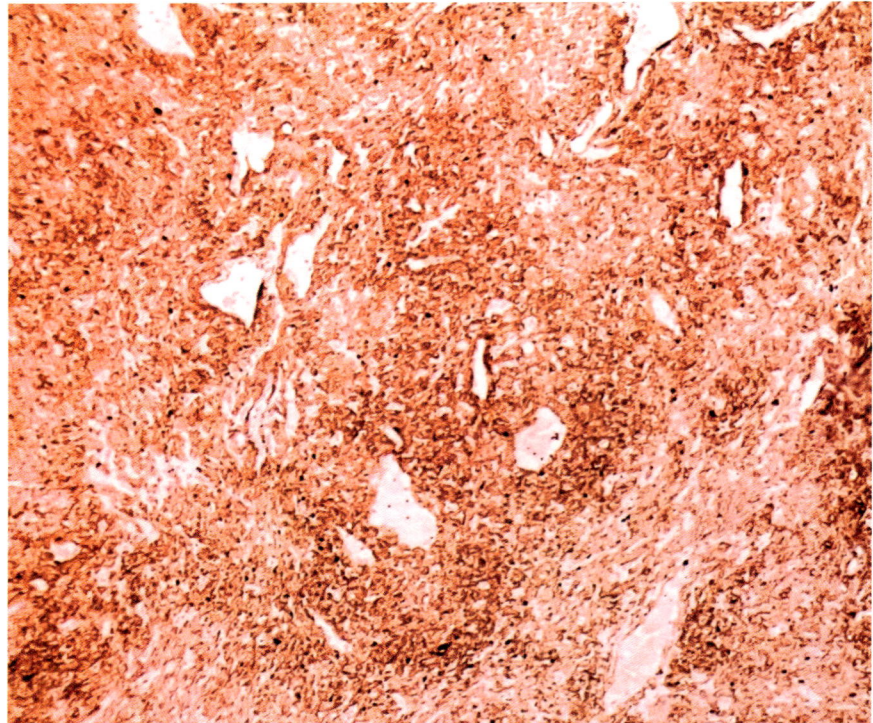

Fig. 106.3: Glomus tumor cells demonstrating smooth muscle actin positivity

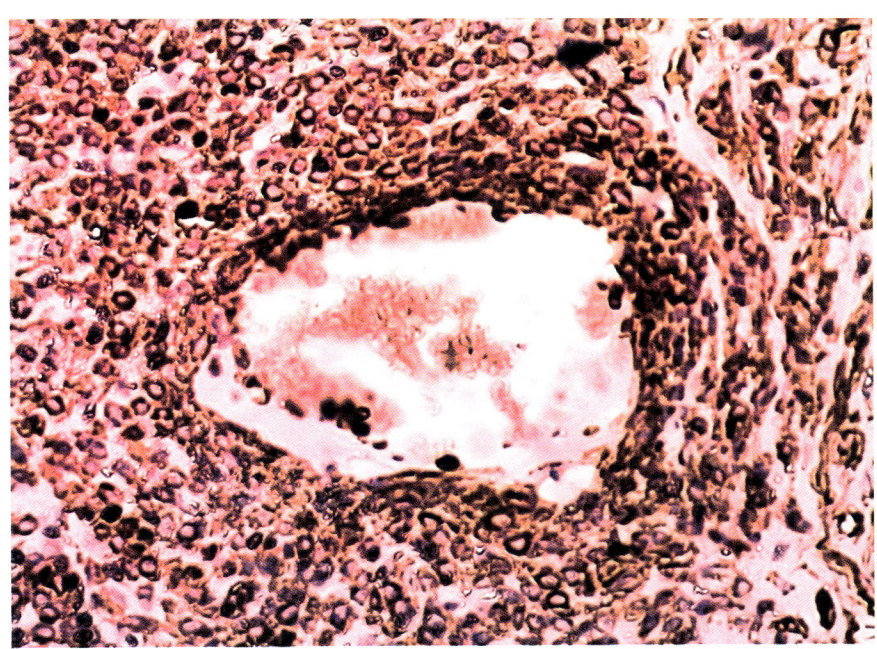

Fig. 106.4: Glomus tumor cells demonstrating cytoplasmic vimentin positivity

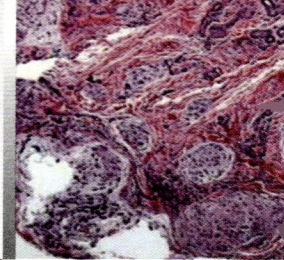

Infantile Hemangioma/ Hemangioendothelioma

INTRODUCTION

- Synonyms—juvenile hemangioma, hemangioma of infancy, strawberry nevus, infantile capillary hemangioma
- Most common tumors of infancy
- Most common sites—head, neck and trunk
- Lesions are raised and appear bright red in color and regress itself by 5–7 years of age

HISTOPATHOLOGY (Figs 107.1 to 107.3)

- Dermis shows vascular channel proliferation, which can extend up to the subcutis
- Vascular lumina of these channels are small, slit-like and are lined by plump endothelial cells

- Lesion shows lobular configuration in the subcutis
- Regression phase shows marked reduction in vessel number and interstitial fibrosis
- Immunohistochemical marker—endothelial cells of the vessel wall show CD31 positivity and GLUT-1 expression

DIFFERENTIAL DIAGNOSIS

Vascular Malformations

- Infantile (juvenile) hemangioma shows diffuse GLUT-1 (glucose transporter-1) positivity
- Vascular malformations are negative for GLUT-1 stain

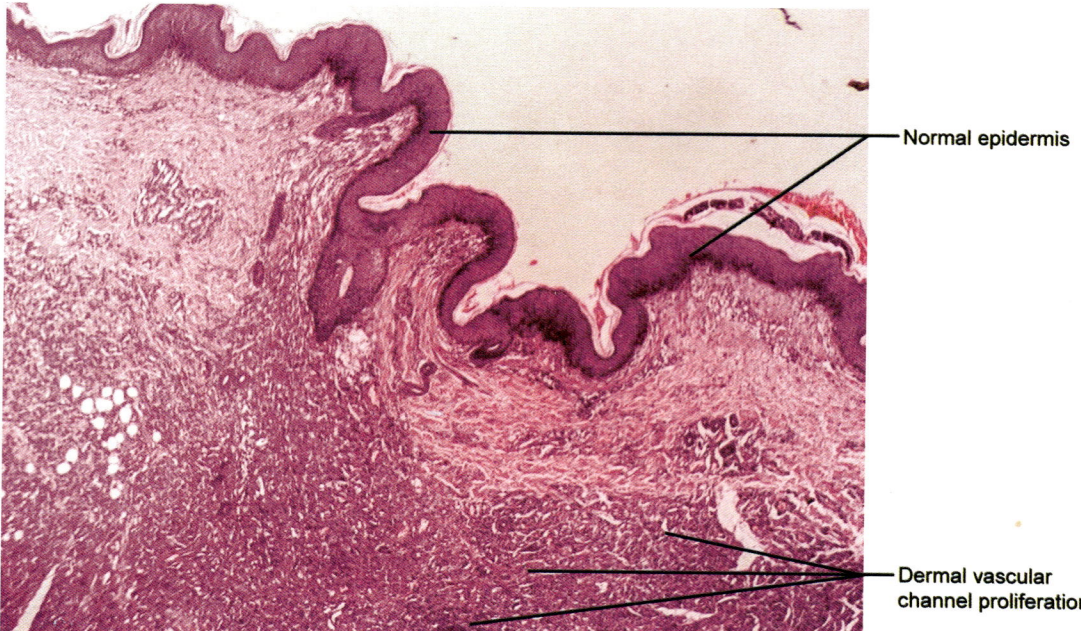

Normal epidermis

Dermal vascular channel proliferation

Fig. 107.1: Infantile hemangioendothelioma

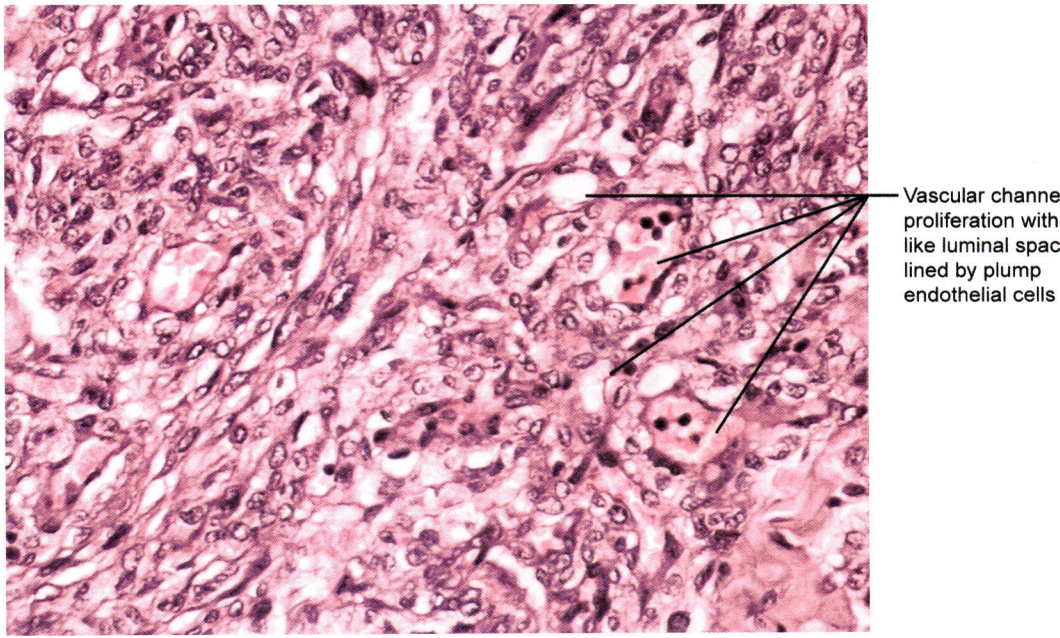

Vascular channel proliferation with slit-like luminal spaces lined by plump endothelial cells

Fig. 107.2: Infantile hemangioendothelioma

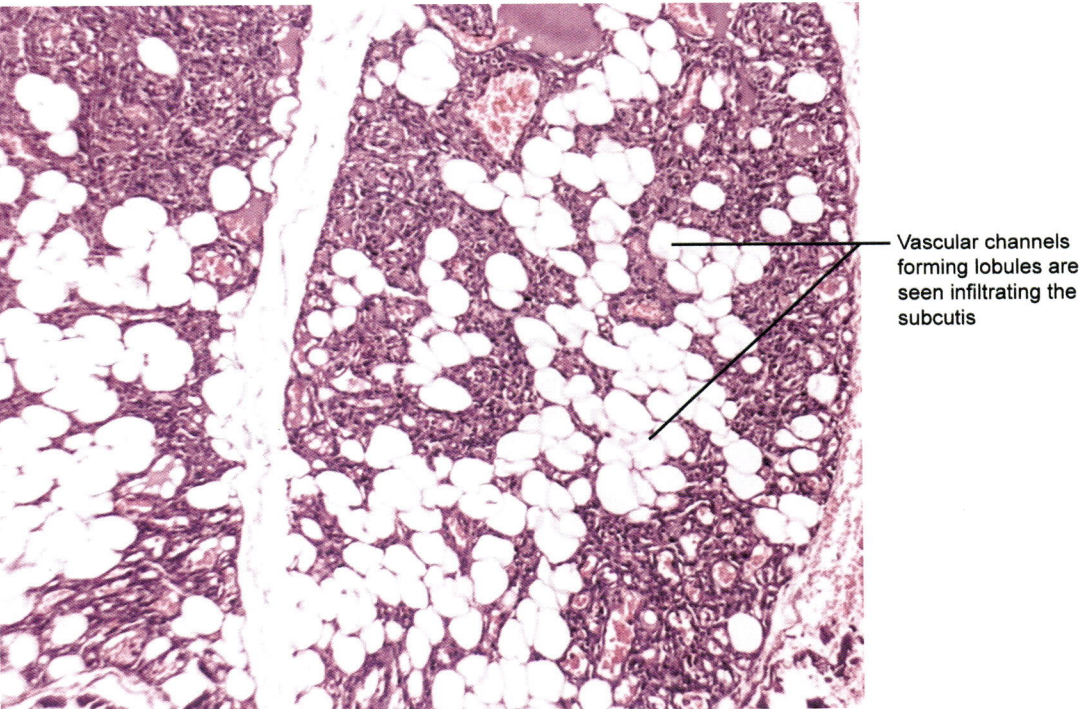

Vascular channels forming lobules are seen infiltrating the subcutis

Fig. 107.3: Infantile hemangioendothelioma

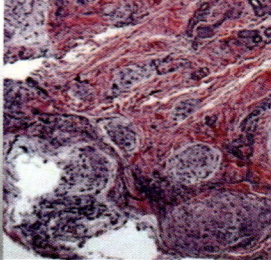

Lymphangioma Circumscriptum

INTRODUCTION

- Developmental malformation
- Age group—affect infants
- Site—most commonly affect extremities
- Clinical presentation—vesicles with clear fluid
- Recurrence is common

HISTOPATHOLOGY (Figs 108.1 and 108.2)

- Epidermis shows acanthosis and hyperkeratosis
- Superficial dermis and papillary dermis show numerous dilated lymphatic channels
- Lymphatic channels show clear fluid or rarely RBCs in their lumen
- Stroma shows lymphocytes

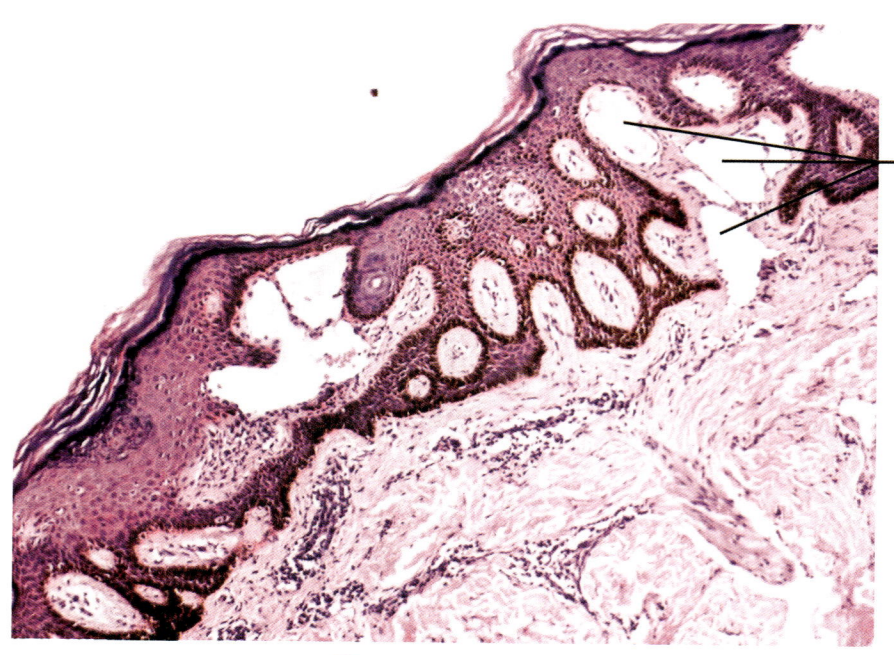

Dilated lymphatic channels in superficial and papillary dermis

Fig. 108.1: Lymphangioma circumscriptum

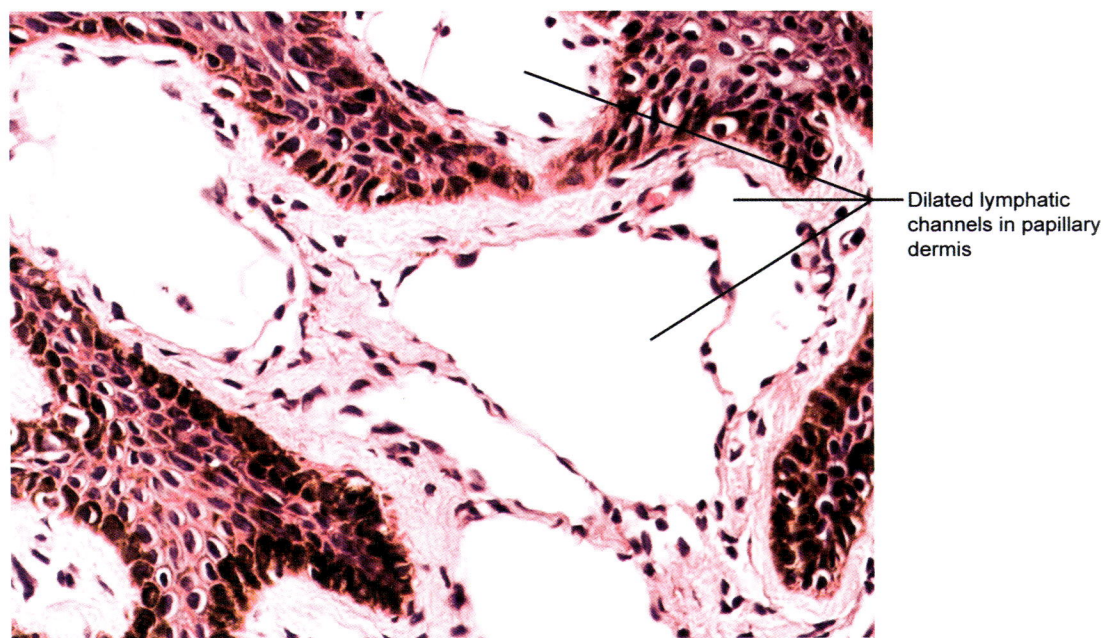

Dilated lymphatic channels in papillary dermis

Fig. 108.2: Lymphangioma circumscriptum

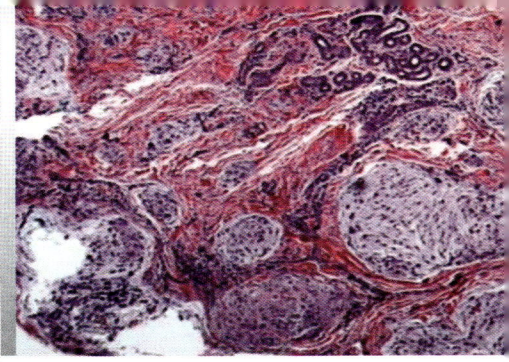

Lymphomas and Pseudolymphomas

Part 17

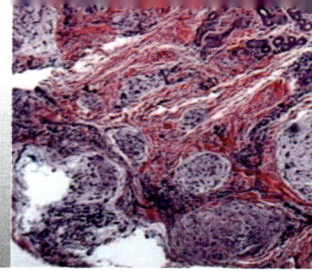

Mycosis Fungoides

INTRODUCTION

- Commonest cutaneous T-cell lymphoma
- Age group—affect individuals of 5th to 6th decade, with males being more commonly affected than females
- Sites—trunk, thighs (lower part) and breasts in females

CLINICAL FEATURES

- Any part of the skin can be involved
- In advanced stage, tumor cells can infiltrate the peripheral blood, and involvement of lymph nodes, bone marrow and other organs can be seen

PRECURSOR LESION

Large Plaque Para-psoriasis (LPP)

- Can progress into mycosis fungoides

- Considered as early mycosis fungoides
- Site—trunk and flexure aspect of extremities
- Presents as large erythematous patches and can measure more than 6 cm in diameter

Lesion Evolutes Through the Following Three Stages

1. **Patch stage**—circumscribed lesions, showing discoloration
2. **Plaque stage**—patches evolve into plaques with infiltration of the surrounding skin
3. **Tumor stage**—formation of nodules, which can show ulceration

HISTOPATHOLOGY (Figs 109.1 to 109.3)

Patch and Plaque Stage

- Early patch stage shows non-specific changes
- In later stages, epidermis shows acanthosis and hyperkeratosis

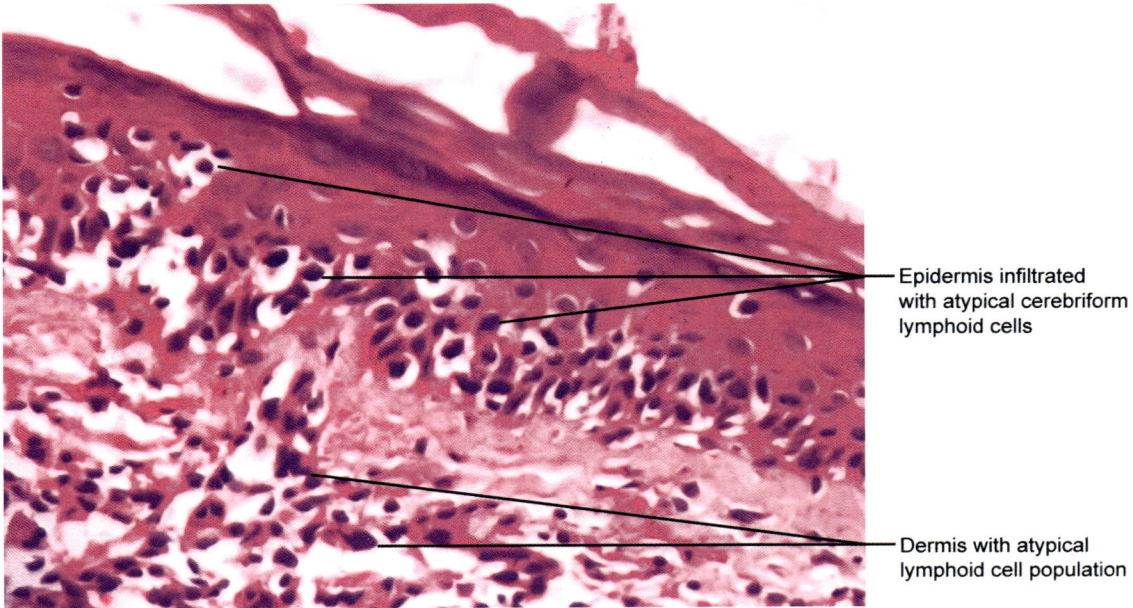

Epidermis infiltrated with atypical cerebriform lymphoid cells

Dermis with atypical lymphoid cell population

Fig. 109.1: Mycosis fungoides

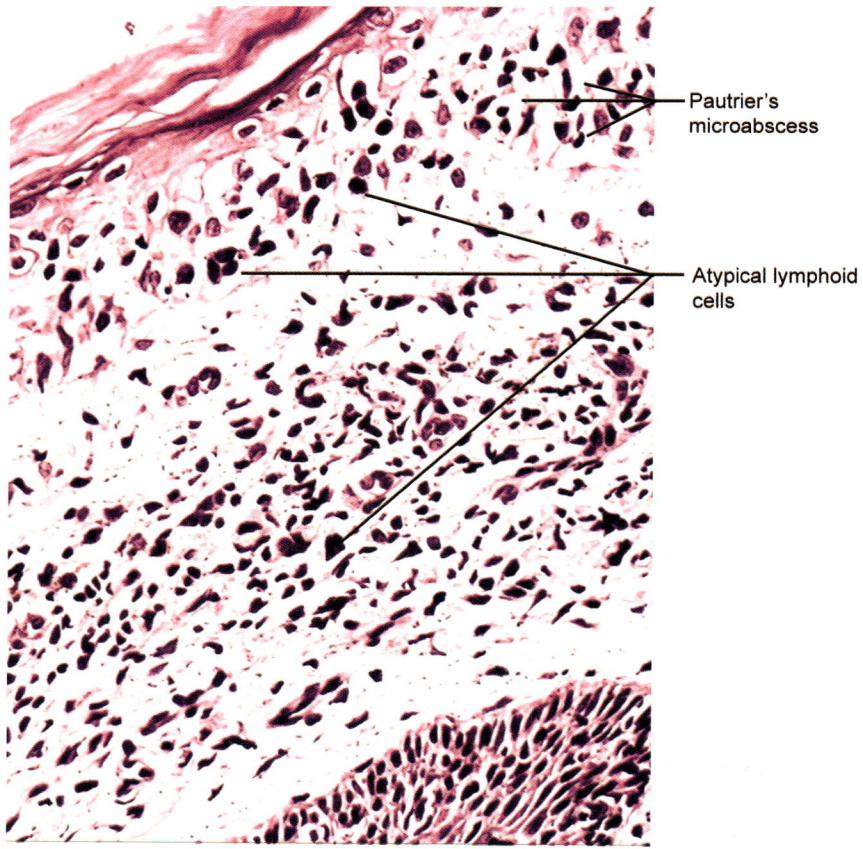

Fig. 109.2: Mycosis fungoides

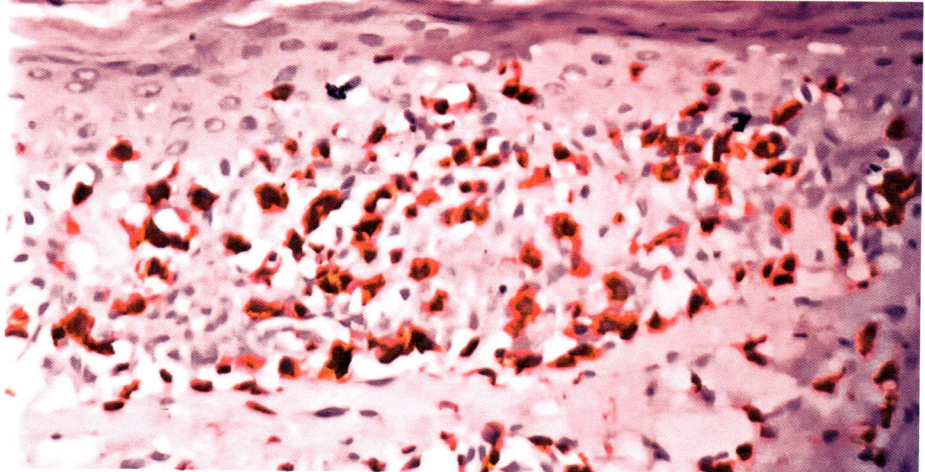

Fig. 109.3: Mycosis fungoides. Atypical lymphoid cells demonstrating CD3 positivity

- Epidermotropism of atypical lymphocytes (lymphocytes arranged throughout the dermoepidermal junction) is seen
- These atypical lymphocytes have cerebriform, indented nuclei, scant eosinophilic cytoplasm and are surrounded by a clear halo

- Pautrier's microabscesses—intraepidermal discrete clusters of atypical lymphocytes
- Dense infiltrate is a feature of plaque stage

Tumor Stage

- Diffuse dermal infiltrate of atypical lymphocytes

- These atypical lymphocytes are of medium to large size and show nuclear pleomorphism
- Epidermotropism and Pautrier's microabscesses are rarely seen
- Transformation to large T-cell lymphoma can occur

ADDITIONAL STUDIES

- Intraepidermal lymphocytes show CD3 and CD4 positivity
- Transformed T-cells of large T-cell lymphoma show CD30 positivity

PROGNOSIS

- In patients with early stage (patch and thin plaque stage), the disease follows an indolent course
- Advanced stage indicates poor prognosis
- Transformation to large T-cell lymphoma signifies worse prognosis

VARIANTS

Pagetoid Reticulosis

- Presents as solitary slow growing patch or plaque, and affects distal limb
- Epidermis shows atypical lymphocytes, arranged in a pagetoid fashion
- These cells have eosinophilic cytoplasm with vesicular chromatin and prominent nucleoli
- Cells show CD3, CD4, and CD30 positivity and are negative for CD8

Syringotropic Mycosis Fungoides

- Atypical lymphocytes involving the eccrine sweat glands

Folliculotropic or Pilotropic Mycosis Fungoides

- Sites—head and neck
- Atypical lymphocytes with cerebriform nuclei are seen around and within the epithelium of hair follicles
- Follicular dilatation and cyst formation can be seen

- These cells are positive for CD3, CD4 and are negative for CD8

Granulomatous Mycosis Fungoides

- An accompanying granulomatous reaction is seen

DIFFERENTIAL DIAGNOSIS

Dermatitis

- Spongiosis
- Acanthosis
- Exocytosis of lymphocytes (in epidermis)
- Lymphocyte does not show atypical features

Pityriasis Lichenoides

- Spongiosis
- Parakeratosis
- Apoptotic keratinocytes and basal cell vacuolization at the dermo-epidermal junction

SÉZARY SYNDROME

- Cutaneous T-cell lymphoma presenting with erythroderma
- Peripheral blood smear shows neoplastic lymphocytes
- Neoplastic T-cells have characteristic cerebriform nuclei
- Age group—more than 60 years with males more commonly affected than females
- Clinical features—presents as a triad of pruritus, erythroderma and lymphadenopathy
- Immunoprofile—Sézary cells show CD2, 3, 4, 5 and CD45-RO positivity and CD8 negativity
- Prognosis—Sézary syndrome has poor prognosis
- **Criteria for diagnosis**
  1. Absolute Sézary cell count of 1000 cells/mm^3
  2. Increased CD4+ T-cell population, with CD4+/CD8+ T-cell ratio >10
  3. Demonstration of abnormal T-cells in the peripheral blood

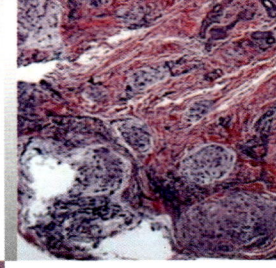

Primary Cutaneous CD30-positive Lymphoproliferative Diseases

Includes
1. Lymphomatoid papulosis (LyP)
2. Primary cutaneous anaplastic large cell lymphoma

LYMPHOMATOID PAPULOSIS (LYP)

INTRODUCTION

- Lymphoproliferative disease affecting the skin
- Age group—affect individuals in third to fourth decade of life
- Presents as erythematous to red-brown papules, nodules or plaque
- Site—trunk and extremities
- Can show spontaneous regression and prognosis is good
- Characterized by atypical lymphoid cells in a polymorphous inflammatory background
- Can progress to malignant lymphoma (Hodgkin disease or Mycosis fungoides)

HISTOPATHOLOGY

Type A

- Dermal infiltrate of anaplastic lymphocytes showing marked nuclear pleomorphism and mitosis
- Background shows neutrophils and eosinophils

Type B

- Band-like infiltrate of atypical lymphocytes in the upper dermis

Type C

- Nodular collection of anaplastic lymphoid cells

IMMUNOHISTOCHEMISTRY

- Atypical lymphoid cells show T-cell marker positivity (i.e. CD3, CD4)

- Tumor cells in Type A and C LyP show CD30 positivity, which is negative in tumor cells of Type B LyP

PRIMARY CUTANEOUS ANAPLASTIC LARGE CELL LYMPHOMA (C-ALCL)

INTRODUCTION

- Large atypical lymphoid cells, which show CD30 positivity
- Age group—sixth decade
- Clinical presentation—solitary firm nodule, that grows rapidly and ulcerates
- Site—most commonly affects extremities and head
- Predisposing factors—most commonly affects HIV patients
- Spontaneous regression can occur, and has good prognosis
- C-ALCL is negative for anaplastic lymphoma related tyrosine kinase (ALK) gene

HISTOPATHOLOGY

- Nodular infiltrate of anaplastic, pleomorphic lymphoid cells
- Tumor cells have round, oval or indented nuclei and are called as "hallmark" or "buttock cells"
- Frequent mitotic figures can be seen
- Infiltrate of small lymphocytes and eosinophils surround these atypical cells

IMMUNOHISTOCHEMISTRY

- Atypical lymphoid cells show CD2, CD3, CD4 positivity
- Anaplastic tumor cells show CD30 positivity (in 75% of cases)

DIFFERENTIAL DIAGNOSIS

Mycosis Fungoides

- Pleomorphic tumor cells resemble type LyP B

Hodgkin Lymphoma

- Cutaneous form is very rare
- Tumor cells demonstrate CD-30 positivity

Keratoacanthoma

- Can resemble lymphoma grossly
- Can be easily differentiated on histopathological examination

Verruca Vulgaris, Molluscum Contagiosum, Scabies and PLEVA

- Show CD30 positive lymphocytes

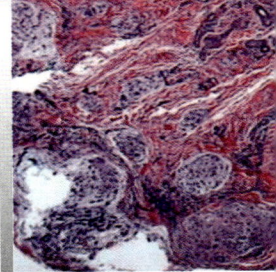

Primary Cutaneous Follicle Center B-cell Lymphoma

INTRODUCTION

- Low grade cutaneous B-cell lymphoma
- Age group—middle age adults
- Most favored sites—trunk, head and neck
- Clinical features—presents as red-brown to blue nodules or plaques (Fig. 111.1)
- t (14;18) chromosomal translocation or bcl-2 gene rearrangements are absent

HISTOPATHOLOGY (Figs 111.2 and 111.3)

- Grenz zone—present between the normal epidermis and tumor cells
- Dermis and subcutaneous tissue show lymphoid follicles (follicular pattern) with monotonous population of tumor cells
- Follicles do not show tingible body macrophages
- Other patterns of arrangement—mixed follicular and diffuse pattern or diffuse pattern

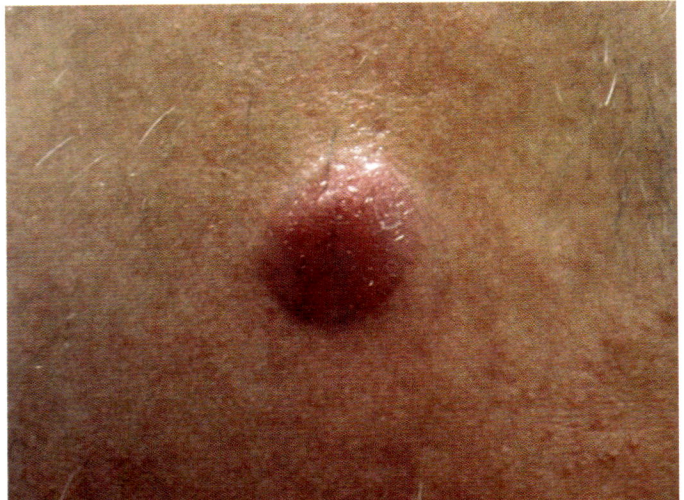

Fig. 111.1: Cutaneous B-cell lymphoma. Solitary firm, erythematous plaque

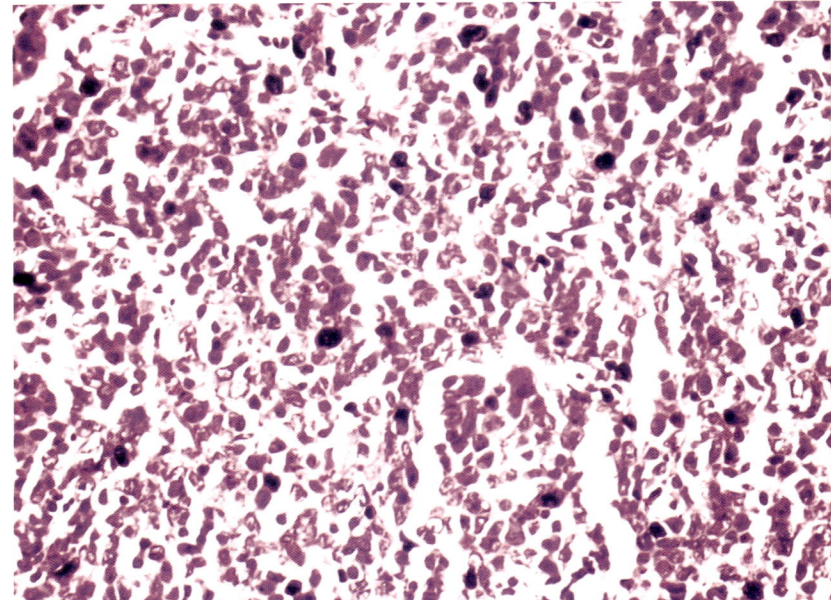

Fig. 111.2: Cutaneous lymphoma. Dermal infiltrate comprising of monotonous population of lymphoid cells

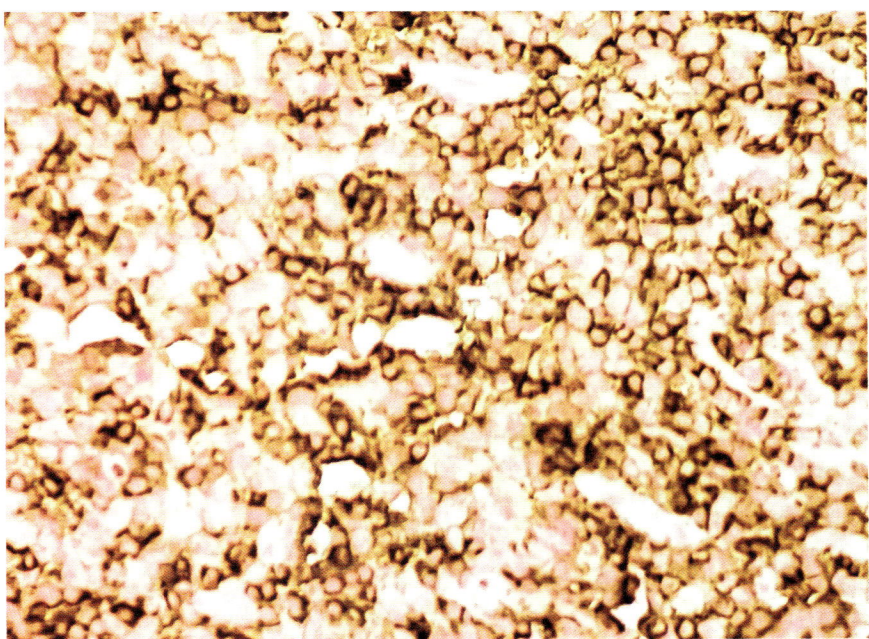

Fig. 111.3: Lymphoid cells demonstrating CD45/leucocyte common antigen (LCA) marker positivity

- Tumor cells are composed of mixture of cleaved cells (centrocytes) and non-cleaved cells (centroblasts)

IMMUNOHISTOCHEMISTRY

- Tumor cells express B-cell markers, i.e. CD19, CD 20, CD 79a and bcl-6
- Interfollicular zones show presence of small clusters of CD10+/bcl-6+ cells
- Tumor cells are negative for bcl-2

PROGNOSIS

- Excellent prognosis
- Local recurrences can occur

DIFFERENTIAL DIAGNOSIS

Primary Cutaneous Marginal Zone B-cell Lymphoma

- In between the follicles, there occurs monocytoid cells or poorly differentiated tumor cells
- Tumor cells demonstrate bcl-2, CD-5 positivity and are negative for bcl-6 and CD-20

Cutaneous B-cell Pseudolymphoma

- Presence of uniform germinal centers with tingible body macrophages

Diffuse Large Cell B-cell Lymphoma, Leg Type

- Tumor cells demonstrate bcl-2 positivity

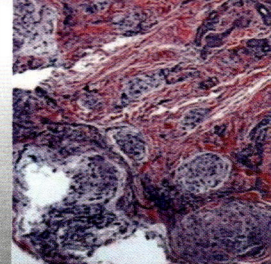

Cutaneous B-cell Pseudolymphoma

INTRODUCTION

- Also commonly known as lymphocytoma cutis or lymphadenosis benigna cutis
- Etiology—*Borrelia burgdoferi* infection (children and young adults), physical and chemical agents, microbes, drugs and tattoos
- Clinical presentation—presents as solitary, reddish brown nodules
- In cases of *Borrelia burgdorferi* infection, skin of ear lobes, nose, nipples, inguinal region and scrotum are commonly involved

HISTOPATHOLOGY

- Dermis shows nodules of reactive follicles
- Follicles show tingible body macrophages
- At the periphery of lesions, lymphoid follicles between collagen bundles can be seen
- Infiltrate of T-cells, histiocytes, eosinophils and plasma cells can be seen

IMMUNOHISTOCHEMISTRY

- Tumor cells demonstrate B-cell marker positivity, i.e. CD20 and CD79a
- CD21 positive follicular dendritic cells are also present

DIFFERENTIAL DIAGNOSIS

Primary Cutaneous Follicle Center B-cell Lymphoma

- Accumulation of B-cells with centrocytic differentiation

Primary Cutaneous Marginal Zone B-cell Lymphoma

- In between the follicles, there occurs monocytoid cells or poorly differentiated tumor cells
- Tumor cells demonstrate bcl-2 positivity and are negative for bcl-6

Prognosis

- Excellent, and it regresses spontaneously

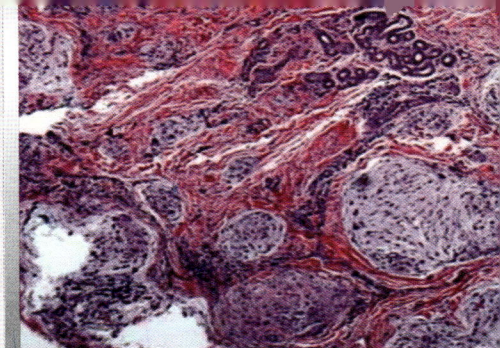

Histiocytosis and Mastocytosis

Part 18

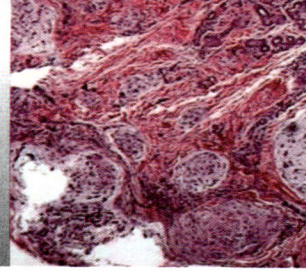

Langerhans Cell Histiocytosis 113

INTRODUCTION

- Disorder characterized by proliferation of dendritic cells, which morphologically resembles Langerhans cells
- Cell of origin—dendritic cells
- Age group—less than 5 years of age
- Spontaneous regression can occur
- Affects skin, bones, ears, liver, lungs and lymph nodes

CLINICAL FEATURES

Four Clinical Forms

Letterer-Siwe Disease

- Most severe form
- Age group—affect infants and children
- Can present as diffuse skin papules or pustules or plaques
- Sites—scalp, face, trunk, and buttocks (Fig. 113.1)

- Clinical features—fever, weight loss, enlarged lymph nodes, hepatosplenomegaly and bone lesions can be seen
- High mortality rate

Hand-Schüller-Christian Disease

- Age group—affects children and adults
- Clinical features—triad of osteolytic bone lesions, diabetes insipidus (due to involvement of pituitary) and exophthalmos; otitis media, hepatosplenomegaly, pulmonary, bone and skin involvement can be seen
- Has better prognosis than Letterer-Siwe disease

Eosinophilic Granuloma

- Age group—most commonly affect adults
- Clinical features—solitary bone or skin lesions involving deep dermis or subcutis
- Has favorable prognosis

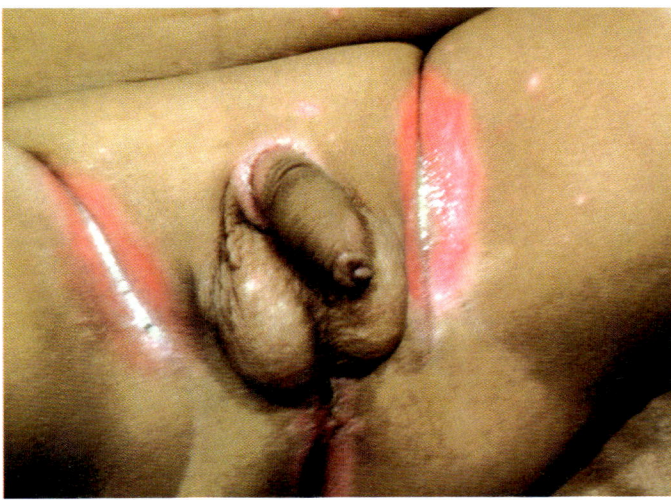

Fig. 113.1: Langerhans cell histiocytosis (Letterer-Siwe disease). Erythematous papular rash in groin, resembling a diaper rash

Congenital Self-healing Reticulohistiocytosis

- Self-limited disease
- Age group—seen congenitally after birth or in neonatal period
- Clinical features—skin lesions in the form of papules, vesicles, plaques or nodules
- Can present as blueberry muffin syndrome
- Has excellent prognosis

HISTOPATHOLOGY (Figs 113.2 and 113.4)

- Langerhans cell appears kidney-shaped with pale eosinophilic cytoplasm
- Accompanying eosinophils, xanthocytes, granulomas or giant cells can be seen
- Epidermotropism of Langerhans cells, with a band-like infiltrate around the dermoepidermal junction can be seen

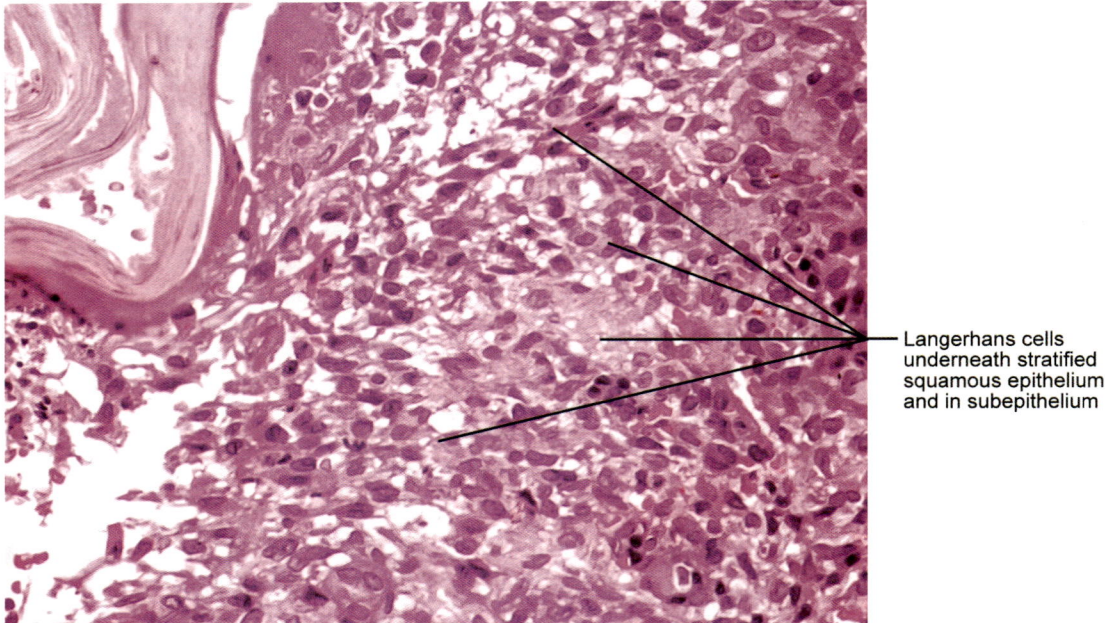

Langerhans cells underneath stratified squamous epithelium and in subepithelium

Fig. 113.2: Langerhans cell histiocytosis

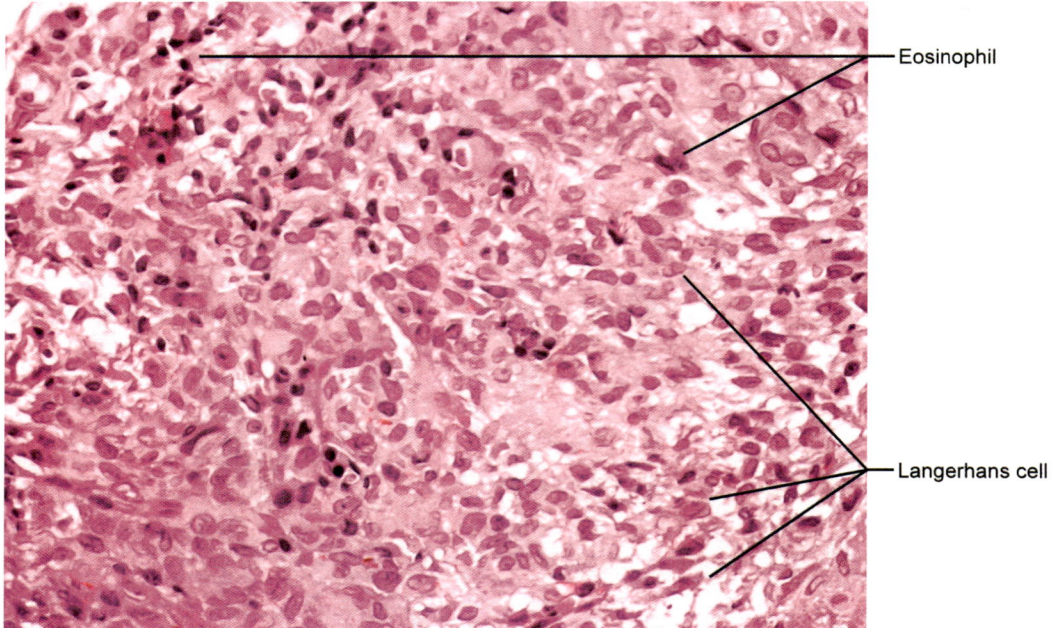

Eosinophil

Langerhans cell

Fig. 113.3: Langerhans cell histiocytosis

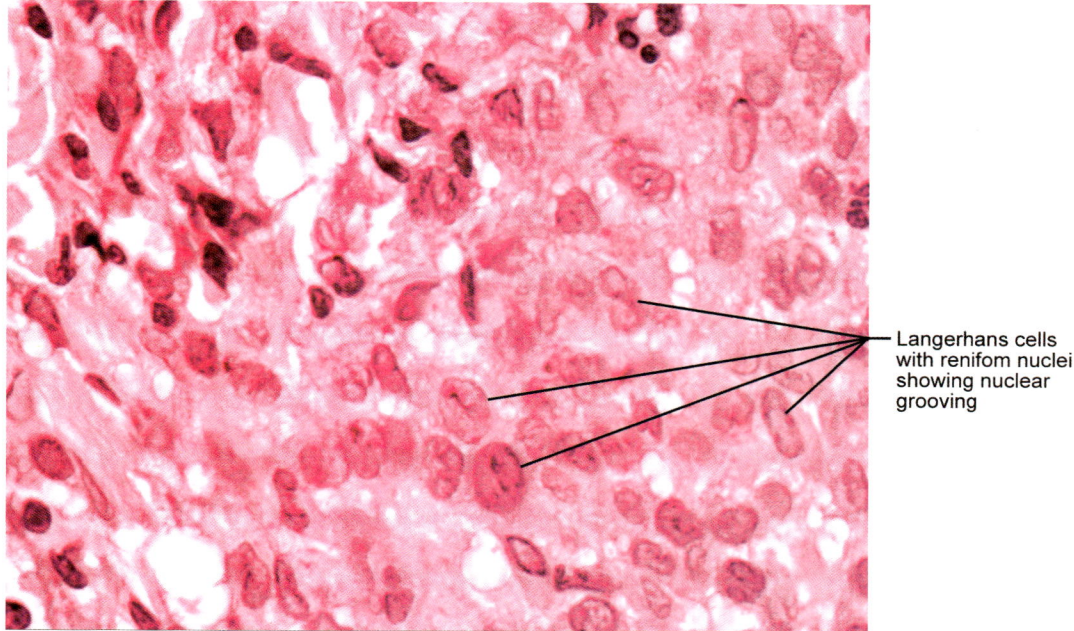

Langerhans cells with renifom nuclei showing nuclear grooving

Fig. 113.4: Langerhans cell histiocytosis

ADDITIONAL STUDIES

- Immunohistochemistry—Langerhans cells express CD-1a, S-100 and langerin
- Electron-microscopy—Birbeck granules, which appear rod or racket shaped
- Genetics—BRAF–V600E mutations can be seen

PROGNOSIS

- Children under 2 years of age with multi-system disease and organ dysfunction have poor prognosis

DIFFERENTIAL DIAGNOSIS

1. *Dermatitis*
   - Acanthosis, spongiosis and exocytosis of lymphocytes are seen

2. *Mycosis fungoides*
   - Intraepidermal collection of T-cells (Pautrier's microabscesses) are seen

3. *Paget disease*
   - Clear tumor cells in the epidermis, showing cytokeratin-7, Her-2-neu and EMA positivity

4. *Superficial spreading melanoma*
   - Atypical melanocytes scattered in the epidermis, showing S-100 and Melan A positivity

5. *Juvenile Xanthogranuloma*
   - Touton giant cells with proliferation of xanthocytes

6. *Rosai-Dorfman disease*
   - Sinus histiocytosis with massive lymphadenopathy

7. *Dermatopathic lymphadenopathy*

8. *Malignant lymphomas*

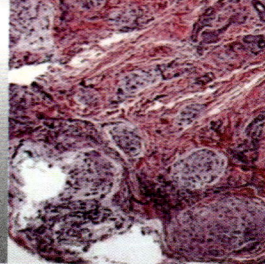

Juvenile Xanthogranuloma

INTRODUCTION

- Benign lesion
- Characterized by localized proliferation of macrophages, foam cells and giant cells
- Age group—affects children with median age of diagnosis being 2 years
- Males are more commonly affected than females
- Can present as single or multiple nodules
- Sites—head and neck (most commonly scalp), upper trunk, upper limbs
- Other sites—eyes, lungs, bones, kidney, pericardium, colon, ovaries, testes and central nervous system

ETIOLOGY

- Increased uptake of low-density lipoprotein (LDL) cholesterol
- Genetics—has an association with Neurofibromatosis 1 and 2

CLINICAL FEATURES

Clinical features can present as:
1. **Papular form:** Characterized by numerous red-brown papules
2. **Nodular form:** Characterized by yellow, round to oval nodules, measuring 1–2 cm in diameter

HISTOPATHOLOGY (Figs 114.1 to 114.4)

- **Early lesions**—macrophages with abundant eosinophilic cytoplasm, in upper and mid-dermis
- **Late lesions**—macrophages with lipid laden cytoplasm (foam cells), multinucleated giant cells (Touton type) with wreath of nuclei surrounding the center

ADDITIONAL STUDIES

- Immunohistochemistry—macrophages show CD 68 positivity

PROGNOSIS

- Cutaneous disease—good prognosis, and lesions can heal spontaneously
- Central nervous involvement—if present, can be fatal
- Peripheral smear—should be done periodically during first two years of life, because of increased risk of juvenile chronic myeloid leukemia

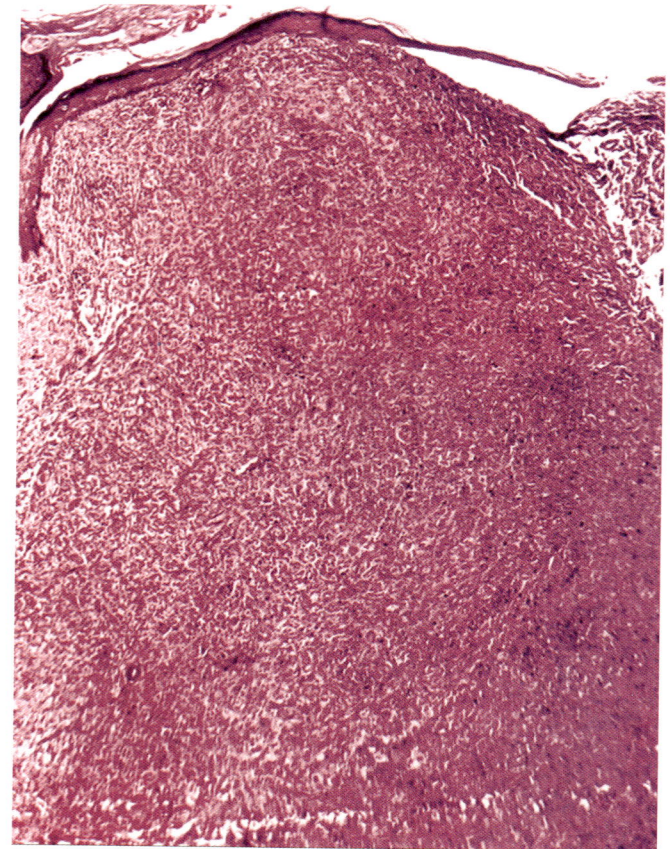

Fig. 114.1: Juvenile xanthogranuloma. Dermis shows foamy macrophages, multinucleated giant cells

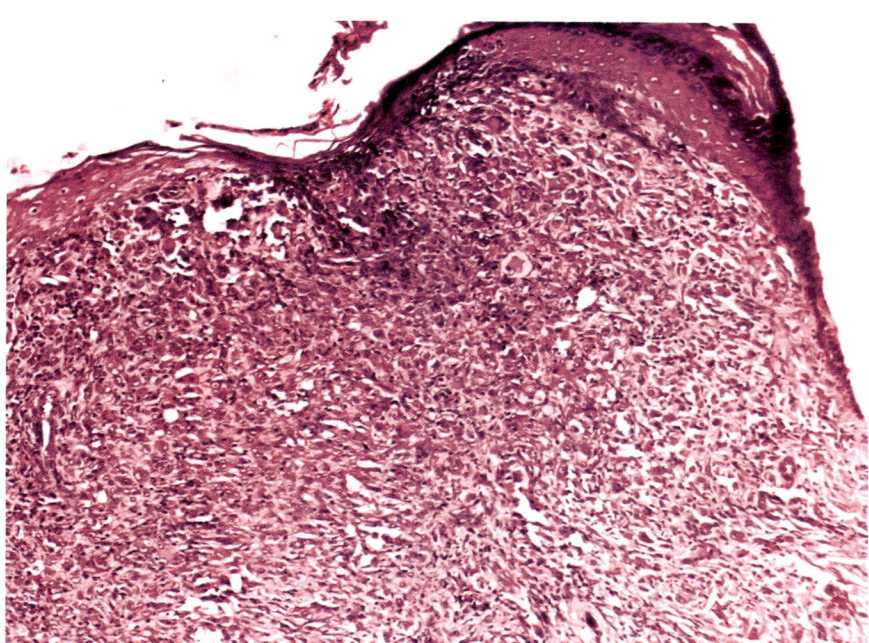

Fig. 114.2: Juvenile xanthogranuloma. High power view of Figure 114.1

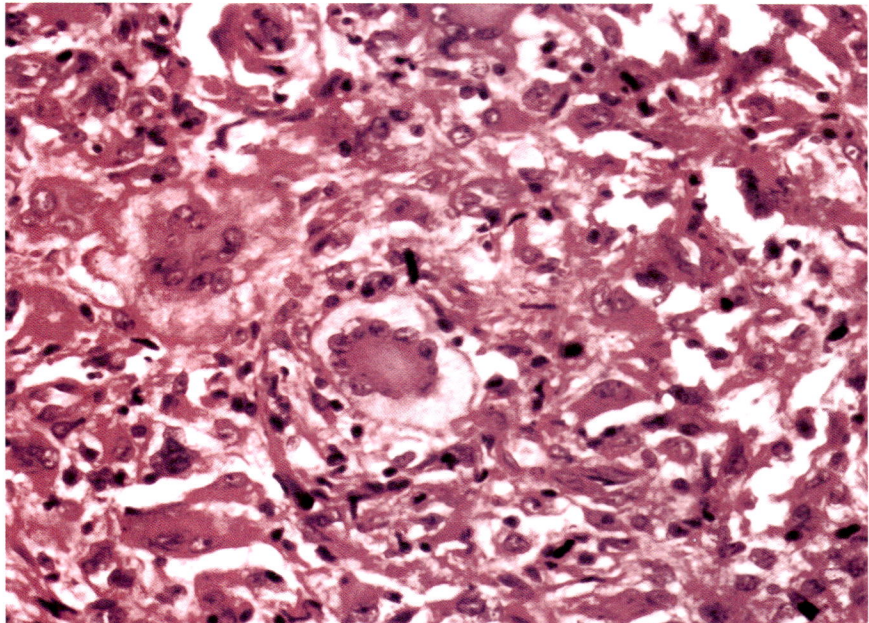

Fig. 114.3: Juvenile Xanthogranuloma. Touton giant cells in dermis

DIFFERENTIAL DIAGNOSIS

1. *Foreign body granuloma*
   - Granuloma comprising of foreign body and multinucleated giant cells

2. *Benign fibrous histiocytoma/dermatofibroma*
   - Acanthotic epidermis

   - Proliferation of macrophages and fibroblasts, which entraps the peripheral collagen bundles

3. *Langerhans cell histiocytosis*
   - Cells show CD1a and S-100 positivity

4. *Reticulohistiocytoma*

5. *Hemangioendothelioma*

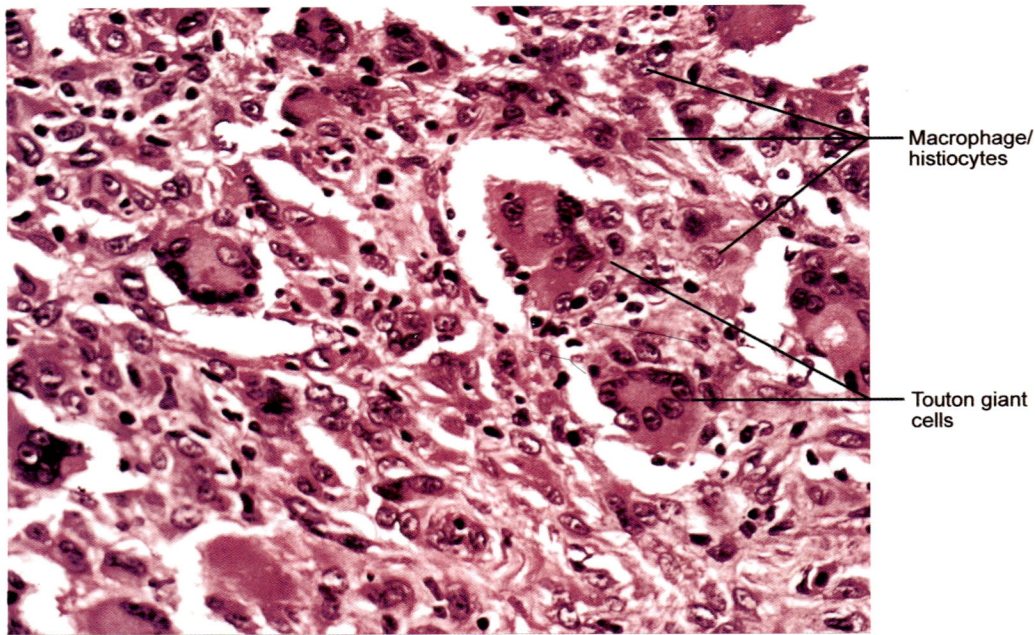

Fig. 114.4: Juvenile xanthogranuloma. Another case demonstrating multinucleated giant cells (Touton type)

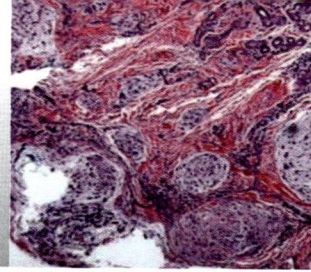

Cutaneous Mastocytosis

INTRODUCTION

- Disorder characterized by an abnormal growth and accumulation of mast cells in skin
- Disease follows an indolent course and lesions can regress spontaneously
- Age group—affects children
- In adults, an association with systemic mastocytosis is seen and disease is aggressive with worse prognosis

ETIOLOGY

- Disease is associated with c-kit proto-oncogene mutations
- Association with gastrointestinal stromal tumor is seen

CLINICAL FEATURES

- Lesions can be
  1. Solitary
  2. Numerous macular—papular or plaque like (resembling urticaria pigmentosa)
  3. Disseminated macules with telangiectasia [Telangiectasia macularis eruptiva perstans (TMEP)]
- **Darier sign**—stroking of the lesion, results in localized swelling or urticaria, due to mast cell degranulation

HISTOPATHOLOGY (Figs 115.1 to 115.4)

- Upper and mid-dermis—circumscribed infiltrate of the mast cells is seen

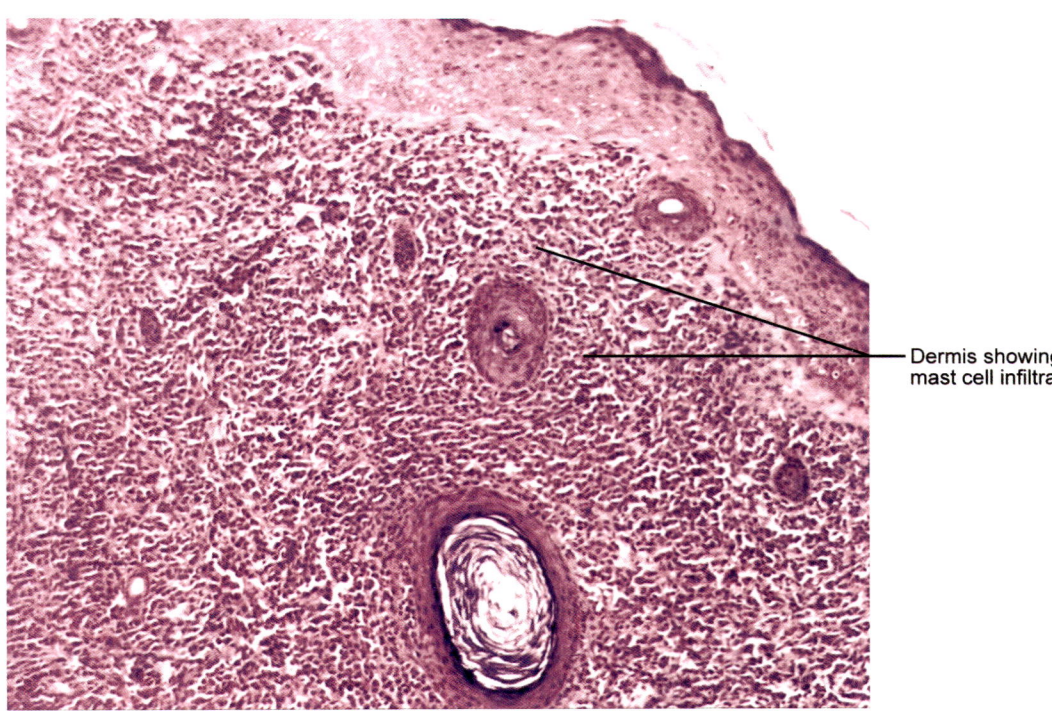

Dermis showing mast cell infiltrate

Fig. 115.1: Cutaneous mastocytosis

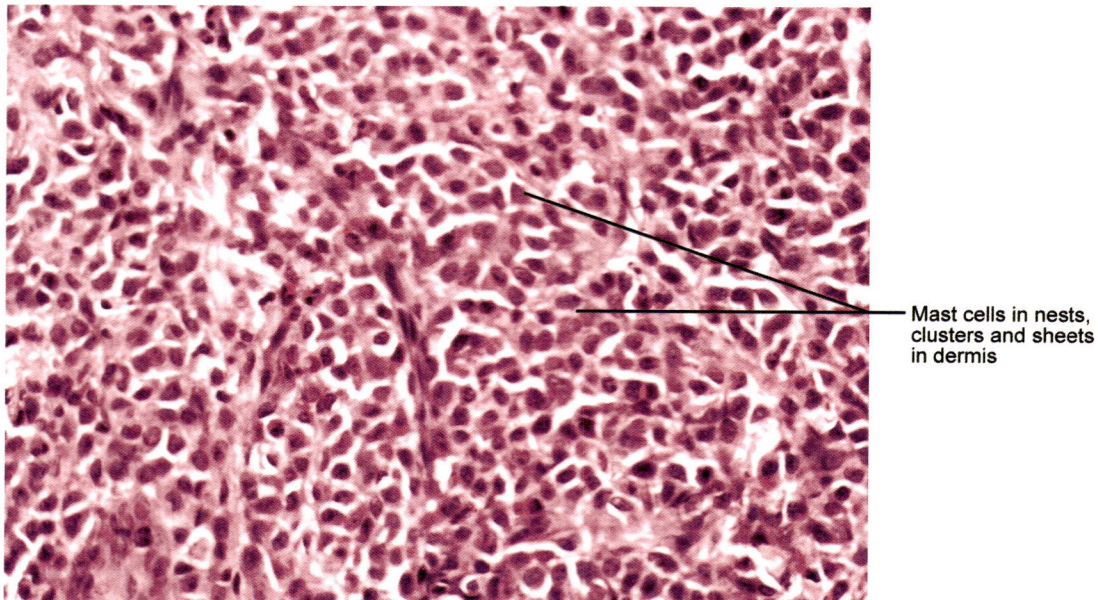

Fig. 115.2: Cutaneous mastocytosis

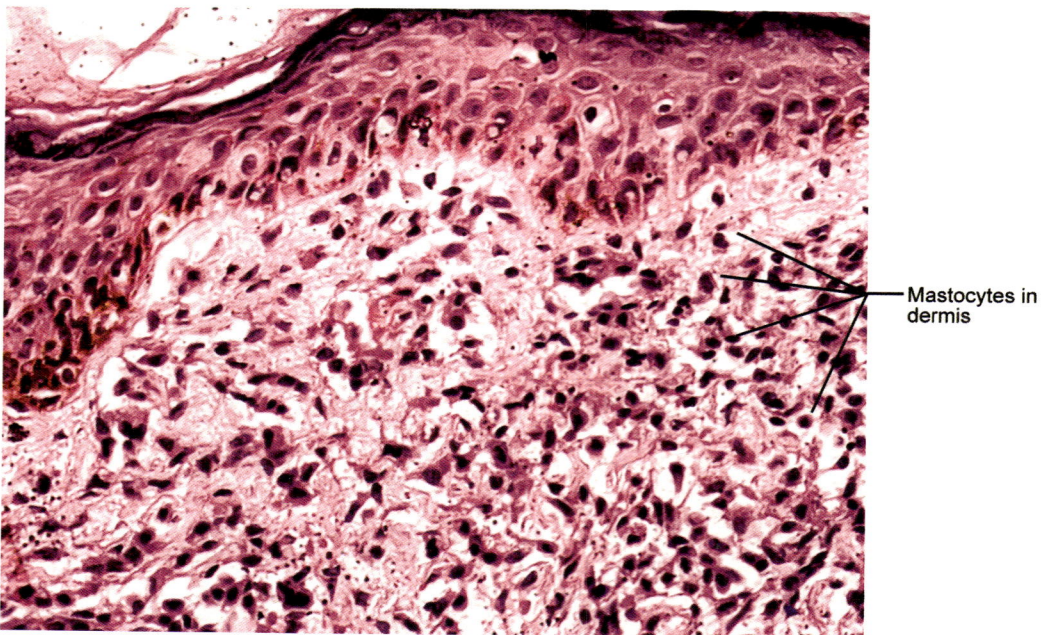

Fig. 115.3: Cutaneous mastocytosis

- Mast cells on hematoxylin and eosin stain, have moderate amount of eosinophilic cytoplasm and round to oval nuclei
- In urticaria pigmentosa, epidermis shows increased basal layer melanin, with peri-vascular lymphocytes, mast cells and eosinophils in the upper dermis
- Telangiectasia macularis eruptiva perstans (TMEP) —mast cells surround dilated blood vessels of the upper dermis (Fig. 115.5)

ADDITIONAL STUDIES

- Mast cells show Giemsa or Toluidine blue stain positivity and CD-117 (c-kit) positivity

DIFFERENTIAL DIAGNOSIS

Granular Cell Tumors

- Tumor cells demonstrate S-100 positivity
- Granules of tumor cells do not stain with Giemsa and Toluidine blue

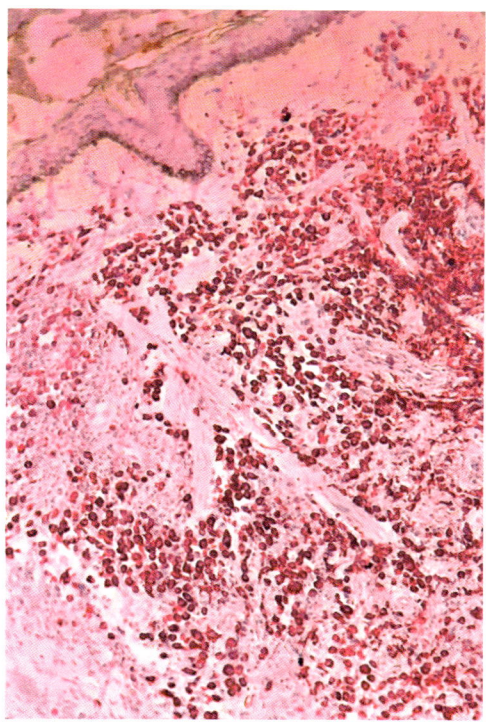

Fig. 115.4: Mast cells demonstrate toluidine blue positivity

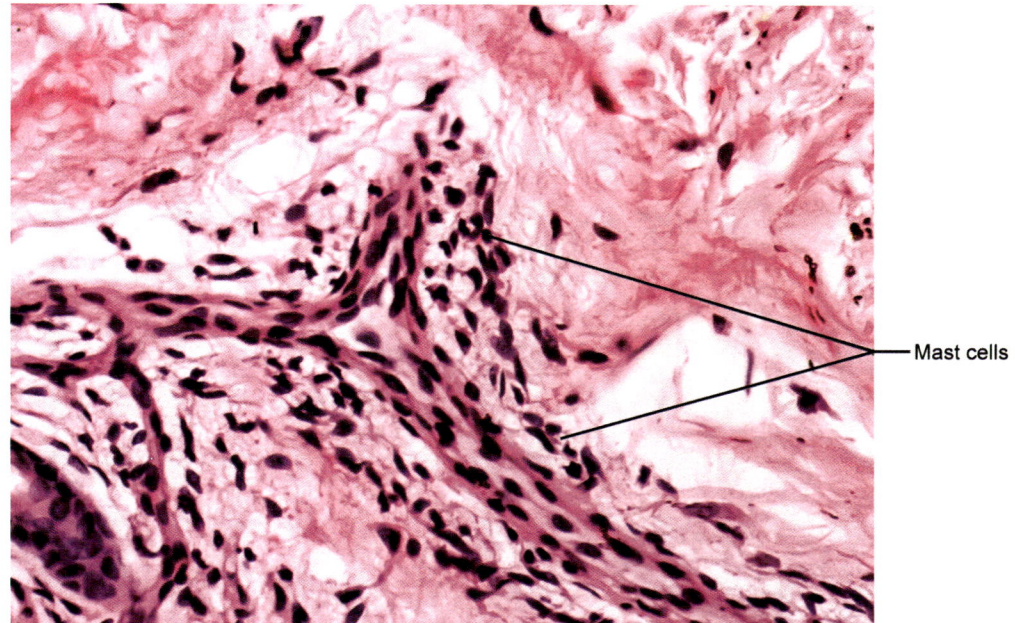

Mast cells

Fig. 115.5: Telangiectasia macularis eruptiva perstans (TMEP). Mast cells are seen surrounding the blood vessels

Lymphoproliferative Disorder

- Shows lymphoid marker positivity

Urticaria

- Increase number of eosinophils with only few mast cells

PROGNOSIS

- Lesions confined to the skin have good prognosis
- Spontaneous regression of localized cutaneous mastocytosis can occur
- Adults with aggressive systemic mastocytosis have poor prognosis

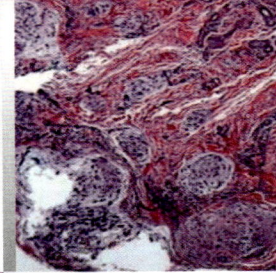

Cutaneous Reticulohistiocytosis

INTRODUCTION

- Two types—giant cell and multi-centric
- **Multi-centric type**—most commonly affect females in fourth decade of life; with face and distal extremities, being most commonly involved; and presents as papulonodular lesions

HISTOPATHOLOGY (Figs 116.1 to 116.4)

- Dermal proliferation of mono-nuclear and multi-nucleated histiocytes is seen
- These histiocytes have eosinophilic finely granular ground glass cytoplasm
- Histiocytes are PAS-positive but diastase resistant

- Admixed amongst the histiocytes, lymphocytes can also be seen
- Dermis also shows perivascular lymphocytic infiltrate

IMMUNOHISTOCHEMISTRY

- Histiocytes are CD68 and TRAP (tartrate resistant acid phosphatase) positive
- Histiocytes are negative for S-100 and CD1a

DIFFERENTIAL DIAGNOSIS

Juvenile Xanthogranuloma

- Age of diagnosis—2 years
- Presence of Touton giant cells

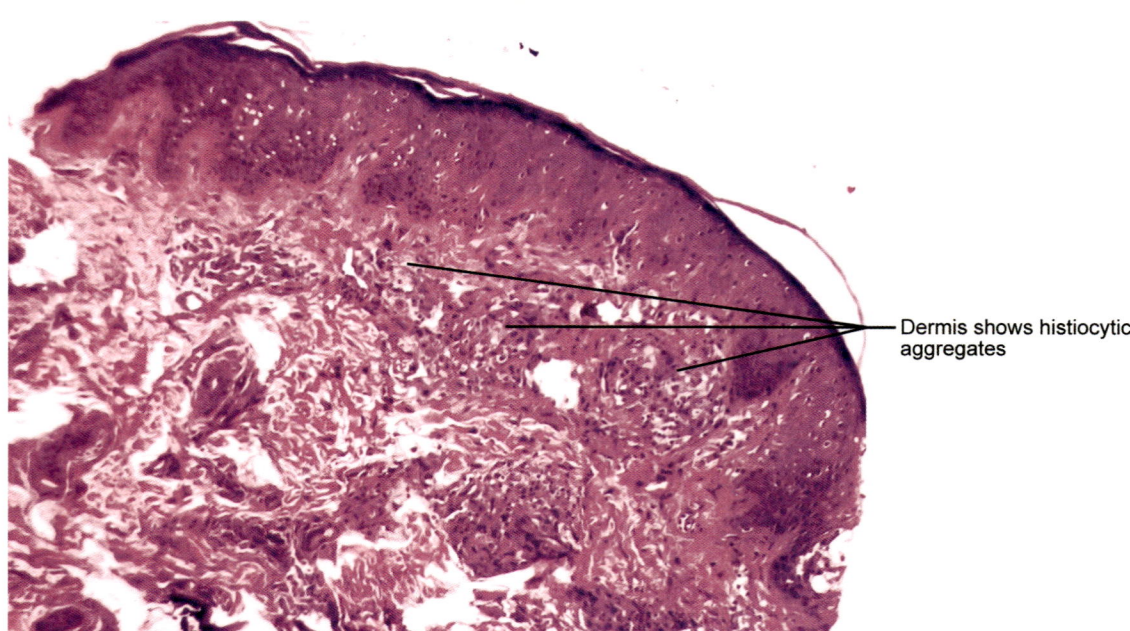

Dermis shows histiocytic aggregates

Fig. 116.1: Cutaneous reticulohistiocytosis. Dermis shows histiocytic aggregates

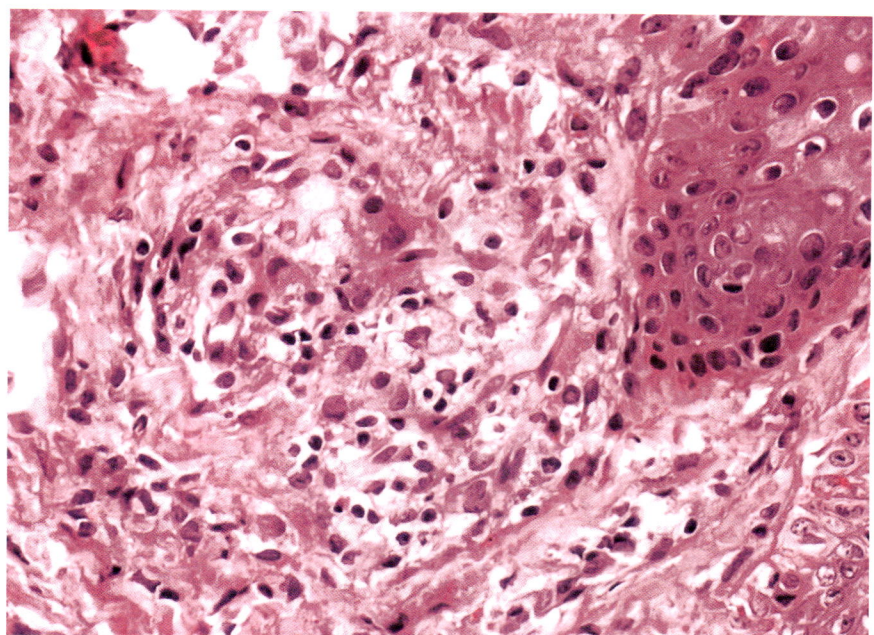

Fig. 116.2: Dermal histiocytic aggregates in reticulohistiocytosis

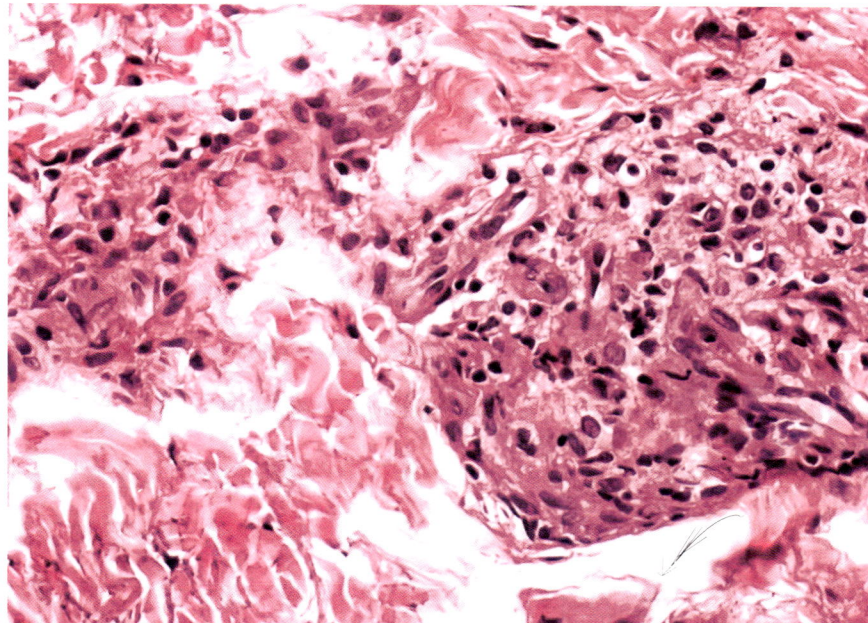

Fig. 116.3: Histiocytic aggregates and lymphocytes in deeper dermis

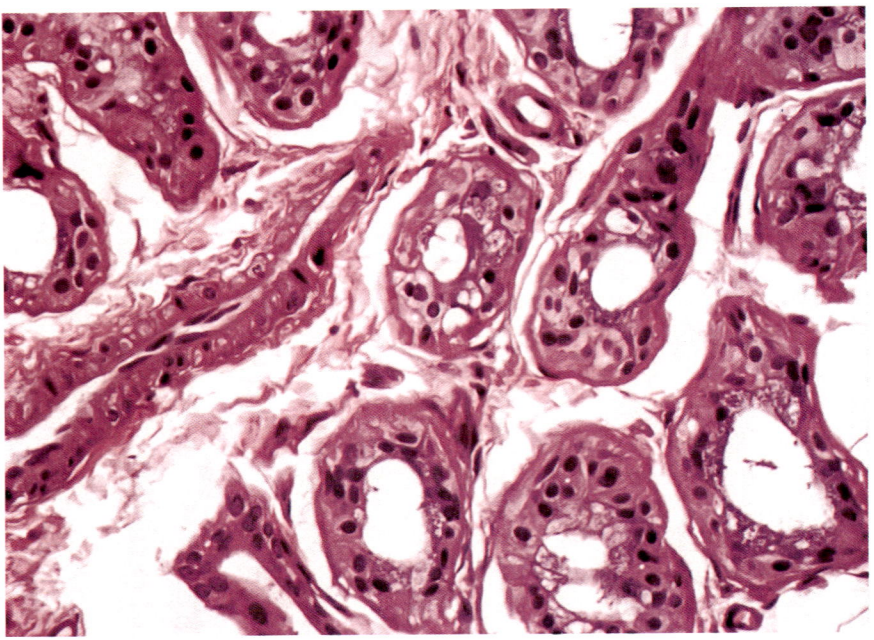

Fig. 116.4: Reticulohistiocytosis. Histiocytes within the dermal eccrine ducts

Index